Dietary Intake and Type 2 Diabetes

Dietary Intake and Type 2 Diabetes

Special Issue Editor

Omorogieva Ojo

MDPI • Basel • Beijing • Wuhan • Barcelona • Belgrade

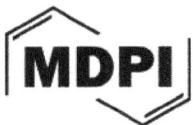

MDPI

Special Issue Editor
Omorogieva Ojo
University of Greenwich
UK

Editorial Office
MDPI
St. Alban-Anlage 66
4052 Basel, Switzerland

This is a reprint of articles from the Special Issue published online in the open access journal *Nutrients* (ISSN 2072-6643) from 2018 to 2019 (available at: https://www.mdpi.com/journal/nutrients/special_issues/dietary_intake_type2_diabetes).

For citation purposes, cite each article independently as indicated on the article page online and as indicated below:

LastName, A.A.; LastName, B.B.; LastName, C.C. Article Title. *Journal Name* **Year**, *Article Number, Page Range.*

ISBN 978-3-03921-704-5 (Pbk)
ISBN 978-3-03921-705-2 (PDF)

Contents

About the Special Issue Editor

Omorogieva Ojo has a Ph.D. in Nutrition from the University of Greenwich, London, and a Postgraduate Diploma in Diabetes from the University of Surrey, Roehampton, UK. He is an Associate Professor in Diabetes Care and Management, School of Health Sciences, University of Greenwich, London. UK. He is also a Senior Fellow of the Higher Education Academy and a Registered Nutritionist.

Dr. Ojo is an internationally acclaimed expert in nutrition and diabetes. He teaches across a range of courses and programmes, has published widely in the areas of nutrition and diabetes, and his articles are widely cited internationally. He is also involved in many postgraduate research activities, including Ph.D. supervision.

Dr. Ojo is the leader of the International Nutrition and Diabetes Research Group with members from the UK, China, and Nigeria, and is on the Editorial Board of many international journals including *Nutrients*.

Dr. Ojo is a principal investigator and a reviewer for a range of international journals. He has been a keynote speaker at conferences and also a member of the scientific and organising committee of many international conferences.

nutrients

MDPI

Editorial

Dietary Intake and Type 2 Diabetes

Omorogieva Ojo

School of Health Sciences, University of Greenwich, London SE9 2UG, UK; o.ojo@greenwich.ac.uk;
Tel.: +44-020-8331-8626; Fax: +44-020-8331-8060

Received: 4 September 2019; Accepted: 6 September 2019; Published: 11 September 2019

Abstract: This editorial aims to examine the risk factors associated with type 2 diabetes and to discuss the evidence relating to dietary strategies for managing people with this condition. It is clear from the evidence presented that a range of dietary interventions can provide useful approaches for managing people with type 2 diabetes, including the regulation of blood glucose and lipid parameters, and for reducing the risks of acute and chronic diabetic complications.

Keywords: type 2 diabetes; dietary intake; glycaemic control; dietary management approaches; micronutrients; macronutrients; nutrition; chronic conditions; lipid parameters

---

Diabetes is a metabolic condition that is characterized by chronic hyperglycemia and results from an interplay of genetic and environmental factors [1–4]. Its prevalence is on the increase in the UK and worldwide, partly due to changes in lifestyle that predispose individuals to obesity and being overweight [1,3–6]. It is estimated that about 90% of adults currently diagnosed with diabetes have type 2 diabetes and, based on a World Health Organisation (WHO) report, about 422 million adults were living with diabetes in 2014 compared with 108 million in 1980 and this condition caused about 1.5 million deaths in 2012 [7,8]. The United States of America has about 30.3 million adults living with diabetes, and 1.5 million estimated new diabetes cases are diagnosed every year, representing an increasing prevalence of this condition [9]. Diabetes presents a major public health challenge despite the developments in technology and the pharmaceutical industry [9]. These problems may be in the form of acute or chronic complications and changes in body composition can be profound. In this regard, Almusaylim et al. [10] conducted a cross-sectional and longitudinal study to evaluate the associations between variations in glycaemic status and changes in total body, trunk, appendicular fat mass, and lean mass in men. The longitudinal analyses demonstrated that changes in total body, fat mass and lean mass, and appendicular lean mass differed among glycaemic groups [10]. In addition, glucose dysregulation was found to be related to adverse changes in total body and appendicular lean mass.

Therefore, in order to attenuate the problems of diabetes, management strategies usually include lifestyle changes such as increased physical activities and dietary interventions. Studies that evaluate the role of nutrition in the management of type 2 diabetes often involve human and animal models as these approaches enable us to have a broader and more in-depth understanding of the condition. Sometimes, diabetes may co-exist with other conditions such as stroke and these may present unique challenges in relation to nutritional interventions.

The current editorial aims to evaluate the risk factors associated with type 2 diabetes and the role of diet in the management of people with the condition. It involves evidence drawn from human and animal studies.

In one of the studies, Muñoz-Garach et al. [11] examined the role of vitamin D status, calcium intake, and the risk of developing type 2 diabetes. According to the authors, the role of vitamin D in glucose homeostasis appears to be its association with insulin secretion, insulin resistance, and systemic inflammation and this is one of its important non-skeletal functions [11]. In addition, there seems to be a link between the consumption of dairy products and a lower risk of type 2 diabetes and this has been demonstrated in many observational studies although the mechanism and the role of calcium intake in the risk of developing this condition have not been well established [11]. Therefore, a randomized controlled trial on the role of vitamin D and calcium in the development of type 2 diabetes will further elucidate our understanding of the mechanisms of action of these micronutrients [11]. In a related study, Contreras-Manzano et al. [12] explored cardiovascular risk factors and their association with vitamin D deficiency based on a nationally representative sample of 3260 young Mexican women. The authors found that the prevalence of vitamin D deficiency among the women aged 20 to 49 years old was a public health problem and that obesity, type 2 diabetes, and high total cholesterol were found to be associated with vitamin D deficiency.

On the other hand, Fernández-Cao et al. [13] conducted a systematic review and meta-analysis in order to evaluate the effect of dietary, supplementary, and total zinc intake and status on the risk of developing type 2 diabetes. This was based on the understanding that zinc may have a protective role against type 2 diabetes [13]. The results showed that a moderately high dietary zinc intake based on the 'Dietary Reference Intake' may reduce the risk of type 2 diabetes by 13% and up to 41% in rural settings [13]. In contrast, elevated serum/plasma zinc concentration was found to be associated with an increased risk of type 2 diabetes in the general population, although no relationship was established between total or supplementary zinc intake and type 2 diabetes [13]. Brandão-Lima et al. [14] also explored the relationship between the dietary intake of zinc, potassium, calcium, and magnesium and glycaemic control in patients with diabetes. The authors used multiple linear regression and binary logistic regression analysis to evaluate the effects of individual and combination intake of these micronutrients on glycated hemoglobin (HbA1c) and found a high likelihood of inadequate intake of the micronutrients. In addition, it was noted that the group with a lower micronutrient intake demonstrated higher % HbA1c ($p = 0.006$) and triglyceride ($p = 0.010$) levels [14].

Apart from evaluating the association between micronutrients and the risk of type 2 diabetes, the role of macronutrients and other metabolites in the development of this condition have been studied extensively. Song et al. [15] sought to examine whether dietary patterns that explain the variation of the triglyceride (TG) to high-density lipoprotein cholesterol (HDL-C) ratio were associated with the incidence of type 2 diabetes in Korean men and women. The authors found evidence that suggests that dietary patterns associated with low levels of TG/HDL-C ratio may have the potential to reduce the risk of type 2 diabetes.

Based on the above, it is essential that dietary management approaches that are tailored to meet the needs of people with type 2 diabetes reflect these elements that are aimed at reducing the risk of acute and chronic complications. In this regard, Hallberg et al. [9] noted in their narrative review that there is evidence that suggests the possible reversal of this condition through interventions and these have been incorporated into guidelines. These approaches may involve the use of bariatric surgery, low-calorie diets, or carbohydrate restriction [9]. In particular, the American Diabetes Association and the European Association for the Study of Diabetes have recommended a low carbohydrate diet and support the use of short-term low-calorie diets for weight loss.

A low carbohydrate diet (LCD), replacing some staple foods with nuts such as tree nuts and groundnuts, has been shown to reduce weight, improve blood glucose, and regulate blood lipid in patients with type 2 diabetes [16]. However, the consumption of tree nuts is difficult to promote in patients with diabetes because they are relatively more expensive compared to groundnuts [16]. It remains unclear whether peanuts and tree nuts, including almonds, in combination with LCD have similar benefits in patients with type 2 diabetes. Therefore, Hou et al. [16] conducted a randomized controlled trial to compare the effect of peanuts and almonds on the cardio-metabolic and inflammatory parameters in patients with type 2 diabetes. This was a parallel design involving 32 patients with type 2 diabetes [16]. The patients consumed a LCD with part of the starchy staple food being replaced with peanuts (peanut group) or almonds (almond group) and involved a follow-up period of three months [16]. The findings showed that the fasting blood glucose (FBG) and postprandial 2-h blood glucose (PPG) decreased in both the peanut and almond groups ($p < 0.05$) compared with the baseline, and, following the intervention, there was no significant difference between the peanut group and the almond group with respect to the FBG and PPG levels [16]. However, compared to the baseline value, there was a decrease in the glycated hemoglobin level in the almond group ($p < 0.05$) and no significant difference was found between the peanut and almond groups with respect to the HbA1c level at the third month. The authors concluded that when incorporated into a LCD, almonds and peanuts have a similar effect on improving fasting and postprandial blood glucose among patients with type 2 diabetes.

In a separate study, Yamada et al. [17] conducted a systematic review of dietary approaches for Japanese patients with diabetes. The main focus of the review was to elucidate the effect of an energy-restricted and carbohydrate-restricted diet on the management of Japanese patients with diabetes [17]. All the randomized controlled trials included in the review showed better glucose management with the carbohydrate-restricted diet. It was found that carbohydrate-restricted diet, not the energy-restricted diet, might have short term benefits for managing Japanese patients with diabetes although the low number of studies included in the review was a limitation [17].

Burch et al. [18] also developed a protocol for a longitudinal study on evaluating how diet changes with the diagnosis of diabetes. It has been observed that the quality of diets plays a significant role in assisting people with type 2 diabetes to manage their condition and thus reduce the risk of developing diabetes-related complications [18,19]. This is because diet quality is the extent to which food intake complies with national or international dietary guidelines or a priori diet quality score and it influences glycaemic control in people with type 2 diabetes and has a significant impact on the risk of complications [18,20]. It often includes the macronutrient components of the diet. Thus, Telle-Hansen et al. [21] summarized the research evidence on randomized controlled trials of the effect of dietary polyunsaturated fatty acids (PUFAs) on glycaemic control in people with type 2 diabetes. This study was based on the fact that replacing saturated fatty acids (SFAs) with PUFAs decreases blood cholesterol levels and prevents cardiovascular diseases and that fat quality may also affect insulin sensitivity and increase the risk of type 2 diabetes [21]. Evidence from prospective studies has also shown that a high intake of SFAs can increase the risk of type 2 diabetes, while a high intake of PUFAs reduces the risk of the condition [21]. Based on this review, while about half of the studies that examined the effect of fish, fish oils, vegetable oils, or nuts found changes related to glycaemic control in people with type 2 diabetes, the other half found no effects [21]. In addition, it remains unclear whether PUFAs from marine or vegetable sources affect glycaemic regulation differently and this is a potential area for future research [21].

What is clear, however, is that a low glycaemic index (GI) diet is more effective in controlling glycated hemoglobin and fasting blood glucose than a high GI diet in patients with type 2 diabetes [22]. In a further systematic review and meta-analysis, Ojo et al. [23] sought to evaluate the effects of a low GI diet on the cardio-metabolic and inflammatory parameters in patients with type 2 diabetes and in women with gestational diabetes mellitus (GDM) and examine whether the effects are different in these conditions. While 10 randomized controlled studies were included in the systematic review, only 9 were selected for the meta-analysis [23]. The results of the meta-analysis found no significant differences ($p > 0.05$) between the low GI and higher GI diets with respect to total cholesterol, high-density lipoprotein (HDL), and low-density lipoprotein (LDL) cholesterol in patients with type 2 diabetes. With respect to the triglyceride, it increased by a mean of 0.06 mmol/L (0.01, 0.11) in patients with type 2 diabetes on a high GI diet and the difference compared with the low GI diet group was significant ($p = 0.027$) [23]. The results from the systematic review were not consistent in terms of the effect of a low GI diet on the lipid profile in women with GDM [23]. Furthermore, the low GI diet significantly decreased interleukin–6 ($p = 0.001$) in patients with type 2 diabetes compared to the high GI diet [23].

Nutritional approaches employed in managing patients with type 2 diabetes may also involve the use of enteral nutrition, including oral nutritional supplements (ONS) [3]. The effectiveness of these diabetes-specific formula (DSF) and standard formulas on glycaemic control and lipid profile in patients with type 2 diabetes continues to generate interest. Based on this, Ojo et al. [1] used a systematic review and meta-analysis of randomized controlled trials to evaluate the effect of diabetes-specific enteral nutrition formula on cardiometabolic parameters in patients with type 2 diabetes. On the other hand, Angarita Dávila et al. [3], conducted a randomized cross-over study to explore the effect of oral diabetes-specific nutritional supplements with sucromalt and isomaltulose compared with the standard formula (SF) on glycaemic index, entero-insular axis peptides, and subjective appetite in patients with type 2 diabetes.

In the review by Ojo et al. [1], it was found that all the fourteen studies included in the systematic review showed that DSF was effective in lowering blood glucose parameters in patients with type 2 diabetes compared with SF. The results of the meta-analysis confirmed the findings of the systematic review with respect to the fasting blood glucose, which was significantly lower ($p = 0.01$) in the DSF group compared to SF, and the glycated hemoglobin, which was significantly lower ($p = 0.005$) in the DSF group compared to the SF group [1]. Based on the systematic review, the outcomes of the studies selected to evaluate the effect of DSF on lipid profile were variable. The authors concluded that the results provided evidence to suggest that DSF is effective in controlling fasting blood glucose and glycated hemoglobin and in increasing HDL cholesterol, but has no significant effect on other lipid parameters. They further noted that the presence of low glycaemic index (GI) carbohydrates, a lower amount of carbohydrates and a higher amount protein, the presence of mono-unsaturated fatty acids, and different amounts and types of fiber in the DSF compared with SF may be responsible for the observed differences in cardiometabolic parameters in both groups [1].

Angarita Dávila et al. [3] also compared the postprandial effects of oral diabetes-specific nutritional supplements with isomaltulose and sucromalt versus the standard formula (SF) on the glycaemic index (GI), insulin, glucose-dependent insulinotropic polypeptide (GIP), glucagon-like peptide 1 (GLP-1), and subjective appetite in people with type 2 diabetes. The subjects were given a portion of supplements containing 25 g of carbohydrates or reference food following overnight fasting [3]. The glycaemic index values were low for oral diabetes-specific nutritional supplements and intermediate for SF ($p < 0.001$). The area under the curve for insulin and GIP were lower ($p < 0.02$ and $p < 0.02$ respectively) after oral diabetes-specific nutritional supplements and higher ($p < 0.05$) for GLP-1 when compared with SF [3]. In addition, the subjective appetite area under the curve was greater ($p < 0.05$) after SF than oral diabetes-specific nutritional supplements [3].

The management of type 2 diabetes may also include the administration of insulin. But questions remain whether the dose of insulin before a meal should be based on glycemia or meal content [24]. Krzymien et al. [24] reviewed existing guidelines and scientific evidence on insulin dosage in people with type 1 and type 2 diabetes and explored the effect of the meal composition such as carbohydrate, protein and fat on postprandial glucose. The authors found that in most current guidelines aimed at establishing prandial insulin doses in type 1 diabetes, only carbohydrates are counted, whereas in type 2 diabetes the meal content is often not taken into consideration. Therefore, it was concluded that prandial insulin doses in managing people with diabetes should take into account the pre-meal glycemia, as well as the size and composition of the meals [24].

Apart from human studies, research based on the effects of different extracts on animal models have been conducted in an attempt to further elucidate our understanding of their role in diabetes. Tse et al. [25] assessed the glycemic lowering effect of an aqueous extract of *Hedychium coronarium* leaves in diabetic rodents. The study involved streptozotocin-induced type 2 diabetes Wistar rats and C57BKSdb/db mice. After treatment with *Hedychium coronarium* for 28 days, glucose tolerance improved in both of the diabetic animal models. The *Hedychium coronarium* also significantly improved the lipid profile in streptozotocin-induced type 2 diabetic rats [25]. On the other hand, Vlavcheski and Tsiani [26] explored the reduction of free fatty acid-induced muscle insulin resistance by Rosemary extract. It was found that Rosemary extract has the potential to counteract the palmitate-induced muscle cell insulin resistance [26].

In another study, Huang et al. [27] examined the effects of Tempeh fermentation with *Lactobacillus plantarum* and *Rhizopus oligosporus* on streptozotocin-induced type 2 diabetes rats. The results

4

demonstrated that the modulation of serum glucose and lipid levels by lactic acid bacteria occurs via alterations in the internal microbiota, leading to the inhibition of cholesterol synthesis and promotion of lipolysis [27]. Furthermore, it was suggested that Tempeh, might be a beneficial dietary supplement for individuals with abnormal carbohydrate metabolism [27].

Yang et al. [28] also evaluated the combination of freeze-dried *Aronia*, red ginseng, ultraviolet-irradiated shiitake mushroom, and nattokinase in order to examine its effects on insulin resistance, insulin secretion, and the gut microbiome in a non-obese type 2 diabetic animal model. It was concluded that the combination of freeze-dried *Aronia*, red ginseng, ultraviolet-irradiated shiitake mushroom, and nattokinase improved glucose metabolism by potentiating insulin secretion and reducing insulin resistance in insulin-deficient type 2 diabetic rats [28]. The improvement of diabetic status ameliorated body composition changes and prevented changes in gut microbiome composition [28].

Overall, this editorial has demonstrated that a range of dietary interventions can provide useful approaches for managing people with type 2 diabetes including regulating blood glucose parameters and lipid profiles and for reducing the risks of acute and chronic diabetic complications.

Funding: This research received no external funding.

Conflicts of Interest: The author declares no conflict of interest.

References

1. Ojo, O.; Weldon, S.M.; Thompson, T.; Crockett, R.; Wang, X.-H. The Effect of Diabetes-Specific Enteral Nutrition Formula on Cardiometabolic Parameters in Patients with Type 2 Diabetes: A Systematic Review and Meta–Analysis of Randomised Controlled Trials. *Nutrients* **2019**, *11*, 1905. [CrossRef] [PubMed]
2. DeFronzo, R.A.; Ratner, R.E.; Han, J.; Kim, D.D.; Fineman, M.S.; Baron, A.D. Effects of exenatide (exendin-4) on glycemic control and weight over 30 weeks in metformin-treated patients with type 2 diabetes. *Diabetes Care* **2005**, *28*, 1092–1100. [CrossRef] [PubMed]
3. Angarita Dávila, L.; Bermúdez, V.; Aparicio, D.; Céspedes, V.; Escobar, M.C.; Durán-Agüero, S.; Cisternas, S.; de Assis Costa, J.; Rojas-Gómez, D.; Reyna, N.; et al. Effect of Oral Nutritional Supplements with Sucromalt and Isomaltulose versus Standard Formula on Glycaemic Index, Entero-Insular Axis Peptides and Subjective Appetite in Patients with Type 2 Diabetes: A Randomised Cross-Over Study. *Nutrients* **2019**, *11*, 1477. [CrossRef] [PubMed]
4. Rosen, E.D.; Kaestner, K.H.; Natarajan, R.; Patti, M.-E.; Sallari, R.; Sander, M.; Susztak, K. Epigenetics and Epigenomics: Implications for Diabetes and Obesity. *Diabetes* **2018**, *67*, 1923–1931. [CrossRef] [PubMed]
5. Public Health England. 3.8 Million People in England Now Have Diabetes. 2016. Available online: https://www.gov.uk/government/news/38-million-people-in-england-now-have-diabetes (accessed on 1 September 2019).
6. National Health Service (NHS) Digital and Healthcare Quality Improvement Partnership. National Diabetes Audit, 2015–2016 Report 1: Care Processes and Treatment Targets. 2017. Available online: http://www.content.digital.nhs.uk/catalogue/PUB23241/nati-diab-rep1-audi-2015-16.pdf (accessed on 1 September 2019).
7. National Institute for Health and Care Excellence (NICE). Type 2 Diabetes in Adults: Management. 2015. Available online: Nice.org.uk/guidance/ng28 (accessed on 1 September 2019).
8. World Health Organization. Global Report on Diabetes. 2016. Available online: https://www.who.int/diabetes/publications/grd-2016/en/ (accessed on 1 September 2019).
9. Hallberg, S.J.; Gershuni, V.M.; Hazbun, T.L.; Athinarayanan, S.J. Reversing Type 2 Diabetes: A Narrative Review of the Evidence. *Nutrients* **2019**, *11*, 766. [CrossRef] [PubMed]
10. Almusaylim, K.; Minett, M.; Binkley, T.L.; Beare, T.M.; Specker, B. Cross-Sectional and Longitudinal Association between Glycemic Status and Body Composition in Men: A Population-Based Study. *Nutrients* **2018**, *10*, 1878. [CrossRef]
11. Muñoz-Garach, A.; García-Fontana, B.; Muñoz-Torres, M. Vitamin D Status, Calcium Intake and Risk of Developing Type 2 Diabetes: An Unresolved Issue. *Nutrients* **2019**, *11*, 642. [CrossRef]

12. Contreras-Manzano, A.; Villalpando, S.; García-Díaz, C.; Flores-Aldana, M. Cardiovascular Risk Factors and Their Association with Vitamin D Deficiency in Mexican Women of Reproductive Age. *Nutrients* **2019**, *11*, 1211. [CrossRef] [PubMed]
13. Fernández-Cao, J.C.; Warthon-Medina, M.; Moran, V.H.; Arija, V.; Doepking, C.; Serra-Majem, L.; Lowe, N.M. Zinc Intake and Status and Risk of Type 2 Diabetes Mellitus: A Systematic Review and Meta-Analysis. *Nutrients* **2019**, *11*, 1027. [CrossRef]
14. Brandão-Lima, P.N.; Carvalho, G.B.; Santos, R.K.F.; Santos, B.D.C.; Dias-Vasconcelos, N.L.; Rocha, V.D.S.; Barbosa, K.B.F.; Pires, L.V. Intakes of Zinc, Potassium, Calcium, and Magnesium of Individuals with Type 2 Diabetes Mellitus and the Relationship with Glycemic Control. *Nutrients* **2018**, *10*, 1948. [CrossRef]
15. Song, S.; Lee, J.E. Dietary Patterns Related to Triglyceride and High-Density Lipoprotein Cholesterol and the Incidence of Type 2 Diabetes in Korean Men and Women. *Nutrients* **2019**, *11*, 8. [CrossRef] [PubMed]
16. Hou, Y.-Y.; Ojo, O.; Wang, L.-L.; Wang, Q.; Jiang, Q.; Shao, X.-Y.; Wang, X.-H. A Randomized Controlled Trial to Compare the Effect of Peanuts and Almonds on the Cardio-Metabolic and Inflammatory Parameters in Patients with Type 2 Diabetes Mellitus. *Nutrients* **2018**, *10*, 1565. [CrossRef] [PubMed]
17. Yamada, S.; Kabeya, Y.; Noto, H. Dietary Approaches for Japanese Patients with Diabetes: A Systematic Review. *Nutrients* **2018**, *10*, 1080. [CrossRef] [PubMed]
18. Burch, E.; Williams, L.T.; Makepeace, H.; Alston-Knox, C.; Ball, L. How Does Diet Change with A Diagnosis of Diabetes? Protocol of the 3D Longitudinal Study. *Nutrients* **2019**, *11*, 158. [CrossRef] [PubMed]
19. Coppell, K.J.; Kataoka, M.; Williams, S.M.; Chisholm, A.W.; Vorgers, S.M.; Mann, J.I. Nutritional intervention in patients with type 2 diabetes who are hyperglycaemic despite optimised drug treatment—Lifestyle Over and Above Drugs in Diabetes (LOADD) study: Randomised controlled trial. *BMJ* **2010**, *341*, c3337. [CrossRef] [PubMed]
20. Leech, R.M.; Worsley, A.; Timperio, A.; McNaughton, S.A. Understanding meal patterns: Definitions, methodology and impact on nutrient intake and diet quality. *Nutr. Res. Rev.* **2015**, *28*, 1–21. [CrossRef] [PubMed]
21. Telle-Hansen, V.H.; Gaundal, L.; Myhrstad, M.C. Polyunsaturated Fatty Acids and Glycemic Control in Type 2 Diabetes. *Nutrients* **2019**, *11*, 1067. [CrossRef]
22. Ojo, O.; Ojo, O.O.; Adebowale, F.; Wang, X.-H. The Effect of Dietary Glycaemic Index on Glycaemia in Patients with Type 2 Diabetes: A Systematic Review and Meta-Analysis of Randomized Controlled Trials. *Nutrients* **2018**, *10*, 373. [CrossRef]
23. Ojo, O.; Ojo, O.O.; Wang, X.-H.; Adegboye, A.R.A. The Effects of a Low GI Diet on Cardiometabolic and Inflammatory Parameters in Patients with Type 2 and Gestational Diabetes: A Systematic Review and Meta-Analysis of Randomised Controlled Trials. *Nutrients* **2019**, *11*, 1584. [CrossRef]
24. Krzymien, J.; Ladyzynski, P. Insulin in Type 1 and Type 2 Diabetes—Should the Dose of Insulin Before a Meal be Based on Glycemia or Meal Content? *Nutrients* **2019**, *11*, 607. [CrossRef]
25. Tse, L.-S.; Liao, P.-L.; Tsai, C.-H.; Li, C.-H.; Liao, J.-W.; Kang, J.-J.; Cheng, Y.-W. Glycemia Lowering Effect of an Aqueous Extract of *Hedychium coronarium* Leaves in Diabetic Rodent Models. *Nutrients* **2019**, *11*, 629. [CrossRef] [PubMed]
26. Vlavcheski, F.; Tsiani, E. Attenuation of Free Fatty Acid-Induced Muscle Insulin Resistance by Rosemary Extract. *Nutrients* **2018**, *10*, 1623. [CrossRef] [PubMed]
27. Huang, Y.-C.; Wu, B.-H.; Chu, Y.-L.; Chang, W.-C.; Wu, M.-C. Effects of Tempeh Fermentation with *Lactobacillus plantarum* and *Rhizopus oligosporus* on Streptozotocin-Induced Type II Diabetes Mellitus in Rats. *Nutrients* **2018**, *10*, 1143. [CrossRef] [PubMed]
28. Yang, H.J.; Kim, M.J.; Kwon, D.Y.; Kim, D.S.; Zhang, T.; Ha, C.; Park, S. Combination of Aronia, Red Ginseng, Shiitake Mushroom and Nattokinase Potentiated Insulin Secretion and Reduced Insulin Resistance with Improving Gut Microbiome Dysbiosis in Insulin Deficient Type 2 Diabetic Rats. *Nutrients* **2018**, *10*, 948. [CrossRef] [PubMed]

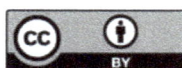

nutrients

MDPI

Review

The Effect of Diabetes-Specific Enteral Nutrition Formula on Cardiometabolic Parameters in Patients with Type 2 Diabetes: A Systematic Review and Meta–Analysis of Randomised Controlled Trials

Omorogieva Ojo [1,*], Sharon Marie Weldon [1,2], Trevor Thompson [3], Rachel Crockett [4] and Xiao-Hua Wang [5]

1   Department of Adult Nursing and Paramedic Science, University of Greenwich, London SE9 2UG, UK
2   Barts Health NHS Trust, The Royal London Hospital, Whitechapel Rd, Whitechapel E1 1BB, UK
3   Department of Psychology, University of Greenwich, London SE10 9LS, UK
4   Division of Psychology, Faculty of Natural Sciences, University of Stirling, Scotland FK9 4LA, UK
5   The School of Nursing, Soochow University, Suzhou 215006, China
*   Correspondence: o.ojo@greenwich.ac.uk; Tel.: +44-20-8331-8626; Fax: +44-20-8331-8060

Received: 24 May 2019; Accepted: 12 August 2019; Published: 15 August 2019

Abstract: Background: The prevalence of diabetes is on the increase in the UK and worldwide, partly due to unhealthy lifestyles, including poor dietary regimes. Patients with diabetes and other co-morbidities such as stroke, which may affect swallowing ability and lead to malnutrition, could benefit from enteral nutrition, including the standard formula (SF) and diabetes-specific formulas (DSF). However, enteral nutrition presents its challenges due to its effect on glycaemic control and lipid profile. Aim: The aim of this review was to evaluate the effectiveness of diabetes-specific enteral nutrition formula versus SF in managing cardiometabolic parameters in patients with type 2 diabetes. Method: This review was conducted in accordance with the preferred reporting items for systematic reviews and meta-analyses. Three databases (Pubmed, EMBASE, PSYCInfo) and Google scholar were searched for relevant articles from inception to 2 January 2019 based on Population, Intervention, Comparator, Outcomes and Study designs (PICOS) framework. Key words, Medical Subject Heading (MeSH) terms, and Boolean operators (AND/OR) formed part of the search strategy. Articles were evaluated for quality and risks of bias. Results: Fourteen articles were included in the systematic review and five articles were selected for the meta-analysis. Based on the findings of the review and meta-analysis, two distinct areas were evident: the effect of DSF on blood glucose parameters and the effect of DSF on lipid profile. All fourteen studies included in the systematic review showed that DSF was effective in lowering blood glucose parameters in patients with type 2 diabetes compared with SF. The results of the meta-analysis confirmed the findings of the systematic review with respect to the fasting blood glucose, which was significantly lower ($p = 0.01$) in the DSF group compared to SF, with a mean difference of −1.15 (95% CI −2.07, −0.23) and glycated haemoglobin, which was significantly lower ($p = 0.005$) in the DSF group compared to the SF group following meta-analysis and sensitivity analysis. However, in relation to the sensitivity analysis for the fasting blood glucose, differences were not significant between the two groups when some of the studies were removed. Based on the systematic review, the outcomes of the studies selected to evaluate the effect of DSF on lipid profile were variable. Following the meta-analysis, no significant differences ($p > 0.05$) were found between the DSF and SF groups with respect to total cholesterol, LDL cholesterol and triglyceride. The level of the HDL cholesterol was significantly higher ($p = 0.04$) in the DSF group compared to the SF group after the intervention, with a mean difference of 0.09 (95% CI, 0.00, 0.18), although this was not consistent based on the sensitivity analysis. The presence of low glycaemic index (GI) carbohydrate, the lower amount of carbohydrate and the higher protein, the presence of mono-unsaturated fatty acids and the different amounts and types of fibre in the DSF compared with SF may be responsible for the observed differences in cardiometabolic parameters in both groups.

Conclusion: The results provide evidence to suggest that DSF is effective in controlling fasting blood glucose and glycated haemoglobin and in increasing HDL cholesterol, but has no significant effect on other lipid parameters. However, our confidence in these findings would be increased by additional data from further studies.

Keywords: diabetes specific formula; standard formula; type 2 diabetes; enteral nutrition; enteral tube feeding; lipids; fasting blood glucose; glycated haemoglobin

1. Introduction

Diabetes is a metabolic condition which is characterised by chronic hyperglycaemia and is caused by a range of factors including genetic inheritance and environmental influences [1]. The prevalence of diabetes is on the increase in the UK and worldwide, partly due to the changes in lifestyle, including lack of physical activity and unhealthy diets, which lead to overweight and obesity [2–5]. In addition, improvements in technology and the greater awareness of the condition have meant that diabetes is now better detected and more people are engaging in screening programmes. About 90% of patients with diabetes are diagnosed with type 2 diabetes [6–8]. The impact of diabetes on the people living with the condition can be profound in terms of morbidity and mortality, as well as a cost burden to the National Health Service (NHS). Individuals with diabetes are more likely to be admitted to hospital and it can have a significant effect on the quality of life of patients [9,10]. Diabetes is a major risk factor for kidney dysfunction, lower limb amputations, retinopathy, cardiovascular disease and other co-morbidities such as stroke, which can lead to swallowing problems and malnutrition. Based on these issues, diabetes continues to be a major public health concern in the UK and globally, and strategies for managing the condition continue to evolve. Often, management relies on lifestyle modifications such as increased physical activity levels and the use of dietary interventions in order to prevent the onset of type 2 diabetes and ultimately reduce the possibility of diabetic complications [11]. However, in patients who are sedentary and immobile, the use of physical activity as a strategy for managing the condition is sometimes impracticable.

Therefore, individuals with diabetes and other conditions, such as stroke, which could affect mobility and swallowing ability, may benefit from enteral nutrition such as oral nutrition supplements and the use of a nasogastric feeding tube (for short-term feeding) or a percutaneous endoscopic gastrostomy tube for long-term intervention to deliver enteral feeds and formulas [12]. Usually, these individuals have functional guts and the essence is to provide adequate nutrition, hydration and medication to these patients in order to improve their nutritional status and clinical outcomes, including quality of life.

Why it is important to do this review:

The current review focuses mainly on patients with type 2 diabetes from a range of backgrounds, including those attending diabetes centre/outpatient diabetic clinics, rehabilitation departments, ambulatory patients, nursing homes and long-term care facilities, and intensive care units. Patients with diabetes are at a greater risk of developing stroke, peripheral vascular disease, renal impairment and dementia compared with those without the condition due to chronic hyperglycaemia [13]. The long-term complications of diabetes, including its co-morbidities, have implications for the length of hospital stay. Thus, while the average length of hospital stay in patients with diabetes as the primary diagnosis has been estimated to be 4.3 days, it is 8 days in patients with additional diagnoses and 3.1 days in all hospitalisations [14]. The use of enteral feeding in patients with diabetes can present a range of challenges in the control of blood glucose levels and other cardiometabolic parameters [15]. These parameters, including lipid profile, such as total cholesterol, high density lipoprotein cholesterol, low density lipoprotein cholesterol and triglyceride, are important biomarkers in patients with type 2 diabetes as they have implications for insulin resistance and cardiovascular mortality.

In patients with diabetes who are on enteral nutrition, the enteral feeds provided can be in the form of either Standard Formulas (SF) or Diabetes Specific Formulas (DSF). Enteral feeding formulas have a tendency to promote hyperglycaemia and insulinemic responses in patients with diabetes and in healthy subjects [16,17]. In addition, the effect of enteral nutrition on blood glucose parameters may be due to the fact that continuous enteral feeding is a source of continuous supply of glucose, providing 10–20 g of carbohydrates per hour, which is not the same during normal eating [15]. The absence of the normal postprandial glucose peak in patients with diabetes on enteral nutrition makes the management of hyperglycaemia difficult [15]. On the other hand, the effect of different types and amounts of fibre and mono-unsaturated fatty acids in various enteral feeds may influence lipid profile and other cardiometabolic parameters such as fasting blood glucose and glycated haemoglobin in patients with type 2 diabetes [18]. The role of the different enteral feeding formulas such as SF and DSF and their impact on cardiometabolic parameters in patients with diabetes continues to generate interest and controversy, and there appears to be no consensus among researchers on the most effective management strategy for these patients.

DSFs usually contain carbohydrates with low GI such as fructose and large amounts of monounsaturated fatty acids in varying amounts, which have effect on glycaemic control [17–20]. On the other hand, SFs are often high in carbohydrate and contain only low to moderate levels of lipids and do not have dietetic fibre [17].

Previous reviews on the use of enteral nutrition in patients with diabetes [16,17,21–23] either lacked consensus in the recommendations, were based only on glycaemic control or did not involve meta-analysis. In addition, concerns remain with the use of DSF in terms of the safety and tolerance of relatively high levels of fat and fructose with respect to lipid metabolism and lactic acidosis, despite its advantage in improving blood glucose compared with SFs [16,19]. Therefore, this review provides a quantitative assessment of the relative effectiveness of DSF compared with SF.

Aim: The aim was to evaluate the effectiveness of diabetes specific enteral nutrition formula versus SF in managing cardiometabolic parameters in patients with type 2 diabetes.

2. Methods

This study was conducted in accordance with the preferred reporting items for systematic reviews and meta-analyses (PRISMA) [24].

2.1. Types of Studies and Participants

Only randomised controlled studies were included in this review and participants were patients with type 2 diabetes.

Inclusion and Exclusion Criteria.

The criteria for considering studies for the review are outlined in Table 1.

Table 1. Criteria for considering studies for the review based on the Population, Intervention, Comparator, Outcomes and Study designs (PICOS) Structure.

	Inclusion Criteria	Exclusion Criteria
Population	Patients with type 2 diabetes and on enteral nutrition irrespective of type of feeding tube.	Patients with type 1 diabetes. Pregnant women with gestational diabetes. Healthy individuals without diabetes on enteral nutrition. Patients with diabetes on parenteral nutrition and parenteral plus enteral nutrition. Studies involving animals
Intervention	Diabetes specific formulas (Oral nutrition supplement or enteral tube feeding)	Parenteral nutrition, parenteral plus enteral nutrition.
Comparator	Standard formulas (Oral nutrition supplement or enteral tube feeding)	Parenteral nutrition and parenteral plus enteral nutrition.
Outcomes	Cardiometabolic parameters	Qualitative outcomes such as patient feelings.
Study Design:	Randomised Controlled Trials	Letters, comments, reviews, qualitative studies

2.2. Type of Intervention

The intervention for this review was based on diabetes-specific enteral formula, irrespective of the type of feeding tube, mode and rate of delivery of the enteral feed and clinical settings.

2.3. Types of Outcome Measures

The following were the outcome measures of interest;

- Blood glucose parameters—Fasting blood glucose and glycated haemoglobin.
- Lipid profile: Total cholesterol, low density lipoprotein (LDL) cholesterol, high density lipoprotein (HDL) cholesterol and triglycerides.

2.4. Search Strategy

Databases encompassing Pubmed, EMBASE, PSYCInfo and Google scholar were searched for relevant articles based on the Population (Patients with diabetes), Intervention (Diabetes Specific Formula), Comparator (Standard enteral formulas), Outcomes (outcome measures) and Study designs (Randomised controlled studies)—PICOS framework (Table 2) [25]. The use of key words, truncation symbols, Medical Subject Heading (MeSH) terms and Boolean operators (AND/OR) formed part of the search strategy. Searches were conducted from the date of inception of databases until 2 January 2019.

The screening of studies and the evaluation of their eligibility and inclusion were in line with PRISMA [24] guidelines (Figure 1). These procedures were conducted by five researchers (OO, SMW, TT, RC, X-HW) and differences were resolved through consensus.

Table 2. Search method for identification of studies.

Patient/Population	Intervention	Comparator	Study Designs	Combining Search Terms
Patients with type 2 diabetes	Diabetes specific formulas	Standard formulas	Randomised Controlled Trial	
Type 2 diabetes OR type 2 diabetes mellitus OR Diabetes complications OR diabetes mellitus, type 2	Diabetes specific formula OR Diabetes specific form* OR Enteral nutrition OR Enteral* OR Enteral feed OR Enteral feed* OR Enteral form* OR Diabetes formula OR tube feeding OR enteral feeding		Randomised Controlled Trial OR Randomized Controlled Trial OR Randomized Controlled study OR RCT OR Randomized* OR controlled clinical trial OR placebo OR randomly OR trial OR groups	Column 1 AND Column 2 AND Column 3

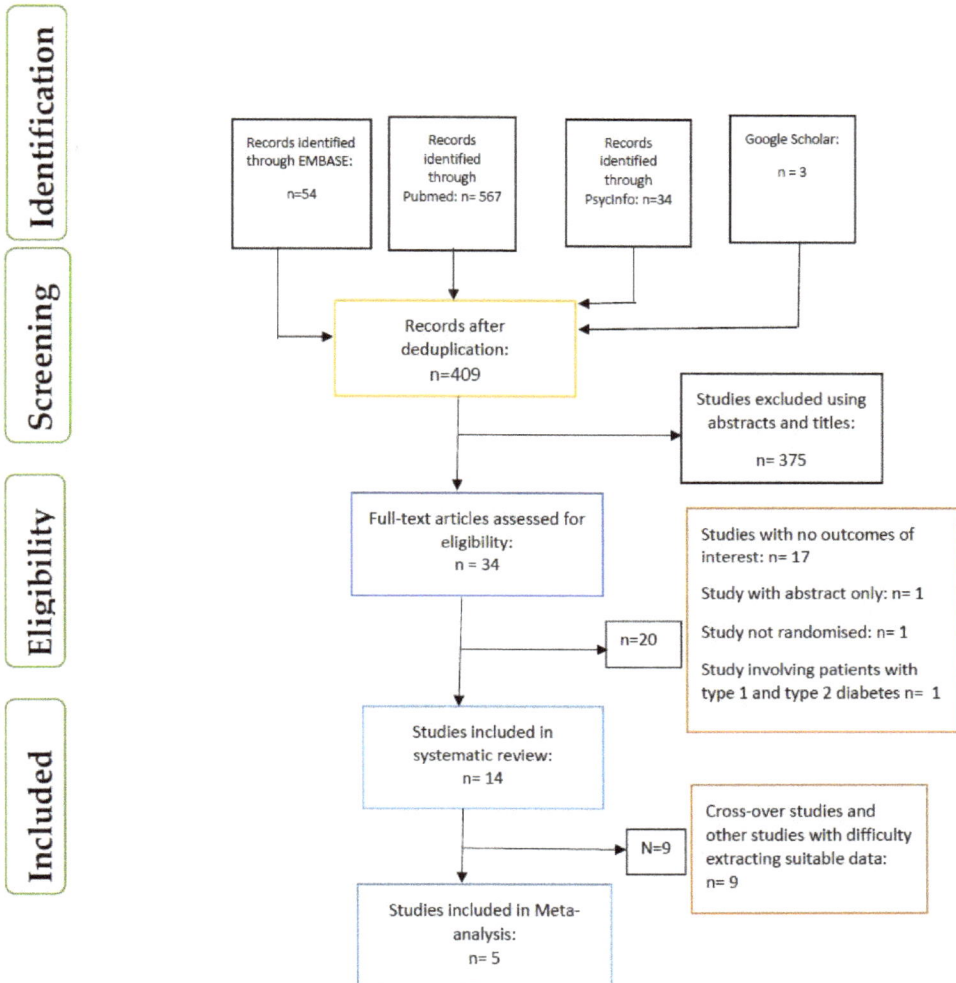

Figure 1. PRISMA flow chart on selection and inclusion of studies.

2.5. Data Extraction

All the articles from different databases were exported to ENDNote (Analytics, Philadelphia, PA, USA) for de-duplication. Data extraction was carried out by one researcher (OO) and cross-checked by the other four researchers (SMW, TT, RC, X-HW).

2.6. Assessment of Risk of Bias and Evaluation of Quality

A critical appraisal skills programme (CASP) tool was used to appraise the quality of the articles [26]. In addition, the researchers carried out an assessment of the risk of bias using the domain-based tool (random sequence generation, allocation concealment, blinding of participants, personnel and outcome assessment, reporting bias and selective reporting) to evaluate the studies included [27].

2.7. Statistical Analysis

Articles that met the inclusion criteria for meta-analysis were exported to RevMan (Review Manager, 5.3) [28] for data analysis. Therefore, cross-over studies and other studies which presented with difficulty in extracting suitable data were excluded from the meta-analysis. The data analysis included both meta-analysis and sensitivity analysis, the latter being conducted to test the consistency of the effect of DSFs on the different cardiometabolic paramters. The random effects model was used for the parameters of interest due to the high level of heterogeneity measured by the statistic I^2 with values ranging from 34% to 100%. A p value of 0.10 was used to determine the statistical significance of heterogeneity.

2.8. Effect Size

A forest plot was used to present the results of the meta-analysis and statistical significance for the overall effect of the intervention was determined by a *p* value of <0.05.

3. Results

3.1. Data Inclusion Decisions

Fasting blood glucose in the studies included was measured after overnight fasting, using standard measuring instruments. This is the standard method of measuring fasting blood glucose: the blood glucose concentrations were expressed as Means. However, the studies by Pohl et al. [29,30] were expressed as median and interquartile ranges and these were converted to means and standard deviations [27]. Fourteen studies were included in the systematic review (Table 3) while only five studies [29–33] were selected for the meta-analysis (Table 4).

Table 3. Characteristics of the articles included in this review ($n = 14$).

Citation	Country	Length of Study	Study Type/Design	Sample Size/Description	Age (Years)	Type of Enteral Formula/Feeding Method	Duration of Diabetes (Years)	Study Results/Conclusion
Ceriello et al. [18]	Netherlands	24 h	Randomized, controlled, double-blind, cross-over	$n = 11$	Mean ± SEM 67.2 ± 1.3	The DSF had 1 kcal/mL and low GI and/or slowly digestible CHO. The SF was isocaloric fibre containing formula. Bolus Feeding	Mean ± SEM 6.6 ± 1.4 years	Administration of DSF lowered glucose profiles. Using DSF resulted in significantly lower 24 h and postprandial glucose profiles than fibre-containing SF after bolus administration.
Buranapin et al. [21]	Thailand	180 min	Single centre, prospective, randomized, double blind, cross-over study. Administration of oral DSF and SF	$n = 30$	Mean ± SD 60.93 ± 11.71	55% CHO, 15% protein, 30% fat for DSF and SF. However, DSF substituted sucrose for combination of fructose, polydextrose and FOS. Bolus Feeding	More than 6 months.	DSF resulted in significantly lower postprandial blood glucose concentration than SF.
Pohl et al. [29]	Germany	12 weeks	Randomized, double-blind, controlled, multi-centre trial.	$n = 78$	Median (Range) Test group (DSF): 71 (42–86) Control group (SF): 72 (51–87)	DSF contained 37% energy as CHO, 45% as fat, 18% as protein, SF contained 52% energy as CHO, 30% of energy as total fat and 18% as protein. Continuous Feeding.	No data	DSF formula resulted in a more effective glycaemia control than SF, and was comparable in DSF significantly decreased triglycerides compared with SF, but differences were not significant in relation to total cholesterol, HDL, and LDL cholesterols.
Pohl et al. [30]	Germany	84 days	Stage two of a randomized, prospective, double-blind, controlled, multicentre, parallel group study Parallel design.	$n = 97$	Median (Range) DSF: 74 (44–91) SF: 69 (53–86)	DSF contained 37% energy as CHO, 45% as fat, 18% as protein, SF contained 52% energy as CHO, 30% of energy as total fat and 18% as protein. Continuous Feeding.	No data	Compared to SF, DSF significantly lowered FBG and improved glycaemic control. There were no significant differences between the two groups with respect to TG, TC, HDL, and LDL cholesterols.

13

Table 3. *Cont.*

Citation	Country	Length of Study	Study Type/Design	Sample Size/Description	Age (Years)	Type of Enteral Formula/Feeding Method	Duration of Diabetes (Years)	Study Results/Conclusion
Craig et al. [31]	USA–New York State	3 months	Randomized, double-blind, controlled, parallel group 3 months pilot trial.	n = 34	DSF: 82 ± 3 (range 52–94) 80 ± 2 (range-SF: 52–100)	Per 1000 mL, DSF contained 1000 kcal, 41.8 g protein, 93.7 g CHO, 55.7 g fat. SF contained 1060 kcal, 44.4 g protein, 151.7 CHO, 35.9 g fat. Continuous or intermittent feeding.	No data	DSF resulted in lower fasting serum glucose and HbA1c than SF. No significant differences between the DSF and SF groups with respect to LDL cholesterol and TG 3 months post intervention, but the DSF group had significantly higher level of HDL cholesterol than the SF group.
Lansink et al. [32]	Netherlands	4 weeks	Randomized, controlled, double-blind, parallel-group study.	n = 44	Mean ± SD DSF: 65.2 ± 7.4 SF: 64.2 ± 5.9	DSF contained 1 kcal/mL, 47 Energy% CHO, 19 Energy% protein, 34 Energy% fat and 2 g fibres/100 mL. The SF contained 50 Energy% CHO, 16 Energy% protein, 34 Energy% fat and 1.5 g fibres/100 mL. Bolus Feeding	Mean (Range) DSF: 84 (18–216) months SF: 66 (10–504) months	DSF significantly lowered postprandial glucose compared with SF. Levels of TG, TC, HDL and LDL cholesterols were not significantly different between the two groups at baseline and 4 weeks post intervention.
Vaisman et al. [33]	No data	12 weeks	Randomized, controlled, double-blind, parallel group study.	n = 25	Total: 76.2 ± 12.8 years DSF: 73.0 ± 14.7 SF: 79.2 ± 10.4	DSF contained 100 kcal, 45 Energy% CHO, 38 Energy% fat, 17 Energy% protein and 1.5 g/100 kcal fibre. SF contained 100 kcal, 55 Energy% CHO, 30 Energy% fat, 15 Energy% protein, 2 g/100 kcal fibre. Bolus, Continuous or intermittent feeding.	Mean ± SD Total: 8.6 ± 7.6 years DSF: 5.0 ± 4.9 SF: 12.6 ± 8.4	The DSF significantly reduced HbA1c compared to SF. No significant effect was found with respect to fasting blood glucose. DSF significantly increased HDL cholesterol, but differences were not significant in relation to TG, TC and LDL cholesterol compared with SF.

Table 3. *Cont.*

Citation	Country	Length of Study	Study Type/Design	Sample Size/Description	Age (Years)	Type of Enteral Formula/Feeding Method	Duration of Diabetes (Years)	Study Results/Conclusion
Alish et al. [34]	USA	10 days	Randomized, double blind, two treatment, crossover design. DSF (Postprandial response protocol) vs. SF (Continuous glucose monitoring).	n = 12	Mean ± SEM Postprandial: 63.1 ± 1.9 Continuous feed: 74.1 ± 4.0	DSF had 1.2 kcal/mL, 114.5 g CHO, 17 g/L fibre, 60 g/L protein, 60 g/L fat. SF had 1.2 kcal/mL, 169.4 g CHO, 18 g/L fibre, 55.5 g/L protein, 39.3 g/L fat. Continuous Feeding.	NS	Use of DSF produced lower postprandial glycaemic and insulinemic responses, reduced glycaemic variability, and resulted in less hyperglycaemia, reduced short acting insulin requirements.
Gulati et al. [35]	India	8 months	Open-label, randomized, crossover, pilot single centre study.	n = 40	35–60 years	DSF administered was 55 g in 210 mL of water to make 250 mL at standard reconstitution (1 kcal/mL) which can be used as tube feed or oral nutrition supplement. The SF was isocaloric Meal. Bolus Feeding	No data	DSF demonstrated lower blood glucose and insulin post meal levels than SF. The level of HDL cholesterol was significantly higher in the DSF group compared with the SF group after intervention, but differences were not significant in relation to TG, TC and LDL cholesterol.
Hofman et al. [36]	Netherlands	360 min	Randomized, double blind, cross over study involving SF (A), DSF with moderate amount of carbohydrate and MUFA (B) and Test feed with low amount of carbohydrate and high amount of fat (C)	n = 12	63 ± 9.4 years	DSF (45 Energy% CHO, 26 Energy% MUFA), SF (49 Energy% CHO, 21 Energy% MUFA). Continuous Feeding.	No data	DSF showed significantly lower glucose levels compared with SF. With respect to TG level, the DSF B with a lower amount of fat showed significantly lower levels than test feed C.

Table 3. Cont.

Citation	Country	Length of Study	Study Type/Design	Sample Size/Description	Age (Years)	Type of Enteral Formula/Feeding Method	Duration of Diabetes (Years)	Study Results/Conclusion
Lansink et al. [37]	Netherlands	8 h	Randomized, controlled, double-blind cross-over study	n = 24	Mean ± SD 64.6 ± 10.7	The DSF had 1.5 kcal/mL, high protein, a mixture of 6 different dietary fibre and low GI CHO. SF was isocaloric fibre containing formula. Continuous Feeding.	Median (Minimum and Maximum) 76.5 months (13, 303)	Administration of a new, high-protein DSF during 4 h of continuous feeding resulted in lower glucose and insulin levels compared with a fiber-containing SF. DSF may contribute to lower glucose levels in these patients.
Mesejo et al. [38]	Spain	2 years	Prospective, open-label, randomized study	n = 157	Median (Q1–Q3) New generation DSF: 57 (43–70) SF: 60 (45–71) Control DSF: 58 (46–68)	Per 100 mL, DSF had 100 kcal, 5.7 g protein, 8.2 g CHO, 4.4 g fat. SF had 100 kcal. 57 g protein, 10.93/15.3 g CHO, 3.79/5.3 g fat. Continuous Feeding.	No data	DSFs lowered insulin requirements, improved glycaemic control and reduced the risk of acquired infections relative to SF. Plasma levels of cholesterol and TG were similar across the three treatment groups.
Voss et al. [39]	USA	240 min	Randomized cross over-study Double-blinded with three-treatments	n = 48	Mean ± SEM 56 ± 1.4 years	DSF had 1 kcal/mL, 47.8 g CHO, 7.2 g fibre, 20.9 g protein, 27.2 g fat. SF had 1.06 kcal/mL, 73 g CHO, 7.2 g fibre, 20.9 g protein, 16.4 g fat. Bolus Feeding		DSF resulted in lower postprandial blood glucose response compared with SF.
Vanschoonbeek et al. [40]	Netherlands	10 days	Randomized, double-blind, cross over study.	n = 15	Mean ± SEM 63 ± 1 years	Per 100 mL, DSF had 98 kcal, 1.44 g fibre and 5.44/50 (g/energy%) of fat. SF had 100 kcal, 1.4 g of fibre, 3.4/30 (g/energy%) of fat.). Bolus Feeding	Mean ± SEM 9 ± 2 years	DSF rich in lowly digestible carbohydrate sources can be equally effective in lowering the postprandial blood glucose response as low-carbohydrate, high-fat enteral formulas without elevating the plasma triglyceride response.

Abbreviations: NS (Not stated); DSF (Diabetes Specific Formula); CHO (Carbohydrate); FOS (Fructo-oligosaccharide); GI (Glycaemic Index); HbA1c (Glycated haemoglobin); SF (Standard Formula); LDL (low density lipoprotein) Cholesterol; HDL (high density lipoprotein)Cholesterol; MUFA (mono-unsaturated fatty acid); FBG (fasting blood glucose); TC (total cholesterol); TG (triglycerides); T2DM (type 2 diabetes mellitus).

Table 4. Blood glucose parameters among individuals with diabetes (Meta-analysis Data Extraction Table).

Study Reference	Interventions	Pre-and Post Intervention	Fasting Blood Glucose mmol/L Mean ± SD/Median (Quartiles)	Glycated Haemoglobin % Mean ± SD/Median (Quartiles)	Total Cholesterol mmol/L Mean ± SD/Median (Quartiles)	LDL Cholesterol mmol/L Mean ± SD/Median (Quartiles)	HDL Cholesterol mmol/L Mean ± SD/Median (Quartiles)	Triglycerides mmol/L Mean ± SD/Median (Quartiles)
Pohl. et al. [29]	DSF, n = 39	Change from baseline	** Δ−1.59 (−3.38 to −0.06)	** Δ−0.8 (−1.5 to −0.5)	** Δ−0.37 (−1.00 to 0.56)	** Δ−0.28 (−1.46 to 0.53)	** Δ0.08 (−0.06 to 0.28)	** Δ−0.37 (−0.36 to 0.38)
	SF, n = 39	Change from baseline	** Δ−0.08 (−1.34 to 0.79)	** Δ0.0 (−0.4 to 0.3)	** Δ−0.23 (−1.22 to 0.46)	** Δ−0.52 (−1.48 to 0.04)	** Δ0.05 (−0.10 to 0.32)	** Δ0.203 (−0.07 to 0.84)
Pohl et al. [30]	DSF, n = 48	Change from baseline	** Δ−2.17 (−2.55/−1.33)	** Δ−1.30 (−2.60/−0.10)	** Δ0.30 (−1.22/1.06)	** Δ0.27 (−0.71/1.40)	** Δ0.03 (−0.26/0.4)	** Δ−0.45 (−1.65/0.27)
	SF, n = 49	Change from baseline	** Δ−0.67 (−0.90/−0.10)	** Δ−1.20 (−2.35/−0.55)	** Δ0.21 (−1.02/0.48)	** Δ−0.33 (−1.03/0.56)	** Δ0.00 (−0.22/0.28)	** Δ−0.70 (−1.50/1.73)
Craig et al. [31]	DSF, n = 14	Baseline	* 7.3 ± 0.4	* 6.9 ± 0.3	* 4.16 ± 0.31	* 2.66 ± 0.23	* 1.01 ± 0.05	* 0.97 ± 0.13
		Final	6.7 ± 0.7	6.5 ± 0.4	3.96 ± 0.31	2.51 ± 0.28	0.98 ± 0.05	0.91 ± 0.17g/L
	SF, n = 13	Baseline	* 6.9 ± 0.6	* 6.9 ± 0.5	* 4.21 ± 0.18	* 2.69 ± 0.15	* 0.98 ± 0.05	* 0.9 ± 0.07
		Final	8.3 ± 1.7	6.9 ± 0.14	3.96 ± 0.23	2.53 ± 0.21	0.83 ± 0.05	1.06 ± 0.12 g/L
Lansink et al. [32]	DSF, n = 21	Baseline	* 8.32 ± 0.33	No data	No data	No data	No data	No data
		Final	8.13 ± 0.33					
	SF, n = 22	Baseline	* 7.73 ± 0.22	No data	No data	No data	No data	No data
		Final	8.22 ± 0.26					
Vaisman et al. [33]	DSF, n = 12	Baseline	No data	*** 6.9 ± 0.3	No data	No data	*** 1.04 ± 0.08	No data
		Final		6.2 ± 0.4			1.23 ± 0.10	
	SF, n = 13	Baseline	No data	*** 7.9 ± 0.3	No data	No data	*** 1.06 ± 0.08	No data
		Final		8.7 ± 0.4			0.94 ± 0.09	

Abbreviations: NS (Not stated); SD (Standard deviation); SEM (Standard Error of Mean); Δ (Change from baseline) * Mean ± SD; ** Median (Quartiles); *** Mean ± SEM.

3.2. Assessment of Risk of Bias in Included Studies

Figure 2 shows the risk of bias summary of the various studies included in the meta-analysis. All the studies demonstrated low risk of bias in all the areas, except with respect to incomplete outcome data (attrition bias) where two studies [29,33] showed high risk of bias.

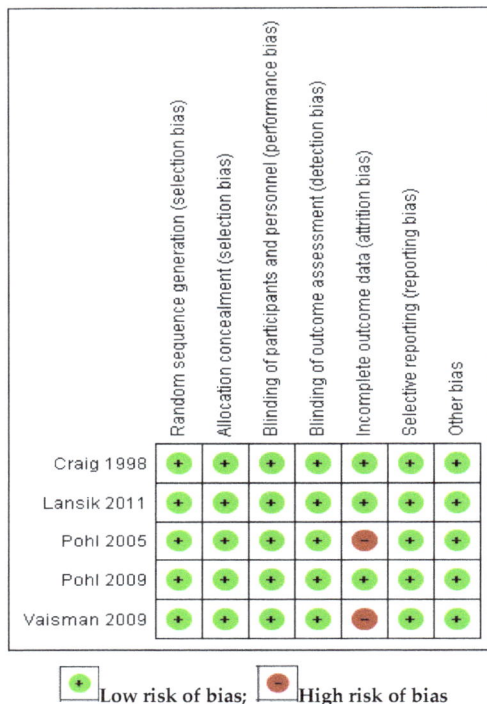

Figure 2. Risk of bias summary.

Based on the findings of the review and the meta-analysis, two distinct areas were evident: the effect of DSF on blood glucose parameters and the effect of DSF on lipid profile.

The effect DSF on blood glucose parameters:

All the fourteen studies included in the systematic review showed that DSF was effective in lowering blood glucose parameters in patients with type 2 diabetes compared with SF. In particular, DSF improved glycaemic control and lowered insulin requirements [18,29,31,35–39]. It provided better clinical outcomes, including reducing the risk of acquired infections and pressure ulcer, reduced body weight and was safer compared to SF [29,31,32]. In addition, the use of DSF was shown to be effective in lowering postprandial blood glucose levels compared to SF [20,32,34,40].

Pohl et al. [30] observed that long-term tube feeding with a DSF significantly lowered fasting blood glucose and improved glycaemic control. Similarly, Vaisman et al. [33] reported that DSF significantly improved longer-term glycaemic control in diabetic patients compared to SF. The results of the meta-analysis confirmed the findings of the systematic review. With respect to the fasting blood glucose, it was significantly lower ($p = 0.01$) in the DSF group compared to SF, with a mean difference of -1.15 (95% CI -2.07, -0.23) (Figure 3). However, in relation to the sensitivity analysis, there were no significant differences ($p > 0.05$) between the two groups with the removal of Pohl et al. [29,30] studies.

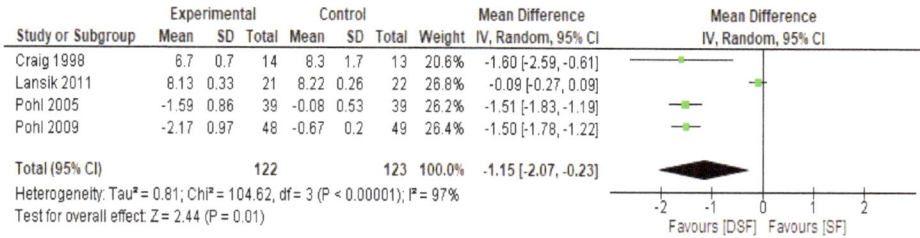

| Study or Subgroup | Experimental | | | Control | | | | Mean Difference | Mean Difference |
	Mean	SD	Total	Mean	SD	Total	Weight	IV, Random, 95% CI	IV, Random, 95% CI
Craig 1998	6.7	0.7	14	8.3	1.7	13	20.6%	-1.60 [-2.59, -0.61]	
Lansik 2011	8.13	0.33	21	8.22	0.26	22	26.8%	-0.09 [-0.27, 0.09]	
Pohl 2005	-1.59	0.86	39	-0.08	0.53	39	26.2%	-1.51 [-1.83, -1.19]	
Pohl 2009	-2.17	0.97	48	-0.67	0.2	49	26.4%	-1.50 [-1.78, -1.22]	
Total (95% CI)			122			123	100.0%	-1.15 [-2.07, -0.23]	

Heterogeneity: Tau² = 0.81; Chi² = 104.62, df = 3 (P < 0.00001); I² = 97%
Test for overall effect: Z = 2.44 (P = 0.01)

Favours [DSF]   Favours [SF]

Figure 3. The effect of DSF on fasting blood glucose (mmol/L).

The glycated haemoglobin was significantly lower (*p* = 0.005) in the DSF group compared to the SF group following meta-analysis (Figure 4) and sensitivity analysis.

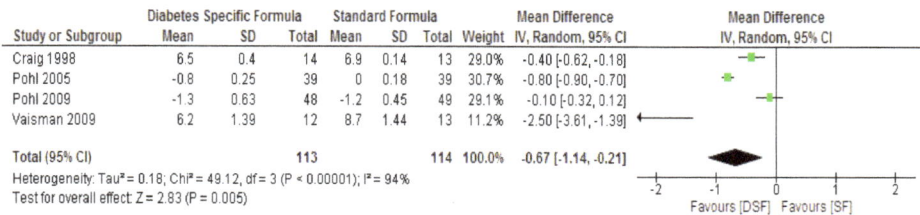

| Study or Subgroup | Diabetes Specific Formula | | | Standard Formula | | | | Mean Difference | Mean Difference |
	Mean	SD	Total	Mean	SD	Total	Weight	IV, Random, 95% CI	IV, Random, 95% CI
Craig 1998	6.5	0.4	14	6.9	0.14	13	29.0%	-0.40 [-0.62, -0.18]	
Pohl 2005	-0.8	0.25	39	0	0.18	39	30.7%	-0.80 [-0.90, -0.70]	
Pohl 2009	-1.3	0.63	48	-1.2	0.45	49	29.1%	-0.10 [-0.32, 0.12]	
Vaisman 2009	6.2	1.39	12	8.7	1.44	13	11.2%	-2.50 [-3.61, -1.39]	
Total (95% CI)			113			114	100.0%	-0.67 [-1.14, -0.21]	

Heterogeneity: Tau² = 0.18; Chi² = 49.12, df = 3 (P < 0.00001); I² = 94%
Test for overall effect: Z = 2.83 (P = 0.005)

Favours [DSF]   Favours [SF]

Figure 4. The effect of DSF on Glycated Haemoglobin %.

3.3. The Effect of DSF on Lipid Profile

Based on the systematic review, the outcomes of the studies selected to evaluate the effect of DSF on lipid profile were variable. Craig et al. [31] did not find significant differences with respect to LDL cholesterol and triglyceride between the DSF and the SF groups, but differences were significantly higher (*p* < 0.05) in the DSF group in relation to HDL cholesterol. In two other studies [33,35], the level of HDL cholesterol was significantly higher (*p* < 0.05) in the DSF group compared with the SF group after intervention, but differences were not significant (*p* > 0.05) in relation to triglycerides, total cholesterol and LDL cholesterols. Differences between DSF and SF were also not significant (*p* > 0.05) in terms of triglyceride, total cholesterol, HDL cholesterol and LDL cholesterol in other studies [30,32,38]. In contrast, Pohl et al. [29] reported that there was a significant difference (*p* < 0.05) between the DSF group and the SF group with respect to triglycerides, but differences were not significant (*p* > 0.05) in relation to total cholesterol, HDL and LDL cholesterol. Other studies [36,40] have also shown that DSF is effective in controlling plasma triglyceride.

Following meta-analysis, no significant differences (*p* > 0.05) were found between the DSF and SF groups with respect to total cholesterol, LDL cholesterol and triglyceride (Figures 5–7). However, the DSF group had a significantly higher level (*p* = 0.04) of HDL cholesterol compared to the SF group after the intervention, with a mean difference of 0.09 (95% CI, 0.00, 0.18) (Figure 8). The results of the sensitivity test for HDL cholesterol demonstrated no significant differences (*p* > 0.05) between the two groups when the Craig et al. [31] and Vaisman et al. [33] studies were removed from the analysis. In addition, the sensitivity analysis showed no significant differences (*p* > 0.05) between the two groups with respect to total cholesterol and triglyceride, while significant differences (<0.05) were observed in relation to LDL cholesterol when the Craig et al. [31] study was removed.

Study or Subgroup	Diabetes Specific Formula			Standard Formula			Weight	Mean Difference IV, Random, 95% CI
	Mean	SD	Total	Mean	SD	Total		
Craig 1998	3.96	0.31	14	3.96	0.23	13	30.4%	0.00 [-0.20, 0.20]
Pohl 2005	-0.37	0.39	39	-0.23	0.42	39	36.1%	-0.14 [-0.32, 0.04]
Pohl 2009	0.3	0.57	48	0.21	0.36	49	33.6%	0.09 [-0.10, 0.28]
Total (95% CI)			101			101	100.0%	-0.02 [-0.16, 0.12]

Heterogeneity: Tau² = 0.00; Chi² = 3.03, df = 2 (P = 0.22); I² = 34%
Test for overall effect Z = 0.29 (P = 0.77)

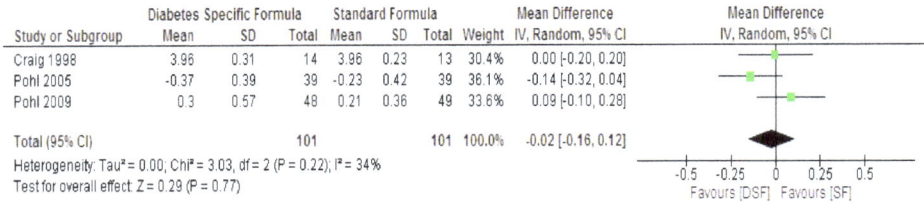

Figure 5. The effect of DSF on total cholesterol (mmol/L).

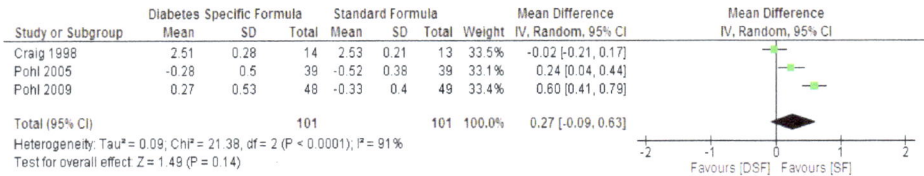

Study or Subgroup	Diabetes Specific Formula			Standard Formula			Weight	Mean Difference IV, Random, 95% CI
	Mean	SD	Total	Mean	SD	Total		
Craig 1998	2.51	0.28	14	2.53	0.21	13	33.5%	-0.02 [-0.21, 0.17]
Pohl 2005	-0.28	0.5	39	-0.52	0.38	39	33.1%	0.24 [0.04, 0.44]
Pohl 2009	0.27	0.53	48	-0.33	0.4	49	33.4%	0.60 [0.41, 0.79]
Total (95% CI)			101			101	100.0%	0.27 [-0.09, 0.63]

Heterogeneity: Tau² = 0.09; Chi² = 21.38, df = 2 (P < 0.0001); I² = 91%
Test for overall effect Z = 1.49 (P = 0.14)

Figure 6. The effect of DSF on LDL cholesterol (mmol/L).

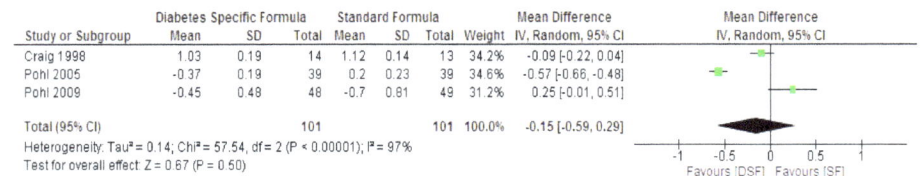

Study or Subgroup	Diabetes Specific Formula			Standard Formula			Weight	Mean Difference IV, Random, 95% CI
	Mean	SD	Total	Mean	SD	Total		
Craig 1998	1.03	0.19	14	1.12	0.14	13	34.2%	-0.09 [-0.22, 0.04]
Pohl 2005	-0.37	0.19	39	0.2	0.23	39	34.6%	-0.57 [-0.66, -0.48]
Pohl 2009	-0.45	0.48	48	-0.7	0.81	49	31.2%	0.25 [-0.01, 0.51]
Total (95% CI)			101			101	100.0%	-0.15 [-0.59, 0.29]

Heterogeneity: Tau² = 0.14; Chi² = 57.54, df = 2 (P < 0.00001); I² = 97%
Test for overall effect Z = 0.67 (P = 0.50)

Figure 7. The effect of DSF on Triglycerides (mmol/L).

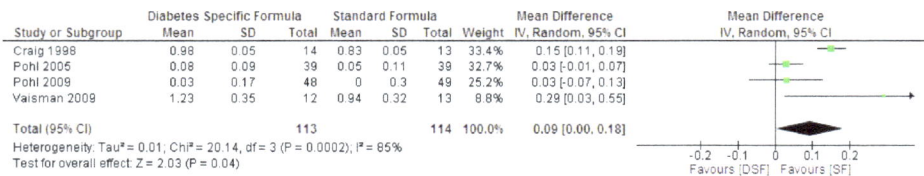

Study or Subgroup	Diabetes Specific Formula			Standard Formula			Weight	Mean Difference IV, Random, 95% CI
	Mean	SD	Total	Mean	SD	Total		
Craig 1998	0.98	0.05	14	0.83	0.05	13	33.4%	0.15 [0.11, 0.19]
Pohl 2005	0.08	0.09	39	0.05	0.11	39	32.7%	0.03 [-0.01, 0.07]
Pohl 2009	0.03	0.17	48	0	0.3	49	25.2%	0.03 [-0.07, 0.13]
Vaisman 2009	1.23	0.35	12	0.94	0.32	13	8.8%	0.29 [0.03, 0.55]
Total (95% CI)			113			114	100.0%	0.09 [0.00, 0.18]

Heterogeneity: Tau² = 0.01; Chi² = 20.14, df = 3 (P = 0.0002); I² = 85%
Test for overall effect Z = 2.03 (P = 0.04)

Figure 8. The effect of DSF on HDL cholesterol (mmol/L).

4. Discussion

The findings of the systematic review and meta-analysis revealed that DSF was effective in lowering blood glucose (fasting blood glucose and glycated haemoglobin) compared with SF in patients with type 2 diabetes. However, the sensitivity analysis for the fasting blood glucose did not demonstrate a significant difference ($p > 0.05$) with the removal of the Pohl et al. [29,30] studies. In addition, there were no significant differences ($p > 0.05$) between the DSF and SF groups with respect to total cholesterol, LDL cholesterol and triglyceride (although a few studies reported significant differences with respect to triglyceride). Differences in the outcomes of studies in the systematic review were observed with respect to the effect of DSF on HDL cholesterol and the meta-analysis also showed significantly higher levels for the DSF group compared with the SF group. The high level of heterogeneity in the studies included in the meta-analyses may explain why the results of the meta-analysis and the sensitivity analysis were not consistent with respect to HDL cholesterol and fasting blood glucose.

The presence of low glycaemic index (GI) carbohydrate in the form of isomaltulose, the lower amount of carbohydrate and the higher protein content in the DSF may have contributed to the findings of this review [37]. In addition, the presence of mono-unsaturated fatty acids (MUFA) and the different amounts and types of fibre in the DSF compared with SF may be responsible for the observed differences in the fasting blood glucose, glycated haemoglobin and lipid profiles in both groups [18,41]. DSFs are usually higher in fat (40–50% of energy with a significant portion of MUFA) and have a lower carbohydrate level (30–40% of energy) and about 15% of energy is derived from fructose and soluble fibre [20]. DSFs contain carbohydrates with low GI such as non-hydrolysed starches, disaccharides, fibre and fructose in varying amounts which are aimed at controlling postprandial glucose [17–20]. In contrast, SFs are high in carbohydrate (about 50%) and have low–moderate levels of lipids (about 30%) and do not contain dietetic fibre [17]. A study by Hofman et al. [42] demonstrated that, in 12 enteral formulas examined, the GI ranged from 12 for DSFs up to 61 for SFs. The GI of food is a measure of how quickly the food is digested and the glucose reaches the blood stream [22,43]. Foods with high GI rapidly increase blood glucose and insulin responses after consumption [43,44]. The results from meta-analysis showed that the intake of a low GI diet was associated with reductions in blood glucose parameters [35,43]. In addition, high soluble fibre-containing foods can improve glycaemic control partly due to delayed absorption [36].

Therefore, DSFs may improve glycaemic control through delay in gastric emptying, delayed intestinal absorption of carbohydrate and lower glycaemic response [20]. In the study by Alish et al. [34], the blend of DSF was made up of low glycaemic and slowly digestible carbohydrates, resistant maltodextrin, isomaltulose, sucromalt and prebiotic fibres, including fructo-oligosaccharides. These constituents collectively produce a slow and consistent release of glucose into the blood stream [34]. Isomaltulose is a naturally occurring low GI slowly digestible carbohydrate [18]. The slower hydrolysation of isomaltulose during digestion may be responsible for the slower rise in blood glucose in patients with diabetes on DSF [18]. In addition, the higher protein content of the DSF may have contributed to the lowering of blood glucose parameters by delaying gastric emptying [18].

The use of high fat content, including MUFA, in the DSF may slow the transit time in the gastrointestinal tract and slow the absorption of sugars which could help improve glycaemic control [35,41]. Diets that are high in MUFA have been shown to increase HDL cholesterol and reduce other components of the lipid profiles [35,41]. HDL cholesterol is useful for reducing the risk of cardiovascular disease [35]. The result of the meta-analysis of the current review confirmed the positive role of DSF in increasing HDL cholesterol. However, the sensitivity tests did not demonstrate consistency in terms of the effect of DSF on HDL cholesterol, which could explain why researchers may be reluctant to recommend the use of high fat content in DSF due to the risk of alterations in lipid profiles [41]. This may also be due to the fact that there have been differences in the outcomes of studies on the effect of DSF on lipid profile [41].

5. Limitation

The limitation of this review was that only five studies were included in the meta-analysis. In particular, there were fewer studies included for lipid outcomes (three for several parameters) and there was substantial variability in the studies. Therefore, the differences between the meta-analysis and the sensitivity analysis in some of the parameters suggest that those results were not quite consistent, which may be due to the high level of heterogeneity of the studies. Therefore, more studies are needed to address this problem.

6. Conclusions

The results provide evidence to suggest that DSF is effective in controlling fasting blood glucose and glycated haemoglobin. In addition, DSF was effective in increasing HDL cholesterol but had no significant effect on other lipid parameters. However, our confidence in these findings would be increased by additional data from further studies. Additional research would also provide the opportunity to refine our understanding of the effect of DSF on cardiometabolic parameters.

Author Contributions: Conceptualization, O.O., S.M.W., T.T., R.C., X.-H.W.; methodology, O.O., S.M.W., T.T., R.C., X.-H.W.; validation, O.O., S.M.W., T.T., R.C., X.-H.W.; formal analysis, O.O. and reviewed by S.M.W., T.T., R.C., X.-H.W.; writing—original draft preparation, O.O.; writing—review and editing, O.O., S.M.W., T.T., R.C., X.-H.W.

Funding: This research received no external funding.

Conflicts of Interest: The authors declare no conflicts of interest.

References

1. DeFronzo, R.A.; Ratner, R.E.; Han, J.; Kim, D.D.; Fineman, M.S.; Baron, A.D. Effects of exenatide (exendin-4) on glycemic control and weight over 30 weeks in metformin-treated patients with type 2 diabetes. *Diabetes Care* **2005**, *28*, 1092–1100. [CrossRef] [PubMed]
2. Jansink, R.; Braspenning, J.; Laurant, M.; Keizer, E.; Elwyn, G.; Weijden, T.D.; Grol, R. Minimal improvement of nurses' motivational interviewing skills in routine diabetes care one year after training: A cluster randomized trial. *BMC Fam. Pract.* **2013**, *14*, 44. [CrossRef] [PubMed]
3. National Collaborating Centre for Chronic Conditions (NCCCC). *Type 2 Diabetes: National Clinical Guideline for Management in Primary and Secondary Care (Update)*; Royal College of Physicians: London, UK, 2008.
4. Public Health England. 3.8 Million People in England Now Have Diabetes. 2016. Available online: https://www.gov.uk/government/news/38-million-people-in-england-now-have-diabetes (accessed on 1 February 2019).
5. National Health Service (NHS) Digital and Healthcare Quality Improvement Partnership. National diabetes audit, 2015–2016 Report 1: Care Processes and Treatment Targets. 2017. Available online: http://www.content.digital.nhs.uk/catalogue/PUB23241/nati-diab-rep1-audi-2015-16.pdf (accessed on 1 February 2019).
6. Diabetes UK. State of the Nation Report. 2015. Available online: https://www.diabetes.org.uk/Documents/About%20Us/What%20we%20say/State%20of%20the%20nation%202014.pdf (accessed on 1 February 2019).
7. Holman, N.; Young, B.; Gadsby, R. What is the current prevalence of diagnosed and yet to be diagnosed diabetes in the UK. *Diabetes Med.* **2014**, *31*, 510–511. [CrossRef] [PubMed]
8. Diabetes UK. Diabetes in the UK 2012: Key Statistics on Diabetes. 2012. Available online: http://tinyurl.com/owcyr7b (accessed on 1 February 2019).
9. Holmes, C.; Dyer, P. Diabetes training for nurses: The effectiveness of an inpatient diabetes half-day workshop. *J. Diabetes Nurs.* **2013**, *17*, 86–94.
10. Pereira, D.A.; da Silva Campos Costa, N.M.; Lima Sousa, A.L.; Veiga Jardim, P.B.; de Oliveira Zanini, C.R. The effect of educational intervention on the disease knowledge of diabetes mellitus patients. *Rev. Lat. Am. De Enferm.* **2012**, *20*, 478–485. [CrossRef] [PubMed]
11. Wyness, L. Understanding the role of diet in type 2 diabetes prevention. *Br. J. Commun. Nurs.* **2009**, *14*, 374–379. [CrossRef] [PubMed]
12. Ojo, O. The role of nutrition and hydration in disease prevention and patient safety. *Br. J. Nurs.* **2017**, *26*, 1020–1022. [CrossRef] [PubMed]
13. Arinzon, Z.; Shabat, S.; Shuval, I.; Peisakh, A.; Berner, Y. Prevalence of diabetes mellitus in elderly patients received enteral nutrition long-term care service. *Arch. Gerontol. Geriatr.* **2008**, *47*, 383–393. [CrossRef]
14. Wong, V.W.; Manoharan, M.; Mak, M. Managing hyperglycaemia in patients with diabetes on enteral nutrition: The role of a specialized diabetes team. *Eur. J. Clin. Nutr.* **2014**, *68*, 1305–1308. [CrossRef]
15. Oyibo, S.; Sagi, S.; Home, C. Glycaemic control during enteral tube feeding in patients with diabetes who have had a stroke: A twice-daily insulin regimen. *Pract. Diabetes* **2012**, *29*, 135–139. [CrossRef]
16. Elia, M.; Ceriello, A.; Laube, H.; Sinclair, A.J.; Engfer, M.; Stratton, R.J. Enteral nutritional support and use of diabetes specific formulas for patients with diabetes. *Diabetes Care* **2005**, *28*, 2267–2279. [CrossRef] [PubMed]
17. Sanz-Paris, A.; Álvarez Hernández, J.; Ballesteros-Pomar, M.D.; Botella-Romero, F.; León-Sanz, M.; Martín-Palmero, Á.; Oliveira, G. Evidence-based recommendations and expert consensus on enteral nutrition in the adult patient with diabetes mellitus or hyperglycemia. *Nutrition* **2017**, *41*, 58–67. [CrossRef] [PubMed]
18. Ceriello, A.; Lansink, M.; Rouws, C.H.F.C.; van Laere, K.M.J.; Frost, G.S. Administration of a new diabetes specific enteral formula results in an improved 24 h glucose profile in type 2 diabetic patients. *Diabetes Res. Clin. Pract.* **2009**, *84*, 259–266. [CrossRef] [PubMed]
19. Hise, M.E.; Fuhrman, M.P. *The Effect of Diabetes Specific Enteral Formulae on Clinical and Glycaemic Indicators*; Parrish, C.R., Ed.; Nutrition Issues in Gastroenterology Series 74; Shugar Publishing: New York, NY, USA, 2009; pp. 20–36.

20. Buranapin, S.; Siangruangsang, S.; Chantapanich, V.; Hengjeerajarus, N. The comparative study of diabetic specific formula and standard formula on postprandial plasma glucose control in type 2 DM patients. *J. Med. Assoc. Thail.* **2014**, *97*, 582–588.
21. McMahon, M.M.; Nystrom, E.; Braunschweig, C.; Miles, J.; Compher, C. The American Society of Parenteral and Enteral Nutrition (ASPEN) Clinical Guidelines: Nutrition support of adult patients with hyperglycaemia. *J. Parenter. Enter. Nutr.* **2013**, *37*, 23–36. [CrossRef] [PubMed]
22. Ojo O and Brooke J Evaluation of the role of enteral nutrition in managing patients with Diabetes: A systematic review. *Nutrients* **2014**, *6*, 5142–5152. [CrossRef]
23. Jones, S.; Honnor, M.; Castro, E.; Alsmadi, A. Management of people with diabetes receiving artificial nutrition: A review. *J. Diabetes Nurs.* **2017**, *21*, 179–183.
24. Moher, D.; Liberati, A.; Tetzlaff, J.; Altman, D.G.; Prisma, G. Preferred reporting items for systematic reviews and meta-analyses: The PRISMA statement. *BMJ* **2009**, *339*, b2535. [CrossRef]
25. Methley, A.M.; Campbell, S.; Chew-Graham, C.; McNally, R.; Cheraghi-Sohi, S. PICO, PICOS and SPIDER: A comparison study of specificity and sensitivity in three search tools for qualitative systematic reviews. *BMC Health Serv. Res.* **2014**, *14*, 579. [CrossRef]
26. Critical Appraisal Skills Programme (CASP) Case Control Study Checklist. Available online: http://docs.wixstatic.com/ugd/dded87_afbfc99848f64537a53826e1f5b30b5c.pdf (accessed on 29 January 2019).
27. Higgins, J.P.T.; Green, S. *Cochrane Handbook for Systematic Reviews of Interventions*; Wiley-Blackwell: Hoboken, NJ, USA, 2009.
28. The Nordic Cochrane Centre. Review Manager (RevMan). In *Computer Program*; Version 5.3; The Nordic Cochrane Centre, The Cochrane Collaboration: Copenhagen, Denmark, 2014.
29. Pohl, M.; Mayr, P.; Mertl-Roetzer, M.; Lauster, F.; Lerch, M.; Eriksen, J.; Haslbeck, M.; Rahlfs, V.W. Glycaemic control in type II diabetic tube-fed patients with a new enteral formula low in carbohydrates and high in monounsaturated fatty acids: A randomised controlled trial. *Eur. J. Clin. Nutr.* **2005**, *59*, 1221–1232. [CrossRef]
30. Pohl, M.; Mayr, P.; Mertl-Roetzer, M.; Lauster, F.; Haslbeck, M.; Hipper, B.; Steube, D.; Tietjen, M.; Eriksen, J.; Rahlfs, V.W. Glycemic control in patients with type 2 diabetes mellitus with a disease-specific enteral formula: Stage II of a randomized, controlled multicenter trial. *J. Parenter. Enter. Nutr.* **2009**, *33*, 37–49. [CrossRef] [PubMed]
31. Craig, L.D.; Nicholson, S.; Silverstone, F.A.; Kennedy, R.D.; Coble Voss, A.; Allison, S. Use of a reduced-carbohydrate, modified-fat enteral formula for improving metabolic control and clinical outcomes in long-term care residents with type 2 diabetes: Results of a pilot trial. *Nutrition* **1998**, *14*, 529–534. [CrossRef]
32. Lansink, M.; van Laere, K.M.; Vendrig, L.; Rutten, G.E. Lower postprandial glucose responses at baseline and after 4 weeks use of a diabetes-specific formula in diabetes type 2 patients. *Diabetes Res. Clin. Pract.* **2011**, *93*, 421–429. [CrossRef] [PubMed]
33. Vaisman, N.; Lansink, M.; Rouws, C.H.; van Laere, K.M.; Segal, R.; Niv, E.; Bowling, T.E.; Waitzberg, D.L.; Morleyf, J.E. Tube feeding with a diabetes-specific feed for 12 weeks improves glycaemic control in type 2 diabetes patients. *Clin. Nutr.* **2009**, *28*, 549–555. [CrossRef] [PubMed]
34. Alish, C.J.; Garvey, W.T.; Maki, K.C.; Sacks, G.S.; Hustead, D.S.; Hegazi, R.A.; Mustad, V.A. A diabetes-specific enteral formula improves glycemic variability in patients with type 2 diabetes. *Diabetes Technol. Ther.* **2010**, *12*, 419–425. [CrossRef] [PubMed]
35. Gulati, S.; Misra, A.; Nanda, K.; Pandey, R.M.; Garg, V.; Ganguly, S.; Cheung, L. Efficacy and tolerance of a diabetes specific formula in patients with type 2 diabetes mellitus: An open label, randomized, crossover study. *Diabetes Metab. Syndr. Clin. Res. Rev.* **2015**, *9*, 252–257. [CrossRef] [PubMed]
36. Hofman, Z.; Lansink, M.; Rouws, C.; van Drunen, J.D.E.; Kuipers, H. Diabetes specific tube feed results in improved glycaemic and triglyceridaemic control during 6 h continuous feeding in diabetes patients. *e-SPEN* **2007**, *2*, 44–50. [CrossRef]
37. Lansink, M.; Hofman, Z.; Genovese, S.; Rouws, C.H.F.C.; Ceriello, A. Improved Glucose Profile in Patients with Type 2 Diabetes with a New, High-Protein, Diabetes-Specific Tube Feed During 4 Hours of Continuous Feeding. *JPEN J. Parenter. Enter. Nutr.* **2017**, *41*, 968–975. [CrossRef]

38. Mesejo, A.; Montejo-Gonzalez, J.C.; Vaquerizo-Alonso, C.; Lobo-Tamer, G.; Zabarte-Martinez, M.; Herrero-Meseguer, J.I.; Escirbano, J.A.; Malpica, A.B.; Lozano, F.M. Diabetes-specific enteral nutrition formula in hyperglycemic, mechanically ventilated, critically ill patients: A prospective, open-label, blind-randomized, multicenter study. *Crit. Care* **2015**, *19*, 390. [CrossRef]
39. Voss, A.C.; Maki, K.C.; Garvey, W.T.; Hustead, D.S.; Alish, C.; Fix, B.; Mustad, V.A. Effect of two carbohydrate-modified tube-feeding formulas on metabolic responses in patients with type 2 diabetes. *Nutrition* **2008**, *24*, 990–997. [CrossRef]
40. Vanschoonbeek, K.; Lansink, M.; van Laere, K.M.; Senden, J.M.; Verdijk, L.B.; van Loon, L.J. Slowly digestible carbohydrate sources can be used to attenuate the postprandial glycemic response to the ingestion of diabetes-specific enteral formulas. *Diabetes Educ.* **2009**, *35*, 631–640. [CrossRef] [PubMed]
41. Vahabzadeh, D.; Valizadeh Hasanloei, M.A.; Vahdat Shariatpanahi, Z. Effect of high-fat, low-carbohydrate enteral formula versus standard enteral formula in hyperglycemic critically ill patients: A randomized clinical trial. *Int. J. Diabetes Dev. Ctries* **2019**, *39*, 173–180. [CrossRef]
42. Hofman, Z.; van Drunen, J.D.E.; de Later, C.; Kuipers, H. The Glycaemic index of standard and diabetes specific enteral formulas. *Asia Pac. J. Clin. Nutr.* **2006**, *15*, 412–417. [PubMed]
43. Ojo, O.; Ojo, O.O.; Adebowale, F.; Wang, X.H. The Effect of Dietary Glycaemic Index on Glycaemia in Patients with Type 2 Diabetes: A Systematic Review and Meta-Analysis of Randomized Controlled Trials. *Nutrients* **2018**, *10*, 373. [CrossRef] [PubMed]
44. Chang, K.T.; Lampe, J.W.; Schwarz, Y.; Breymeyer, K.L.; Noar, K.A.; Song, X.; Neuhouser, M.L. Low Glycemic Load Experimental Diet More Satiating Than High Glycemic Load Diet. *Nutr. Cancer* **2012**, *64*, 666–673. [CrossRef] [PubMed]

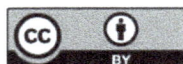

nutrients

MDPI

Article

Effect of Oral Nutritional Supplements with Sucromalt and Isomaltulose versus Standard Formula on Glycaemic Index, Entero-Insular Axis Peptides and Subjective Appetite in Patients with Type 2 Diabetes: A Randomised Cross-Over Study

Lisse Angarita Dávila [1,*], Valmore Bermúdez [2], Daniel Aparicio [3], Virginia Céspedes [4], Ma. Cristina Escobar [1], Samuel Durán-Agüero [5], Silvana Cisternas [6], Jorge de Assis Costa [7,8], Diana Rojas-Gómez [9], Nadia Reyna [3] and Jose López-Miranda [10,11]

[1] Escuela de Nutrición y Dietética, Facultad de Medicina, Universidad Andres Bello, Sede Concepción 4260000, Chile
[2] Facultad de Ciencias de la Salud, Universidad Simón Bolívar, Barranquilla 080003, Colombia
[3] Centro de Investigaciones Endocrino-Metabólicas "Dr. Félix Gómez", Escuela de Medicina. Facultad de Medicina, Universidad del Zulia, Maracaibo 4001, Venezuela
[4] Departamento de Medicina Física y Rehabilitación, Hospital "12 de Octubre", Madrid 28041, Spain
[5] Escuela de Nutrición y Dietética, Facultad de Ciencias para el Cuidado de la Salud, Universidad San Sebastián, Santiago 7500000, Chile
[6] Escuela de Salud, Universidad Tecnológica de Chile, INACAP, Sede Concepción, Talcahuano 4260000, Chile
[7] Faculty of Medicine/UniFAGOC, Ubá 36506-022, Minas Gerais, Brazil
[8] Universidade do Estado de Minas Gerais (UEMG), Barbacena 36202-284, Minas Gerais, Brazil
[9] Escuela de Nutrición y Dietética, Facultad de Medicina, Universidad Andres Bello, Santiago 8370321, Chile
[10] Lipids and Atherosclerosis Unit, Maimonides Institute for Biomedical Research in Cordoba, Reina Sofía University Hospital, University of Córdoba, 14004 Córdoba, Spain
[11] CIBER Physiopathology of Obesity and Nutrition (CIBEROBN), Institute of Health Carlos III, 28029 Madrid, Spain
* Correspondence: lisse.angarita@unab.cl; Tel.: +56412662147

Received: 19 April 2019; Accepted: 24 June 2019; Published: 28 June 2019

Abstract: Oral diabetes-specific nutritional supplements (ONS-D) induce favourable postprandial responses in subjects with type 2 diabetes (DM2), but they have not been correlated yet with incretin release and subjective appetite (SA). This randomised, double-blind, cross-over study compared postprandial effects of ONS-D with isomaltulose and sucromalt versus standard formula (ET) on glycaemic index (GI), insulin, glucose-dependent insulinotropic polypeptide (GIP), glucagon-like peptide 1 (GLP-1) and SA in 16 individuals with DM2. After overnight fasting, subjects consumed a portion of supplements containing 25 g of carbohydrates or reference food. Blood samples were collected at baseline and at 30, 60, 90, 120, 150 and 180 min; and SA sensations were assessed by a visual analogue scale on separate days. Glycaemic index values were low for ONS-D and intermediate for ET ($p < 0.001$). The insulin area under the curve ($AUC_{0–180\ min}$) ($p < 0.02$) and GIP AUC ($p < 0.02$) were lower after ONS-D and higher GLP-1 AUC when compared with ET ($p < 0.05$). Subjective appetite AUC was greater after ET than ONS-D ($p < 0.05$). Interactions between hormones, hunger, fullness and GI were found, but not within the ratings of SA; isomaltulose and sucromalt may have influenced these factors.

Keywords: glycaemic index; incretins; subjective appetite; isomaltulose; sucromalt; nutritional supplement

1. Introduction

Diabetes mellitus (DM) is a complex metabolic disorder associated with long-term complications as a result of the interplay of genetic, epigenetic, environmental and lifestyle factors [1]. Nowadays, DM is considered a pandemic health problem and one of the top 10 killers, responsible for 1.6 million deaths in 2016 [2]. According to International Diabetes Federation projections, by 2045, 629 million people will be afflicted by DM, exhibiting the fastest rising prevalence of this phenomenon in the history of humanity, which the highest prevalence rates in North America and the Caribbean [3]. Thus, the epidemiological impact of this disease is translated into higher public health expenditures worldwide [4,5].

One of the most important strategies for the prevention and treatment of DM has been correct management of carbohydrate consumption, having been reviewed in dietary guidelines and recommendations stated by many scientific organisations worldwide [6]. The American Diabetes Association (ADA) has highlighted this need, considering nutritional therapy as the fundamental basis of glycaemic control in DM patients [7]. Besides that, the European Association for the Study of Diabetes (EASD) has also focused its recommendations on the amount and type of carbohydrates consumed [8], generating considerable interest in low glycaemic index (LGI) food prescription for management of DM2 [9]. Indeed, a recent international expert consensus debated about the clinical role of GI and glycaemic load (GL) in DM management [10], concluding that low GI and low GL diets have been associated with a reduction in the glycaemic response variability [11], and better appetite control [12,13]. This phenomenon leads us to hypothesise that lower insulin responses exhibited by these supplements could promote satiety and fullness [10,12–14].

Nutritional approaches to type 2 diabetes usually include novel strategies in dietary advice, especially in oral nutritional supplements (ONS) prescription as part of the management of some DM comorbidities or as a complement for daily diet [15,16]. Any ONS designed for people with diabetes (ONS-D) provides better control in postprandial glucose and glycated haemoglobin (HbA$_1$c) when compared with standard supplements [17], since they are lower in total carbohydrate content (with a variety of sugar substitutes) and enriched with fibre and monounsaturated fatty acids [16,18,19]. Dietary fat and carbohydrate modifications modulate postprandial glycaemic responses by a reduction in glucose absorption rate [20].

The increase in peripheral glucose uptake via entero-insular axis peptides (EIAPs) such as the glucose-dependent insulinotropic peptide (GIP), glucagon-like peptide 1 (GLP-1), and insulin are a group of synergistic pathways counteracting undesirable glucose postprandial peaks [21]. Furthermore, a decrease in GIP secretion drives to adipocyte hypertrophy arrest and insulin resistance amelioration [22]. By contrast, GLP-1 has a direct suppression effect on appetite and protects pancreatic β-cells from programmed cell death [22,23]. It is well known that beverages have a faster gastric emptying and intestinal transit speed than solid food, which results in a rapid glycaemic response and lower perception of satiety [13,23]. For these reasons, the strategies of specific oral supplements designed for people with diabetes should include adaptation in the overall nutrients content [18,19]. Therefore, variations in both EIAP action and gastric emptying modulation by diet could play a fundamental role in short-time appetite regulation and energy intake [24,25].

Use of ONS-Ds in malnourished or sarcopenic diabetic patients enhances energy intake and overall nutritional status, improving glycaemic control, and thus, cause indirect economic benefits [19]. A meta-analysis by Elia et al. [15] on a total of 23 studies and 784 patients receiving oral supplements or tube feeding showed that when compared with standard supplements, ONS-D significantly reduced postprandial rise in blood glucose, peak blood glucose concentration and glucose area under the curve (AUCG) with no significant effects on HDL, total cholesterol, or triglyceride levels. Furthermore, this study reported a reduced insulin requirement (26–71% lower) and fewer complications in patients with ONS-D therapy when compared with standard nutritional supplements [15]. Therefore, in order to tighten glycaemic control, starch modification and sugar substitution [16,26] has become a primary strategy in the formulation of these supplements [15,16]. However, there is a compelling need to conduct more studies in special situations such as hospitalised patients, older people with DM2 or end-stage kidney disease and patients with cancer [27,28].

Recent evidence suggests a favourable glycaemic response after nutritional supplement intake with sucromalt (a natural analogue of sucrose with a lower glycaemic response) in diabetic patients [18,29,30]. Isomaltulose, another sucrose replacer, is a disaccharide composed of glucose and fructose linked by an alpha-1,6-glycosidic bond exhibiting prolonged absorption, LGI (GI = 32), and a 20–25% lower hydrolyzation rate when compared with sucrose [31]. Interestingly, GIP and GLP-1 secretion are affected by this disaccharide [32], resulting in a better insulin secretion profile [33] and a possible reduction in postprandial appetite [34].

Moreover, a study by Pfeiffer et al. [32] gave evidence on the relationship between high-glycaemic index carbohydrates and a faster GIP release pattern in patients with fatty liver disease, subclinical inflammation, DM2 and cardiovascular diseases. On the other hand, LGI carbohydrate consumption would induce a lower GIP release and a higher release of GLP-1 [32], promoting a better metabolic markers profile in both healthy and type DM2 individuals [18]. Therefore, these authors propose the GIP release rate as a determining factor in the "metabolic quality" and in consequence, relevant criteria for the selection of dietary carbohydrates [32].

Several studies in DM-2 subjects have explored incretin release after consumption of oral nutritional supplements with sucromalt or isomaltulose [18,35]; however, GI and GL have only been studied in healthy subjects [35,36] and not in diabetic patients. Likewise, the correlation between the glycaemic response (GI/GL) and SA as well as EIAP behaviour is not sufficiently well described to date, especially during ONS-D intake, digestion and absorption time.

Based on available literature, we hypothesised that an ONS-D that contains slow-digesting carbohydrates (isomaltulose or sucromalt) resulting in a significant release of GLP-1 and lower secretion of both GIP and insulin. As consequence, a reduction in GI/GL index and subjective postprandial appetite ratings would be found when compared with standard nutritional supplements. Thus, the aim of this study was to assess sucromalt/isomaltulose ONS-D effects on the glycaemic response (GI/GL), EIAP release and postprandial SA in type 2 diabetic individuals.

2. Materials and Methods

2.1. Study Design

2.1.1. Design and Ethics Issues

A randomised, double-blind, cross-over study was conducted according to Good Clinical Practice Guidelines, applicable Food and Drug privacy regulations and ethical principles based on the World Medical Association-Helsinki Declaration [37]. This research was approved by the Human Research Ethics Committee of the Endocrine and Metabolic Diseases Research Centre (EMDRC), "Dr. Félix Gómez", School of Medicine at the University of Zulia, Venezuela, and then registered in Clinical Trials.gov (https://clinicaltrials.gov/ct2/show/NCT03829800).

2.1.2. Inclusion and Exclusion Criteria

This study included both male and female DM2 subjects over 50 years old who attended the outpatient diabetes medical clinic at EMDRC [37]. The only antidiabetic therapies allowed were diet/physical activity and/or metformin monotherapy. Body mass index (BMI) between 18.5 kg/m^2–35 kg/m^2 was the only compelling anthropometric marker in order to be included in this trial. Patients with diabetes mellitus type 1 (DM1), diabetic ketoacidosis, hypothyroidism/thyrotoxicosis congestive heart failure, gastric, kidney or hepatic diseases, myocardial infarction, stroke and subjects with insulin therapy or sulfonylureas, antibiotic therapy or corticosteroids, end-stage organ failure, or individuals with organ transplantation, coagulation disorder, bleeding disorders, chronic infectious disease (such as tuberculosis, hepatitis B or C or HIV) were excluded.

2.1.3. Population, Sample Size, and Patient's Selection

Taking into account the criteria mentioned above, the whole EMDRC electronic medical record database was filtered obtaining a population of 57 eligible patients. Literature regarding GI and GL suggests 8 to 10 subjects for a proper meal/supplement assessment [10,36,38]. Thus, a random selection of 23 DM2 patients was made with the purpose of obtaining a sample size with a reasonable accuracy in determining the ONS-D glycaemic impact, GI and GL [36,38]. Since postprandial glycaemia and glycaemic index was our primary outcome, this study was powered to detect the difference among the AUCGs after consuming three oral nutritional supplements (effect size = 0.79) [20,24,35,36,38]. Based on our calculation, at least 15 participants were needed to detect this effect size at 80% statistical power using a cross-over study design [24]. Assuming an attrition rate of 30%, 23 participants were recruited in this study. Eligible subjects were contacted by phone and invited to attend a medical screening visit in order to: (1) be invited to participate in the study, (2) verify if the participant met the inclusion criteria and, (3) asked to give their written consent before beginning the study.

2.1.4. Anthropometric Assessment

Anthropometric data were obtained in fasting state, using light clothing and no shoes. For weight determination and electric bioimpedance study, an UM-018 Digital Scale (Tanita, Tokyo, Japan) was used. Height was measured using a SECA 216 stadiometer (Hamburg, Germany). Body mass index was calculated using the equation: BMI (kg/m^2) = mass (Kg)/height (m^2).

2.2. Study Protocol

2.2.1. Oral Nutritional Supplements Composition

In this study, three oral nutritional supplements were examined: (1) non-diabetes-specific standard oral nutritional supplements (ET; Ensure® Abbott Nutrition, Columbus, OH, USA); (2) oral supplements with a blend of slow-digesting carbohydrates including resistant maltodextrin and sucromalt (GS; Glucerna SR® Abbott Nutrition, Columbus, OH, USA); and (3) oral supplements composed of lactose, isomaltulose, and resistant starch (DI; Diasip® Nutricia Advanced, Medical Nutrition, Dublin, Ireland).

The macronutrient composition of these formulas per 100 mL is shown in Table 1. Considering that two of the supplements contained a relatively low amount of total carbohydrates, a standardised portion with 25 g of this nutrient was administered in each patient for all tests. This criterion is recommended when the carbohydrate load in the food is low, in order not to overestimate portion size [35,38]. Therefore, all supplements were compared with a glucose load of 25 g (GB), as a reference food (anhydrous glucose dissolved in 250 mL plain water) (100 Kcal) [35,38]. It is important to mention that there was no significant difference in the volume of formulations supplied in this study (Table 2).

Table 1. Macronutrient composition of the oral nutritional supplements per 100 mL.

Composition	ET	DI	GS
Calories (kcal)	105	104	93
Protein (g)	3.8	4.9	4.3
Fat (g)	2.5	3.8	3.5
Saturates (g)	0.4	0.5	0.3
Monounsaturates (g)	0.8	2.2	2.1
Polyunsaturates (g)	1.3	1.1	0.9
Total carbohydrate (g)	17.3	11.7	10.9
Sugar (g)	10.0	8.3	1.7
Dietary Fibre (g)	1.0	2.0	1.8

Table 1. *Cont.*

Composition	ET	DI	GS
Soluble (g)	0.0	1.6	1.8
Non-soluble (g)	0.0	0.4	0.0
Chromium (μg)	12.7	12.0	5.0
Portion size (mL)	100	100	100

Ensure® (ET): A standard oral nutritional supplement which is non-specific for diabetic patients. Diasip® (DI): Isomaltulose and resistant starch oral nutritional supplement. Glucerna® (GS): Resistant maltodextrin and sucromalt oral nutritional supplement.

Table 2. Nutrient composition of oral nutritional supplements based on 25 g available carbohydrate.

Composition	ET	DI	GS
Calories (kcal)	149	223	214
Protein (g)	5.3	10.5	9.9
Fat (g)	3.5	8.1	8.1
Saturates (g)	0.5	1.0	0.6
Monounsaturated (g)	1.1	4.7	4.9
Polyunsaturated (g)	1.8	2.3	2.0
Total carbohydrate (g)	25.0	25.0	25.0
Sugar (g)	14.1	8.3	0.0
Dietary Fibre (g)	0.9	4.3	4.1
Soluble (g)	0.0	3.4	4.1
Non-soluble (g)	0.0	0.8	0.0
Chromium (μg)	12.4	25.8	11.5
Portion size (mL)	141	214	230

Ensure® (ET): A standard oral nutritional supplement not specific for diabetic patients. Diasip® (DI): Isomaltulose and resistant starch oral nutritional supplement. Glucerna® (GS): Resistant maltodextrin and sucromalt oral nutritional supplement.

The three oral nutritional supplements delivered energy ranging from 149 to 223 kcal (Table 2). Both DI and GS contained 208 kcal per 200 mL versus 205 Kcal per 220 mL, respectively (recommended daily serving size). Supplement DI had a lower percentage of carbohydrate (47 energy%) and protein (19%) but higher percentage of fat (32 energy%, of which 18.5% was monounsaturated fatty acids (MUFAs). On the other hand, the composition of GS was more comparable with DI; a lower percentage of carbohydrate 47.7% and protein 18.42%, and higher percentage of fat 33.81% (MUFA: 20.5%), while the composition of ET had a higher percentage of carbohydrate: 55.68%; lower percentage of fat: 29.45%; and protein: 14.87%; with 250 Kcal per 237 mL. The GI values were calculated according to the information reported in the nutritional labelling of each supplement.

2.2.2. Experimental Protocol

Background Diet, Physical Activities and Other Measurements

Subjects were informed about diet and physical activity restrictions to be followed before each session, which included: (1) 10–12 h fasting, (2) abstinence from alcohol, caffeine or smoking and not exercising excessively 24 h before each session; (3) avoiding the metformin morning dose or other medications allowed on trial days until instructed, and to do so at the health centre. Participants were evaluated before each treatment by a licenced nutritionist. In this evaluation, patients had to submit a 3 day food record in order to confirm adherence to the meal plan. The day before the administration of supplements, the nutritionist recommended a standardised dinner before 21:00 and were asked not to consume anything before arriving at the laboratory except water, which was allowed until midnight [14,39]. In order to ensure that participants complied with established protocols, they had to complete a compliance survey. In case they did not comply with the previous test protocols, the test sessions were rescheduled.

During the appetite test sessions, patients engaged in 60 min of sedentary activities (word puzzles, reading, board games, etc.) [14,39]. The activities were performed in a friendly, non-competitive manner to avoid emotional excitement or stress. Any food-related topics were avoided for the duration of the sessions [14]. Research team members evaluated the compliance of the experimental protocol verifying the correct administration to all patients in each visit. Participants had access to water during the day of the trial. The leading investigator reviewed these records before performing the food tolerance test. During each test day subjects were allowed to drink water each hour (maximum 150 mL each hour) immediately after filling in the appetite questionnaires. Water consumed during the test session on the first day was recorded and repeated on the other test days [14,39].

Randomisation

All participants were randomly assigned to eight consumption tests: two for the standard glucose solutions and two for each of the three nutritional supplements. This scheme was carried out with an interval of 1 week between tests in random sequences. The test supplement selection was randomised using a computerized randomisation matrix. The order of supplement was further randomised for each subject. The number of tests in each patient was done according to methodological considerations for glycaemic index protocols [38]. Appetite was assessed twice for the same subject before and after supplement intake on two different occasions [14,39].

Previous-evening lunch standardisation: the dinner consumed by all participants the night before each session day consisted of meat with boiled rice and a fruit cake for dessert ~505 kcal [14]. The energy content of this meal was 35% of the daily estimated energy needs of each participant [40]. The distribution of energy in the evening meal was 50% from carbohydrate, 37% from fat and 13% from protein [14,39].

2.3. Measurement of EIAP/GI and Subjective Appetite Evaluation

2.3.1. EIAP and Glycaemic Index

Participants attended the EMDRC following 10–12 h fasting at 07:00. Both duplicated blood capillary samples (0.5 mL) and venous samples were taken in basal state, and then each patient was randomly assigned to drink one of both the ONS (ET DI or GS) supplement or the reference food (glucose 25 g in plain water) during a period not exceeding 15 min [35,36,38]. The reference food (GB) (glucose solution) was used for glucose and insulin AUC determination only. Subsequently, samples of capillary and venous blood were obtained at 30, 60, 90, 120 and 180 min for serum glucose, insulin, GIP and GLP-1 measurement. During this phase, subjects were comfortably seated in a room with a quiet environment [38]. This process was repeated seven more times, on different days, with one week interval until all consumption tests were done [36,38].

2.3.2. Subjective Appetite Assessment

The appetite sensations measured in this study were: hunger, desire to eat, prospective food consumption and fullness assessed on different days from those in which the GI was determined. The visual analogue scale (VAS) chart was supplied in every session [39] and the subjects were asked to fill this instrument at baseline (0 min), 30, 60, 90, 120, 150 and 180 min after the ingestion of each supplement. This instrument contemplates four questions: What is your feeling of fullness? How hungry are you? How intense is your desire to eat? And how much food do you think you could eat? [14,39].

The VAS structure consisted of 100 mm lines anchored at each end with opposite statements with a scale of 0 to 100 mm, in which 0 means absence of perception and 100 maximum perception. The distance between 0 and the marked point (an "x" placed by the participants on the line to indicate their assessment at that time) was measured to quantify the perceived sensations. The score was calculated by measuring the distance in millimetres from the beginning of the line to the "x" position (from left to right) [39].

The following equation was used to calculate the ratings of subjective appetite [41]: "Subjective appetite = (desire to eat + hunger + (100 − fullness) + prospective food consumption)/4".

2.3.3. Laboratory Determinations

Capillary glycaemia was determined by the glucose oxidase method using a portable glucometer (Optium Xceed, Abbott Laboratories, Dallas, TX, USA) Both intra-assay and inter-assay coefficients of variation were 3.2 and 10.8%, respectively. Plasma Insulin (mU/L) was measured by an enzyme-linked immunosorbent assay (10-1113; Mercodia, Uppsala, Sweden) with a minimum detectable limit of 1.0 mU/L, and an intra- and inter-assay variation coefficients of 3.0% and 8.7%. Glycated haemoglobin HbA1c was determined using a cationic exchange resin separation method (SIGMA, St. Louis, MO, USA). Plasma total GIP (pg/mL) and GLP-1 (pmol/L) were measured by radioimmunoassay (RIA) (SIGMA, St. Louis, MO, USA). The minimum detectable limits were 2 pmol/L and 3 pmol/L with an intra- and inter-assay coefficient of variation for GIP of 3.9% and 9%, and for GLP-1 6.3% and 10.3%, respectively. Total cholesterol, triacylglycerides, and HDL-C were determined by commercial enzymatic-colorimetric kits (Human Gesellschaft für Biochemica und Diagnostica MBH, Wiesbaden, HE, Germany). Serum LDL-C levels were calculated according to Friedewald's equation.

2.4. Data Processing and Statistical Analyses

Statistical analyses were performed using IBM SPSS Statistics for Windows, version 23.0 (IBM Corp., 2015, Armonk, NY, USA). Shapiro–Wilk test was used for the normality distribution assessment of quantitative variables.

Incremental areas under the curves (IAUCs) were determined according to the trapezoidal method for all variables using NCSS statistical software version 12.0 (NCSS, LLC, 2018, Kaysville, UT, USA). A 2 h glycaemic response curve was generated for each subject for test foods. Any area below the baseline fasting value was ignored. The calculated median of AUCG for three test foods from 16 participants was compared with the response to reference food or glucose solution (median of two measurements), and the GI value of the glucose solution was set as 100.

The GI was calculated using the following equation [36,38]: GI = (AUCG value for the test food/AUCG value for the reference food) × 100.

Data obtained was classified in low GI (≤55), intermediate (55–69) and high (≥70) [41]. Glycaemic load (GL) was represented by a derivative measure of the GI of the nutritional supplement tested and calculated by the following formula: GL = (GI × grams of carbohydrate per food portion)/100 [36,38].

All quantitative variables were presented as mean ± standard error of the mean (SEM). Plasma glucose, insulin, GIP, GLP-1, perceptions of hunger, desire to eat, prospective food consumption, fullness and SA had a normal distribution and its arithmetic means were analysed using ANOVA for repeated measures with the Tukey's HSD (honestly significant difference) test. Significant statistical differences between ONS were evaluated through one-way ANOVA. The bivariate relation between variables such as the AUC, blood glucose, EIAP and SA was analysed by correlation coefficients for each oral test. Statistical significance was accepted at $p < 0.05$.

3. Results

At the beginning of the study, the initial sample was 23 individuals (12 women, 11 men), but seven subjects did not complete the trial for different reasons: (1) two subjects needed both corticosteroid and antibiotic therapy; (2) two subjects initiated a vigorous physical activity program by medical prescription; and (3) three voluntarily withdrew from the study. At the end of the study, only 16 subjects (seven women and nine men) completed all the test protocols. Table 3 shows the general characteristics of the sample.

Table 3. General characteristics of the enrolled patients.

	Sex					
	Female		Male		Total	
	Mean	SEM *	Mean	SEM	Mean	SEM
Age (years)	54.75	1. 65	57.83	1.35	56.0	1.11
Weight (cm)	87.75	3.73	90.17	1.22	89.0	1.58
Height (m)	1.68	0.04	1.69	0.01	1.68	0.01
BMC (kg/m^2)	30.90	0.44	31.04	0.36	30.8	0.26
Waist circumference (cm)	106.00	1.58	111.00	0.89	106	0.77
Base glycaemia (mmol/L)	7.51	0.40	6.75	0.30	7.05	0.26
Total cholesterol (mg/dL)	209.60	5.71	213.77	8.84	212.10	5.56
High-density lipoprotein (mg/dL)	44.70	4.63	44.30	2.32	44.46	2.16
Low-density lipoprotein (mg/dL)	130.95	4.37	133.28	1.54	132.35	1.87
Triglycerides (mg/dL)	161.70	2.56	158.06	4.45	159.52	2.80
Glycated haemoglobin HbA1c (%)	6.95	0.30	6.98	0.30	6.97	0.20

* Standard error of the mean. There were no significant differences between sexes.

The protocol was well tolerated by all subjects. No individual reported nausea, dizziness or vomiting after taking the nutritional supplements or the reference product. Basal concentrations of serum glucose, insulin, GLP-1 and GIP (Table 4 and Figure 1) did not show significant differences according to sex or among weekly visits. Similarly, hunger perception, fullness, desire to eat, prospective food consumption in fasting state and SA ratings (Table 5 and Figure 2) did not show significant differences among gender or study session ($p > 0.05$).

Table 4. Serum glucose concentration and EIAP according to each treatment.

Supplement	Time (min)	Serum Glucose (mmol/L)	Insulin (mU/L)	GLP-1 (pmol/L)	GIP (pg/mL)
ET	0	6.52 ± 0.07	6.44 ± 0.32	6.26 ± 0.28	29.64 ± 0.50
	30	10.14 ± 0.07 [bc]	22.84 ± 1.00 [bc]	12.93 ± 0.21 [bc]	55.44 ± 0.58 [bc]
	60	10.80 ± 0.12 [bd]	33.91 ± 0.97 [bc]	8.35 ± 0.22 [bc]	62.27 ± 0.89 [bc]
	90	9.39 ± 0.16 [b]	36.20 ± 0.64 [bc]	7.78 ± 0.15 [b]	74.68 ± 0.72 [bc]
	120	8.76 ± 0.17 [b]	25.90 ± 0.70 [bc]	7.16 ± 0.27 [b]	71.23 ± 0.36 [bc]
	150	8.14 ± 0.21 [bc]	16.80 ± 0.56 [bc]	6.55 ± 0.12 [b]	67.77 ± 0.50 [bc]
	180	7.13 ± 0.21 [b]	9.91 ± 0.81	5.99 ± 0.21 [b]	62.86 ± 1.26 [bc]
GS	0	6.64 ± 0.08	6.49 ± 0.11	6.95 ± 0.36 [c]	29.97 ± 0.40
	30	6.68 ± 0.13 [ac]	17.24 ± 0.31 [a]	18.16 ± 0.26 [ac]	45.57 ± 0.42 [a]
	60	9.10 ± 0.06 [ac]	18.16 ± 0.24 [ac]	14.75 ± 0.24 [ac]	50.85 ± 0.15 [ac]
	90	8.53 ± 0.07 [ac]	19.09 ± 0.20 [a]	12.73 ± 0.24 [ac]	54.23 ± 0.21 [ac]
	120	7.92 ± 0.05 [ac]	14.38 ± 0.16 [ac]	11.63 ± 0.14 [ac]	55.99 ± 1.09 [ac]
	150	6.98 ± 0.12 [a]	12.93 ± 0.19 [a]	10.86 ± 0.19 [ac]	57.87 ± 0.31 [a]
	180	6.16±0.10 [a]	10.87 ± 0.18	8.91 ± 0.21 [ac]	52.85 ± 1.69 [ac]
DI	0	6.66 ± 0.10	6.50 ± 0.40	6.20 ± 0.53	28.70 ± 1.07
	30	7.47 ± 0.12 [ab]	19.04 ± 0.27 [a]	14.51 ± 0.22 [ab]	46.00 ± 0.71 [a]
	60	10.17 ± 0.05 [ab]	24.86 ± 0.35 [ab]	10.26 ± 0.11 [ab]	56.51 ± 1.12 [ab]
	90	9.10 ± 0.05 [b]	21.14 ± 0.36 [a]	8.09 ± 0.17 [b]	63.78 ± 0.63 [ab]
	120	8.56 ± 0.07 [b]	17.98 ± 0.30 [ab]	7.35 ± 0.14 [b]	61.10 ± 0.51 [ab]
	150	7.33 ± 0.07 [a]	13.24 ± 0.25 [a]	6.95 ± 0.09 [b]	57.52 ± 0.50 [a]
	180	6.61 ± 0.12	11.13 ± 0.21	6.56 ± 0.20 [b]	45.19 ± 0.96 [ab]

Treatment groups were defined as a standard nutritional supplement not specific for people with diabetes (ET); resistant maltodextrin and sucromalt supplement (GS); isomaltulose and resistant starch supplement (DI). GIP: glucose-dependent insulinotropic polypeptide; GLP-1: glucagon-like peptide 1; SEM: standard error of the mean. [a] $p < 0.05$ versus ET. [b] $p < 0.05$ versus GS. [c] $p < 0.05$ versus DI.

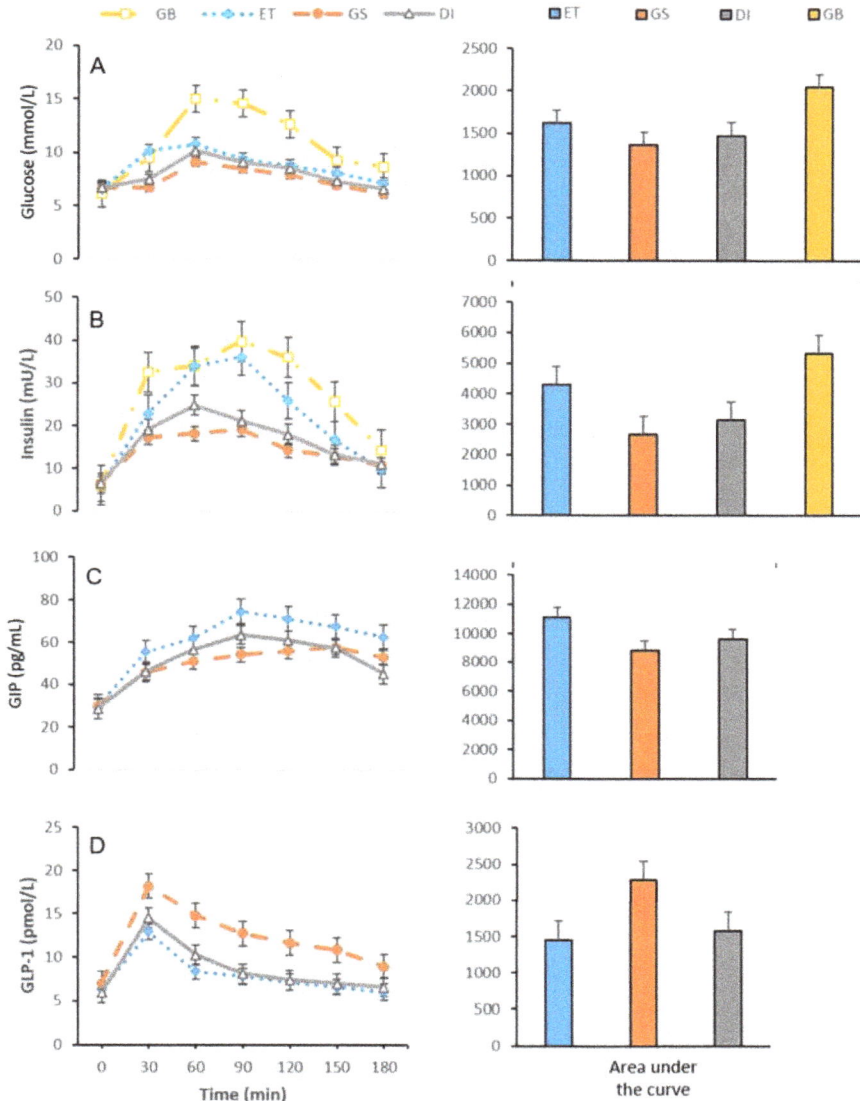

Figure 1. Time course and AUC$_{0-180\text{ min}}$ of serum glucose, insulin GIP and GPL-1 concentrations following ingestions of GB, ET, GS and DI. (**A**) Glucose in relation with time and AUC$_{0-180\text{ min}}$, (**B**) insulin in relation with time and AUC$_{0-180\text{ min}}$, (**C**) GIP in relation with time and AUC$_{0-180\text{ min}}$, and (**D**) GLP-1 in relation with time and AUC$_{0-180\text{ min}}$ for all the different types of treatments. Data are expressed as means ± SEM; n = 16. The same colour scheme was used for all the graphs. All AUC$_{0-180\text{ min}}$ means significant differences ($p < 0.02$) in each group. Treatment groups: (GB) Glucose solution or reference product; (ET) standard nutritional supplement not specific for diabetics; (GS) resistant maltodextrin and sucromalt supplement; (DI) isomaltulose and resistant starch supplement. GIP: glucose-dependent insulinotropic polypeptide; GLP-1: glucagon-like peptide 1.

Table 5. Subjective appetite measurements according to each treatment.

Supplement	Time (min)	Hunger(mm)	Fullness(mm)	Desire to Eat(mm)	Prospective Food Consumption (mm)	SA (mm)
ET	0	63.80 ± 1.70	34.30 ± 0.88	61.80 ± 1.14	21.40 ± 1.88	53.18 ± 0.40
	30	33.60 ± 2.45	62.50 ± 1.60 [b]	32.10 ± 1.19	28.90 ± 2.04 [b]	33.03 ± 0.91 [bc]
	60	37.10 ± 1.10 [bc]	55.70 ± 2.32 [b]	42.60 ± 1.11 [bc]	35.50 ± 0.91 [bc]	40.08 ± 0.56 [bc]
	90	46.00 ± 1.00 [bc]	38.40 ± 3.14 [bc]	43.40 ± 0.82 [bc]	38.00 ± 1.97 [b]	47.05 ± 1.08 [bc]
	120	47.20 ± 1.58 [bc]	32.60 ± 2.02 [bc]	46.00 ± 1.00 [bc]	41.80 ± 0.95 [bc]	50.60 ± 0.53 [bc]
	150	56.60 ± 1.41 [bc]	30.40 ± 2.10 [bc]	54.30 ± 1.39 [bc]	46.80 ± 1.44 [b]	56.83 ± 0.74 [bc]
	180	70.60 ± 1.92 [bc]	20.50 ± 1.71 [bc]	73.60 ± 1.06 [bc]	55.90 ± 1.27 [b]	69.90 ± 0.91 [bc]
GS	0	66.40 ± 1.42	32.50 ± 1.76	63.50 ± 0.93	19.20 ± 0.80	54.15 ± 0.62
	30	30.80 ± 1.78	70.10 ± 2.12 [a]	30.80 ± 1.65	20.60 ± 0.69 [a]	28.03 ± 0.85 [a]
	60	28.50 ± 1.66 [a]	65.90 ± 1.57 [a]	27.80 ± 1.80 [ac]	22.00 ± 1.09 [ac]	28.10 ± 0.58 [ac]
	90	27.30 ± 1.95 [ac]	63.70 ± 1.92 [ac]	31.00 ± 1.69 [a]	24.40 ± 1.75 [ac]	29.75 ± 0.93 [ac]
	120	29.80 ± 1.70 [ac]	58.60 ± 1.99 [ac]	35.60 ± 0.83 [a]	33.30 ± 1.12 [a]	35.03 ± 0.77 [ac]
	150	34.30 ± 1.16 [ac]	46.00 ± 1.74 [ac]	43.90 ± 1.16 [a]	36.60 ± 0.90 [ac]	40.20 ± 0.42 [ac]
	180	62.30 ± 1.51 [a]	34.90 ± 1.47 [ac]	58.80 ± 1.90 [a]	45.00 ± 1.32 [ac]	57.80 ± 0.64 [ac]
DI	0	63.20 ± 1.30	32.80 ± 1.18	65.20 ± 1.24	21.40 ± 127	54.25 ± 0.59
	30	32.30 ± 1.50 [a]	68.40 ± 1.38	29.60 ± 1.97	23.90 ± 1.30	29.35 ± 0.85 [a]
	60	28.60 ± 2.03 [ab]	60.60 ± 1.35	34.60 ± 1.48 [ab]	25.50 ± 0.91 [ab]	32.03 ± 0.68 [ab]
	90	33.90 ± 1.38 [ab]	54.80 ± 1.17 [ab]	35.00 ± 1.22 [a]	35.00 ± 1.02 [b]	37.28 ± 0.64 [ab]
	120	39.00 ± 1.13 [ab]	45.90 ± 1.49 [ab]	36.90 ± 1.17 [a]	36.70 ± 1.27 [a]	40.93 ± 0.58 [ab]
	150	44.90 ± 0.99 [ab]	38.30 ± 2.39 [ab]	47.40 ± 1.97 [a]	44.90 ± 1.50 [b]	49.73 ± 0.63 [ab]
	180	60.60 ± 2.02 [a]	27.00 ± 1.71 [ab]	61.90 ± 2.36 [a]	52.00 ± 1.21 [b]	61.88 ± 076 [ab]

Treatment groups were defined as a standard nutritional supplement not specifically for people with diabetes (ET); resistant maltodextrin and sucromalt supplement (GS); isomaltulose and resistant starch supplement (DI). GIP: glucose-dependent insulinotropic polypeptide; GLP-1: glucagon-like peptide 1; SEM: standard error of the mean. [a] $p < 0.05$ versus ET. [b] $p < 0.05$ versus GS. [c] $p < 0.05$ versus DI. SA: Subjective appetite.

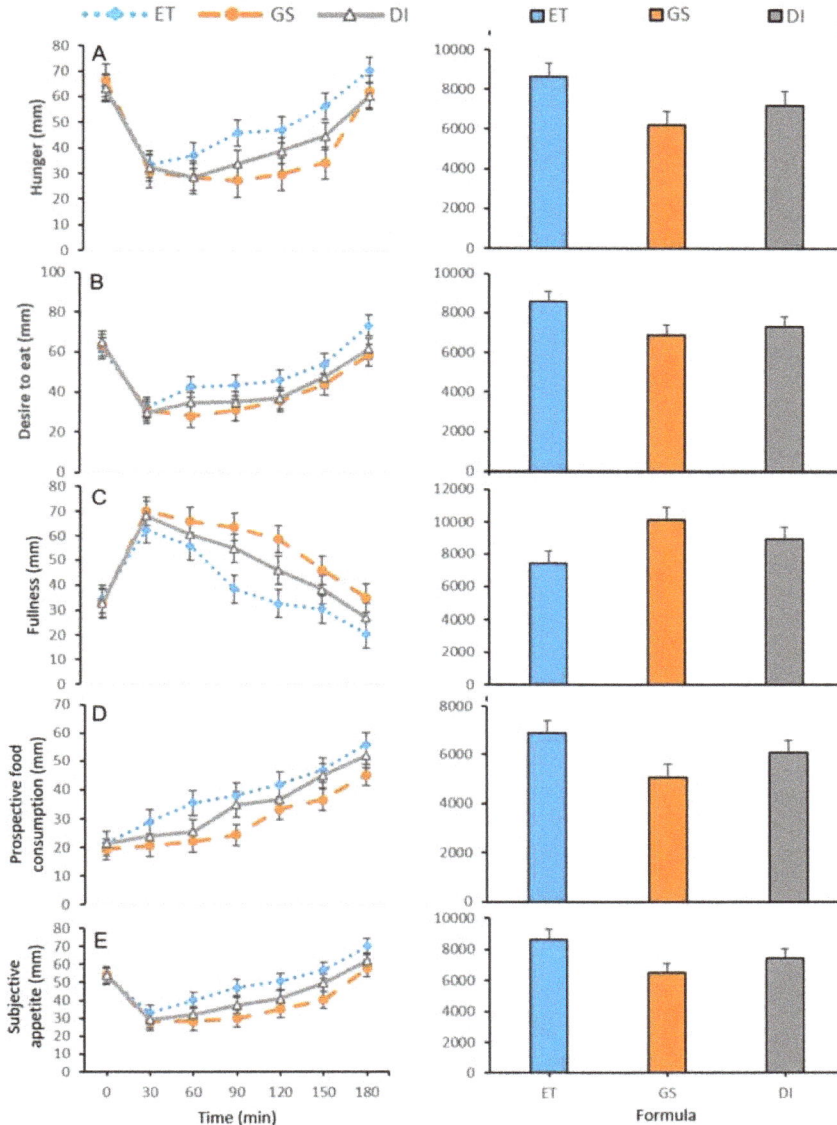

Figure 2. Time course and formula of postprandial perception of hunger, desire to eat, fullness, prospective food consumption, subjective appetite and $AUC_{0-180\ min}$ values following ingestions of GB, ET, GS and DI. (**A**) hunger in relation with time and formula; (**B**) desire to eat in relation with time and formula, (**C**) fullness in relation to time and formula, (**D**) prospective food consumption in relation with time and formula and (**E**) subjective appetite in relation with time and formula. Data are expressed as means ± SEM, (*n* = 16). Data comparisons about differences in subjective measurements of appetite according to consumption tests are described in Table 5. The same colour scheme was used for all graphs. All means of $AUC_{0-180\ min}$ showed significant differences ($p < 0.02$) in each group. Treatment groups: (ET) standard nutritional supplement not specifically for people with diabetes. (GS) Resistant maltodextrin and sucromalt supplement. (DI) Isomaltulose and resistant starch supplement.

3.1. Glycaemic Response and EIAP Concentrations

Glycaemic curves, as well as the mean and SEM of the glucose $AUC_{0-180\,min}$ after ingestion of both the reference product (glucose) and the nutritional supplements, are shown in Figure 1. Glucose maximum peak was observed at 60 min (Table 4) for all products but significantly higher for GB 15.03 ± 0.20 when compared with ET 10.80 ± 0.12mmol/L ($p < 0.001$), DI 10.17 ± 0.05 ($p < 0.001$) and GS 9.10 ± 0.06 mmol/L ($p < 0.001$). Glucose at 180 min was significantly higher in comparison with both, fasting level for GB ($p < 0.001$) and for ET ($p < 0.024$). The $AUC_{0-180\,min}$ of ET ($p < 0.001$) was significantly higher than DI ($p < 0.001$) and GS ($p < 0.01$) (Figure 1).

3.1.1. Insulin

Plasma insulin concentrations increased after the consumption of all supplements and the reference product, reaching significant differences at 90 min for GB (serum peak) in comparison to ET ($p < 0.05$), GS ($p < 0.001$) and DI ($p < 0.001$), respectively (Figure 1). At 150 min, ET presented a higher glucose concentration than DSF ($p < 0.001$), but no significant differences were found in insulin concentration between DI and GS ($p = 0.976$), see Table 4. The $AUC_{0-180\,min}$ in insulin response was significantly lower in GS when compared with the other supplements ($p < 0.001$) (Figure 1).

3.1.2. GLP-1

Maximum GLP-1 concentration was observed at 30 min after the intake of the three supplements, significantly higher for GS in comparison to ET ($p < 0.05$) and DI ($p < 0.05$). At 150 min, concentrations of GLP-1 in ET and DI supplements were similar ($p = 0.841$), but the value of this incretin was significantly higher for GS when compared with both, ET ($p < 0.001$) and DI ($p < 0.001$), (Table 4). The $AUC_{0-180\,min}$ of the GLP-1 response was significantly higher in GS in contrast to the ET ($p < 0.001$) and DI ($p < 0.001$), (Figure 1).

3.1.3. GIP

The GIP plasma concentration increased after consumption of all supplements. The maximum peak of this incretin was observed at 90 min with ET and DI, which was higher when compared to GS levels ($p < 0.05$). At 150 min, ET presented higher GIP concentrations when compared to GS ($p < 0.001$) and DI ($p < 0.001$), however, DSF levels did not show significant differences ($p = 0.844$), Table 4. The $AUC_{0-180\,min}$ of the GIP response for GS was lower when compared to DI ($p < 0.001$) and ET ($p < 0.001$, (Figure 1).

3.2. Subjective Appetite Measurements

Hunger sensation, fullness, desire to eat, prospective food consumption and SA from baseline to 180 min are shown in Figure 2. Consumption of the different treatments promoted an immediate decrease in hunger and desire to eat accompanied by an increase in the perception of fullness, reversing these sensations over the curve as time passed.

The arithmetic mean of hunger perception decreased after the consumption of all supplements, registering the lowest level at 30 min for E, while the minimum value for GS was evidenced at 90 min, significantly lower when compared to ET ($p < 0.05$) and DI ($p < 0.05$), (Table 5). The $AUC_{0-180\,min}$ of hunger sensation for GS was significantly lower when compared to ET ($p < 0.001$) and DI ($p < 0.001$), (Figure 2).

Regarding fullness sensation, the maximum level was found at 30 min in the three groups, without significant differences between DI and GS, while the peak of fullness sensation was significantly lower with ET ($p < 0.05$), (Table 5). The $AUC_{0-180\,min}$ of this sensation was significantly higher in GS when compared to DI ($p < 0.001$) and ET ($p < 0.05$), (Figure 2). On the other hand, the desire to eat $AUC_{0-180\,min}$ was significantly lower for GS when compared to DI ($p = 0.035$) and ET ($p < 0.001$), (Figure 2).

This same pattern was evidenced in the prospective food consumption, in which the $AUC_{0-180 \, min}$ was significantly lower in GS when compared with ET ($p < 0.001$) and DI ($p < 0.001$), (Figure 2). Subjective appetite SA decreased to a minimum value at 30 min and then increased 60 min after the three treatments for all subjects; this score was higher with ET when compared to GS ($p < 0.01$) and DI ($p < 0.01$), (Table 5). The $AUC_{0-180 \, min}$ of SA was significantly lower with GS than with DI ($p < 0.01$) and ET ($p < 0.001$), (Figure 2).

3.3. Correlation Analysis Between EIAP, Serum Glucose and Subjective Appetite

After ET intake, insulin concentration $AUC_{0-180 \, min}$ and subjective sensation of fullness were directly related ($r = 0.713$, $p = 0.021$), while an inverse relationship between fullness perception and GLP-1 concentration $AUC_{0-180 \, min}$ ($r = -0.756$, $p = 0.011$) and serum glucose ($r = -0.687$; $p = 0.028$) was observed. The value SA was directly correlated with serum glucose ($r = 0.659$, $p = 0.038$), see Table 6. No statistically significant correlations were found for $AUC_{0-180 \, min}$ concentrations of these peptides with DI and GS.

Table 6. Coefficient correlations between AUC values of glycaemia, EIAP and subjective measurements of appetite according to consumption tests.

	Hunger		Fullness		Desire to Eat		Prospective Food Consumption		Subjective Appetite	
	r	p	r	p	r	p	r	p	r	p
ET										
Glycaemia	0.060	0.868	−0.687	0.028	0.217	0.547	−0.025	0.945	0.659	0.038
Insulin	−0.215	0.552	0.713	0.021	−0.046	0.900	0.362	0.304	−0.437	0.321
GLP-1	−0.133	0.714	−0.756	0.011	0.392	0.262	−0.543	0.105	0.321	0.540
GIP	0.219	0.544	−0.082	0.821	0.486	0.155	0.399	0.253	0.540	0.107
DI	r	p	r	p	r	p	r	p	r	p
Glycaemia	0.004	0.992	−0.226	0.530	−0.069	0.849	0.173	0.633	0.357	0.311
Insulin	0.190	0.599	−0.163	0.652	−0.455	0.187	−0.196	0.587	−0.254	0.479
GLP-1	0.483	0.158	0.140	0.700	0.158	0.662	−0.407	0.243	0.098	0.787
GIP	0.294	0.410	0.099	0.785	−0.615	0.058	0.069	0.850	−0.540	0.107
GS	r	p	r	p	r	p	r	p	r	p
Glycaemia	−0.192	0.595	0.019	0.958	−0.152	0.674	0.128	0.726	−0.154	0.672
Insulin	0.466	0.175	−0.020	0.957	0.217	0.548	−0.175	0.628	0.344	0.330
GLP-1	0.308	0.386	0.072	0.843	0.436	0.208	−0.421	0.226	0.191	0.596
GIP	0.231	0.521	−0.046	0.900	−0.135	0.710	−0.076	0.834	0.086	0.813

Treatment groups: (ET) standard nutritional supplement not specifically for diabetes patients; (DI) isomaltulose and resistant starch supplement; (GS) resistant maltodextrin and sucromalt supplement. GIP: glucose-dependent insulinotropic polypeptide; GLP-1: glucagon-like peptide 1; SEM: standard error of the mean. The values presented correspond to *r* coefficients and *p*-value for all subject correlations between subjective perceptions of appetite and concentrations hormones according to the treatment group. *p*-values were significant when $p < 0.05$.

Correlations between baseline and postprandial concentrations at 30, 90 and 120 min of glucose, EIAP and SA measures were accomplished in all treatments. Insulin at 30 min for ET was inversely related to hunger sensation ($r = -0.745$, $p = 0.012$) and SA ($r = -0.849$, $p = 0.002$) (Supplementary Materials Table S1). DI intake was correlated with glycaemia and prospective food consumption at 30 min ($r = 0.775$, $p = 0.008$) and, GLP-1 with the desire to eat at 120 min ($r = 0.667$ $p = 0.035$); whereas, SA was inversely correlated at 30 min with GIP ($r = -0.688$, $p = 0.028$) (Supplementary Materials Table S2).

GS evidenced a direct relationship between glycaemia at 90 min with sensation of fullness ($r = 0.698$, $p = 0.025$) and levels of GIP with sensation of hunger ($r = 0.825$, $p = 0.003$). GLP-1 at 30 min and prospective food consumption were inversely related ($r = -0.722$, $p = 0.018$). SA was directly correlated with blood glucose levels at 30 min ($r = 0.711$, $p = 0.021$) (Supplementary Materials Table S3).

3.4. Glycaemic Index and Glycaemic Load

ET presented a GI mean higher than that calculated for DI ($p < 0.001$) and GS ($p < 0.001$), respectively. Comparing both specific supplements for diabetics, the lowest value for this indicator was evidenced in GS ($p < 0.001$). Concerning GL, ET showed the highest mean compared to the rest of treatments ($p < 0.001$), and the lowest mean value for DI (11.28 ± 0.14, $p < 0.001$), (Table 7).

Table 7. Glycaemic index and glycaemic load according to consumption tests.

Treatment Groups	Mean ± SEM
Glycaemic Index (GI)	
ET	56.40 ± 0.43 [bc]
DI	51.44 ± 0.60 [ab]
GS	47.59 ± 0.49 [ac]
Glycaemic Load (GL)	
ET	23.69 ± 0.18 [bc]
DI	12.04 ± 0.14 [ac]
GS	11.42 ± 0.12 [ab]

Treatment groups: (ET) standard nutritional supplement not specifically for people with diabetes; (DI) isomaltulose and resistant starch supplement; (GS) resistant maltodextrin and sucromalt supplement. SEM: Standard error of the mean. There were no significant differences between sexes. ANOVA and post-hoc Tukey HSD for intragroup comparisons; p-value was significant when $p < 0.05$. [a] $p < 0.001$ versus ET. [b] $p < 0.001$ versus GS. [c] $p < 0.001$ versus DI.

3.5. EIAP and SA Relation with GI and GL

In relation to each supplement, it was found that hunger sensation $AUC_{0-180\,min}$ was directly correlated with GI ($r = 0.777$, $p = 0.008$) and GL ($r = 0.777$, $p = 0.008$) for ET; while DI, both GI and GL were inversely related to GIP ($r = -0.867$, $p = 0.001$). GS, GI and GL were inversely related with fullness sensation ($r = -0.698$, $p = 0.025$). SA ratings did not correlate significantly with any of these indexes ($p > 0.05$), (Supplementary Materials Table S4).

4. Discussion

This study assessed ONS-D with isomaltulose and sucromalt versus a standard oral supplement on GI/GL, insulin response, incretin release and SA in DM2 patients. In this regard, the main finding of this study confirmed that ONS-D intake in diabetic subjects stimulated GLP-1 release, reducing GIP levels with a subsequent decrease in insulin secretion. This particular EIAP pattern promotes a lower IG/CG index when compared with a standard supplement. In spite of the former, there was a reduction of SA and $AUC_{0-180\,min}$ after ONS-D intake; only correlation between hunger perception, fullness and some metabolic variables were found after GS intake.

These findings confirm that ONS-D consumption promotes a better metabolic profile in diabetic subjects than standard supplements, allowing greater control in postprandial appetite. Specifically, this investigation demonstrates that plasma glucose levels and glucose $AUC_{0-180\,min}$ were significantly lower after the ingestion of ONS-D than ET. Our observations are consistent with previous research carried out with slow-digesting carbohydrates supplements [18,29,42,43]. In this study, after the consumption of GS, the mean glycaemic peak was consistent with ADA recommendations for glucose level < 180 mg/dL (9.99 mmol/L), with elevated HbA1c in DM patients [7] and IDF of 160 mg/dL goal, both in the postprandial period [6]. Similar to observations by Mottalib et al. [42] this study shows that serum glucose level after ONS-D ingestion returned to baseline in a shorter period (150 min) when compared with ET (180 min) [42], see Figure 1 and Table 4 [18,29,42]. These differences in glycaemic profile can be attributed, at least in part, to the low GI of ONS-D [18,29,35,42], a point of paramount importance to avoid cardiovascular complications [44] because of pro-inflammatory cytokines and oxygen free radical overproduction [44,45]. In this trial, the consumption of GS produced lower values of GI/GL, a lower increment of GIP/insulin and more significant release of GLP-1.

Among the different factors that influence the GI of a food, the source and carbohydrate type are very relevant aspects. High GI carbohydrates differ from those with LGI, not only in postprandial glycaemic and insulinemic response but also in GIP release [45–47]. In this regard, Pfeiffer et al. [32], suggest a novel concept that encompasses the intake of LGI CHO with a lower release of GIP and a greater GLP-1 secretion results in improvements of metabolic markers in healthy [45], type 2 and insulin-resistant individuals [46].

This concept relates to GI of each food to different secretory responses of GIP and GLP-1, which are released in different segments of the small intestine [21,45–47]. These authors propose that both a fast and pronounced GIP release in the proximal small intestine by high GI carbohydrates programming the intermediary metabolism towards useful energy storage but adversely promoting fatty liver disease [46], insulin resistance [48], obesity [49], subclinical inflammation and hypertriglyceridemia [46]. This program could represent an evolutionary advantage in times that rapid energy storage was required [32,46]. Complete understanding of the pathophysiological mechanisms of foods with a high GI provides a basis for the development of nutritional and therapeutic solutions [10,11,41,46].

Nonetheless, it is essential to differentiate the digestion (di, oligo and polysaccharides) and absorption rate (monosaccharide), from the particular metabolism of each monosaccharide. This is because certain simple sugars, such as fructose, with a relatively low GI (=23) [36], could induce insulin-independent additional metabolic effects [50] on uric acid levels, blood pressure, liver cell triacylglycerides content and hepatic insulin sensitivity when consumed in high amounts [51]. On the other hand, tagatose is a low GI (=3) monosaccharide [36], that promoting a GLP-1 release in a similar extent to fructose without any significant GIP secretion response [52] and exhibiting an interesting glucose-lowering effect [53]. In this study, we assessed two of the most employed slow-digesting carbohydrates in ONS-D: isomaltulose and sucromalt.

Beneficial metabolic effects have been reported when low GI disaccharides = 32, such as isomaltulose [31,36], are added to oral supplements in people with DM2 [29]. This disaccharide has an α-1,6-glycosidic bond replacing the original sucrose´s 1,2-glycosidic linkage by enzymatic isomerisation rearrangement obtained from beet sugar [33]. This molecular reorganisation leads to slower digestion and, in consequence, delayed intestinal uptake of glucose and fructose [33,54]. Unlike sucrose, isomaltulose administration prevents proximal K cells stimulation, secreting less GIP and promoting a smaller insulin release [32,33]. For its part, the low glycaemic response to sucromalt showed a sustained increase in GLP-1 secretion at 4 h post intake, suggesting an almost complete uptake by the small intestine [30]. Thus, it is important to distinguish the effects in GI from those caused by changes in gut microbiota that occur when sugar reaches the colon and alter microbiome composition, affecting long-term carbohydrate metabolism and insulin response [55–57].

In this study, ONS-D insulinemic behaviour interestingly showed a lower $AUC_{0–180\,min}$ level in ET, especially after GS at 90 min, the time when the maximum peak of this hormone occurs. Meanwhile, the maximum insulin concentration after DI intake occurred at the 60 min (Figure 1). The maximum increase in GIP levels after GS occurred after the rest of the treatments (150 min), but it was only statistically different from ET (Table 4). Likewise, the $AUC_{0–180\,min}$ for GIP was lower for ONS-D compared with the ET, and lowest for GS versus DI, (Figure 1). This finding could confirm the theory mentioned above about the effect of slow digestion carbohydrates on the release of insulin and GIP, although insulinemic peak after ET also occurred in 90 min, but with a much higher incretin concentration than that produced by ONS ($p < 0.05$ for both).

It has been proposed that slow-digestion carbohydrates can reach the more distal segments of the small intestine before being absorbed, hence, stimulating a late-plasma increase of GLP-1 [30,52]. In this trial, the $AUC_{0–180\,min}$ of GLP-1 was higher after ONS-D consumption when compared to ET, and higher for GS when compared with DI, (Figure 1). Our results were similar to those reported by Devitt et al. [29] regarding metabolic differences after specific supplement ingestion composed of a variety of carbohydrates like tapioca dextrins, isomaltulose, tapioca starch/fructose and sucromalt in DM2 patients. In this study, patients showed an increase in $AUC_{0–240\,min}$ for GLP-1 after sucromalt-based supplement intake, but it was only significantly higher after supplements made with tapioca dextrin in comparison with the standard ET [29].

Some benefits of increased GLP-1 secretion in DM2 patients are an improvement in insulin–glucagon ratio, suppression of endogenous glucose production and the increase in first-pass splanchnic glucose uptake [47,58]. It is currently unclear whether inhibition of L-cell secretion or GLP-1 enhanced degradation entails to the characteristic blunted-effect of this incretin in DM2. Also, the exact mechanism of GLP-1 effects on glucose control has not yet been elucidated [18,21]. Although there are studies about this incretin for isomaltulose and sucromalt in healthy subjects [46], other studies have reported benefits in individuals with metabolic syndrome, obesity and DM2 after isomaltulose versus sucrose consumption [31,58–60], but few have compared the effects of cross-consumption of pre-loads elaborated with these types of carbohydrates in DM2. To date, only one study has determined a higher release of GLP-1 after the consumption of isomaltulose in individuals with diabetes [58]. Our results showed an $AUC_{0-180 \, min}$ of GLP-1 higher after the consumption of GS versus DI, (Figure 1) exhibiting a synergistic effect of these carbohydrates.

In this sense, it is well-known that GLP-1 secretion is directly related to macronutrients composition, in particular to both carbohydrates and monounsaturated fatty acids (MUFAs) [61,62] without any significant effect on insulin levels [61,63,64]. This is consistent with our results and with the Mottalib et al. work regarding GLP-1 secretion and MUFA content in ONS-D when compared to ET [42]. In a study by Printz [65], adequate glycaemic and insulinemic responses were found after the intake of three enteral supplements for diabetics in subjects with DM2, but no significant differences in the release of GIP and GLP-1 were found [65]. In fact, carbohydrates used in Printz's [65] study, such as glucose, fructose, lactose and maltose [65], probably resulted in both changes in the final place of the intraluminal digestion and the speed of absorption, which could explain these results, especially when comparing the forenamed carbohydrates with those administered in our study. Even though DI also contains disaccharides such as lactose, its metabolic profile could be sufficient to produce a more significant GLP-1 release of and less GIP than ET, but not enough to produce a better effect on incretins and insulin than GS. This observation confirms previous findings that both the amount and type of carbohydrates and fats influence incretin release 18,24,29,45], as well as in the GI and GL.

Our study could be one of the first demonstrating ONS-D effects on GI in DM2 subjects. In fact, when compared with glucose solution, the evaluated supplements turned out to have an intermediate GI value in people with diabetes for ET = 56. Meanwhile for GS = 47 and DI = 51, the result was a low GI. Whereas, GL was high for ET = 23 and intermediate for GS = 11 and DI = 12, (Table 7). The mean of these values is higher than the reported in the international GI and GL tables for healthy subjects [36]: GI for ET = 48, GS = 23, DI = 12; with an intermediate GL: ET = 16, GS = 6 DI = 3. In a randomised cross-over study conducted by Hofman et al. [35], in which the GI of 12 supplements was evaluated in healthy subjects, the mean GI value in the ONS-D was 19.4 ± 1.8, and from 42.1 ± 5.9 in standard supplements [35].

Significant differences have been reported in the GI value of different foods and/or typical foods between healthy subjects and DM2 [66]. It is well known that the subject's characteristics does not have a significant effect on mean IG values [38], but the variation of the values can differ in different groups, being higher in people suffering from type 1 diabetes (29%) than in healthy subjects (22%) or in DM2 patients (15%) [38]. Our results are comparable with a previous study in which the GI for a DM oral specific supplement was assessed in healthy subjects (IG = 27) and DM2 (IG = 54), finding a significant difference between groups [67].

This situation can be explained by a greater relative increase in the glycaemic response after consumption of the reference food (GB) in people with diabetes compared to healthy subjects [38,68]. One possible explanation in that a defective insulin secretion is unable to counteract greater glycaemic excursions in DM2 patients. At the same time [68], healthy people preserve their insulin secretory machinery, preventing a greater glycaemic increase especially for the lowest digestion rates [38,68].

As mentioned above, we found a higher GI for DI, even though a lower GI value has been reported in healthy subjects when compared to the rest of the treatments [35,36]. However, in the study conducted by Hofman et al. [35], both supplements GS and DI contained fructose 1.9 g/100 mL, and a higher amount of MUFAs, DI = 3.6 g/100 mL versus GS = 3.8 g/100 mL than the supplements evaluated in this study, therefore, it is not possible to make an exact comparison [35].

The GI value for DI in DM2 patients could be explained in part by the quantitative sugar content (which has an 8.3 g versus 0.0 g to GS per portion given in this study) (Table 2). The rest of the components like both the amount and type of fibre can also influence these results. Moreover, soluble fibre can decrease the GI by many factors such as postprandial glucose fluctuation cushioning, and, by its action on intestinal motility, on peptide action and gastrointestinal enzymes [29,69,70].

In this study, total fibre concentration in DI was 2 g/100 mL, whose proportion corresponds to the 80:20 ratio of soluble/insoluble fibre compared to GS, whose total amount corresponds to 1.8 g/100 mL soluble (Table 1). In this regard, identical fibre concentrations generated different GI, such is the case of supplements with 1.5 g/100 mL of fibre and with GI = 26 and 17, respectively, in healthy subjects [35,36], constituted by different fibre mixtures based on fructooligosaccharides, inulin, oligofructose, Arabic gum, soybean polysaccharides and cellulose. Furthermore, it has been reported that soluble fibre can stimulate appetite-regulating peptides such as GLP-1 and pancreatic peptide YY (PYY) in rodents as well as in human [69–71]. It is important to note that DI has resistant starch, whereas GS contains a modified and resistant maltodextrin linked to soluble fibre [69]. In a study in healthy subjects, an increase in peptide YY concentrations and GLP-1 was observed alongside a corresponding decrease in the sensation of hunger and an increased satiety perception after the consumption of tea with 10 g of this component [69].

Few investigations about OSF-D intake have correlated SA with incretin concentrations as it has been evaluated in this study. This indicator was quantified through a score that included variables such as perception of hunger, desire to eat, prospective consumption of food and fullness [14]. It was observed in this investigation that plasma insulin, GIP and GLP-1 were related to some of these parameters but observing a lower SA ratings $AUC_{0-180\,min}$ in the ET (Supplementary Materials Table S4). It is known that appetite regulation is a complex process stimulated by several central and peripheral signals in response to energy and, mainly, to food composition, where emotional, sensory and environmental factors can influence the overall response [71,72].

There is a lack of consensus regarding GI/GL usefulness in predicting appetite and food intake [12,73,74]. Although GI is not synonymous with glycaemic response, the debate is anchored to the controversy toward the effect of postprandial glycaemic level and its effects on SA reduction [14,75]. Some authors state that the evidence about these affirmations are not conclusive [73,76], postulating that postprandial glycaemic and appetite are not related and considering that insulin response [74], but not the glycaemic response is the real mediator of the short-term appetite reduction, as shown by Flint et al. [14,76]. Specifically, Flint et al. has reported that the maximum insulinemic peak after meal ingestion was related to a decrease in hunger sensation and a satiety increase.

Likewise, in our study, precisely at 30 min and not at the maximum peak, insulin values were inversely related to the sensation of hunger and the overall of SA rating after ET intake, but not the perception of fullness (Supplementary Materials Table S1). However, the same behaviour for these variables was not evident after the consumption of ONS-D. Possibly, this was due to the higher and faster insulin increase produced by ET at this point of the curve, based on the type and amount of non-extended release carbohydrates of this ONS, and more than half corresponded to free sugars (14.1 g/per portion given in this study) (Table 2). Despite this premise, a relationship between glycaemia concentration and prospective food consumption 30 min after DI intake was found, (Supplementary Materials Table S2) and a direct relationship between glycaemic levels in 90 min with the sensation of fullness after the consumption of GS (Supplementary Materials Table S3). The observed feeling of fullness could be related to another mechanism produced via carbohydrate type and fibre content in GS, a supplement that besides sucromalt also has amylase-resistant maltodextrin, in which fibre-viscosity addition could increase the fullness sensation [69].

It is important to note there was an inverse correlation between GLP-1 levels and prospective consumption of food 30 min after GS ingestion (Supplementary Materials Table S3). In other studies [24,77], a relationship between GLP-1 and delayed gastric emptying has been evidenced. This gastrointestinal response would influence the feeling of fullness after GS intake at this curve time. Niwano [12] showed that high GI foods consumption are associated with increased hunger and short-term satiety reduction in humans, but not over the long-term [74].

It is relevant to highlight the inverse correlation between GIP and GI/GL after ONS-D ingestion (Supplementary Materials Table S4). This finding could confirm the theory proposed by Pfeiffer et al. [32] regarding the role of this incretin as an indicator of "carbohydrate metabolic quality" [32]. On the other hand, we confirmed our hypothesis that ONS-D with slow-digesting carbohydrates strongly stimulates GLP-1 release with a subsequent decrease in GIP and insulin secretion, promoting a lower IG/CG index in DM2 subjects when compared with a standard supplement. Although ONS-D reduced the $AUC_{0-180\ min}$ of subjective appetite, only GS exhibited both a hunger sensation decreasing effect and an increased fullness perception in some points of the postprandial response. Finally, these results were also consistent with Peters et al. [78], who evaluated the digestibility of three carbohydrates on appetite and its relation to blood glucose levels and postprandial insulin, reporting that glycaemic response had minimal effects on appetite when the products only differed in the rate and extension of carbohydrate digestibility [78].

The limitations of our research comprised the lack of evaluation of some variables such as gastric emptying. Although the number of subjects who completed this study was sufficient to assess GI/GL accurately, a higher number of patients is recommended for SA evaluation. On the other hand, one of the strengths of this study is that the results of these indicators, especially GI/GL, could be the first of their kind in the literature done in diabetic individuals from Latin America. It is also one of the first to combine these variables with subjective appetite and incretin levels. It would be a matter of interest to extend the curve's time after consumption in order to evaluate the intake suppression force to the following meal, along with intervention protocols regarding intestinal microbiota in this type of individual.

5. Conclusions

The results of this study showed lower values in postprandial subjective appetite ratings and better metabolic profile after ONS-D intake when compared to standard supplements. A more attenuated glycaemic and insulinemic response along with a lower GIP release and higher levels of GLP-1 confirmed the synergistic effect of slow-digesting carbohydrates along MUFA addition. Isomaltulose and sucromalt may have influenced these factors. In this study, GI/GL in subjects with DM2 after ONS-D consumption were lower than the reference food (glucose solution) and the standard supplement, and lower for GS than DI.

Strategies in food technology, such as intestinal amylase-resistant dextrins along with new functional fibres, need to be considered in low GI product development in order to obtain adequately managed metabolic responses of fullness perception after ONS-D consumption. Our study qualifies two of these supplements as optimal for prescription in people with diabetes when compared with a standard supplement. However, it is necessary to conduct more investigations allowing to correlate long-term appetite suppression with the EG/CG of these supplements.

Supplementary Materials: The following are available online at http://www.mdpi.com/2072-6643/11/7/1477/s1, Table S1: Correlation coefficients between biochemical variables and subjective measurements of appetite in 0, 30, 90 and 120 min at standard oral nutritional supplements not specific for diabetic patients (ET). Table S2: Correlations coefficients between biochemical variables and subjective measurements of appetite in 0, 30, 90 and 120 min at isomaltulose and resistant starch supplement (DI). Table S3: Correlations coefficients between biochemical variables and subjective measurements of appetite in 0, 30, 90 and 120 min at resistant maltodextrin and sucromalt supplement (GS). Table S4: Correlations coefficients between glycaemic index and glycaemia load with AUC values of hormones and subjective measurements of appetite.

Author Contributions: Conceptualization, L.A.D., V.B. and J.L.-M.; methodology, L.A.D., V.B., N.R., J.d.A.C. and J.L.-M.; software, D.A.; validation, V.C. and N.R.; formal analysis, D.A. and V.C.; investigation, J.d.A.C., S.D.-A. and D.R.-G.; resources, V.B., S.D.-A. and S.C.; data handling, D.A. and V.C.; writing—original draft preparation, L.A.D., V.B. and J.L.-M.; writing—review and editing, L.A.D., V.B., J.L.-M. and M.C.E.; visualization, M.C.E., D.R.-G., J.d.A.C. and S.C.; supervision, L.A.D.; project administration, L.A.D. and N.R.; funding acquisition, L.A.D., N.R. and V.B. All authors conducted the drafting of the manuscript and agreed on the final approval of the version to be published.

Funding: This research was funded by University of Zulia, Venezuela "VAC Condes 1457" and Andres Bello University, Chile.

Acknowledgments: The authors thank Valmore Bermúdez and Nadia Reina Villasmil for their laboratory assistance and the Endocrine and Metabolic Diseases Research Centre (EMDRC) and Andres Bello University for this publication.

Conflicts of Interest: The authors declare no competing interests.

Abbreviations

ADA	American Diabetes Association
BMI	Body mass index
DI	Isomaltulose and resistant starch supplement
DM2	Diabetes mellitus type 2
ET	Standard nutritional supplement not specific for diabetics
GB	Glucose solution or reference food
GI	Glycaemic index
GIP	Glucose-dependent insulinotropic polypeptide
GL	Glycaemic load
GLP-1	Glucagon-like peptide 1
GS	Resistant maltodextrin and sucromalt supplement
HbA1c	Glycated haemoglobin (HbA1c)
IDF	International Diabetes Federation
ONS-D	Oral nutritional supplements specific for diabetics
SEM	Standard error of the mean
VAS	Visual analogue scale
LGL	Low glycaemic load
AUCG	Area under the curve glucose

References

1. Rosen, E.D.; Kaestner, K.H.; Natarajan, R.; Patti, M.-E.; Sallari, R.; Sander, M.; Susztak, K. Epigenetics and Epigenomics: Implications for Diabetes and Obesity. *Diabetes* **2018**, *67*, 1923–1931. [CrossRef]
2. World Health Organization. The Top 10 Causes of Death. 2018. Available online: https://www.who.int/news-room/fact-sheets/detail/the-top-10-causes-of-death (accessed on 31 March 2019).
3. World Health Organization. Diabetes. 2018. Available online: https://www.who.int/en/news-room/fact-sheets/detail/diabetes (accessed on 31 March 2019).
4. Unnikrishnan, R.; Pradeepa, R.; Joshi, S.R.; Mohan, V. Type 2 Diabetes: Demystifying the Global Epidemic. *Diabetes* **2017**, *66*, 1432–1442. [CrossRef] [PubMed]
5. International Diabetes Federation (IDF). The 8th Edition of the Diabetes Atlas. 2017. Available online: http://diabetesatlas.org/resources/2017-atlas.html (accessed on 31 March 2019).
6. International Diabetes Federation Guideline Development Group. Guideline for management of postmeal glucose in diabetes. *Diabetes Res. Clin. Pract.* **2014**, *103*, 256–268. [CrossRef]
7. American Diabetes Association. 15. Diabetes Advocacy: Standards of Medical Care in Diabetes—2018. *Diabetes Care* **2018**, *41*, S152–S153. [CrossRef] [PubMed]
8. Diabetes and Nutrition Study Group of the European Association for the Study of Diabetes Recommendations for the nutritional management of patients with diabetes mellitus. *Eur. J. Clin. Nutr.* **2000**, *54*, 353–355. [CrossRef]

9. Willett, W.; Manson, J.; Liu, S. Glycemic index, glycemic load, and risk of type 2 diabetes. *Am. J. Clin. Nutr.* **2002**, *76*, 274S–280S. [CrossRef]
10. Augustin, L.S.A.; Kendall, C.W.C.; Jenkins, D.J.A.; Willett, W.C.; Astrup, A.; Barclay, A.W.; Björck, I.; Brand-Miller, J.C.; Brighenti, F.; Buyken, A.E.; et al. Glycemic index, glycemic load and glycemic response: An International Scientific Consensus Summit from the International Carbohydrate Quality Consortium (ICQC). *Nutr. Metab. Cardiovasc. Dis.* **2015**, *25*, 795–815. [CrossRef] [PubMed]
11. Ojo, O.; Ojo, O.O.; Adebowale, F.; Wang, X.-H. The Effect of Dietary Glycaemic Index on Glycaemia in Patients with Type 2 Diabetes: A Systematic Review and Meta-Analysis of Randomized Controlled Trials. *Nutrients* **2018**, *10*, 373. [CrossRef] [PubMed]
12. Niwano, Y.; Adachi, T.; Kashimura, J.; Sakata, T.; Sasaki, H.; Sekine, K.; Yamamoto, S.; Yonekubo, A.; Kimura, S. Is glycemic index of food a feasible predictor of appetite, hunger, and satiety? *J. Nutr. Sci. Vitaminol. (Tokyo)* **2009**, *55*, 201–207. [CrossRef]
13. Sun, F.-H.; Li, C.; Zhang, Y.-J.; Wong, S.; Wang, L. Effect of Glycemic Index of Breakfast on Energy Intake at Subsequent Meal among Healthy People: A Meta-Analysis. *Nutrients* **2016**, *8*, 37. [CrossRef] [PubMed]
14. Flint, A.; Møller, B.K.; Raben, A.; Sloth, B.; Pedersen, D.; Tetens, I.; Holst, J.J.; Astrup, A. Glycemic and insulinemic responses as determinants of appetite in humans. *Am. J. Clin. Nutr.* **2006**, *84*, 1365–1373. [CrossRef]
15. Elia, M.; Ceriello, A.; Laube, H.; Sinclair, A.J.; Engfer, M.; Stratton, R.J. Enteral nutritional support and use of diabetes-specific formulas for patients with diabetes: A systematic review and meta-analysis. *Diabetes Care* **2005**, *28*, 2267–2279. [CrossRef]
16. Ojo, O.; Brooke, J. Evaluation of the Role of Enteral Nutrition in Managing Patients with Diabetes: A Systematic Review. *Nutrients* **2014**, *6*, 5142–5152. [CrossRef] [PubMed]
17. De Luis DA, D.M. A randomized clinical trial with two enteral diabetes-specific supplements in patients with diabetes mellitus type 2: Metabolic effects. *Eur. Rev. Med. Pharmacol. Sci.* **2008**, *12*, 261–266.
18. Voss, A.C.; Maki, K.C.; Garvey, W.T.; Hustead, D.S.; Alish, C.; Fix, B.; Mustad, V.A. Effect of two carbohydrate-modified tube-feeding formulas on metabolic responses in patients with type 2 diabetes. *Nutrition* **2008**, *24*, 990–997. [CrossRef]
19. Sanz-Paris, A.; Boj-Carceller, D.; Lardies-Sanchez, B.; Perez-Fernandez, L.; Cruz-Jentoft, A. Health-Care Costs, Glycemic Control and Nutritional Status in Malnourished Older Diabetics Treated with a Hypercaloric Diabetes-Specific Enteral Nutritional Formula. *Nutrients* **2016**, *8*, 153. [CrossRef] [PubMed]
20. Tan, S.Y.; Siow, P.C.; Peh, E.; Henry, C.J. Influence of rice, pea and oat proteins in attenuating glycemic response of sugar sweetened beverages. *Eur. J. Nutr.* **2018**, *57*, 2795–2803. [CrossRef] [PubMed]
21. Yabe, D.; Seino, Y.; Seino, Y. Incretin concept revised: The origin of the insulinotropic function of glucagon-like peptide-1 -the gut, the islets or both? *J. Diabetes Investig.* **2018**, *9*, 21–24. [CrossRef]
22. Rojas, J.; Bermudez, V.; Palmar, J.; Martínez, M.S.; Olivar, L.C.; Nava, M.; Tomey, D.; Rojas, M.; Salazar, J.; Garicano, C.; et al. Pancreatic Beta Cell Death: Novel Potential Mechanisms in Diabetes Therapy. *J. Diabetes Res.* **2018**, *2018*, 1–19. [CrossRef]
23. Prinz, P. The role of dietary sugars in health: Molecular composition or just calories? *Eur. J. Clin. Nutr.* **2019**. [CrossRef]
24. Giezenaar, C.; Trahair, L.G.; Luscombe-Marsh, N.D.; Hausken, T.; Standfield, S.; Jones, K.L.; Lange, K.; Horowitz, M.; Chapman, I.; Soenen, S. Effects of randomized whey-protein loads on energy intake, appetite, gastric emptying, and plasma gut-hormone concentrations in older men and women. *Am. J. Clin. Nutr.* **2017**, *106*, 865–877. [CrossRef] [PubMed]
25. Steinert, R.E.; Feinle-Bisset, C.; Asarian, L.; Horowitz, M.; Beglinger, C.; Geary, N. Ghrelin, CCK, GLP-1, and PYY(3-36): Secretory controls and physiological roles in eating and glycemia in health, obesity, and after RYGB. *Physiol. Rev.* **2017**, *97*, 411–463. [CrossRef] [PubMed]
26. Behall, K.M.; Scholfield, D.J.; Canary, J. Effect of starch structure on glucose and insulin responses in adults. *Am. J. Clin. Nutr.* **1988**, *47*, 428–432. [CrossRef] [PubMed]
27. McMahon, M.M.; Nystrom, E.; Braunschweig, C.; Miles, J.; Compher, C.; the American Society for Parenteral and Enteral Nutrition (A.S.P.E.N.) Board of Directors. A.S.P.E.N. Clinical Guidelines: Nutrition Support of Adult Patients with Hyperglycemia. *J. Parenter. Enter. Nutr.* **2013**, *37*, 23–36. [CrossRef] [PubMed]

28. Doola, R.; Todd, A.S.; Forbes, J.M.; Deane, A.M.; Presneill, J.J.; Sturgess, D.J. Diabetes-Specific Formulae Versus Standard Formulae as Enteral Nutrition to Treat Hyperglycemia in Critically Ill Patients: Protocol for a Randomized Controlled Feasibility Trial. *JMIR Res. Protoc.* **2018**, *7*, e90. [CrossRef]

29. Devitt, A.A.; Williams, J.A.; Choe, Y.S.; Hustead, D.S.; Mustad, V.A. Glycemic responses to glycemia-targeted specialized-nutrition beverages with varying carbohydrates compared to a standard nutritional beverage in adults with type 2 diabetes. *Adv. Biosci. Biotechnol.* **2013**, *4*, 1–10. [CrossRef]

30. Grysman, A.; Carlson, T.; Wolever, T.M.S. Effects of sucromalt on postprandial responses in human subjects. *Eur. J. Clin. Nutr.* **2008**, *62*, 1364–1371. [CrossRef]

31. Maresch, C.C.; Petry, S.F.; Theis, S.; Bosy-Westphal, A.; Linn, T. Low Glycemic Index Prototype Isomaltulose-Update of Clinical Trials. *Nutrients* **2017**, *9*, 381. [CrossRef]

32. Pfeiffer, A.F.H.; Keyhani-Nejad, F. High Glycemic Index Metabolic Damage—A Pivotal Role of GIP and GLP-1. *Trends Endocrinol. Metab.* **2018**, *29*, 289–299. [CrossRef]

33. Holub, I.; Gostner, A.; Theis, S.; Nosek, L.; Kudlich, T.; Melcher, R.; Scheppach, W. Novel findings on the metabolic effects of the low glycaemic carbohydrate isomaltulose (Palatinose). *Br. J. Nutr.* **2010**, *103*, 1730–1737. [CrossRef]

34. Kendall, F.E.; Marchand, O.; Haszard, J.J.; Venn, B.J. The Comparative Effect on Satiety and Subsequent Energy Intake of Ingesting Sucrose or Isomaltulose Sweetened Trifle: A Randomized Crossover Trial. *Nutrients* **2018**, *10*, 1504. [CrossRef] [PubMed]

35. Hofman, Z.; De Van Drunen, J.; Kuipers, H. The Glycemic Index of standard and diabetes-specific enteral formulas. *Asia Pac. J. Clin. Nutr.* **2006**, *15*, 412–417. [PubMed]

36. Atkinson, F.S.; Foster-Powell, K.; Brand-Miller, J.C. International Tables of Glycemic Index and Glycemic Load Values: 2008. *Diabetes Care* **2008**, *31*, 2281–2283. [CrossRef] [PubMed]

37. World Medical Association. Ethical Principles for Medical Research Involving Human Subjects. 64ª General Assembly. 2013. Available online: https://www.wma.net/policies-post/wma-declaration-of-helsinki-ethical-principles-for-medical-research-involving-human-subjects/ (accessed on 24 March 2019).

38. Brouns, F.; Bjorck, I.; Frayn, K.N.; Gibbs, A.L.; Lang, V.; Slama, G.; Wolever, T.M. Glycaemic index methodology. *Nutr. Res. Rev.* **2005**, *18*, 145–171. [CrossRef] [PubMed]

39. Parker, B.A.; Sturm, K.; Macintosh, C.G.; Feinle, C.; Horowitz, M.; Chapman, I.M. Relation between food intake and visual analogue scale ratings of appetite and other sensations in healthy older and young subjects. *Eur. J. Clin. Nutr.* **2004**, *58*, 212–218. [CrossRef] [PubMed]

40. World Health Organization. Energy and Protein Requirements: Report of a Joint FAO/WHO/UNU Expert Consultation. 1981. Available online: https://apps.who.int/iris/handle/10665/39527 (accessed on 24 March 2019).

41. Akilen, R.; Deljoomanesh, N.; Hunschede, S.; Smith, C.E.; Arshad, M.U.; Kubant, R.; Anderson, G.H. The effects of potatoes and other carbohydrate side dishes consumed with meat on food intake, glycemia and satiety response in children. *Nutr. Diabetes* **2016**, *6*, e195. [CrossRef]

42. Mottalib, A.; Mohd-Yusof, B.-N.; Shehabeldin, M.; Pober, D.; Mitri, J.; Hamdy, O. Impact of Diabetes-Specific Nutritional Formulas versus Oatmeal on Postprandial Glucose, Insulin, GLP-1 and Postprandial Lipidemia. *Nutrients* **2016**, *8*, 443. [CrossRef]

43. Alish, C.J.; Garvey, W.T.; Maki, K.C.; Sacks, G.S.; Hustead, D.S.; Hegazi, R.A.; Mustad, V.A. A Diabetes-Specific Enteral Formula Improves Glycemic Variability in Patients with Type 2 Diabetes. *Diabetes Technol. Ther.* **2010**, *12*, 419–425. [CrossRef]

44. Ceriello, A.; Davidson, J.; Hanefeld, M.; Leiter, L.; Monnier, L.; Owens, D.; Tajima, N.; Tuomilehto, J. Postprandial hyperglycaemia and cardiovascular complications of diabetes: An update. *Nutr. Metab. Cardiovasc. Dis.* **2006**, *16*, 453–456. [CrossRef]

45. Yoshizane, C.; Mizote, A.; Yamada, M.; Arai, N.; Arai, S.; Maruta, K.; Mitsuzumi, H.; Ariyasu, T.; Ushio, S.; Fukuda, S. Glycemic, insulinemic and incretin responses after oral trehalose ingestion in healthy subjects. *Nutr. J.* **2017**, *16*. [CrossRef]

46. Kawaguchi, T.; Nakano, D.; Oriishi, T.; Torimura, T. Effects of isomaltulose on insulin resistance and metabolites in patients with non-alcoholic fatty liver disease: A metabolomic analysis. *Mol. Med. Rep.* **2018**. [CrossRef] [PubMed]

47. Nauck, M.A.; Meier, J.J. The incretin effect in healthy individuals and those with type 2 diabetes: Physiology, pathophysiology, and response to therapeutic interventions. *Lancet Diabetes Endocrinol.* **2016**, *4*, 525–536. [CrossRef]
48. Holst, J.J. On the Physiology of GIP and GLP-1. *Horm. Metab. Res.* **2004**, *36*, 747–754. [CrossRef] [PubMed]
49. Nasteska, D.; Harada, N.; Suzuki, K.; Yamane, S.; Hamasaki, A.; Joo, E.; Iwasaki, K.; Shibue, K.; Harada, T.; Inagaki, N. Chronic Reduction of GIP Secretion Alleviates Obesity and Insulin Resistance Under High-Fat Diet Conditions. *Diabetes* **2014**, *63*, 2332. [CrossRef] [PubMed]
50. Bray, G.A. Potential health risks from beverages containing fructose found in sugar or high-fructose corn syrup. *Diabetes Care* **2013**, *36*, 11–12. [CrossRef] [PubMed]
51. Herman, M.A.; Samuel, V.T. The Sweet Path to Metabolic Demise: Fructose and Lipid Synthesis. *Trends Endocrinol. Metab.* **2016**, *27*, 719–730. [CrossRef] [PubMed]
52. Donner, T.W.; Wilber, J.F.; Ostrowski, D. D-tagatose, a novel hexose: Acute effects on carbohydrate tolerance in subjects with and without type 2 diabetes. *Diabetes Obes. Metab.* **1999**, *1*, 285–291. [CrossRef]
53. Guerrero-Wyss, M.; Durán Agüero, S.; Angarita Dávila, L. D-Tagatose Is a Promising Sweetener to Control Glycaemia: A New Functional Food. *BioMed Res. Int.* **2018**, *2018*, 8718053. [CrossRef]
54. Maeda, A.; Miyagawa, J.-I.; Miuchi, M.; Nagai, E.; Konishi, K.; Matsuo, T.; Tokuda, M.; Kusunoki, Y.; Ochi, H.; Murai, K.; et al. Effects of the naturally-occurring disaccharides, palatinose and sucrose, on incretin secretion in healthy non-obese subjects. *J. Diabetes Investig.* **2013**, *4*, 281–286. [CrossRef]
55. Ruiz-Ojeda, F.J.; Plaza-Díaz, J.; Sáez-Lara, M.J.; Gil, A. Effects of Sweeteners on the Gut Microbiota: A Review of Experimental Studies and Clinical Trials. *Adv. Nutr. (Bethesda Md.)* **2019**, *10*, S31–S48. [CrossRef]
56. Zeevi, D.; Korem, T.; Zmora, N.; Israeli, D.; Rothschild, D.; Weinberger, A.; Ben-Yacov, O.; Lador, D.; Avnit-Sagi, T.; Lotan-Pompan, M.; et al. Personalized Nutrition by Prediction of Glycemic Responses. *Cell* **2015**, *163*, 1079–1094. [CrossRef] [PubMed]
57. Angarita, L.; Bermudez, V.; Reina, N.; Cisternas, S.; Díaz, W.; Escobar, M.C.; Carrasco, P.; Durán, S.; Buhring, K.; Buhring, R.; et al. New Insights into Alleviating Diabetes Mellitus: Role of Gut Microbiota and a Nutrigenomic Approach. In *Diabetes Food Plan*; Waisundara, V., Ed.; InTech: London, UK, 2018; ISBN 978-1-78923-274-5.
58. Ang, M.; Linn, T. Comparison of the effects of slowly and rapidly absorbed carbohydrates on postprandial glucose metabolism in type 2 diabetes mellitus patients: A randomized trial. *Am. J. Clin. Nutr.* **2014**, *100*, 1059–1068. [CrossRef] [PubMed]
59. König, D.; Theis, S.; Kozianowski, G.; Berg, A. Postprandial substrate use in overweight subjects with the metabolic syndrome after isomaltulose (Palatinose TM) ingestion. *Nutrition* **2012**, *28*, 651–656. [CrossRef] [PubMed]
60. Van Can, J.G.P.; van Loon, L.J.C.; Brouns, F.; Blaak, E.E. Reduced glycaemic and insulinaemic responses following trehalose and isomaltulose ingestion: Implications for postprandial substrate use in impaired glucose-tolerant subjects. *Br. J. Nutr.* **2012**, *108*, 1210–1217. [CrossRef]
61. Sloth, B.; Due, A.; Larsen, T.M.; Holst, J.J.; Heding, A.; Astrup, A. The effect of a high-MUFA, low-glycaemic index diet and a low-fat diet on appetite and glucose metabolism during a 6-month weight maintenance period. *Br. J. Nutr.* **2008**, *101*, 1846–1858. [CrossRef] [PubMed]
62. Drucker, D.J. The biology of incretin hormones. *Cell Metab.* **2006**, *3*, 153–165. [CrossRef]
63. Rocca, A.S.; LaGreca, J.; Kalitsky, J.; Brubaker, P.L. Monounsaturated Fatty Acid Diets Improve Glycemic Tolerance through Increased Secretion of Glucagon-Like Peptide-1*. *Endocrinology* **2001**, *142*, 1148–1155. [CrossRef]
64. Storm, H.; Holst, J.J.; Hermansen, K.; Thomsen, C. Differential effects of saturated and monounsaturated fats on postprandial lipemia and glucagon-like peptide 1 responses in patients with type 2 diabetes. *Am. J. Clin. Nutr.* **2003**, *77*, 605–611. [CrossRef]
65. Printz, H.; Recke, B.; Fehmann, H.C.; Göke, B. No apparent benefit of liquid formula diet in NIDDM. *Exp. Clin. Endocrinol. Diabetes* **2009**, *105*, 134–139. [CrossRef]
66. Noreberg, C.; Indar-Brown, K.; Madar, Z. Glycemic and insulinemic responses after ingestion of ethnic foods by NIDDM and healthy subjects. *Am. J. Clin. Nutr.* **1992**, *55*, 89–95. [CrossRef]
67. Aguirre, P.C.; Galgani, F.J.; Díaz, B.E. Determinación del índice glicémico del alimento nutridiabetic® destinado a diabéticos tipo 2. *Rev. Chil. Nutr.* **2006**, *33*, 14–21. [CrossRef]

68. Rizkalla, S.W.; Laromiguiere, M.; Champ, M.; Bruzzo, F.; Boillot, J.; Slama, G. Effect of baking process on postprandial metabolic consequences: Randomized trials in normal and type 2 diabetic subjects. *Eur. J. Clin. Nutr.* **2006**, *61*, 175. [CrossRef] [PubMed]

69. Ye, Z.; Arumugam, V.; Haugabrooks, E.; Williamson, P.; Hendrich, S. Soluble dietary fibre (Fibersol-2) decreased hunger and increased satiety hormones in humans when ingested with a meal. *Nutr. Res.* **2015**, *35*, 393–400. [CrossRef] [PubMed]

70. Delzenne, N.M.; Cani, P.D.; Daubioul, C.; Neyrinck, A.M. Impact of inulin and oligofructose on gastrointestinal peptides. *Br. J. Nutr.* **2005**, *93*, S157–S161. [CrossRef] [PubMed]

71. Kirkmeyer, S.V.; Mattes, R.D. Effects of food attributes on hunger and food intake. *Int. J. Obes.* **2000**, *24*, 1167–1175. [CrossRef]

72. Stafleu, A.; Hendriks, H.F.; Smeets, P.A.; Blom, W.A.; de Graaf, C. Biomarkers of satiation and satiety. *Am. J. Clin. Nutr.* **2004**, *79*, 946–961.

73. Thomas, D.; Elliott, E.; Baur, L. Low glycaemic index or low glycaemic load diets for overweight and obesity. *Cochrane Database Syst. Rev.* **2007**. [CrossRef]

74. Bornet, F.R.J.; Jardy-Gennetier, A.-E.; Jacquet, N.; Stowell, J. Glycaemic response to foods: Impact on satiety and long-term weight regulation. *Appetite* **2007**, *49*, 535–553. [CrossRef]

75. Van Dam, R.M.; Seidell, J.C. Carbohydrate intake and obesity. *Eur. J. Clin. Nutr.* **2007**, *61*, S75. [CrossRef]

76. Flint, A.; Gregersen, N.T.; Gluud, L.L.; Møller, B.K.; Raben, A.; Tetens, I.; Verdich, C.; Astrup, A. Associations between postprandial insulin and blood glucose responses, appetite sensations and energy intake in normal weight and overweight individuals: A meta-analysis of test meal studies. *Br. J. Nutr.* **2007**, *98*, 17–25. [CrossRef]

77. Giezenaar, C.; van der Burgh, Y.; Lange, K.; Hatzinikolas, S.; Hausken, T.; Jones, K.; Horowitz, M.; Chapman, I.; Soenen, S. Effects of Substitution, and Adding of Carbohydrate and Fat to Whey-Protein on Energy Intake, Appetite, Gastric Emptying, Glucose, Insulin, Ghrelin, CCK and GLP-1 in Healthy Older Men—A Randomized Controlled Trial. *Nutrients* **2018**, *10*, 113. [CrossRef] [PubMed]

78. Peters, H.P.F.; Ravestein, P.; van der Hijden, H.T.W.M.; Boers, H.M.; Mela, D.J. Effect of carbohydrate digestibility on appetite and its relationship to postprandial blood glucose and insulin levels. *Eur. J. Clin. Nutr.* **2010**, *65*, 47. [CrossRef] [PubMed]

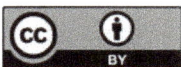

nutrients

MDPI

Review

Reversing Type 2 Diabetes: A Narrative Review of the Evidence

Sarah J Hallberg [1,2,3,*] , **Victoria M Gershuni** [4], **Tamara L Hazbun** [2,3]
and Shaminie J Athinarayanan [1]

1   Virta Health, 535 Mission Street, San Francisco, CA 94105, USA; shaminie@virtahealth.com
2   Indiana University Health Arnett, Lafayette, IN 47904, USA; thazbun@iuhealth.org
3   Indiana University School of Medicine, Indianapolis, IN 46202, USA
4   Department of Surgery, Perelman School of Medicine University of Pennsylvania,
     Philadelphia, PA 19104, USA; victoriagershunimd@gmail.com
*   Correspondence: sarah@virtahealth.com

Received: 27 February 2019; Accepted: 22 March 2019; Published: 1 April 2019

Abstract: Background: Type 2 diabetes (T2D) has long been identified as an incurable chronic disease based on traditional means of treatment. Research now exists that suggests reversal is possible through other means that have only recently been embraced in the guidelines. This narrative review examines the evidence for T2D reversal using each of the three methods, including advantages and limitations for each. Methods: A literature search was performed, and a total of 99 original articles containing information pertaining to diabetes reversal or remission were included. Results: Evidence exists that T2D reversal is achievable using bariatric surgery, low-calorie diets (LCD), or carbohydrate restriction (LC). Bariatric surgery has been recommended for the treatment of T2D since 2016 by an international diabetes consensus group. Both the American Diabetes Association (ADA) and the European Association for the Study of Diabetes (EASD) now recommend a LC eating pattern and support the short-term use of LCD for weight loss. However, only T2D treatment, not reversal, is discussed in their guidelines. Conclusion: Given the state of evidence for T2D reversal, healthcare providers need to be educated on reversal options so they can actively engage in counseling patients who may desire this approach to their disease.

Keywords: diabetes; diabetes reversal; bariatric surgery; very-low-calorie; low-carbohydrate

1. Introduction

According to 2017 International Diabetes Federation (IDF) statistics, there are approximately 425 million people with diabetes worldwide [1]. In the United States, there are an estimated 30.3 million adults living with diabetes, and its prevalence has been rising rapidly, with at least 1.5 million new diabetes cases diagnosed each year [2]. Diabetes is a major public health epidemic despite recent advances in both pharmaceutical and technologic treatment options.

Type 2 diabetes (T2D) has long been identified as an incurable chronic disease. The best outcome that has been expected is amelioration of diabetes symptoms or slowing its inevitable progression. Approximately 50% of T2D patients will need insulin therapy within ten years of diagnosis [3] Although in the past diabetes has been called chronic and irreversible, the paradigm is changing [4,5].

The recent 2016 World Health Organization (WHO) global report on diabetes added a section on diabetes reversal and acknowledged that it can be achieved through weight loss and calorie restriction [4]. "Diabetes reversal" is a term that has found its way into scientific articles and the lay press alike; "remission" has also been used. While the exact criteria are still debated, most agree that a hemoglobin A1c (HbA1c) under the diabetes threshold of 6.5% for an extended period of time without the use of glycemic control medications would qualify [6]. Excluding metformin from the glycemic control medications list, as it has indications beyond diabetes, may also be a consideration [7,8]. Likewise, terms such as "partial" (HbA1c <6.5 without glycemic control medications for 1 year) or "complete" (HbA1c <5.7 without glycemic control medications for 1 year) remission have been defined by an expert panel as more evidence accumulates that points to the possibility of avoiding the presumably progressive nature of T2D [9]. It is important to note that the term "cure" has not been applied to T2D, as there does exist the potential for re-occurrence, which has been well documented in the literature.

Despite the growing evidence that reversal is possible, achieving reversal is not commonly encouraged by our healthcare system. In fact, reversal is not a goal in diabetes guidelines. Specific interventions aimed at reversal all have one thing in common: they are not first-line standard of care. This is important, because there is evidence suggesting that standard of care does not lead to diabetes reversal. This raises the question of whether standard of care is really the best practice. A large study by Kaiser Permanente found a diabetes remission rate of 0.23% with standard of care [10]. The status quo approach will not reverse the health crisis of diabetes.

A significant number of studies indicate that diabetes reversal is achievable using bariatric surgery, while other approaches, such as low-calorie diets (LCD) or carbohydrate restriction (LC), have also shown effectiveness in an increasing number of studies. This review will examine each of these approaches, identifying their beneficial effects, supporting evidence, drawbacks, and degree of sustainability.

2. Materials and Methods

A literature search was performed as appropriate for narrative reviews, including electronic databases of PubMed, EMBASE, and Google Scholar from 1970 through December 2018. We reviewed English-language original and review articles found under the subject headings diabetes, bariatric surgery, metabolic surgery, very low-calorie diet, calorie restriction, low carbohydrate diet, ketogenic diet, diabetes remission, and diabetes reversal. References of the identified publications were searched for more research articles to include in this review. Selected studies were reviewed and evaluated for eligibility for inclusion in this review based on their relevance for diabetes reversal and remission. Either remission or reversal needed to be discussed in the paper or the results were consistent with these terms for inclusion. Randomized clinical trials and intervention-based studies were given emphasis for inclusion.

A total of 99 original articles containing information pertaining to diabetes reversal or remission were included in this narrative review.

3. Results and Discussion

3.1. Bariatric Surgery

Bariatric surgery has long been recognized as a potential treatment for both morbid obesity and the metabolic processes that accompany it, specifically T2D. While the efficacy of T2D reversal depends on the choice of procedure, there is unilateral improvement in glycemia following operation [11], and bariatric surgery has been found to be superior to intensive T2D medical management. Accordingly, in 2016, the second Diabetes Surgery Summit (DSS-II) released recommendations, endorsed by 45 medical and scientific societies worldwide, to use bariatric surgery as a treatment for T2D (bariatric surgery is currently approved by the 2016 recommendations for adults with a body mass index (BMI) >40, or >35 kg/m^2 with obesity-related comorbidities) [12]. Of interest is the consistent finding that glycemic improvements occur rapidly, often within hours to days, and precede weight loss, which likely represents the enteroendocrine responses to altered flow of intestinal contents (i.e., bile acid signaling and changes in microbiota and their metabolome) [13–19].

The most commonly performed bariatric surgeries in the United States include laparoscopic and robotic Roux-en-Y Gastric Bypass (RYGB) or Sleeve Gastrectomy (SG). While surgical treatment is based on the principles of restriction and intestinal malabsorption, evidence suggests that there are more complex mechanisms at play. Bariatric surgery has consistently been shown to dramatically and rapidly improve blood glucose [20] while allowing decreased oral hypoglycemic medications and insulin use, effectively reversing diabetes in up to 80% of patients [21] in the short term. In addition to early post-operative improvement in blood glucose and insulin sensitivity, bariatric surgery has also been shown to cause alterations in GI hormone release, including ghrelin, leptin, cholecystokinin (CCK), peptide-tyrosine-tyrosine (PYY), and glucagon-like peptide 1 (GLP-1), that may impact feeding behavior via the gut–brain axis in addition to modulating euglycemia [22]. Furthermore, microbial changes in the human gut have been linked to obesity, and surgical alterations to gastrointestinal anatomy have been associated with dramatic changes in gut microbiota populations with reversion from an "obesogenic" to a lean bacterial population [13,14,16,19,23,24].

Long-term outcomes from bariatric surgery depend on multiple factors, including type of surgery performed, patient comorbidities, patient readiness for lifelong dietary change, and ongoing surveillance. While bariatric surgery has been demonstrated to be safe and effective overall, it is important to recognize that it is not without risks. Each patient must weigh the risks and benefits associated with untreated morbid obesity versus those associated with surgery or effective dietary management and choose accordingly. Surgery of any type can be associated with complications leading to morbidity or mortality; the complication rates have been stated to be as high as 13% and 21% for SG and RYGB, respectively. The postoperative mortality rate is 0.28–0.34% for SG and 0.35–0.79% for RYGB; in comparison, an elective laparoscopic cholecystectomy is associated with overall complication rates of 9.29% and with a 30-day mortality rate of 0.15–0.6%, depending on the series [25,26]. Significant complications include anastomotic leak or hemorrhage, post-operative readmission, need for reoperation, post-operative hypoglycemia, dumping syndrome, worsening acid reflux, marginal ulceration, and micronutrient deficiencies [25–29].

It is important to consider that while short-duration studies have shown early resolution of comorbidities following bariatric procedures, when followed for multiple decades, there may be decreased efficacy of disease resolution and increased incidence of hospital admission long-term. Long-term reversal of T2D and true glucose homeostasis remain uncertain. Weight loss after surgery is a significant predictor of a return to euglycemia post-operatively. Multiple studies have reported initial T2D remission rates as high as 80% [30,31], however, long-term remission is less durable. The five-year follow-up outcomes of the SLEEVEPASS RCT found complete or partial remission of T2D in 37% of SG and 45% of RYGB patients, which is similar to other studies showing long-term T2D remission in up to a third of patients [32]. In the large prospective cohort study Longitudinal Assessment of Bariatric Surgery 2 (LABS-2), the investigators found that long-term diabetes remission after RYGB was higher than predicted by weight loss alone, which suggests that the surgery itself impacts metabolic factors that contribute to disease management [31]. Similarly, the STAMPEDE trial—an RCT that followed 150 patients with T2D who were randomized to intensive medical intervention (IMT) versus IMT plus RYGB versus IMT plus SG for diabetes resolution (defined as HbA1c <6.0%) and followed for five years—revealed increased rates of T2D resolution with RYGB (29%) and SG (23%) compared to IMT alone (5%) (Figure 1). The surgery cohort also demonstrated greater weight loss and improvements in triglycerides, HDL, need for insulin, and overall quality of life [33–35].

Despite the likelihood of improved glycemic control, there are significant financial costs for the patient, health system, and insurance companies associated with bariatric surgery (U.S. average of $14,389) [36]. Despite the high initial cost of surgery, Pories and colleagues found that prior to surgery, patients spend over $10,000 per year on diabetes medications; after RYGB, the annual cost falls to less than $2000, which represents an $8000 cost savings at the individual level [30]. Furthermore, economic analyses show that surgery is likely to be cost-effective, especially in patients who are obese [37,38]. In a clinical effectiveness review of the literature that included 26 trials extracted from over 5000 references, Picot et al. found that bariatric surgery was a more effective intervention for weight loss than non-surgical options; however, there was extreme heterogeneity and questionable long-term adherence to the non-surgical interventions [39]. After surgery, metabolic syndrome improved, and there were higher rates of T2D remission compared to the non-surgical groups [39]. Further, while there were improvements in comorbidities after surgery independent of bariatric procedure, there was also an increased likelihood of adverse events. While the overall event rate remained low, major adverse events included medication intolerance, need for reoperation, infection, anastomotic leakage, and venous and thromboembolic events [39].

It is imperative to consider that one of the requirements of qualifying for bariatric surgery is demonstration of at least six months of unsuccessful attempts at weight loss using traditional dietary and exercise advice according to the 2016 Recommendations [12]. There are, however, no requirements as to what weight loss strategy is employed, which may represent a time point where dietary intervention, including low-calorie, ketogenic, or carbohydrate-restricted diets, should be utilized. At least two recent clinical trials have demonstrated safety and efficacy in pre-operative very low-carbohydrate ketogenic diets before bariatric surgery for increasing weight loss and decreasing liver volume [40,41].

Furthermore, despite technically adequate surgery, an alarming number of patients may still experience weight regain and/or recurrence of comorbid obesity-associated conditions. In these patients, effective strategies for dietary intervention are even more important. Approximately 10–15% of patients fail to lose adequate weight (failure defined as <50% of excess weight) or demonstrate significant weight regain after bariatric surgery without evidence of an anatomic or technical reason [42]. Additionally, in 25–35% of patients who undergo surgery, significant weight regain (defined as >15% of initial weight loss) occurs within two to five years post-operatively [43]. These patients often require further medical management with weight loss medications, further dietary and behavioral intervention, and, for some, reoperation. Reoperation can be for either revision for further weight loss (narrowing of the gastric sleeve, conversion of VSG to RYGB, and increasing the length of the roux limb) or reversal of RYGB due to health concerns, most commonly associated with malnutrition. A small cohort of patients (4%) may experience severe weight loss with significant malnutrition leading to hospitalization in over 50%, mortality rates of 18%, and need for reversal of RYGB anatomy. While the incidence of RYGB reversal is unknown, based upon a systematic review that included 100 patients spanning 1985–2015, the rate of reversal parallels the increasing rate of bariatric surgery [44].

In the short term, T2D reversal rates with surgery have been reported to be as high as 80%, with an additional 15% demonstrating partial improvement in T2D despite still requiring medication [17]. Within one week after RYGB, patients experience improved fasting hepatic insulin clearance, reduced basal de novo glucose production, and increased hepatic insulin sensitivity; by three months and one year after surgery, patients have improved beta-cell sensitivity to glucose, increased GLP-1 secretion from the gut, and improved insulin sensitivity in muscle and fat cells [45]. Over time, T2D remission rates remain high but do decline; Purnell and colleagues reported three-year remission rates of 68.7% after RYGB [29]. However, Pories published results from a 14-year prospective study with mean follow-up of 7.6 years, and found 10-year remission rates remained around 83% [46]. In a 10-year follow-up study of participants from the Swedish Obese Subjects (SOS) study that prospectively followed patients who underwent bariatric surgery, the authors reported a 72% ($n = 342$) and 36% ($n = 118$) recovery rate from T2D for RYGB at two years and 10 years, respectively [47].

The long-term metabolic impact and risk reduction from surgery remain high in a substantial number of patients and this route to reversal clearly has the most robust data to support its use. As evidenced by the dramatic improvements in metabolic state that precede weight loss, bariatric surgery is far more than merely a restrictive and/or malabsorptive procedure. Large shifts in bile acid signaling in the lumen of the small intestine, gut nutrient sensing, and changes in the microbiota community appear to greatly impact overall host health. Further research is ongoing using both basic and translational science models to identify the role of these various hormones and metabolites; perhaps there will be a way to one day harness the beneficial effects of bariatric surgery without the need for anatomic rearrangement.

3.2. Low-Calorie Diets (LCD)

As diabetes rates have risen to unprecedented levels [1,2], the number of studies examining diabetes reversal using non-surgical techniques has increased. A handful of studies have reported successful weight loss with decreased insulin resistance, plasma glucose, and medication use following a LCD. As early as 1976, Bistrian et al. [48] reported that a very low-calorie protein-sparing modified fast allowed for insulin elimination in all seven obese patients with T2D. The average time to insulin discontinuation was only 6.5 days, and the longest was 19 days. In a study by Bauman et al., a low-calorie diet of 900 kcal, including 115 g of protein, led to significant improvement in glycemic control that was mainly attributed to improvements in insulin sensitivity [49]. Furthermore, a study conducted in obese T2D patients found that a LCD and gastric bypass surgery were equally effective in achieving weight loss and improving glucose and HbA1c levels in the short term [50]. Weight loss, however, persisted in the diet-treated patients only for the first three months, indicating difficulty with long-term maintenance [47]. Similarly, other studies also reported similar pattern of early blood glucose normalization without medication use, but the improvements were not sustained long-term [51–53]. Likewise, the study by Wing et al., even though reported significant and greater improvements of HbA1c at 1 year in the intermittently delivered very low-calorie diet, the HbA1c improvement was not significantly different than what was reported in the patients receiving low-calorie diet (LCD) throughout the one year period [54]. Furthermore, the glycemic improvements observed at 1 year were not maintained through 2-years, even though the group with intermittent very low-calorie diet had less medication requirement than the group in the LCD arm at 2 years [54]. Lastly, micronutrient deficiencies with the use of calorie restricted diets has been shown and supplementation and monitoring for deficiencies is a consideration with their use [55,56].

While these previous studies were not assessing diabetes remission or reversal rate per se, they demonstrated the effectiveness of calorie restriction in achieving weight loss and improved glycemic control, which are the core goals of reversal. In 2003, the Look AHEAD trial randomized 5145 overweight or obese patients with T2D to an intervention group that received either an intensive lifestyle intervention (ILI) including calorie restriction and increased physical activity or to a control group that included diabetes support and education (DSE) [57]. Post hoc analysis of this study revealed that at one year, 11.5% of the participants in the ILI group achieved remission (partial or complete); however, remission rates subsequently decreased over time (9.2% at year two and 7.3% at year four). Nevertheless, the remission rates achieved through ILI were three to six times higher than those achieved in the DSE group. Lower baseline HbA1c, greater level of weight loss, shorter duration of T2D diagnosis, and lack of insulin use at baseline predicted higher remission rate in ILI participants [58].

Following the Look AHEAD study, other studies have evaluated a LCD for diabetes remission [59–61]. Most of these studies assessed remission over a short period of time in a small study sample. Bhatt et al. reported that six of the 12 individuals achieved partial remission at the end of the three-month intervention [61]. Ades et al. studied an intensive lifestyle program including calorie restriction and exercise, and reported that eight of the 10 individuals with recently diagnosed T2D achieved partial remission at six months, including one with complete remission [60]. The study ended at six months, therefore long term sustainability was not assessed. Another study assessing a one-year diabetes remission retrospectively among those undergoing 12 weeks of the intensive weight loss program "Why Wait" had a much lower remission rate of 4.5%, with 2.3% of them achieving partial remission, while another 2.3% had complete remission [59]. This study suggests that long-term maintenance of remission is a challenge. Moreover, diabetes remission was more likely reported in those who had a shorter diabetes duration, lower baseline HbA1c, and were taking fewer hypoglycemic medications [59,61].

An initial 2011 diabetes reversal study by Taylor and colleagues showed that a very low-calorie diet of 600 Kcal/day not only normalized glucose, HbA1c, and hepatic insulin sensitivity levels within a week, but also led to decreased hepatic and pancreatic triacylglycerol content and normalization of the insulin response within eight weeks [62]. At 12 weeks post-intervention, many of the improvements were maintained, but over a quarter of the patients had an early recurrence of diabetes. Further, average weight regain during the 12 weeks post-intervention was 20% [62]. As a follow-up to the 2011 study, the same group performed a larger and longer study with eight weeks of a very low-calorie meal replacement (624–700 kcal/day) followed by two weeks of solid food replacement and a weight maintenance program of up to six months [63]. In this study, those who achieved a fasting blood glucose of <7 mmol/L (<126 mg/dL) were categorized as responders, while others were categorized as non-responders. At six months, 40% of participants who initially responded to the intervention were still in T2D remission which was defined by achieving a fasting plasma glucose of <7mmol/L; the majority of those who remitted (60%) had a shorter diabetes duration (<4 years) [63].

These short-term studies were the foundation for a community-based cluster-randomized clinical trial called DiRECT (Diabetes Remission Clinical Trial). DiRECT enrolled a sample of 306 relatively healthy participants with T2D (people on insulin or with a diabetes duration longer than six years were excluded) [64] (Figure 1). They were cluster randomized to either standard diabetes care or an intervention using low-calorie meal replacement diet (825–853 kcal/day) for three to five months, followed by stepwise food re-introduction and a long-term weight maintenance program. At one-year follow-up, 46% of patients met the study criteria of diabetes remission (HbA1c <6.5% without antiglycemic medications) [64] and at two years the remission rate was 36% [65]. The DiRECT study has extended their follow-up an additional three years to assess the long-term impact on remission.

Taken together, evidence suggests that a LCD is effective in reversing diabetes in the short term up to two years, and its effectiveness was predominantly demonstrated in those with shorter duration since diabetes diagnosis. It is important to note that a substantial level of calorie restriction is needed to generate a sufficient level of weight loss for reversing diabetes. Short-term intervention with moderate energy restriction and metformin for modest weight loss was not as effective in reversing diabetes as compared to standard diabetes care [66]. Lifestyle intervention with severe energy restriction may have some deleterious effect on the body composition and physiology, which poses a concern for long-term health [67]. Furthermore, long-term achievement of diabetes remission, adherence to the diet, and weight loss maintenance after the diet remain a challenge. Studies have also suggested that physiological and metabolic adaptation of the body in response to caloric restriction may shift energy balance and hormonal regulation of weight toward weight regain after weight loss [67,68]. Thus, it is crucial that future studies are directed towards assessing the long-term sustainability of diabetes remission led by LCD and feasibility of this diet on the physiological adaptation and body composition changes.

3.3. Carbohydrate-Restricted Diets (LC)

Before the discovery of insulin in 1921, low carbohydrate (LC) diets were the most frequently prescribed treatment for diabetes [69,70]. The paradigm shifted both with the development of exogenous insulin and later with the emergence of the low-fat diet paradigm. A diet low in fat, which by default is high in carbohydrate, became the standard recommendation in guidelines around the globe [71]. Rather than preventing elevations in glucose, the goal became maintenance of blood sugar control via the increased use of glycemic control medications, including insulin [72]. Over the last decade, clinical studies have begun to resurrect the pre-insulin LC dietary approach. In response to the new evidence on the efficacy of carbohydrate restriction, low-carbohydrate has recently been endorsed as an eating pattern by the ADA and the European Association for the Study of Diabetes (EASD) [5,73]. In addition, the Veterans Affairs/Department of Defense (VA/DOD) guidelines now recommend carbohydrate restriction as low as 14% of energy intake in its most recent guidelines for treatment of diabetes (VA) [74].

LC diets are based on macronutrient changes rather than a focus on calorie restriction [75]. Although the exact definition varies, a low-carbohydrate diet usually restricts total carbohydrates to less than 130 grams per day, while a very low-carbohydrate or ketogenic diet usually restricts total carbohydrates to as low as 20–30 grams per day. Protein consumption is generally unchanged from a standard ADA diet (around 20% of intake), with the remaining energy needs met by fat from either the diet or mobilized body fat stores. Carbohydrate sources are primarily non-starchy vegetables with some nuts, dairy, and limited fruit [75].

A total of 32 separate trials examining carbohydrate restriction as a treatment for T2D were found when our search was performed [76–108]. However, for reasons that may include varied levels of carbohydrate restriction and differing levels of support given, not all studies had results that would be consistent with diabetes reversal. A number of shorter-term trials have found a significant between-group advantage of a low-carbohydrate intervention for T2D [80,84,92,97]. Data from longer-term trials are limited, and in some follow-up studies, the between-group advantage seen initially was lost or reduced, although it often remains significantly improved from baseline. This raises the question of long-term sustainability using this approach. Due to heterogeneity in methodology and definition of carbohydrate restriction, the ability to fully examine T2D reversal based on the existing studies is limited. Based upon a recent systematic review of LC, it appears that the greatest improvements in glycemic control and greatest medication reductions have been associated with the lowest carbohydrate intake [109]. In consideration of these limitations, it appears important to assess the level of carbohydrate restriction, support or other methods given to encourage sustainability, and length of follow-up.

A study comparing an ad libitum very low-carbohydrate (<20 g total) diet to an energy-restricted low-glycemic diet in T2D found greater reduction in HbA1c, weight, and insulin levels in the low-carbohydrate arm [89]. Additionally, 95% of participants in the low-carbohydrate arm reduced or eliminated glycemic control medications, compared to 62% in the low glycemic index arm at 24 weeks. Instruction was given in a one-time session with a dietician and included take-home materials for reference. A slightly longer study (34 weeks) trial [85] found that a very low-carbohydrate ketogenic diet intervention (20–50 g net carbs per day) resulted in HbA1c below the threshold for diabetes in 55% of the patients, compared to 0% of patients in the low-fat arm. The education sessions were all online and included behavior modification strategies and mindful eating which was aimed to address binge eating. New lessons were emailed to the patients weekly for the first 16 weeks and then every two weeks for the remainder of the study.

A small (34 participants) one-year study of an ad libitum, very low-carbohydrate diet compared to a calorie-restricted moderate carbohydrate diet found a significant reduction in HbA1c between groups favoring the low-carbohydrate arm [86]. At one year, 78% of participants who began the trial with a HbA1c above 6.5% no longer met the cutoff for the diagnosis of diabetes, no longer required any non-metformin medication, and significantly reduced or eliminated metformin. Total kilocalorie intake was not significantly different between the two groups, even with moderate carbohydrate restriction. Despite equal energy intake, the low carbohydrate group lost significantly more weight and had improved glycemic control, which indicates a potential mechanistic role for carbohydrate restriction itself. The support given was 19 classes over the 12-month period, tapering in frequency over time.

Another one-year trial [76] found significant HbA1c reduction in the subset of patients with diabetes (*n* = 54) assigned to an ad libitum low-carbohydrate diet (<30 total grams per day), compared to an energy-restricted low-fat diet. These results remained significant after adjusting the model for weight loss, indicating an effect of the carbohydrate reduction itself. The support given was four weekly sessions during the first month, followed by monthly sessions for the remaining 11 months.

A metabolic ward study on 10 patients with T2D [96] found that 24-h glucose curves normalized within two weeks on a very low-carbohydrate diet (<21 g total per day). This was in addition to medication reduction and elimination including insulin and sulfonylureas After accounting for body water changes, the average weight loss during the two-week period was 1.65 kg (average of <2% total body weight which is similar to the results of bariatric surgery, where normoglycemia is seen prior to significant weight loss. Interestingly, despite the diet being ad libitum other than the carbohydrate limit, the average energy intake decreased by 1000 kcal per day. Assuming no further change in glycemic control, HbA1c would be 5.6% after eight weeks, which would represent a reduction of 23%

from baseline. The fact that HbA1c reductions were greater than in other, longer-term outpatient studies may indicate that support of dietary changes is the key to longer-term success.

In our published trial providing significant support through the use of a continuous care intervention (CCI), we examined using a low-carbohydrate diet aimed at inducing nutritional ketosis in patients with T2D (*n* = 262), compared with usual care T2D patients (*n* = 87) [98] (Figure 1). At one year, the HbA1c decreased by 1.3% in the CCI, with 60% of completers achieving a HbA1c below 6.5% without hypoglycemic medication (not including metformin). Overall, medications were significantly reduced, including complete elimination of sulfonylureas and reduction or elimination of insulin therapy in 94% of users. Most cardiovascular risk factors showed significant improvement [110]. The one-year retention rate was 83%, which indicates that a non-calorie-restricted, low-carbohydrate intervention can be sustained. Improvements were not observed in the usual care patients. The newly released two-year results of this trial [106] show sustained improvements in normoglycemia, with 54% of completers maintaining HbA1c below 6.5% without medication or only on metformin. The retention rate at two years was 74%, further supporting the sustainability of this dietary intervention for diabetes reversal. Weight loss of 10% was seen at 2-years despite no intentional caloric restriction instruction. Additionally, this trial involved participants with a much longer duration of diabetes (8.4 years on average) than other nutrition trial interventions [58,64,65] and did not exclude anyone taking exogenous insulin. As duration of T2D and insulin use have both been identified to be negative factors in predicting remission after bariatric surgery [111,112], the 2-year results of this trial may be even more significant.

It is interesting to note that most studies utilize ad libitum intake in the carbohydrate-restricted arm. Despite this, in studies that have tracked energy intake, spontaneous calorie restriction has occurred [113,114]. In many trials where energy intake has been prescribed or weight loss has been equal, an advantage has been seen in glycemic control, weight, or both in the low-carbohydrate arm [86,91,107]. A better understanding of the role that caloric intake, whether prescribed or spontaneous, plays in the overall success is important. In cases of spontaneous energy intake reduction, elucidating the specific mechanism behind this reduction would help in the overall personalization of this approach.

Multiple studies have evaluated side effects or potential complications of carbohydrate restriction. The diet has been found to be safe and well tolerated although long term hard outcome data is lacking and should be a focus of future research. A transient rise in uric acid early in very low-carbohydrate restriction without an associated increase in gout or kidney stones has been documented [84,98,100]. Blood urea nitrogen (BUN) has been found to increase and decrease in different studies without an associated change in kidney function [87,98,100,115,116]. Recently, bone mineral density has been found to be unchanged despite significant weight loss after two years of a ketogenic diet intervention in patients with T2D [108]. While most studies show an improvement or no change in LDL-C levels in patients with T2D on a low-carbohydrate diet, there have been two studies that have found an increase in LDL-C in participants with T2D [99,111]. In one of the studies that found an increase in calculated LDL-C, a non-significant reduction in measured ApoB lipoproteins and unchanged non-HDL cholesterol were seen. Monitoring LDL-C or a measured value of potentially atherogenic lipoproteins such as ApoB should be considered. Lastly, micronutrient deficiency has been seen with a carbohydrate restricted diet, supplementation and monitoring should be given consideration with this intervention [56].

Although the use of very low-carbohydrate diets for diabetes reversal shows promising results, the lack of longer-term follow-up studies remains a limitation. Follow up is limited to two years, and therefore longer-term studies are needed to determine the sustainability of the metabolic improvements. Determining the appropriate method of support may be a key to the overall success with disease reversal.

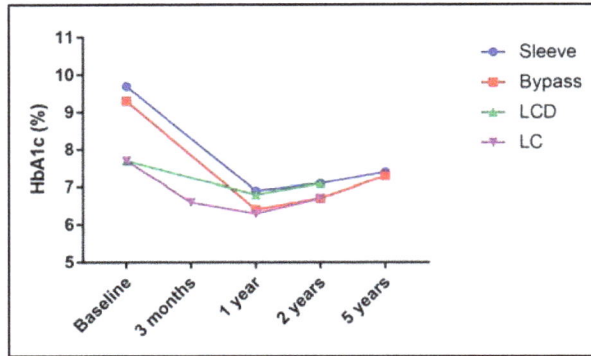

(A)

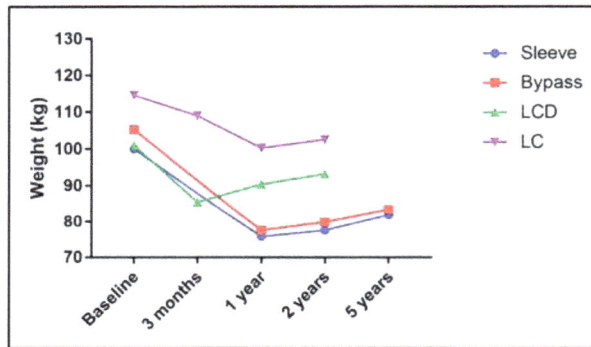

(B)

Figure 1. (**A**) Mean changes of hemoglobin A1c (HbA1c) from baseline to last published date for each study retrieved to represent the three methods of reversal; (**B**) mean changes of weight from baseline to last published date for each studies retrieved to represent the three methods of reversal. Note: We chose these three studies to represent the three methods of reversal based on publication date and relevance to diabetes reversal. Note that baseline characteristics differ. Surgery trial examined by sleeve gastrectomy and Roux-en-Y gastric bypass separately and were represented as sleeve and bypass in the graph. Surgery: STAMPEDE [34,35]. Low-calorie diets (LCD): DIRECT [65,66]; carbohydrate restriction (LC): IUH [99,107].

4. Summary

Additional evidence has become available in recent years suggesting that diabetes reversal is a possible alternative to consider in place of traditional diabetes treatment and management. In this paper, we provide a review of three methods that have been shown to successfully reverse type 2 diabetes. The current body of evidence suggests that bariatric surgery is the most effective method for overall efficacy and prolonged remission, even though concerns associated with surgical complications, treatment cost and complete lifestyle modification after surgery remain challenges for wide adoption of this approach. While both the LCD and LC dietary approaches are convincing for reversing diabetes in the short term (up to two years), long term maintenance of diabetes remission is still unproven. There are limited available data supporting long term maintenance of weight loss and its associated glycemic improvements in response to LCD; similarly, long-term adherence to a low carbohydrate diet will likely remain an obstacle without the development of proper patient education and optimal support for long-term behavioral change. Moreover, research in understanding the mechanism of diabetes reversibility in all three approaches and its overlapping mechanistic pathways are lacking; this is an area for future research emphasis.

There are similar identified negative predictors of remission for all three approaches. These factors include longer diabetes duration and increased severity, lower BMI, advanced age, poor glycemic control, and low C-peptide levels (indicating decreased endogenous insulin production) [117]. Further exploration into the heterogeneity of these factors will help personalize the approach, determine realistic goals for each patient, and should be considered during treatment discussions. Ongoing research into algorithm development will be helpful in this regard.

5. Conclusions

Overall, as a society we can no longer afford or tolerate the continued rising rates of diabetes. Despite many barriers within the healthcare system as a whole, providers are responsible on a daily basis for the lives of patients caught up in this unprecedented epidemic. The current standard of care may be suitable for some, but others would surely choose reversal if they understood there was a choice. The choice can only be offered if providers are not only aware that *reversal is possible* but have the education needed to review these options in a patient-centric discussion.

Author Contributions: Conceptualization, S.J.H. and S.J.A. Investigation, S.J.H., V.M.G., T.L.H., S.J.A. Writing—original draft, S.J.H., V.M.G., S.J.A. Writing—review and editing, S.J.H., V.M.G., T.L.H., S.J.A. All authors approved of the final manuscript.

Acknowledgments: We thank James McCarter and Stephen Phinney for their edits, which greatly improved the manuscript.

Conflicts of Interest: S.J.H. is an employee and shareholder of Virta Health, a for-profit company that provides remote diabetes care using a low-carbohydrate nutrition intervention, and serves as an advisor for Atkins Corp. V.M.G. has no conflicts of interest to declare. T.L.H. is an employee of Virta Health. S.J.A. is an employee and shareholder of Virta Health.

Abbreviations:

C	carbohydrate restriction
DSS-II	Diabetes Surgery Summit
RYGB	Roux-en-Y Gastric Bypass
SG	Sleeve Gastrectomy
CCK	cholecystokinin
PYY	peptide-tyrosine-tyrosine
GLP-1	glucagon-like peptide 1
LABS-2	Longitudinal Assessment of Bariatric Surgery 2
LCD	low-calorie diet
IMT	intensive medical intervention
DiRECT	Diabetes Remission Clinical Trial
ASD	European Association for the Study of Diabetes
VA/DOD	Veterans Affairs/Department of Defense

References

1. International Diabetes Federation. In *IDF Diabetes Atlas*, 8th ed.; International Diabetes Federation: Brussels, Belgium, 2017.
2. Centers for Disease Control and Prevention. National Diabetes Statistics Report, 2017. Available online: https://www.cdc.gov/diabetes/pdfs/data/statistics/national-diabetes-statistics-report.pd (accessed on 1 February 2019).

3. Home, P.; Riddle, M.; Cefalu, W.T.; Bailey, C.J.; Del Prato, S.; Leroith, D.; Schemthaner, G.; van Gaal, L.; Raz, I. Insulin therapy in people with Type 2 diabetes: Opportunities and challenges. *Diabetes Care* **2014**, *37*, 1499–1508. [CrossRef] [PubMed]

4. World Health Organization. Global Report on Diabetes. 2016. Available online: https://www.who.int/diabetes/publications/grd-2016/en/ (accessed on 1 February 2019).

5. Davies, M.J.; D'Alessio, D.A.; Fradkin, J.; Kernan, W.N.; Mathieu, C.; Mingrone, G.; Rossing, P.; Tsapas, A.; Wexler, D.J.; Buse, J.B. Management of hyperglycemia in Type 2 diabetes, 2018. A consensus report by the American Diabetes Association (ADA) and the European Association for the Study of Diabetes (EASD). *Diabetes Care* **2018**, *41*, 2669–2701. [CrossRef] [PubMed]

6. Ramos-Levi, A.M.; Cabrerizo, L.; Matia, P.; Sanchez-Pernaute, A.; Torres, A.J.; Rubio, M.A. Which criteria should be used to define type 2 diabetes remission after bariatric surgery. *BMC Surgery* **2013**, *13*, 8. [CrossRef] [PubMed]

7. Xiang, A.H.; Trigo, E.; Martinez, M.; Katkhouda, N.; Beale, E.; Wang, X.; Wu, J.; Chow, T.; Montgomery, C.; Nayak, K.S.; et al. Impact of gastric banding versus metformin on β-cell function in adults with impaired glucose tolerance or mild type 2 diabetes. *Diabetes Care* **2018**, *41*, 2544–2551. [CrossRef]

8. Diabetes Prevention Program Research Group. Long-term effects of metformin on diabetes prevention: Identification of subgroups that benefited most in the diabetes prevention program and diabetes prevention outcomes study. *Diabetes Care* **2019**, dc181970. [CrossRef]

9. Buse, J.B.; Caprio, S.; Cefalu, W.T.; Ceriello, A.; Del Prato, S.; Inzucchi, S.E.; McLaughlin, S.; Phillips, G.L., II; Robertson, R.P.; Rubino, F.; et al. How do we define cure of diabetes? *Diabetes Care* **2009**, *32*, 2133–2135. [CrossRef]

10. Karter, A.J.; Nundy, S.; Parker, M.M.; Moffet, H.H.; Huang, E.S. Incidence of remission in adults with Type 2 diabetes: The Diabetes & Aging Study. *Diabetes Care* **2014**, *37*, 3188–3195.

11. Steven, S.; Carey, P.E.; Small, P.K.; Taylor, R. Reversal of Type 2 diabetes after bariatric surgery is determined by the degree of achieved weight loss in both short- and long-duration diabetes. *Diabet Med.* **2015**, *32*, 47–53. [CrossRef] [PubMed]

12. Rubino, F.; Nathan, D.; Eckel, R.H.; Schauer, P.R.; Alberti, K.G.; Zimmet, P.Z.; Del Prato, S.; Ji, L.; Sadikot, S.M.; Herman, W.H.; et al. Delegates of the 2nd Diabetes Surgery Summit. Metabolic surgery in the treatment algorithm for type 2 diabetes: A joint statement by International Diabetes Organizations. *Diabetes Care* **2016**, *39*, 861–877. [CrossRef]

13. Anhe, F.F.; Varin, T.V.; Schertzer, J.D.; Marette, A. The Gut Microbiota as a Mediator of Metabolic Benefits after Bariatric Surgery. *Can. J. Diabetes* **2017**, *41*, 439–447. [CrossRef]

14. Medina, D.A.; Pedreros, J.P.; Turiel, D.; Quezada, N.; Pimentel, F.; Escalona, A.; Garrido, D. Distinct patterns in the gut microbiota after surgical or medical therapy in obese patients. *PeerJ* **2017**, *5*, e3443. [CrossRef]

15. Magouliotis, D.E.; Tasiopoulou, V.S.; Sioka, E.; Chatedaki, C.; Zacharoulis, D. Impact of Bariatric Surgery on Metabolic and Gut Microbiota Profile: A Systematic Review and Meta-analysis. *Obes. Surg.* **2017**, *27*, 1345–1357. [CrossRef]

16. Murphy, R.; Tsai, P.; Jullig, M.; Liu, A.; Plank, L.; Booth, M. Differential Changes in Gut Microbiota After Gastric Bypass and Sleeve Gastrectomy Bariatric Surgery Vary According to Diabetes Remission. *Obes. Surg.* **2017**, *27*, 917–925. [CrossRef] [PubMed]

17. Kaska, L.; Sledzinski, T.; Chomiczewska, A.; Dettlaff-Pokora, A.; Swierczynski, J. Improved glucose metabolism following bariatric surgery is associated with increased circulating bile acid concentrations and remodeling of the gut microbiome. *World J. Gastroenterol.* **2016**, *22*, 8698–8719. [CrossRef] [PubMed]

18. Penney, N.C.; Kinross, J.; Newton, R.C.; Purkayastha, S. The role of bile acids in reducing the metabolic complications of obesity after bariatric surgery: a systematic review. *Int. J. Obes. (Lond).* **2015**, *39*, 1565–1574. [CrossRef] [PubMed]

19. Sweeney, T.E.; Morton, J.M. The human gut microbiome: A review of the effect of obesity and surgically induced weight loss. *JAMA Surg.* **2013**, *148*, 563–569. [CrossRef]

20. Rubino, F.; Gagner, M. Potential of surgery for curing type 2 diabetes mellitus. *Ann. Surg.* **2002**, *236*, 554–559. [CrossRef]

21. Cohen, R.; Caravatto, P.P.; Correa, J.L.; Noujaim, P.; Petry, T.Z.; Salles, J.E.; Schiavon, C.A. Glycemic control after stomach-sparing duodenal-jejunal bypass surgery in diabetic patients with low body mass index. *Surg. Obes. Relat. Dis.* **2012**, *8*, 375–380. [CrossRef]

22. Federico, A.; Dallio, M.; Tolone, S.; Gravina, A.G.; Patrone, V.; Romano, M.; Tuccillo, C.; Mozzillo, A.L.; Amoroso, V.; Misso, G.; et al. Gastrointestinal Hormones, Intestinal Microbiota and Metabolic Homeostasis in Obese Patients: Effect of Bariatric Surgery. *In Vivo* **2016**, *30*, 321–330.

23. Peat, C.M.; Kleiman, S.C.; Bulik, C.M.; Carroll, I.M. The Intestinal Microbiome in Bariatric Surgery Patients. *Eur. Eat. Disord. Rev.* **2015**, *23*, 496–503. [CrossRef] [PubMed]

24. Sweeney, T.E.; Morton, J.M. Metabolic surgery: Action via hormonal milieu changes, changes in bile acids or gut microbiota? A summary of the literature. *Best Pract. Res. Clin. Gastroenterol.* **2014**, *28*, 727–740. [CrossRef]

25. Ma, I.T.; Madura, J.A. Gastrointestinal Complications after Bariatric Surgery. *Gastroenterol. Hepatol. (N Y).* **2015**, *11*, 526–535.

26. Rubino, F.; Schauer, P.R.; Kaplan, L.M.; Cummings, D.E. Metabolic surgery to treat type 2 diabetes: Clinical outcome and mechanisms of action. *Annu. Rev. Med.* **2010**, *61*, 393–411. [CrossRef] [PubMed]

27. Abraham, A.; Ikramuddin, S.; Jahansouz, C.; Arafat, F.; Hevelone, N.; Leslie, D. Trends in bariatric surgery: Procedure selection, revisional surgeries, and readmissions. *Obes. Surg.* **2016**, *26*, 1371–1377. [CrossRef] [PubMed]

28. Tack, J.; Deloose, E. Complications of bariatric surgery: Dumping syndrome, reflux and vitamin deficiencies. *Best Prac. Res. Clin. Gastroenterol.* **2014**, *28*, 741–749. [CrossRef] [PubMed]

29. Eisenbarg, D.; Azagury, D.E.; Ghiassi, S.; Grover, B.T.; Ki, J.J. ASMBS position statement on postprandial hyperinsulinemic hypoglycemia after bariatric surgery. *Surg. Obes. Relat. Dis.* **2017**, *13*, 371–378. [CrossRef]

30. Pories, W.J.; Mehaffey, J.H.; Staton, K.M. The surgical treatment of type two diabetes mellitus. *Surg Clin. N. Am.* **2011**, *91*, 821–836. [CrossRef]

31. Purnell, J.Q.; Selzer, F.; Wahed, A.S.; Pender, J.; Pories, W.; Pomp, A.; Dakin, G.; Mitchell, J.; Garcia, L.; Staten, M.A.; et al. Type 2 Diabetes Remission Rates After Laparoscopic Gastric Bypass and Gastric Banding: Results of the Longitudinal Assessment of Bariatric Surgery Study. *Diabetes Care* **2016**, *39*, 1101–1107. [CrossRef] [PubMed]

32. Salminen, P.; Helmio, M.; Ovaska, J.; Juuti, A.; Leivonen, M.; Peromaa-Haavista, P.; Hurme, S.; Soinio, M.; Nuutila, P.; Victorzon, M. Effect of laparoscopic sleeve gastrectomy vs. laparoscopic Roux-en-Y gastric bypass on weight loss at 5 years among patients with morbid obesity: The SLEEVEPASS randomized clinical trial. *JAMA* **2018**, *319*, 241–254. [CrossRef] [PubMed]

33. Schauer, P.R.; Kashyap, S.R.; Wolski, K.; Brethauer, S.A.; Kirwan, J.P.; Pothier, C.E.; Thomas, S.; Abood, B.; Nissen, S.E.; Bhatt, D.L. Bariatric surgery versus medical therapy in obese patients with diabetes. *N. Engl. J. Med.* **2012**, *366*, 1567–1576. [CrossRef]

34. Kashyap, S.R.; Bhatt, D.L.; Wolski, K.; Watanabe, R.M.; Abdul-Ghani, M.; Abood, B.; Pothier, C.E.; Brethauer, S.; Nissen, S.; Gupta, M.; et al. Metabolic effects of bariatric surgery in patients with moderate obesity and type 2 diabetes: Analysis of a randomized control trial comparing surgery with intensive medical treatment. *Diabetes Care* **2013**, *36*, 2175–2182. [CrossRef] [PubMed]

35. Schauer, P.R.; Bhatt, D.L.; Kirwan, J.P.; Wolski, K.; Aminian, A.; Brethauer, S.A.; Navaneethan, S.D.; Singh, R.P.; Pothier, C.E.; Nissen, S.E.; et al. Bariatric surgery versus intensive medical therapy for diabetes: 5-year outcomes. *N. Engl. J. Med.* **2017**, *376*, 641–651. [CrossRef] [PubMed]

36. Doble, B.; Wordsworth, S.; Rogers, C.A.; Welbourn, R.; Byrne, J.; Blazeby, J.M.; By-Band-Sleeve Trial Management Group. What are the real procedural costs of bariatric surgery? A systematic literature review of published cost analyses. *Obes. Surg.* **2017**, *27*, 2179–2192. [CrossRef] [PubMed]

37. Warren, J.A.; Ewing, J.A.; Hale, A.L.; Blackhurst, D.W.; Bour, E.S.; Scott, J.D. Cost-effectiveness of bariatric surgery: Increasing the economic viability of the most effective treatment for type II diabetes mellitus. *Am. Surgeon.* **2015**, *81*, 807–811.

38. Klein, S.; Ghosh, A.; Cremieux, P.Y.; Eapen, S.; McGavock, T.J. Economic impact of the clinical benefits of bariatric surgery in diabetes patients with BMI $\geq$ 35kg/m^2. *Obesity* **2011**, *19*, 581–587. [CrossRef] [PubMed]

39. Picot, J.; Jones, J.; Colquitt, J.L.; Gospodarevskaya, E.; Loveman, E.; Baxter, L.; Clegg, A.J. The clinical effectiveness and cost-effectiveness of bariatric (weight loss) surgery for obesity: A systematic review and economic evaluation. *Health Technol. Assess.* **2009**, *13*, 1–190. [CrossRef]

40. Schiavo, L.; Pilone, V.; Rossetti, G.; Barbarisi, A.; Cesaretti, M.; Iannelli, A. A 4-Week Preoperative Ketogenic Micronutrient-Enriched Diet Is Effective in Reducing Body Weight, Left Hepatic Lobe Volume, and Micronutrient Deficiencies in Patients Undergoing Bariatric Surgery: A Prospective Pilot Study. *Obes. Surg.* **2018**, *28*, 2215–2224. [CrossRef]

41. Leonetti, F.; Campanile, F.C.; Coccia, F.; Capoccia, D.; Alessandroni, L.; Puzziello, A.; Coluzzi, I.; Silecchia, G. Very low-carbohydrate ketogenic diet before bariatric surgery: Prospective evaluation of a sequential diet. *Obes. Surg.* **2015**, *25*, 64–71. [CrossRef]

42. Gumbs, A.A.; Pomp, A.; Gagner, M. Revisional bariatric surgery for inadequate weight loss. *Obes. Surg.* **2007**, *17*, 1137–1145. [CrossRef]

43. Velapati, S.R.; Shah, M.; Kuchkuntla, A.R.; Abu-Dayyeh, B.; Grothe, K.; Hurt, R.T.; Mundi, M.S. Weight Regain After Bariatric Surgery: Prevalence, Etiology, and Treatment. *Curr. Nutr. Rep.* **2018**, *7*, 329–334. [CrossRef] [PubMed]

44. Shoar, S.; Nguyen, T.; Ona, M.A.; Reddy, M.; Anand, S.; Alkuwari, M.J.; Saber, A.A. Roux-end-Y gastric bypass reversal: A systematic review. *Surg. Obes. Relat. Dis.* **2016**, *12*, 1366–1372. [CrossRef]

45. Bojsen-Moller, K.N. Mechanisms of improved glycemic control after Roux-en-Y gastric bypass. *Dan. Med. J.* **2015**, *62*, B5057. [PubMed]

46. Pories, W.J.; Swanson, M.S.; MacDonald, K.G.; Long, S.B.; Morris, P.G.; Brown, B.M.; Barakat, H.A.; de Ramon, R.A.; Israel, G.; Dolezal, J.M. Who would have thought it? An operation proves to be the most effective therapy for adult-onset diabetes mellitus. *Ann. Surg.* **1995**, *222*, 339–350. [CrossRef]

47. Sjostrom, L.; Lindroos, A.K.; Peltonen, M.; Torgerson, J.; Bouchard, C.; Carlsson, B.; Dahlgren, S.; Larsson, B.; Narbro, K.; Sjostrom, D.; et al. Lifestyle, diabetes and cardiovascular risk factors 10 years after bariatric surgery. *N. Engl. J. Med.* **2004**, *351*, 2683–2693. [CrossRef] [PubMed]

48. Bistrian, B.R.; Blackburn, G.L.; Flatt, J.P.; Sizer, J.; Scrimshaw, N.S.; Sherman, M. Nitrogen metabolism and insulin requirements in obese diabetic adults on a protein-sparing modified fast. *Diabetes* **1976**, *25*, 494–504. [CrossRef] [PubMed]

49. Bauman, W.A.; Schwartz, E.; Rose, H.G.; Eisenstein, H.N.; Johnson, D.W. Early and long term effects of acute caloric deprivation in obese diabetic patients. *Am. J. Med.* **1988**, *85*, 38–46. [CrossRef]

50. Hughes, T.A.; Gwynne, J.T.; Switzer, B.R.; Herbst, C.; White, G. Effects of caloric restriction and weight loss on glycemic control, insulin release and resistance, and atherosclerotic risk in obese patients with type II diabetes mellitus. *Am. J. Med.* **1984**, *77*, 7–17. [CrossRef]

51. Hammer, S.; Snel, M.; Lamb, H.J.; Jazet, I.M.; van der Meer, R.W.; Pijl, H.; Meinders, E.A.; Romijn, J.A.; de Roos, A.; Smit, J.W. Prolonged caloric restriction in obese patients with type 2 diabetes mellitus decreases myocardial triglyceride content and improves myocardial function. *J. Am. Coll. Cardiol.* **2008**, *52*, 1006–1012. [CrossRef]

52. Snel, M.; Jonker, J.T.; Hammer, S.; Kerpershoek, G.; Lamb, H.J.; Meinders, A.E.; Pijl, H.; de Roos, A.; Romijn, J.A.; Smit, J.W.A. Long-term beneficial effect of a 16-week very low calorie diet on pericardial fat in obese type 2 diabetes mellitus patients. *Obesity* **2012**, *20*, 1572–1576. [CrossRef]

53. Paisey, R.B.; Harvey, P.; Rice, S.; Belka, I.; Bower, L.; Dunn, M.; Taylor, P.; Paisey, R.M. An intensive weight loss programme in established type 2 diabetes and controls: Effect on weight and atherosclerosis risk factors at 1 year. *Diabet. Med.* **1998**, *15*, 73–79. [CrossRef]

54. Wing, R.R.; Blair, E.; Marcus, M.; Epstein, L.H.; Harvey, J. Year-long weight loss treatment for obese patients with type II diabetes: Does including an intermittent very-low-calorie diet improve outcome? *Am. J. Med.* **1994**, *97*, 354–362. [CrossRef]

55. Damms-Machado, A.; Weser, G.; Bischoff, SC. Micronutrient deficiency in obese subjects undergoing low calorie diet. *Nutr. J.* **2012**, *11*. [CrossRef] [PubMed]

56. Gardner, C.D.; Kim, S.; Bersamin, A.; Dopler-Nelson, M.; Otten, J.; Oelrich, B.; Cherin, R. Micronutrient quality of weight-loss diets that focus on macronutrients: Results from the A to Z study. *Am. J. Clin. Nutr.* **2010**, *92*, 304–312. [CrossRef] [PubMed]

57. Ryan, D.H.; Espeland, M.A.; Foster, G.D.; Haffner, S.M.; Hubbard, V.S.; Johnson, K.C.; Kahn, S.E.; Knowler, W.C.; Yanovski, S.Z.; Look AHEAD Research Group. Look AHEAD (Action for Health in Diabetes): Design and methods for a clinical trial of weight loss for the prevention of cardiovascular disease in type 2 diabetes. *Control Clin Trials.* **2003**, *24*, 610–628. [PubMed]

58. Gregg, E.W.; Chen, H.; Wagenknecht, L.E.; Clark, J.M.; Delahanty, L.M.; Bantle, J.; Pownall, H.J.; Johnson, K.C.; Safford, M.M.; Kitabchi, A.E.; et al. Association of an intensive lifestyle intervention with remission of type 2 diabetes. *JAMA.* **2012**, *308*, 2489–2496. [CrossRef] [PubMed]

59. Mottalib, A.; Sakr, M.; Shehabeldin, M.; Hamdy, O. Diabetes remission after nonsurgical intensive lifestyle intervention in obese patients with Type 2 diabetes. *J. Diabetes Res.* **2015**, 468704. [CrossRef]

60. Ades, P.A.; Savage, P.D.; Marney, A.M.; Harvey, J.; Evans, K.A. Remission of recently diagnosed type 2 diabetes mellitus with weight loss and exercise. *J. Cardiopulm. Rehabil. Prev.* **2015**, *35*, 193–197. [CrossRef] [PubMed]

61. Bhatt, A.A.; Choudhari, P.K.; Mahajan, R.R.; Sayyad, M.G.; Pratyush, D.D.; Hasan, I.; Javherani, R.S.; Bothale, M.M.; Purandare, V.B.; Unnikrishnan, A.G. Effect of a low-calorie diet on restoration of normoglycemia in obese subjects with Type 2 diabetes. *Indian J. Endocrinol. Metab.* **2017**, *21*, 776–780. [PubMed]

62. Lim, E.L.; Hollingsworth, K.G.; Aribisala, B.S.; Chen, M.J.; Mathers, J.C.; Taylor, R. Reversal of type 2 diabetes: Normalisation of beta cell function in association with decreased pancreas and liver triacylglycerol. *Diabetol* **2011**, *54*, 2506–2514. [CrossRef]

63. Steven, S.; Hollingsworth, K.G.; Al-Mrabeh, A.; Avery, L.; Aribisala, B.; Caslake, M.; Taylor, R. Very low-calorie diet and 6 months of weight stability in type 2 diabetes: Pathophysiological changes in responders and nonresponders. *Diabetes Care* **2016**, *39*, 808–815. [CrossRef]

64. Lean, M.J.; Leslie, W.S.; Barnes, A.C.; Brosnahan, N.; Thom, G.; McCombie, L.; Peters, C.; Zhyzhneuskaya, S.; Al-Mrabeh, A.; Hollingsworth, K.G.; et al. Primary care-led weight management for remission of type 2 diabetes (DiRECT): An open-label, cluster-randomised trial. *Lancet.* **2018**, *391*, 541–551. [CrossRef]

65. Lean, M.E.J.; Leslie, W.S.; Barnes, A.C.; Brosnahan, N.; Thom, G.; McCombie, L.; Peters, C.; Zhyzhneuskaya, S.; Al-Mrabeh, A.; Hollingsworth, K.G.; et al. Durability of a primary care-led weight-management intervention for remission of type 2 diabetes: 2-year results of the DiRECT open-label, cluster-randomised trial. *Lancet Diabetes Endocrinol.* 2019. [CrossRef]

66. McInnes, N.; Smith, A.; Otto, R.; Vandermey, J.; Punthakee, Z.; Sherifali, D.; Balasubramaniam, K.; Hall, S.; Gerstein, HC. Piloting a remission strategy in type 2 diabetes: Results of a randomized controlled trial. *J. Clin. Endocrinol. Metab.* **2017**, *102*, 1596–1605. [CrossRef]

67. Fothergill, E.; Guo, J.; Howard, L.; Kerns, J.C.; Knuth, N.D.; Brychta, R.; Chen, K.Y.; Skarulis, M.C.; Walter, M.; Walter, P.J.; et al. Persistent metabolic adaptation 6 years after "The Biggest Loser" competition. *Obesity* **2016**, *24*, 1612–1619. [CrossRef] [PubMed]

68. Greenway, F.L. Physiological adaptations to weight loss and factors favouring weight regain. *Int. J. Obes.* **2015**, *39*, 1188–1196. [CrossRef]

69. Campbell, W.R. Dietetic treatment in diabetes mellitus. *Can. Med. Assoc. J.* **1923**, *13*, 487–492. [PubMed]

70. Westman, E.C.; Yancy, W.S.; Humphreys, M. Dietary treatment of diabetes mellitus in the pre-insulin era (1914–1922). *Perspect. Biol. Med.* **2006**, *49*, 77–83. [CrossRef]

71. Arky, R.; Wylie-Rosett, J.; El-Beheri, B. Examination of current dietary recommendations for individuals with diabetes mellitus. *Diabetes Care* **1982**, *5*, 59–63. [CrossRef]

72. Anderson, J.W.; Geil, P.B. New perspectives in nutrition management of diabetes mellitus. *Am. J. Med.* **1988**, *85*, 159–165. [CrossRef]

73. American Diabetes Association. Summary of Revisions: Standards of Medical Care in Diabetes-2019. *Diabetes Care* **2019**, *42*, S4–S6.

74. Department of Veteran Affairs and Department of Defense. VA/DoD Clinical Practice Guideline for the Management of Type 2 Diabetes Mellitus in Primary Care. Version 5.0. Available online: https://www.healthquality.va.gov/guidelines/cd/diabetes/ (accessed on 20 January 2019).

75. Westman, E.C.; Feinman, R.D.; Mavropoulos, J.C.; Vernon, M.C.; Volek, J.S.; Wortman, J.A.; Yancy, W.S.; Phinney, S.D. Low carbohydrate nutrition and metabolism. *Am. J. Clin. Nutr.* **2007**, *86*, 276–284. [CrossRef] [PubMed]

76. Stern, L.; Iqbal, N.; Seshadri, P.; Chicano, K.L.; Daily, D.A.; McGrory, J.; Williams, M.; Gracely, E.J.; Samaha, F.F. The effects of low-carbohydrate versus conventional weight loss diets in severely obese adults: One-year follow-up of a randomized trial. *Ann. Intern. Med.* **2004**, *140*, 778–785. [CrossRef]

77. Miyashita, Y.; Koide, N.; Ohtsuka, M.; Ozaki, H.; Itoh, Y.; Oyama, T.; Uetake, T.; Ariga, K.; Shirai, K. Beneficial effect of low carbohydrate in low calorie diets on visceral fat reduction in type 2 diabetic patients with obesity. *Diabetes Res. Clin. Pract.* **2004**, *65*, 235–241. [CrossRef] [PubMed]

78. Jönsson, T.; Granfeldt, Y.; Ahren, B.; Branell, U.C.; Pålsson, G.; Hansson, A.; Söderström, M.; Lindeberg, S. Beneficial effects of a Paleolithic diet on cardiovascular risk factors in type 2 diabetes: A randomized cross-over pilot study. *Cardiovasc. Diabetol.* **2009**, *8*, 3. [CrossRef] [PubMed]

79. Davis, N.J.; Tomuta, N.; Schechter, C.; Isasi, C.R.; Segal-Isaacson, C.J.; Stein, D.; Zonszein, J.; Wylie-Rosett, J. Comparative study of the effects of a 1-year dietary intervention of a low- carbohydrate diet versus a low-fat diet on weight and glycemic control in type 2 diabetes. *Diabetes Care* **2009**, *32*, 1147–1152. [CrossRef]

80. Daly, M.E.; Paisey, R.; Paisey, R.; Millward, B.A.; Eccles, C.; Williams, K.; Hammersley, S.; MacLeod, K.M.; Gale, T.J. Short-term effects of severe dietary carbohydrate-restriction advice in type 2 diabetes: A randomized controlled trial. *Diabet. Med.* **2006**, *23*, 15–20. [CrossRef]

81. Dyson, P.A.; Beatty, S.; Matthews, D.R. A low-carbohydrate diet is more effective in reducing body weight than healthy eating in both diabetic and non-diabetic subjects. *Diabet. Med.* **2007**, *24*, 1430–1435. [CrossRef]

82. Wolever, T.M.; Gibbs, A.L.; Mehling, C.; Chiasson, J.L.; Connelly, P.W.; Josse, R.G.; Leiter, L.A.; Maheux, P.; Rabasa-Lhoret, R.; Rodger, N.W.; et al. The Canadian trial of carbohydrates in diabetes (CCD), a 1-yr controlled of low-glycemic index dietary carbohydrate in type 2 diabetes: No effect on glycated hemoglobin but reduction in C-reactive protein. *Am. J. Clin. Nutr.* **2008**, *87*, 114–125. [CrossRef] [PubMed]

83. Iqbal, N.; Vetter, M.L.; Moore, R.H.; Chittams, J.L.; Dalton-Bakes, C.V.; Dowd, M.; Williams-Smith, C.; Cardillo, S.; Wadden, T.A. Effects of a low-intensity intervention that prescribed a low-carbohydrate vs. a low-fat diet in obese, diabetic participants. *Obesity (Silver Spring)* **2010**, *18*, 1733–1738. [CrossRef] [PubMed]

84. Goday, A.; Bellido, D.; Sajoux, I.; Crujeiras, A.B.; Burguera, B.; García-Luna, P.P.; Casanueva, F.F. Short-term safety, tolerability and efficacy of a very low-calorie ketogenic diet interventional weight loss program versus hypocaloric diet in patients with type 2 diabetes mellitus. *Nutr. Diabetes.* **2016**, *6*, e230. [CrossRef]

85. Saslow, L.R.; Mason, A.E.; Kim, S.; Goldman, V.; Ploutz-Snyder, R.; Bayandorian, H.; Daubenmier, J.; Hecht, F.M.; Moskowitz, J.T. An online intervention comparing a very low-carbohydrate ketogenic diet and lifestyle recommendations versus a plate method diet in overweight individuals with type 2 diabetes: A randomized controlled trial. *J. Med. Int. Res.* **2017**, *19*, e36. [CrossRef] [PubMed]

86. Saslow, L.R.; Daubenmier, J.J.; Moskowitz, J.T.; Kim, S.; Murphy, E.J.; Phinney, S.D.; Ploutz-Snyder, R.; Goldman, V.; Cox, R.M.; Mason, A.E.; et al. Twelve-month outcomes of a randomized trial of a moderate-carbohydrate versus very low-carbohydrate diet in overweight adults with type 2 diabetes mellitus or prediabetes. *Nutr. Diabetes.* **2017**, *7*, 304. [CrossRef]

87. Yamada, Y.; Uchida, J.; Izumi, H.; Tsukamoto, Y.; Inoue, G.; Watanabe, Y.; Irie, J.; Yamada, S. A non-calorie-restricted low-carbohydrate diet is effective as an alternative therapy for patients with type 2 diabetes. *Int. Med.* **2014**, *53*, 13–19. [CrossRef]

88. Guldbrand, H.; Dizdar, B.; Bunjaku, B.; Lindström, T.; Bachrach-Lindström, M.; Fredrikson, M.; Östgren, C.J.; Nystrom, F.H. In type 2 diabetes, randomisation to advice to follow a low-carbohydrate diet transiently improves glycaemic control compared with advice to follow a low-fat diet producing a similar weight loss. *Diabetologi.* **2012**, *55*, 2118–2127. [CrossRef]

89. Westman, E.C.; Yancy, W.S.; Mavropoulos, J.C.; Marquart, M.; McDuffie, J.R. The effect of a low-carbohydrate, ketogenic diet versus a low-glycemic index diet on glycemic control in type 2 diabetes mellitus. *Nutr. Metab.* **2008**, *19*, 36. [CrossRef]

90. Haimoto, H.; Iwata, M.; Wakai, K.; Umegaki, H. Long-term effects of a diet loosely restricting carbohydrates on HbA1c levels, BMI and tapering of sulfonylureas in type 2 diabetes: A 2-year follow-up study. *Diabetes Res. Clin. Pract.* **2008**, *79*, 350–356. [CrossRef] [PubMed]

91. Tay, J.; Thompson, C.H.; Luscombe-Marsh, N.D.; Wycherley, T.P.; Noakes, M.; Buckley, J.D.; Wittert, G.A.; Yancy, W.S., Jr.; Brinkworth, G.D. Effects of an energy-restricted low-carbohydrate, high unsaturated fat/low saturated fat diet versus a high-carbohydrate, low-fat diet in type 2 diabetes: A 2-year randomized clinical trial. *Diabetes Obes. Metab.* **2018**, *20*, 858–871. [CrossRef] [PubMed]

92. Wang, L.L.; Wang, Q.; Hong, Y.; Ojo, O.; Jiang, Q.; Hou, Y.Y.; Huang, Y.-H.; Wang, X.H. The effect of low-carbohydrate diet on glycemic control in patients with type 2 diabetes mellitus. *Nutrients* **2018**, *10*, 661. [CrossRef] [PubMed]

93. Larsen, R.N.; Mann, N.J.; Maclean, E.; Shaw, J.E. The effect of high-protein, low-carbohydrate diets in the treatment of type 2 diabetes: A 12 month randomised controlled trial. *Diabetologia* **2011**, *54*, 731–740. [CrossRef] [PubMed]

94. Sato, J.; Kanazawa, A.; Makita, S.; Hatae, C.; Komiya, K.; Shimizu, T.; Ikeda, F.; Tamura, Y.; Ogihara, T.; Mita, T.; et al. A randomized controlled trial of 130g/day low-carbohydrate diet in type 2 diabetes with poor glycemic control. *Clin. Nutr.* **2017**, *36*, 992–1000. [CrossRef]

95. Sanada, M.; Kabe, C.; Hata, H.; Uchida, J.; Inoue, G.; Tsukamoto, Y.; Yamada, Y.; Irie, J.; Tabata, S.; Tabata, M.; et al. Efficacy of a moderately low carbohydrate diet in a 36-month observational study of Japanese patients with Type 2 diabetes. *Nutrients* **2018**, *10*, 528. [CrossRef] [PubMed]

96. Boden, G.; Sargrad, K.; Homko, C.; Mozzoli, M.; Stein, T.P. Effect of a low carbohydrate diet on appetite, blood glucose levels, and insulin resistance in obese patients with type 2 diabetes. *Ann. Intern. Med.* **2005**, *142*, 403–411. [CrossRef] [PubMed]

97. Gannon, M.C.; Nuttall, F.Q. Effect of a high-protein, low-carbohydrate diet on blood glucose control in people with type 2 diabetes. *Diabetes* **2004**, *53*, 2375–2382. [CrossRef] [PubMed]

98. Hallberg, S.J.; McKenzie, A.L.; Williams, P.T.; Bhanpuri, N.H.; Peters, A.L.; Campbell, W.W.; Hazbun, T.L.; Volk, B.M.; McCarter, J.P.; Phinney, S.D.; et al. Effectiveness and safety of a novel care model for the management of type 2 diabetes at 1 year: An open-label, non-randomized, controlled study. *Diabetes Ther.* **2018**, *9*, 583–612. [CrossRef] [PubMed]

99. Krebs, J.D.; Bell, D.; Hall, R.; Parry-Strong, A.; Docherty, P.D.; Clarke, K.; Chase, J.G. Improvements in glucose metabolism and insulin sensitivity with a low-carbohydrate diet in obese patients with type 2 diabetes. *J. Am. Coll. Nutr.* **2013**, *32*, 11–17. [CrossRef] [PubMed]

100. Hussain, T.A.; Matthew, T.C.; Dashti, A.A.; Asfar, S.; Al-Zaid, N.; Dashti, H.M. Effect of low-calorie versus low-carbohydrate ketogenic diet in type 2 diabetes. *Nutrition* **2012**, *28*, 1016–1021. [CrossRef]

101. Sasakabe, T.; Haimoto, H.; Umegaki, H.; Wakai, K. Effects of a moderate low-carbohydrate diet on preferential abdominal fat loss and cardiovascular risk factors in patients with type 2 diabetes. *Diabetes Metab. Syndr. Obes.* **2011**, *4*, 167–174. [CrossRef] [PubMed]

102. Nielsen, J.V.; Joensson, E.A. Low carbohydrate diet in type 2 diabetes: Stable improvement of bodyweight and glycemic control during 44 months follow-up. *Nutr. Metab.* **2008**, *5*, 14. [CrossRef] [PubMed]

103. Dashti, H.M.; Mathew, T.C.; Khadada, M.; Al-Mousawi, M.; Talib, H.; Asfar, S.K.; Behbahani, A.I.; Al-Zaid, N.S. Beneficial effects of ketogenic diet in obese diabetic subjects. *Mol. Cell Biochem.* **2007**, *302*, 249–256. [CrossRef] [PubMed]

104. Yancy, W.S.; Foy, M.; Chalecki, A.M.; Vernon, A.C.; Westman, E.C. A low carbohydrate, ketogenic diet to treat type 2 diabetes. *Nutr. Metab.* **2005**, *2*, 34. [CrossRef] [PubMed]

105. Dashti, H.M.; Mathew, T.C.; Hussein, T.; Asfar, S.K.; Behbahani, A.; Khoursheed, M.A.; Al-Sayer, H.M.; Bo-Abbas, Y.Y.; Al-Zaid, N.S. Long-term effects of a ketogenic diet in obese patients. *Exp. Clin. Cardiol.* **2004**, *9*, 200–205.

106. Shai, I.; Schwarzfuchs, D.; Henkin, Y.; Shahar, D.R.; Witkow, S.; Greenberg, I.; Golan, R.; Fraser, D.; Bolotin, A.; Vardi, H.; et al. Weight loss with a low-carbohydrate, Mediterranean, or low-fat diet. *N. Engl. J. Med.* **2008**, *359*, 229–241. [CrossRef] [PubMed]

107. Elhayany, A.; Lustman, A.; Abel, R.; Attal-Singer, J.; Vinker, S. A low carbohydrate Mediterranean diet improves cardiovascular risk factors and diabetes control among overweight patients with type 2 diabetes mellitus: A 1-year prospective randomized intervention study. *Diabetes Obes. Metab.* **2010**, *12*, 204–209. [CrossRef]

108. Athinarayanan, S.J.; Adams, R.N.; Hallberg, S.J.; McKenzie, A.L.; Bhanpuri, N.H.; Campbell, W.W.; Volek, J.S.; Phinney, S.D.; McCarter, J.P. Long-term effects of a novel continuous remote care intervention including nutritional ketosis for the management of type 2 diabetes: A 2-year non-randomized clinical trial. *bioRxiv* **2018**, *476275*. [CrossRef]

109. Snorgaard, O.; Poulsen, G.M.; Andersen, H.K.; Astrup, A. Systematic review and meta-analysis of dietary carbohydrate restriction in patients with type 2 diabetes. *BMJ Open Diabetes Res. Care.* **2017**, *5*, e000354. [CrossRef] [PubMed]

110. Bhanpuri, N.H.; Hallberg, S.J.; Williams, P.T.; McKenzie, A.L.; Ballard, K.D.; Campbell, W.W.; McCarter, J.P.; Phinney, S.D.; Volek, J.S. Cardiovascular disease risk factor responses to a type 2 diabetes care model including nutritional ketosis induced by sustained carbohydrate restriction at one year: An open label, non-randomized, controlled study. *Cardiovasc. Diabetol.* **2018**, *17*, 56. [CrossRef]

111. Wang, G.F.; Yan, Y.X.; Yin, D.; Hui, Y.; Zhang, J.P.; Han, G.J.; Ma, N.; Wu, Y.; Xu, J.Z.; Yang, T. Predictive factors of Type 2 diabetes mellitus remission following bariatric surgery: A Meta-analysis. *Obes. Surg.* **2015**, *25*, 199–208. [CrossRef]

112. Yan, W.; Bai, R.; Li, Y.; Xu, J.; Zhong, Z.; Xing, Y.; Yan, M.; Lin, Y.; Song, M. Analysis of predictors of type 2 diabetes mellitus remission after roux-en-Y gastric bypass in 101 Chinese patients. *Obes. Surg.* **2019**. [CrossRef]

113. Brehm, B.J.; Seeley, R.J.; Daniels, S.R.; D'Alessio, D.A. A Randomized Trial Comparing a Very Low Carbohydrate Diet and a Calorie-Restricted Low Fat Diet on Body Weight and Cardiovascular Risk Factors in Healthy Women. *J. Clin. Endocrinol. Metab.* **2003**, *88*, 1617–1623. [CrossRef]

114. Nordmann, A.J.; Nordmann, A.; Briel, M.; Keller, U.; Yancy, W.S.; Brehm, B.J.; Bucher, H.C. Effects of a low-carbohydrate vs. low-fat diets on weight loss and cardiovascular risk factors. *Arch. Intern. Med.* **2006**, *166*, 285–293. [CrossRef] [PubMed]

115. Westman, E.C.; Yancy, W.S.; Edman, J.S.; Tomlin, K.F.; Perkins, CE. Effect of 6-month adherence to a very low carbohydrate diet program. *Am. J. Med.* **2002**, *113*, 30–36. [CrossRef]

116. Nuttall, F.Q.; Gannon, M.C. The metabolic response to a high-protein, low-carbohydrate diet in men with type 2 diabetes mellitus. *Metabolism* **2006**, *55*, 243–251. [CrossRef] [PubMed]

117. Min, T.; Barry, J.D.; Stephens, J.W. Predicting the Resolution of Type 2 Diabetes after Bariatric Surgical Procedures: A Concise Review. *J. Diabetes Metab.* **2015**, *6*, 617.

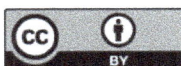

nutrients

MDPI

Article

Cross-Sectional and Longitudinal Association between Glycemic Status and Body Composition in Men: A Population-Based Study

Khaleal Almusaylim, Maggie Minett, Teresa L. Binkley, Tianna M. Beare and Bonny Specker *

EA Martin Program in Human Nutrition, South Dakota State University, SWC, Box 506,
Brookings, SD 57007, USA; khalealabdulha.almusaylim@jacks.sdstate.edu (K.A.);
maggie.minett@sdstate.edu (M.M.); teresa.binkley@sdstate.edu (T.L.B.); tianna.beare@sdstate.edu (T.M.B.)
* Correspondence: Bonny.Specker@sdstate.edu; Tel.: +1-605-688-4661

Received: 29 October 2018; Accepted: 23 November 2018; Published: 3 December 2018

Abstract: This study sought to evaluate the associations between changes in glycemic status and changes in total body (TB), trunk, and appendicular fat (FM) and lean mass (LM) in men. A population-based study of men aged 20–66 years at baseline were included in cross-sectional ($n = 430$) and three-year longitudinal ($n = 411$) analyses. Prediabetes was defined as fasting glucose 100–125 mg/dL. Type 2 diabetes (T2D) was determined by: self-reported diabetes, current anti-diabetic drug use (insulin/oral hypoglycemic agents), fasting glucose ($\geq$126 mg/dL), or non-fasting glucose ($\geq$200 mg/dL). Body composition was evaluated by dual-energy X-ray absorptiometry. Longitudinal analyses showed that changes in TB FM and LM, and appendicular LM differed among glycemic groups. Normoglycemic men who converted to prediabetes lost more TB and appendicular LM than men who remained normoglycemic (all, $p < 0.05$). Normoglycemic or prediabetic men who developed T2D had a greater loss of TB and appendicular LM than men who remained normoglycemic (both, $p < 0.05$). T2D men had greater gains in TB FM and greater losses in TB and appendicular LM than men who remained normoglycemic (all, $p < 0.05$). Dysglycemia is associated with adverse changes in TB and appendicular LM.

Keywords: prediabetes; type 2 diabetes; total body fat; total body lean; appendicular fat; appendicular lean; body composition; cohort study

---

1. Introduction

Prediabetes and type 2 diabetes (T2D) are major public health issues in the United States. The national prevalence of prediabetes and T2D among adults aged $\geq$20 years has increased over time, with the prevalence of prediabetes rising from 26% in 1988–1994 [1] to 37% in 2009–2012 [2]. Recent estimates from the Centers for Disease Control and Prevention indicate that 15–30% of prediabetic cases progress from impaired fasting glucose or impaired glucose tolerance to T2D within five years. There are currently 25.8 million adults in the United States with prediabetes that will develop T2D by 2020, which will double the number of individuals affected by T2D [3]. The prevalence of T2D rose from 7% in 2005 to 12% in 2011 [4], and is projected to increase 165% by 2050 [5].

Case-control and cross-sectional studies have reported inconsistent associations of total body (TB), trunk, and appendicular fat mass (FM) and lean mass (LM) with prediabetes and T2D diabetes in middle-aged and older adults, including a positive association [6], an inverse association [7–10], and no association [6,8,9]. Prospective studies aimed at investigating the relationship between baseline glycemic status and subsequent changes in TB and regional distribution of FM and LM are sparse and inconclusive. Some studies reported differences in body composition measurements among glycemic groups [11–14], but others did not find differences [15,16]. The possible explanation for inconsistent findings includes different durations of follow-up period, sample size, and other covariates that were not adjusted for when investigating the association between various measures of body composition and glycemic status. We found no epidemiological studies that investigated the association between glycemic status (men with prediabetes who revert to normoglycemia, or men who are normoglycemic or prediabetic at baseline and convert to T2D) and changes in the TB and regional distribution of FM and LM.

The objective of the present analysis was to examine the associations between baseline and changes in glycemic status with baseline and changes over three years in TB, trunk, and appendicular FM and LM. The following *a priori* hypotheses were tested: (1) men with prediabetes or T2D at baseline would have higher TB and trunk fat measurements but lower appendicular fat than normoglycemic men; (2) men who were normoglycemic at baseline and developed either prediabetes or T2D would have increases in TB and trunk FM, and decreases in TB and appendicular LM over the three-year study compared with men who remained normoglycemic; (3) among men with prediabetes at baseline, the changes in TB and trunk FM and LM would differ over the three-year study depending on whether they remained prediabetic or developed T2D versus reverting to a normoglycemic state. Those who develop T2D would gain TB FM and lose LM, while those reverting to normoglycemia would lose FM and maintain or gain LM; and (4) men with T2D at baseline would have decreases in TB and trunk LM over the three-year study compared to normoglycemic men.

2. Materials and Methods

2.1. Study Population

The South Dakota Rural Bone Health Study is a population-based longitudinal study designed to investigate the impact of lifestyle factors on bone and body composition. The design and rationale of the study have been described elsewhere [17]. Briefly, adults aged 20 to 66 years, from eight counties in eastern South Dakota, were eligible for enrollment. A total of 1271 participants were recruited between 2001–2004 (baseline), and followed for an average of 3.0 years (range of 2.8 to 3.8 years), and the current analysis was limited to men (*n* = 544). Among those participants, 410 men farmed at least 75% of their lives (rural) and 134 men never lived on an active farm (non-rural). The rural population was divided into Hutterites and non-Hutterites. A Hutterite was defined as a participant of Hutterite descent who resided on a Hutterite colony. Hutterites are an Anabaptist religious group who believe in isolated communal living and self-sufficiency through an agriculturally advanced lifestyle. Non-Hutterites were randomly selected from the eight-county region as described elsewhere [17].

Men with chronic use (> six months) of immunosuppressants, anticonvulsants, or steroids or a diagnosis of type 1 diabetes mellitus at baseline were not eligible for inclusion in the original cohort. For baseline analyses, we excluded men with missing glucose measures at either baseline (*n* = 12) or follow-up (*n* = 34), baseline body composition measurements (*n* = 23), or men who withdrew from the study (*n* = 45) (Figure 1). For follow-up analyses, we further excluded men who did not have body composition measurements at follow-up (*n* = 19). These exclusions led to 430 men in the baseline analyses and 411 in the follow-up analyses. The study was approved by the South Dakota State University Institutional Review Board (IRB#1406004), and informed consent was obtained from all of the participants.

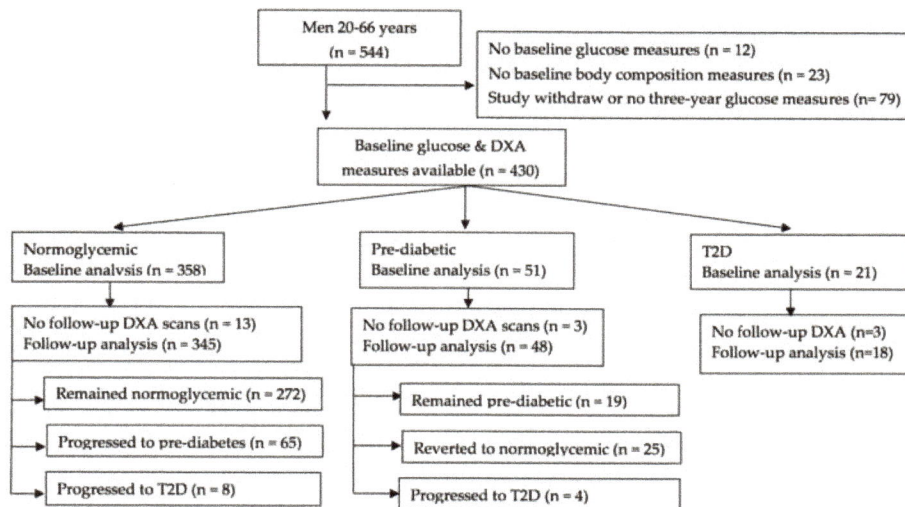

Figure 1. Flowchart of participants. Abbreviations: DXA, dual-energy X-ray absorptiometry; T2D, type 2 diabetic. Individuals who were unable to be categorized into glycemic groups were excluded.

2.2. Assessment of Covariates

Questionnaires were administered at study enrollment and at three years to obtain information on demographic and lifestyle characteristics as well as quarterly physical activity and dietary intake recalls. Information on smoking status and specific details regarding the use of prescription drugs was not collected at baseline; however, an 18-month survey was used to obtain this information. Participants were asked to provide information on types of smoking, such as cigarettes, cigars, and pipes, and were classified as smokers or non-smokers. The presence or absence of hypertension at 18 months was based on self-reported information on the use of antihypertensive medication.

2.2.1. Anthropometric Measures

Body height and weight were measured in lightweight clothes without shoes using a calibrated stadiometer and scale. Standing height was measured to the nearest 0.5 cm in duplicate with a stadiometer (Seca, Chino, CA, USA). A third measurement was taken if the discrepancy between the duplicate height measurements was more than 0.5 cm. Weight was measured to the nearest 0.1 kg with a digital scale (Seca Model 770, Chino, CA, USA).

2.2.2. Physical Activity Assessment

The Paffenbarger Physical Activity Questionnaire (PPAQ) was used to measure the average amount of time spent in sedentary behaviors and different intensity levels of physical activity during the past week [18]. Participants were asked to recall how many hours on their usual weekday and weekend day they spent sleeping, sitting, and engaging in moderate or vigorous intensity activity. Since the time spent in sleeping, sitting, and participating in moderate plus vigorous activity was measured, the remaining time was considered light activity. The PPAQ was administered quarterly over the first three years of the study. To properly report participants' physical activity, trained personnel administered the PPAQ by interview. The average time spent in sitting and moderate-plus-vigorous activity, as well as the average sleeping time, was calculated. The validity and reliability of the PPAQ have been established to measure physical activity intensities in men [19] and rural populations [20].

2.2.3. Dietary Assessment

Dietary intake was assessed using 24-h dietary recalls that were conducted at similar times as the activity recall. Trained interviewers administered 24-h dietary recalls, and dietary recall data were analyzed using Nutritionist Pro software (version 2.3.1, 2004, First DataBank, Inc., San Bruno, CA, USA) to estimate macronutrient and micronutrient intakes. For foods not available in the Nutritionist Pro software, the nutrient composition of the foods was obtained from recipes and entered into the diet analysis software. Activity levels and nutrient intakes at baseline were the averages of the baseline, three-month and six-month recalls, and measures at the 36-month visit were the averages of the 30-month, 33-month, and 36-month recalls.

2.3. Ascertainment of Glycemic Status

According to American Diabetes Association classifications, individuals with a fasting blood glucose of 100 mg/dL to 125 mg/dL were classified as having prediabetes [21]. T2D was determined by one of the following criteria: self-reported T2D, current use of an anti-diabetic drug (insulin or oral hypoglycemic agents), or a fasting blood glucose concentration $\geq$126 mg/dL or a non-fasting blood glucose concentration $\geq$200 mg/dL [21]. The same criteria for the diagnosis of prediabetes and T2D were applied at both the baseline and three-year visits. Attempts were made to obtain fasting blood samples at each visit, and measurements were made in the field from a sample of venous whole blood (with added ethylenediaminetetraacetic acid) using an Accu-Check Advantage glucometer (Roche Diagnostics, Indianapolis, IN, USA).

2.4. Body Composition Measurements

Body composition was assessed using dual-energy x-ray absorptiometry (DXA) (Discovery, Software Version 12.01, Hologic, Waltham, MA, USA). A TB scan was completed with boundaries for the various anatomical regions set according to manufacturer's specifications. The step phantom scan for body composition calibration was completed weekly as suggested by the manufacturer. Prior to DXA measurements, the Hologic spine phantom was scanned for quality control. All of the scans were analyzed by the same technician who was certified by the International Society of Clinical Densitometry. Scan results were deleted for obese participants with an equivalent epoxy thickness greater than 12 inches, as determined by the Hologic software, per manufacturer recommendations ($n = 16$ men: $n =$ seven Hutterite, $n =$ four rural, $n =$ five non-rural). DXA-derived measurements of TB, trunk and appendicular FM and LM were expressed in kilograms. Our coefficients of variation for TB FM and LM assessed in 15 adults (one male) using triplicate scans with repositioning between each scan are <1.5%.

2.5. Statistical Analysis

All of the continuous variables were tested for normality before performing the analyses. Analysis of variance adjusting for multiple comparisons for continuous variables and a Fisher's exact test for categorical variables were used to determine statistical significance in baseline characteristics among the glycemic categories. The annual absolute change in each body composition measure was calculated as the follow-up value minus baseline value divided by length of follow-up in years.

Multiple regression models were used to estimate marginal means $\pm$ standard error of the mean (sem) for baseline body composition parameters and changes in outcome measures by different categories of glycemic status. Differences in marginal means among glycemic groups were evaluated using post hoc contrast tests based on the hypotheses. A priori determined covariates (age at baseline, height, population group, percent time in moderate-plus-vigorous activity, and total daily caloric intake) were included in all of the models, since they were found to be associated with at least one body composition measure. The multiple regression models that were used for baseline analyses included these covariates, and the FM model included the LM of the same compartment (TB, trunk, or appendicular), and the LM model included covariates plus the FM of the same compartment. Multiple regression models for the longitudinal analyses were adjusted for the same covariates, as well as changes in percent time in moderate-plus-vigorous activity and total daily caloric intake between baseline and three-year follow-up, baseline measure of the specific body compartment (TB, trunk, or appendicular), and baseline and annual changes in the FM or LM of same compartment. Due to issues with multicollinearity and the problem of body composition measures being components of both body mass index (BMI) and weight, neither BMI nor weight was included as covariates. The assumptions of linearity, normality, and homoscedasticity were evaluated visually to ensure no violation of assumptions. All of the analyses were performed using JMP software (version 13, SAS Institute, Cary, NC, USA), and the statistical significance level was set at $p < 0.05$ (two-tailed).

3. Results

3.1. Subject Characteristics

At the baseline visit, 358 (83.2%) of the men were normoglycemic, 51 (11.9%) were prediabetic based on fasting glucose concentrations, and 21 (4.9%) had T2D (14 self-reported a medical diagnosis, six based on fasting glucose, and one based on non-fasting glucose). Of the 345 men who were normoglycemic at baseline and for whom glucose and body composition measurements were available at three years, 272 (78.9%) remained normoglycemic, 65 (18.8%) progressed to prediabetes, and eight (2.3%) progressed to T2D (five based on fasting glucose, one based on non-fasting glucose, one self-reported a medical diagnosis, and one taking anti-diabetic medication). Among the 48 prediabetic men, 19 (39.6%) remained prediabetic, 25 (52.1%) reverted to normoglycemic, and four (8.3%) progressed to T2D based on fasting glucose concentrations. Of the 18 T2D men who were diabetic throughout the study, four (22.2%) self-reported a medical diagnosis, 11 (61.1%) were taking anti-diabetic medication, and three (16.7%) had T2D based on fasting glucose concentrations.

Participant characteristics by glycemic categories at baseline and follow-up are summarized in Tables 1 and 2. The mean age (+ sem) was 42.7 ± 0.6 years (range: 20 to 66 years), and men with T2D at baseline were older than those who were normoglycemic. The study population was 37.4% Hutterite, 37.2% rural non-Hutterite, and 25.4% non-rural. Hutterites and married men had a higher prevalence of prediabetes and T2D than non-Hutterites and single men. Men with prediabetes weighed more than normoglycemic men. A higher percentage of prediabetic and T2D men were taking antihypertensive medication than normoglycemic men, and carbohydrate intake was greater in normoglycemic men than in prediabetic and T2D men. At follow-up, men with T2D had lower caloric and carbohydrate intake than men who remained normoglycemic throughout the study or men who were normoglycemic and developed prediabetes (Table 2). Prediabetic men who remained prediabetic at three years increased their carbohydrate intake, and men who remained normoglycemic throughout the study increased their weight, time spent in moderate-plus-vigorous activity, and average daily fat intake. The overall mean changes over the three-year study in percent time in moderate-plus-vigorous activity and average dietary intake of calories, carbohydrates, fat, and protein were not significant (mean changes were 0.6 ± 0.4%, 10 ± 28 kcal, 1.0 ± 3.8 g, 3.0 ± 1.6 g, and 0.0 ± 1.5 g, respectively), and changes in caloric and macronutrient intakes did not differ by glycemic categories (data not shown).

Table 1. Baseline characteristics of the 430 men from the South Dakota Rural Bone Health Study cohort. NH: non-Hutterite.

	Normoglycemic	Prediabetic	T2D	p-Value [1]
Participants (n)	358	51	21	
Demographics				
Age (years)	41.6 ± 0.6 [a]	45.8 ± 1.7	53.0 ± 2.6 [a]	<0.001
Population Group (%)				0.001
Hutterite (n = 161)	73.3	18.0	8.7	
NH Rural (n = 160)	89.3	8.8	1.9	
NH Non-rural (n = 109)	89.0	7.3	3.7	
Ever Married (%)	81.3	92.2	95.2	0.06
Anthropometrics				
Height (cm)	177.9 ± 0.4	177.9 ± 0.9	174.3 ± 1.5	0.06
Weight (kg)	91.1 ± 0.8 [a]	98.5 ± 2.1 [a]	95.9 ± 3.3	0.003
Lifestyle Variables				
Smokers (%)	33.2	24.0	38.1	0.43
BP Meds (%)	8.7	23.5	47.6	<0.001
% Time in MVPA [2]	21.8 ± 0.5	23.1 ± 1.4	19.3 ± 2.1	0.32
Daily Macronutrient Intake [2]				
Total energy (kcal)	2373 ± 33	2218 ± 87	2060 ± 135	0.03 [3]
Carbohydrate (g)	265 ± 5 [ab]	224 ± 12 [b]	202 ± 19 [a]	<0.001
Fat (g)	97 ± 2	98 ± 4	90 ± 7	0.55
Protein (g)	105 ± 2	102 ± 4	102 ± 7	0.80

Values are means $\pm$ sem or n (percentages). [1] Significance based on ANOVA for continuous variables and Fisher's exact test for categorical variables; means with similar superscripts are different using a *post hoc* Tukey test. [2] Physical activity levels and nutrient intakes at baseline were the average of the baseline, 3-and 6-month recalls. [3] No means differed by post-hoc Tukey test for multiple comparisons. Abbreviations: T2D, type 2 diabetic; NH, non-Hutterite; BP Meds, hypertensive medications; MVPA, moderate-plus-vigorous physical activity.

Table 2. Anthropometrics, activity levels, and diet intake of the 411 men from the South Dakota Rural Bone Health Study cohort, according to glycemic categories after three years of follow-up.

Baseline:	Normoglycemic		Prediabetic		Normoglycemic or Prediabetic	T2D	
Follow-Up:	Normoglycemic	Prediabetic	Normoglycemic	Prediabetic	T2D	T2D	p-Value [1]
Participants (n)	272	65	25	19	12	18	
Baseline Age (years)	41.0 ± 0.7 [ab]	42.6 ± 1.5 [c]	43.9 ± 2.6	47.1 ± 2.3	51.9 ± 2.3 [b]	53.0 ± 2.2 [ac]	<0.001
Baseline Height (cm)	177.9 ± 0.4	177.0 ± 0.8	179.4 ± 1.0	176.9 ± 2.0	175.3 ± 1.7	175.1 ± 1.7	0.17
Weight (kg)							
Baseline	90.3 ± 0.9 ‡	92.5 ± 2.0	96.1 ± 3.3	98.8 ± 3.9	100.4 ± 4.1	96.0 ± 3.1	0.01 [3]
Follow-Up	91.5 ± 0.9	93.3 ± 2.0	95.2 ± 3.4	100.1 ± 4.3	98.3 ± 4.0	96.0 ± 3.3	0.08
% Time MVPA [2]							
Baseline	21.0 ± 0.6 ‡	23.7 ± 1.2	22.6 ± 1.7	24.4 ± 2.3	26.2 ± 3.0	19.8 ± 2.1	0.11
Follow-Up	22.5 ± 0.6	22.1 ± 1.1	19.9 ± 1.6	21.9 ± 2.1	24.5 ± 2.5	22.8 ± 2.4	0.77
Daily Intake [2]							
Total Energy (kcal)							
Baseline	2344 ± 38	2435 ± 75	2284 ± 130	2140 ± 106	2248 ± 183	2067 ± 108	0.18
Follow-Up	2382 ± 38 [a]	2386 ± 81 [b]	2268 ± 102	2211 ± 95	2176 ± 189	1898 ± 132 [ab]	0.02
Carbohydrate (g)							
Baseline	263 ± 5 [a]	268 ± 11	239 ± 17	208 ± 14 ‡	233 ± 21	204 ± 15 [a]	0.003
Follow-Up	265 ± 5 [a]	267 ± 13 [b]	248 ± 16	232 ± 14	208 ± 19	186 ± 16 [ab]	0.001
Fat (g)							
Baseline	95 ± 2	102 ± 4	101 ± 7	94 ± 6	94 ± 10	91 ± 8	0.57
Follow-Up	101 ± 2 ‡	100 ± 3	95 ± 5	98 ± 6	99 ± 11	90 ± 8	0.75
Protein (g)							
Baseline	103 ± 2	107 ± 4	105 ± 7	96 ± 5	101 ± 11	101 ± 6	0.79
Follow-Up	104 ± 2	106 ± 3	105 ± 5	98 ± 5	107 ± 11	93 ± 8	0.50

Values are unadjusted means ± sem or *n* (percentages). ‡ Significant change from baseline to follow-up based on paired *t*-test. [1] Significance among glycemic categories based on ANOVA for continuous variables and Fisher's exact test for categorical variables; means with similar superscripts are different using a post hoc Tukey test. [2] Physical activity (PA) levels and nutrient intakes at baseline were the averages of the baseline, three-month, and six-month recalls, and at follow-up were the averages of 30-month, 33-month, and 36-month recalls. [3] No means differed by post hoc Tukey test for multiple comparisons. Abbreviations: T2D, type 2 diabetic; MVPA, moderate-plus-vigorous physical activity.

3.2. Cross-Sectional Assessment of Baseline Body Composition in Men with Prediabetes or Type 2 Diabetes

There were no differences in TB, trunk, or appendicular FM or LM among the three glycemic groups at baseline when covariates were included in the analyses (Table 3). Prediabetic men weighed more than normoglycemic men.

Table 3. Total body and regional body composition in the 430 men from the South Dakota Rural Bone Health Study cohort, according to glycemic status at baseline.

	Normoglycemic	Prediabetic	T2D	*p*-Value [1]
Participants (*n*)	358	51	21	
Body Weight (kg)				
Unadjusted Model	91.1 ± 0.8 [a]	98.5 ± 2.1 [a]	95.9 ± 3.3	0.003
Basic Model [2]	91.0 ± 0.8 [a]	97.0 ± 3.2 [a]	95.9 ± 3.2	0.01
Fat Mass (kg)				
Total Body				
Unadjusted Model	22.1 ± 0.5 [ab]	26.4 ± 1.2 [b]	26.7 ± 1.9 [a]	0.001
Full Model [3]	22.6 ± 0.3	24.0 ± 0.9	23.3 ± 1.5	0.38
Trunk				
Unadjusted Model	11.4 ± 0.3 [ab]	14.2 ± 0.8 [b]	15.1 ± 1.2 [a]	<0.001
Full Model [3]	11.8 ± 0.2	12.6 ± 0.5	11.8 ± 0.9	0.38
Appendicular				
Unadjusted Model	9.6 ± 0.2 [a]	11.1 ± 0.5 [a]	10.4 ± 0.8	0.01
Full Model [3]	9.7 ± 0.2	10.3 ± 0.4	10.1 ± 0.7	0.66
Lean Mass (kg)				
Total Body				
Unadjusted Model	67.0 ± 0.4	69.9 ± 1.2	66.8 ± 1.8	0.07
Full Model [4]	67.1 ± 0.3	67.9 ± 0.8	67.9 ± 1.2	0.56
Trunk				
Unadjusted Model	32.7 ± 0.2 [a]	34.5 ± 0.6 [a]	34.1 ± 0.9	0.01
Full Model [4]	32.7 ± 0.1	33.1 ± 0.4	33.8 ± 0.6	0.24
Appendicular				
Unadjusted Model	30.5 ± 0.2	31.6 ± 0.6 [a]	28.9 ± 0.9 [a]	0.04
Full Model [4]	30.5 ± 0.2	31.0 ± 0.4	30.3 ± 0.7	0.44

Data are means and marginal means ± sem. [1] *p*-values are from multiple regression models. Means with similar superscripts are different using a post hoc contrast test. [2] Basic model adjusted for age, height, population group, percent time in moderate-plus-vigorous activity, and average daily calories. [3] Fat mass models included covariates in basic model plus lean mass of same compartment (total body, trunk, or appendicular). [4] Lean mass models included covariates in basic model plus fat mass of same compartment. Abbreviations: T2D, type 2 diabetic.

3.3. Association between Development of Prediabetes and Type 2 Diabetes and Changes in Body Composition

Changes in body composition for the six glycemic groups are shown in Figures 2 and 3. There were differences among men who developed prediabetes or T2D and men who remained normoglycemic regarding the annual change in TB and appendicular LM. Among men who were normoglycemic at baseline, those who progressed to prediabetic lost more TB and appendicular LM than those who remained normoglycemic (Figure 3). Normoglycemic or prediabetic men who developed T2D also had greater losses in TB and appendicular LM than men who remained normoglycemic (Figure 3).

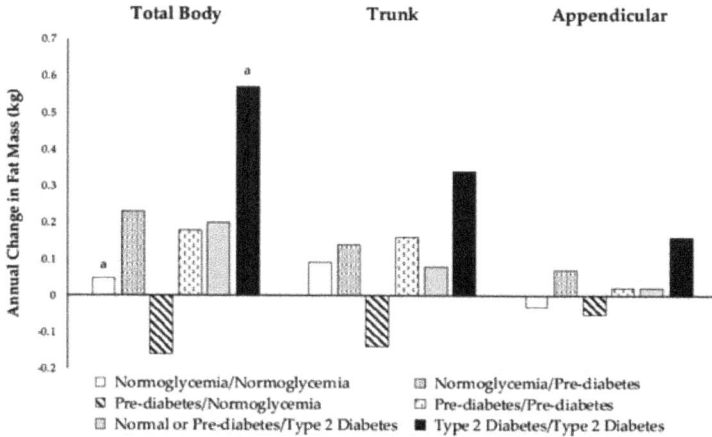

Figure 2. Adjusted marginal means of annual change from baseline in total body (*p* = 0.02), trunk (*p* = 0.06), and appendicular (*p* = 0.06) fat mass according to categories of glycemic status during the three-year follow-up. Model included baseline age, height, population group, percent time in moderate-plus-vigorous activity, average caloric intake, baseline measures of fat and lean mass in the specific body compartment (total body, trunk, or appendicular), changes in percent time in moderate-plus-vigorous activity and average caloric intake, and annual change in lean mass of the same compartment. Means with similar superscripts are different using post hoc contrast tests based on hypotheses.

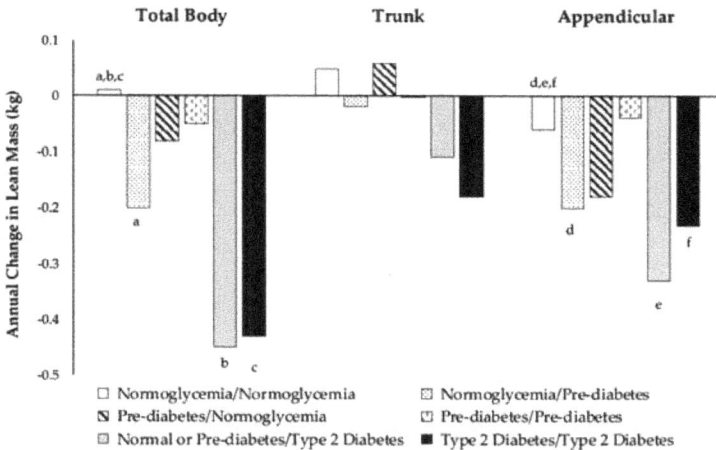

Figure 3. Adjusted marginal means of annual change from baseline in total body (*p* = 0.004), trunk (*p* = 0.24), and appendicular (*p* < 0.001) lean mass according to categories of glycemic status during the three-year follow-up. Model included baseline age, height, population group, percent time in moderate-plus-vigorous activity, average caloric intake, baseline measures of fat and lean mass in the specific body compartment (total body, trunk, or appendicular), changes in percent time in moderate-plus-vigorous activity and average caloric intake, and annual change in the fat mass of the same compartment. Means with similar superscripts are different using post hoc contrast tests based on hypotheses.

3.4. Changes in Body Composition among Prediabetic Men Depending on Reversion to Normoglycemia

There were no differences in the FM or LM between prediabetic men who remained prediabetic and those that reverted to normoglycemia (Figures 2 and 3). In general, prediabetic men who reverted to normoglycemia had negative changes in FM, whereas men who remained prediabetic had positive changes.

3.5. Changes in Body Composition among Type 2 Diabetic Men

Men who were T2D at baseline had greater gains in TB FM (Figure 2) and greater losses in TB and appendicular LM (Figure 3) than men who remained normoglycemic over the three-year follow-up.

4. Discussion

This is the first prospective population-based cohort study investigating the association of baseline glycemic status and changes in glycemic status over time with changes in TB, trunk, and appendicular FM and LM. Consequently, the findings of prior observational longitudinal studies cannot be compared to our findings. The findings of the current study indicate that there were no baseline differences among glycemic groups in TB, trunk, or appendicular FM and LM. Normoglycemic men who developed prediabetes or T2D had greater losses in TB and appendicular LM than men who remained normoglycemic. Men who had T2D throughout the study period had greater gains in TB FM, and greater losses in TB and appendicular LM, than men who were normoglycemic throughout the study. No differences were observed in changes in weight or body composition measures among prediabetic men who reverted to normoglycemia compared to those who remained prediabetic.

Contrary to our first hypothesis, we did not find differences in TB and regional FM and LM at baseline among the glycemic groups. The present study differs from other studies [6–8,10,22,23] due to the adjustment for covariates and inclusion of other body composition compartments (e.g., when determining whether TB FM was associated with glycemic status, TB LM was included in the statistical model). The inclusion of these covariates resulted in the relationships becoming non-significant.

Consistent with our hypothesis, normoglycemic men who developed prediabetes or T2D had greater losses in TB and appendicular LM than men who remained normoglycemic, but we found no association with changes in FM. A positive association between glucose concentrations and intermuscular adipose tissue has been reported [24], and it has been suggested that hyperglycemia stimulates the differentiation of mesenchymal stem cells derived from adipose and muscle tissues into adipocytes by activating the protein kinase C β pathway [25]. Other studies also have reported an association between hyperglycemia and reduced TB and appendicular LM in men [10]. The underlying mechanisms of the decline in LM may include elevated circulating concentrations of inflammatory markers and oxidative stress. Biomarkers of inflammation, tumor necrosis factor alpha, and C-reactive protein stimulate the loss of skeletal muscle through the activation of nuclear factor kappa B [26] and the inhibition of protein synthesis [27]. Oxidative stress contributes to a catabolic and anabolic imbalance in skeletal muscle, mitochondrial damage, and muscle atrophy and apoptosis [28]. These findings indicate that elevated inflammation markers in the presence of oxidative stress in prediabetic and T2D men can induce the loss of TB and appendicular LM. The present findings from the study support these reports.

The association of changes in prediabetes status over time with changes in body composition by compartments have not been previously investigated. A few prospective studies have examined changes in TB and appendicular FM and LM in prediabetic individuals compared to normoglycemic controls. Our findings are similar to other studies reporting no difference in longitudinal changes in TB and lower extremity LM between individuals with and without prediabetes [14,16,29]. On the contrary, others have reported a loss in TB FM and appendicular LM that was greater in prediabetics compared to their normoglycemic counterparts [14,29].

In addition to greater gains in TB FM among men with T2D than among normoglycemic men, we found a significant loss in TB and appendicular LM among men who either had T2D at baseline or developed T2D during the study compared to men who remained normoglycemic. By contrast, Park et al. [15] reported no differences in longitudinal changes in TB and appendicular FM and LM between older adults with normoglycemia and those diagnosed T2D. Our findings are consistent with longitudinal studies that have found T2D men gained TB FM and lost TB and appendicular LM [12–14]. The mechanism for fat gain and muscle loss may stem from insulin resistance in T2D. An excessive influx of free fatty acids into the systemic circulation resulting from the adipose tissue contributes to insulin resistance by increasing fat accumulation in the liver leading to decreased insulin clearance, and increasing fat accumulation in skeletal muscle by impairing glucose transport, decreasing muscle protein synthesis, and inducing muscle protein breakdown, leading to a reduced muscle surface area and insulin signaling [30,31].

The strengths of our study include the first prospective population-based study of the association between changes in glycemic status and changes in TB and regional body composition measured by DXA, our low dropout rate, and our statistical adjustment for the same body composition compartments. Our study has several limitations. The present study included predominantly white men, and our findings may not be generalizable to women or other races. The majority of the men were farmers who may have different activity patterns and dietary intake than non-farmers, which may influence the relationship between dysglycemia and body composition. However, a study conducted on a representative sample of the United States (U.S.) population reported a similar association between dysglycemia and reduced lean mass [10]. Another limitation is the sample size of some of the glycemic categories. We did not observe differences between those men who were prediabetic at baseline and remained prediabetic, or reverted to normoglycemia as we hypothesized. It is likely that our sample size (n = 19 and 25, respectively) was too small. Based on the observed means and standard deviations in changes in TB FM, we estimate that 72 men per group would be needed (α = 0.05, β = 0.20). Despite the small sample size in some categories, we did observe other differences that we hypothesized, including differences in changes in TB and appendicular LM between normoglycemic men who developed prediabetes or T2D and those who remained normoglycemic throughout the study. We relied on participants' recall of diagnosis of T2D, antidiabetic medication usage, dietary intake, and physical activity. A self-reported diagnosis of T2D or the use of antidiabetic medication can lead to misclassification due to recall or reporting errors. Dietary and physical activity recalls may result in overestimation or underestimation. However, dietary intake and physical activity assessments were performed quarterly to consider seasonality. The 24-h diet recall [32] and PPAQ [19] are valid measures of dietary intake and physical activity in adults. Although this was a longitudinal study, given the period of time between measurements (three years), it is not possible to determine whether changes in glycemic status preceded changes in body composition or vice versa. Future studies should be over longer periods of time with more frequent measures of glycemic status and body composition in order to determine which factor comes first: dysglycemia or body composition changes. Only one fasting or non-fasting blood glucose measurement per visit was obtained for defining prediabetes and T2D. Although the American Diabetes Association recommends different criteria for screening for prediabetes and T2D using glycated hemoglobin, fasting blood glucose, and two-hour plasma glucose after an oral glucose tolerance test [21], numerous studies have reported that using two-hour plasma glucose test detects more cases of prediabetes and diabetes than using glycated hemoglobin or a fasting blood glucose test [33–38]; thus, we might have missed men with prediabetes and T2D using only one fasting blood glucose measurement, which would have made it more difficult to identify group differences in changes in body composition.

5. Conclusions

In conclusion, (1) there were no differences among glycemic groups in baseline TB and regional distribution of FM and LM; (2) men who were normoglycemic at baseline and developed prediabetes or

T2D had greater losses in TB and appendicular LM than men who remained normoglycemic; (3) there were no differences in changes in body weight or composition among men who were prediabetic at baseline and remained prediabetic compared to those who reverted back to normoglycemia; and (4) men who had T2D at baseline had greater gains in TB FM and greater losses in TB and appendicular LM than normoglycemic men. These findings add to a growing body of literature on the associations between changes in glycemic status and body composition.

Author Contributions: Conceptualization, K.A. and B.S.; Data curation, M.M., T.L.B., T.M.B. and B.S.; Formal analysis, K.A. and B.S.; Funding acquisition, B.S.; Investigation, M.M., T.L.B., T.M.B. and B.S.; Methodology, T.L.B. and B.S.; Project administration, M.M., T.L.B., T.M.B. and B.S.; Resources, B.S.; Software, T.L.B., T.M.B. and B.S.; Supervision, M.M., T.L.B., T.M.B. and B.S.; Validation, M.M. and T.L.B.; Visualization, K.A. and B.S.; Writing—original draft, K.A. and B.S.; Writing—review & editing, M.M., T.L.B., T.M.B. and B.S. All authors read and approved the final manuscript.

Funding: This research was funded in part by a grant from the National Institutes of Health (R01-AR47852) and the Ethel Austin Martin Endowment at South Dakota State University.

Acknowledgments: We would like to acknowledge the willingness and time the participants contributed to this research.

Conflicts of Interest: The authors declare no conflict of interest.

References

1. Cowie, C.C.; Rust, K.F.; Ford, E.S.; Eberhardt, M.S.; Byrd-Holt, D.D.; Li, C.; Williams, D.E.; Gregg, E.W.; Bainbridge, K.E.; Saydah, S.H. Full accounting of diabetes and pre-diabetes in the US population in 1988–1994 and 2005–2006. *Diabetes Care* **2009**, *32*, 287–294. [CrossRef] [PubMed]
2. Centers for Disease Control and Prevention. *National Diabetes Statistics Report: Estimates of Diabetes and its Burden in the United States, 2014*; US Department of Health and Human Services: Atlanta, GA, USA, 2014.
3. Centers for Disease Control and Prevention. Prediabetes: Could It Be You? Available online: http://www.cdc.gov/diabetes/pubs/images/prediabetes-inforgraphic.jpg (accessed on 12 July 2017).
4. O'Brien, M.J.; Whitaker, R.C.; Yu, D.; Ackermann, R.T. The comparative efficacy of lifestyle intervention and metformin by educational attainment in the Diabetes Prevention Program. *Prev. Med.* **2015**, *77*, 125–130. [CrossRef] [PubMed]
5. Steeves, J.A.; Murphy, R.A.; Crainiceanu, C.M.; Zipunnikov, V.; Van Domelen, D.R.; Harris, T.B. Daily patterns of physical activity by type 2 diabetes definition: Comparing diabetes, prediabetes, and participants with normal glucose levels in nhanes 2003–2006. *Prev. Med. Rep.* **2015**, *2*, 152–157. [CrossRef] [PubMed]
6. Rabijewski, M.; Papierska, L.; Piątkiewicz, P. The relationships between anabolic hormones and body composition in middle-aged and elderly men with prediabetes: A cross-sectional study. *J. Diabetes Res.* **2016**, *2016*. [CrossRef] [PubMed]
7. Heshka, S.; Ruggiero, A.; Bray, G.A.; Foreyt, J.; Kahn, S.E.; Lewis, C.E.; Saad, M.; Schwartz, A.V. Altered body composition in type 2 diabetes mellitus. *Int. J. Obes. (Lond.)* **2008**, *32*, 780–787. [CrossRef] [PubMed]
8. Azuma, K.; Heilbronn, L.K.; Albu, J.B.; Smith, S.R.; Ravussin, E.; Kelley, D.E. Adipose tissue distribution in relation to insulin resistance in type 2 diabetes mellitus. *Am. J. Physiol. Endocrinol. Metab.* **2007**, *293*, E435–E442. [CrossRef] [PubMed]
9. Leenders, M.; Verdijk, L.B.; van der Hoeven, L.; Adam, J.J.; van Kranenburg, J.; Nilwik, R.; van Loon, L.J. Patients with type 2 diabetes show a greater decline in muscle mass, muscle strength, and functional capacity with aging. *J. Am. Med. Dir. Assoc.* **2013**, *14*, 585–592. [CrossRef] [PubMed]
10. Kalyani, R.R.; Tra, Y.; Egan, J.; Ferrucci, L.; Brancati, F. Hyperglycemia is associated with relatively lower lean body mass in older adults. *J. Nutr. Health Aging* **2014**, *18*, 737–743. [CrossRef] [PubMed]
11. Lee, C.G.; Boyko, E.J.; Strotmeyer, E.S.; Lewis, C.E.; Cawthon, P.M.; Hoffman, A.R.; Everson-Rose, S.A.; Barrett-Connor, E.; Orwoll, E.S. Association between insulin resistance and lean mass loss and fat mass gain in older men without diabetes mellitus. *J. Am. Geriatr. Soc.* **2011**, *59*, 1217–1224. [CrossRef] [PubMed]
12. Pownall, H.J.; Bray, G.A.; Wagenknecht, L.E.; Walkup, M.P.; Heshka, S.; Hubbard, V.S.; Hill, J.; Kahn, S.E.; Nathan, D.M.; Schwartz, A.V. Changes in body composition over 8 years in a randomized trial of a lifestyle intervention: The Look Ahead Study. *Obesity* **2015**, *23*, 565–572. [CrossRef] [PubMed]

13. Pownall, H.J.; Schwartz, A.V.; Bray, G.A.; Berkowitz, R.I.; Lewis, C.E.; Boyko, E.J.; Jakicic, J.M.; Chen, H.; Heshka, S.; Gregg, E.W. Changes in regional body composition over 8 years in a randomized lifestyle trial: The Look Ahead Study. *Obesity* **2016**, *24*, 1899–1905. [CrossRef] [PubMed]

14. Lee, C.G.; Boyko, E.J.; Barrett-Connor, E.; Miljkovic, I.; Hoffman, A.R.; Everson-Rose, S.A.; Lewis, C.E.; Cawthon, P.M.; Strotmeyer, E.S.; Orwoll, E.S. Insulin sensitizers may attenuate lean mass loss in older men with diabetes. *Diabetes Care* **2011**, *34*, 2381–2386. [CrossRef] [PubMed]

15. Park, S.W.; Goodpaster, B.H.; Lee, J.S.; Kuller, L.H.; Boudreau, R.; De Rekeneire, N.; Harris, T.B.; Kritchevsky, S.; Tylavsky, F.A.; Nevitt, M. Excessive loss of skeletal muscle mass in older adults with type 2 diabetes. *Diabetes Care* **2009**, *32*, 1993–1997. [CrossRef] [PubMed]

16. Kalyani, R.R.; Metter, E.J.; Egan, J.; Golden, S.H.; Ferrucci, L. Hyperglycemia predicts persistently lower muscle strength with aging. *Diabetes Care* **2015**, *38*, 82–90. [CrossRef] [PubMed]

17. Specker, B.; Binkley, T.; Fahrenwald, N. Rural versus nonrural differences in BMC, volumetric BMD, and bone size: A population-based cross-sectional study. *Bone* **2004**, *35*, 1389–1398. [CrossRef] [PubMed]

18. Paffenbarger, R.S.; Wing, A.L.; Hyde, R.T. Physical activity as an index of heart attack risk in college alumni. *Am. J. Epidemiol.* **1978**, *108*, 161–175. [CrossRef] [PubMed]

19. Simpson, K.; Parker, B.; Capizzi, J.; Thompson, P.; Clarkson, P.; Freedson, P.; Pescatello, L.S. Validity and reliability question 8 of the Paffenbarger physical activity questionnaire among healthy adults. *J. Phys. Act. Health* **2015**, *12*, 116–123. [CrossRef] [PubMed]

20. Samra, H.A.; Beare, T.; Specker, B. Pedometer readings and self-reported walking distances in a rural Hutterite population. *J. Rural Health* **2008**, *24*, 99–100. [CrossRef] [PubMed]

21. American Diabetes Association. Classification and diagnosis of diabetes. Sec. 2. In standards of medical care in diabetes—2015. *Diabetes Care* **2015**, *38*, S8–S16.

22. Kim, T.N.; Park, M.S.; Yang, S.J.; Yoo, H.J.; Kang, H.J.; Song, W.; Seo, J.A.; Kim, S.G.; Kim, N.H.; Baik, S.H. Prevalence and determinant factors of sarcopenia in patients with type 2 diabetes: The Korean Sarcopenic Obesity Study (KSOS). *Diabetes Care* **2010**, *33*, 1497–1499. [CrossRef] [PubMed]

23. Julian, V.; Blondel, R.; Pereira, B.; Thivel, D.; Boirie, Y.; Duclos, M. Body composition is altered in pre-diabetic patients with impaired fasting glucose tolerance: Results from the NHANES survey. *J. Clin. Med. Res.* **2017**, *9*, 917–925. [CrossRef] [PubMed]

24. Yim, J.; Heshka, S.; Albu, J.; Heymsfield, S.; Kuznia, P.; Harris, T.; Gallagher, D. Intermuscular adipose tissue rivals visceral adipose tissue in independent associations with cardiovascular risk. *Int. J. Obes. (Lond.)* **2007**, *31*, 1400–1405. [CrossRef] [PubMed]

25. Aguiari, P.; Leo, S.; Zavan, B.; Vindigni, V.; Rimessi, A.; Bianchi, K.; Franzin, C.; Cortivo, R.; Rossato, M.; Vettor, R. High glucose induces adipogenic differentiation of muscle-derived stem cells. *Proc. Natl. Acad. Sci. USA* **2008**, *105*, 1226–1231. [CrossRef] [PubMed]

26. Li, Y.-P.; Reid, M.B. Nf-κb mediates the protein loss induced by TNF-α in differentiated skeletal muscle myotubes. *Am. J. Physiol. Regul. Integr. Comp. Physiol.* **2000**, *279*, R1165–R1170. [CrossRef] [PubMed]

27. Wåhlin-Larsson, B.; Wilkinson, D.J.; Strandberg, E.; Hosford-Donovan, A.; Atherton, P.J.; Kadi, F. Mechanistic links underlying the impact of c-reactive protein on muscle mass in elderly. *Cell Physiol. Biochem.* **2017**, *44*, 267–278. [CrossRef] [PubMed]

28. Bianchi, L.; Volpato, S. Muscle dysfunction in type 2 diabetes: A major threat to patient's mobility and independence. *Acta Diabetol.* **2016**, *53*, 879–889. [CrossRef] [PubMed]

29. Piaggi, P.; Thearle, M.S.; Bogardus, C.; Krakoff, J. Fasting hyperglycemia predicts lower rates of weight gain by increased energy expenditure and fat oxidation rate. *J. Clin. Endocrinol. Metab.* **2015**, *100*, 1078–1087. [CrossRef] [PubMed]

30. Frayn, K.N. Visceral fat and insulin resistance—causative or correlative? *Br. J. Nutr.* **2000**, *83*, S71–S77. [CrossRef] [PubMed]

31. Brøns, C.; Grunnet, L.G. Mechanisms in endocrinology: Skeletal muscle lipotoxicity in insulin resistance and type 2 diabetes: A causal mechanism or an innocent bystander? *Eur. J. Endocrinol.* **2017**, *176*, R67–R78. [CrossRef] [PubMed]

32. Conway, J.M.; Ingwersen, L.A.; Moshfegh, A.J. Accuracy of dietary recall using the USDA five-step multiple-pass method in men: An observational validation study. *J. Am. Diet. Assoc.* **2004**, *104*, 595–603. [CrossRef] [PubMed]

33. Menke, A.; Casagrande, S.; Geiss, L.; Cowie, C.C. Prevalence of and trends in diabetes among adults in the United States, 1988–2012. *JAMA* **2015**, *314*, 1021–1029. [CrossRef] [PubMed]

34. Menke, A.; Rust, K.F.; Cowie, C.C. Diabetes based on 2-h plasma glucose among those classified as having prediabetes based on fasting plasma glucose or A1c. *Diab. Vasc. Dis. Res.* **2018**, *15*, 46–54. [CrossRef] [PubMed]

35. Cowie, C.C.; Rust, K.F.; Byrd-Holt, D.D.; Eberhardt, M.S.; Flegal, K.M.; Engelgau, M.M.; Saydah, S.H.; Williams, D.E.; Geiss, L.S.; Gregg, E.W. Prevalence of diabetes and impaired fasting glucose in adults in the US population. *Diabetes Care* **2006**, *29*, 1263–1268. [CrossRef] [PubMed]

36. Cowie, C.C.; Rust, K.F.; Byrd-Holt, D.D.; Gregg, E.W.; Ford, E.S.; Geiss, L.S.; Bainbridge, K.E.; Fradkin, J.E. Prevalence of diabetes and high risk for diabetes using A1c criteria in the US population in 1988–2006. *Diabetes Care* **2010**, *33*, 562–568. [CrossRef] [PubMed]

37. DECODE Study Group. Age-and sex-specific prevalences of diabetes and impaired glucose regulation in 13 European cohorts1. *Diabetes Care* **2003**, *26*, 61–69. [CrossRef]

38. NCD Risk Factor Collaboration. Effects of diabetes definition on global surveillance of diabetes prevalence and diagnosis: A pooled analysis of 96 population-based studies with 331 288 participants. *Lancet Diabetes Endocrinol.* **2015**, *3*, 624–637. [CrossRef]

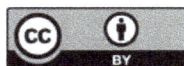

nutrients

MDPI

Communication

Vitamin D Status, Calcium Intake and Risk of Developing Type 2 Diabetes: An Unresolved Issue

Araceli Muñoz-Garach [1,2,*], **Beatriz García-Fontana** [3,4] **and Manuel Muñoz-Torres** [3,4,5,6,*]

1   Department of Endocrinology and Nutrition, Virgen de la Victoria University Hospital,
    Institute of Biomedical Research in Malaga (IBIMA), 29010 Malaga, Spain
2   Instituto de Salud Carlos III, 28029 Madrid, Spain
3   Instituto de Investigación Biosanitaria (Ibs.GRANADA), 18106 Granada, Spain; bgfontana@fibao.es
4   Centro de Investigación Biomédica en Red sobre Fragilidad y Envejecimiento Saludable (CIBERFES),
    Instituto de Salud Carlos III, 28029 Madrid, Spain
5   Unidad de Gestión Clínica Endocrinología y Nutrición, Hospital Universitario San Cecilio de Granada,
    Avenida de la Innovacion, 18016 Granada, Spain
6   Department of Medicine, University of Granada, 18016 Granada, Spain
*   Correspondence: aracelimugar@gmail.com (A.M.-G.); mmt@mamuto.es (M.M.-T.);
    Tel.: +34-646032764 (A.M.-G.); +34-678481018 (M.M.-T.)

Received: 27 February 2019; Accepted: 12 March 2019; Published: 16 March 2019

Abstract: The relationship between vitamin D status, calcium intake and the risk of developing type 2 diabetes (T2D) is a topic of growing interest. One of the most interesting non-skeletal functions of vitamin D is its potential role in glucose homeostasis. This possible association is related to the secretion of insulin by pancreatic beta cells, insulin resistance in different tissues and its influence on systemic inflammation. However, despite multiple observational studies and several meta-analyses that have shown a positive association between circulating 25-hydroxyvitamin D concentrations and the risk of T2D, no randomized clinical trials supplementing with different doses of vitamin D have confirmed this hypothesis definitively. An important question is the identification of what 25-hydroxyvitamin D levels are necessary to influence glycemic homeostasis and the risk of developing T2D. These values of vitamin D can be significantly higher than vitamin D levels required for bone health, but the currently available data do not allow us to answer this question adequately. Furthermore, a large number of observational studies show that dairy consumption is linked to a lower risk of T2D, but the components responsible for this relationship are not well established. Therefore, the importance of calcium intake in the risk of developing T2D has not yet been established. Although there is a biological plausibility linking the status of vitamin D and calcium intake with the risk of T2D, well-designed randomized clinical trials are necessary to answer this important question.

Keywords: calcium intake; dairy products; vitamin D; type 2 diabetes

---

1. Introduction

The incidence of type 2 diabetes (T2D) has increased substantially in recent years related, in part, to higher obesity rates. If current trends continue, more than 642 million people will have diabetes by 2040 [1]. The management and early treatment of T2D are essential to prevent further complications involving loss of quality of life and premature death. It is unclear whether vitamin D deficiency might be contributing to an increased T2D risk [2].

A vast body of evidence associates vitamin D deficiency and T2D [3]. This relationship could be mediated by the direct and indirect effects of vitamin D on glucose homeostasis such as insulin secretion, insulin sensitivity, and systemic inflammation. However, the extent of this relationship and its clinical relevance are not well established.

There is no doubt that vitamin D homeostasis is of vital importance for skeletal health, being especially important for bone mineralization. Moreover, recent studies have demonstrated that low vitamin D concentrations are related to other pathologic conditions that were not previously considered, such as insulin resistance, T2D, metabolic syndrome and cardiovascular diseases. All these diseases could potentially be developed as a result of vitamin D deficiency [4–6].

Moreover, the evidence linking milk and, in particular, calcium intake, insulin secretion and sensitivity has been related to glucose homeostasis in both prediabetes and T2D [7–9]. However, the main clinical studies conducted to confirm this hypothesis have yielded inconsistent results.

The aim of the present review is to summarize the recent evidence linking vitamin D and calcium intake with the development of T2D. We also analyzed different intervention studies with vitamin D supplements to determine their influence on glucose metabolism.

2. Methods

We performed a comprehensive literature search on PubMed to identify peer-reviewed articles on vitamin D levels, vitamin D supplementation and T2D prevention published until December 2018. Search strategies included the following search terms: vitamin D intake, vitamin D supplementation, 25-hydroxyvitamin D, calcium intake, dairy products, type 2 diabetes, impaired glucose tolerance, insulin resistance, insulin sensitivity, β-cell function and obesity.

We included a selection of papers that showed original research articles in humans mainly published in English language; and also in vitro studies, observational studies (prospective and retrospective) and randomized controlled trials. Finally, we reviewed meta-analyses published compiling all studies information. Priority was given to larger studies (according to number of patients included) and the most recent and strongest available evidence.

3. Vitamin D and Type 2 Diabetes (T2D)

3.1. Vitamin D Physiology and Glucose Homeostasis

The term vitamin D includes vitamin D2 or ergocalciferol and vitamin D3 or cholecalciferol. The main metabolites of vitamin D, which differ in their hydroxylation patterns, are 25-hydroxyvitamin D or calcidiol (25(OH)D) and 1,25-dihydroxyvitamin D3 or calcitriol (1,25-$(OH)_2D_3$). In humans, the main sources of vitamin D come from the skin through the cutaneous synthesis of vitamin D3 and, to a lesser extent, from the intake of foods rich in vitamins D2 and D3 or supplements. Circulating vitamin D is bound to vitamin D binding protein (DBP), which transports it to the liver, there vitamin D25-hydroxylase converts it to 25(OH)D. This form of vitamin D is primarily converted to the most biologically active form, 1,25-$(OH)_2D$ in the kidneys. This transformation is done by the enzyme 25-hydroxyvitamin D-1alpha-hydroxylase (CYP27B1). The presence of CYP27B1 in multiple tissues, which also express the vitamin D receptor, suggests that vitamin D could play an important function beyond bone metabolism.

Both in vitro and in vivo studies have reported that vitamin D may play an important role in the maintenance of pancreatic beta cell function [10]. This effect could have different explanations. It could be induced by the activation of the vitamin D receptor (VDR) located in pancreatic beta cells. It was suggested by the study results that showed how mice without VDR have impaired insulin secretion [11] and the addition of calcitriol to the culture medium stimulated pancreatic islets and resulted in an increased insulin secretion [12].

Moreover, vitamin D could also influence insulin secretion by regulating calcium channel opening and closure. Calcitriol participates as a chemical messenger interacting with different receptors regulating calcium flux in beta cells. They are located on the phospholipid layers of plasma membranes. For this reason, calcium is essential for appropriate insulin secretion by pancreatic beta cells; and, therefore, insufficient vitamin D may alter normal insulin secretion through alterations in calcium flux in beta cells [13,14]. In relation to this, the regulation of the protein calbindin, a calcium-binding protein, by vitamin D may be another mechanism influencing insulin secretion. In addition, preclinical studies show that vitamin D can reduce the hyperactivity of the renin angiotensin system and, thus, improve the functioning of beta cells (Leung PS. Nutrients 2016 [15]).

An adequate vitamin D level can also improve insulin resistance pathways associated with diabetes. It is caused mainly by alterations in calcium flux and concentration through the cell membranes of insulin-responsive tissues [16]. The regulation of extracellular and intracellular calcium concentrations may promote dephosphorylation of glucose transporter-4 (GLUT-4) driving a reduced insulin-stimulated glucose transport [14,17]. The 1,25-$(OH)_2$D stimulates the expression of insulin receptors and, therefore, stimulates insulin sensitivity. In addition, calcitriol could also improve insulin sensitivity activating the peroxisome proliferator-activated delta receptor (PPAR-d), a transcription factor that regulates fatty acids metabolism in adipose tissue and the skeletal muscle. Another interesting study indicates that insulin resistance may also be reduced by the specific effects of calcitriol on hepatic lipid synthesis and glucose output, and on skeletal muscle (Leung PS. Nutrients 2016 [15]).

Calcitriol has a central role in a wide variety of metabolic pathways by binding to the VDR, and the measurement of its substrate 25(OH)D is an important marker for health risks. This receptor is expressed in an assortment of cells, such as in the pancreatic beta cells of Langerhans, but also in liver, adipose tissue, and muscle cells [18,19]. The VDR and the 1α-hydroxylase, the enzyme catalyzing calcidiol to calcitriol conversion, are expressed in primary preadipocytes and recently differentiated adipocytes [18]. Therefore, in vitro studies suggest that calcitriol regulates the growth of human adipose tissue and its remodeling. Moreover, fat tissue is a storage site for vitamin D [19]. In contrast, a higher body mass index (BMI) is associated to lower vitamin D concentrations. Vitamin D, a fat-soluble hormone, is sequestered in the adipose tissue and, consequently, only small quantities are available for circulation [20]. On the other hand, since the concentrations of 25(OH)D in serum and adipose tissue are closely related, obesity can reduce serum 25(OH)D through volumetric dilution and the distribution of 25(OH)D in larger fat volumes [21].

Vitamin D could also shorten the effects of chronic inflammation, and it is well established that it plays a key role in the pathogenesis of T2D. Therefore, 1,25$(OH)_2$D can protect against cytokine-induced apoptosis of beta cells directly regulating the activity and expression of cytokines, with an improvement in insulin sensitivity [22]. Moreover, vitamin D demonstrated the possibility of deactivating inflammatory cytokines associated with insulin resistance and promoting calbindin expression which involves protection from apoptosis [23]. Finally, vitamin D also reduces the accumulation of advanced glycation products in experimental studies [24]. These products are related with the development of T2D complications and have been involved with insulin resistance. Vitamin D functions related with glucose homeostasis are summarized in Figure 1.

3.2. Vitamin D Status and Its Relationship with T2D in Cross-Sectional and Longitudinal Studies

Serum 25(OH)D concentrations have been noticed to be inversely associated with glucose homeostasis, insulin resistance, and beta cell function, and forecast lower risks of both metabolic syndrome and T2D [25–27]. Numerous clinical studies have associated vitamin D inadequacy with the development of insulin resistance in different populations, not only in adults [5,28,29] but also in children [30,31].

Consistently, higher baseline 25(OH)D levels have been found to predict better beta cell function and lower glucose levels in subjects at risk for T2D in longitudinal studies [32]. Overall, data from observational studies strongly support an association between low vitamin D status and incidence of T2D [33–35].

We discuss in this review the largest prospective articles and some meta-analyses. In 2013, Afzal et al. published the results of a prospective cohort study that included 9841 participants who were followed-up for 29 years. They found an odds ratio for the development of T2D of 1.5 (95% CI 1.33–1.70) between the lowest and the highest quartile of 25(OH)D [34]. More recently, Park et al. measured 25(OH)D levels in a cohort of 903 adults without diabetes or prediabetes, these authors found an inverse dose-response association between 25(OH)D concentration and risk of diabetes. They proposed a target 25(OH)D of 50 ng/mL; higher than the levels previously suggested in other studies, in the attempt to influence and reduce the incidence rate of diabetes [36]. These data are consistent with the levels published recently by Avila-Rubio et al. in postmenopausal women, the authors link values of 25(OH)D > 45 ng/dL in these women with better glycemic indexes measured by homeostasis model assessment (HOMA) [37].

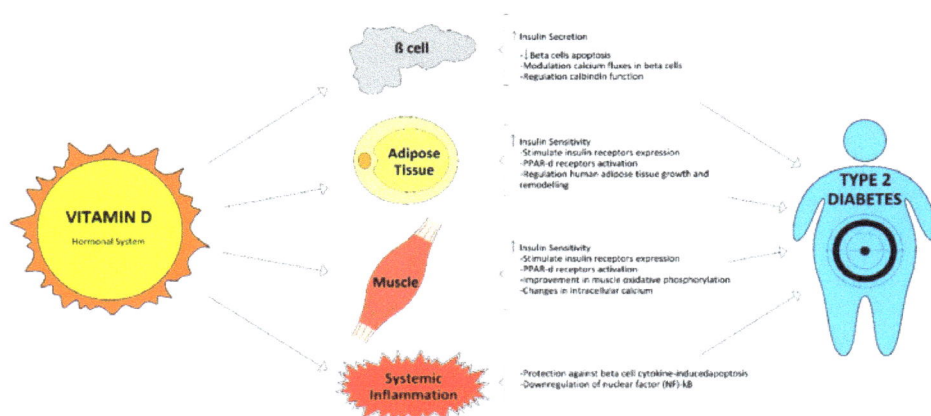

Figure 1. Vitamin D functions related with glucose homeostasis.

The multicenter EPIC-InterAct study measured plasma 25(OH)D metabolites: non-epimeric 25(OH)D$_3$, 3-epi-25(OH)D$_3$ and 25(OH)D$_2$. They identified that plasma non-epimeric 25(OH)D$_3$ (the major component of total 25(OH)D) was inversely associated with T2D, whereas 3-epi-25(OH)D$_3$ was positively associated with the incidence of T2D, and 25(OH)D$_2$ was not associated with T2D [38].

Another large cohort was The Melbourne cohort, which included a sample of middle-aged Australians, the authors showed how vitamin D status was inversely associated with the risk of T2D and, apparently, this association cannot be explained by reverse causality [39]. If the association was due to reverse causality, then a much stronger association would be expected to be observed in the first few years of follow-up.

The meta-analysis conducted by Song et al. included 21 observational studies with 76,220 subjects in total; the authors found a 38% lesser risk of developing T2D in the highest baseline reference category of 25(OH)D compared to the lowest one (95% CI 0.54–0.70) [35].

Despite the consistency of these results, all these were observational studies and estimation of causality cannot be completely excluded because of residual confounding agents.

3.3. Vitamin D Supplementation and Risk of T2D: Randomized Trials and Meta-Analysis

In the last decade, more than ten well-designed, randomized trials evaluated the effect of vitamin D3 supplementation on glucose homeostasis in subjects at risk for T2D and showed inconsistent results. We have selected a set of studies that analyzed outcomes related to the objectives of this review. Table 1 summarizes the main results of these studies.

In Table 1 we describe the main findings of the largest trials. Sollid et al. [40] conducted a randomized clinical trial with approximately 500 prediabetes subjects comparing vitamin D versus placebo for the prevention of T2D. They supplemented with 20,000 IU cholecalciferol weekly and after one year, no significant differences were reported between those receiving vitamin D and those taking placebo in any of the glycemic or inflammatory markers and blood pressure, regardless of baseline serum 25(OH)D concentrations.

Two years later, Forouhi et al. [41] compared, in another large randomized trial including 340 prediabetes or at risk of developing T2D subjects, the effect of supplementation with cholecalciferol or ergocalciferol (both 100,000 IU/month) versus placebo, for four months. Prediabetes was estimated by the Cambridge Risk Score [42]. Despite vitamin D supplementation, neither ergocalciferol or cholecalciferol, resulted in increased 25(OH)D$_2$ and 25(OH)D$_3$ concentrations. No differences in HbA1c concentration were found between groups. It is important to point out that only half of the subjects had concentrations of 25(OH)D < 50 nmol/L. This data could influence the results.

Their results are in accordance with previous findings by Davidson et al. [43]. They supplemented a cohort of Latino and African Americans subjects with prediabetes and hypovitaminosis D at baseline for one year. They used a cholecalciferol dose sufficient to raise serum 25(OH)D levels into the upper-normal range versus placebo. They did not find any effect on insulin secretion or sensitivity, nor the proportion of subjects who developed T2D or whose oral glucose tolerance test became normal [43].

However, it is possible to find some positive effect on glycemic markers in some studies. In this line, Gagnon et al. [44] reported when they performed a post hoc analysis only including subjects with prediabetes, an improvement in insulin sensitivity indices was observed. Previously, they gave a supplement of calcium carbonate 1200 mg and cholecalciferol 2000–6000 UI daily to subjects with glucose intolerance or recently diagnosed diabetes, but they found no effect on insulin sensitivity or secretion, and beta cell function. So, despite most clinical randomized trials failing to show a favorable effect of vitamin D supplementation on glycemic control, insulin sensitivity indices, and incident T2D [40,41,43–49] in subjects at risk for diabetes, there is some interesting evidence supporting a beneficial effect of vitamin D on beta cell function. In fact, Mitri et al. [50] reported in 2011 a significant improvement in insulin secretion in 92 prediabetic subjects who were overweight or obese and at risk for T2D. They were supplemented with cholecalciferol 2000 IU daily and calcium carbonate versus placebo for four months. An important restriction of the above described studies is that they were not designed specifically to assess glycemic homeostasis and the results found correspond to post hoc analyses.

Although not being designed for this purpose, we would like to point out the results of the Vitamin D and Omega-3 Trial (VITAL), a large-scale trial that evaluated high-dose vitamin D supplementation. This study was designed to evaluate the effect of supplementation with vitamin D on incidence of invasive cancer or cardiovascular events versus placebo. Overall, no differences were found between groups. However, in Black Americans a potential beneficial effect was found in cancer mortality [51].

A recent meta-analysis conducted by Rafiq et al. showed an inverse relationship; higher vitamin D concentrations were associated with lower BMI in T2D patients and non-diabetic subjects at risk for T2D. But this association was more pronounced in T2D patients. Moreover, the correlation was directly associated to the BMI quartiles, so the highest BMI quartile had the greatest correlations in both populations, both T2D and non-diabetic [52].

Tang et al. [53] published a meta-analysis and did not find an effect of vitamin D supplementation on the incidence of T2D. However, the authors suggested a possible dose-response effect of vitamin D supplementation to improve glucose and insulin metabolism among non-diabetic adults. They postulated a possible benefit of taking vitamin D supplements in higher doses for the primary prevention of T2D.

In summary, studies were very heterogeneous in terms of design, duration, and type of supplement administered and participants characteristics. It is noteworthy that adherence to the treatment would have played a major role in arguing these results.

Table 1. Clinical trials investigating the association between vitamin D supplementation and risk of type 2 diabetes (T2D).

Study, Year	Country	Population Characteristics (Mean age/age range (years))	Type of Treatment	N	Duration (months)	Main Outcomes
LeBlanc et al. D2d Research Group [53] 2018	US	Prediabetes (59)	4000 IU D3/day vs. placebo	2423	36	Not yet published
Forouhi et al. [41] 2016	UK	Prediabetes IFG or IGT or positive diabetes risk score (53)	100,000 IU D2/month or 100,000 IU D3/month vs. placebo	340	4	No effect on HbA1c. Improve pulse wave velocity (arterial stiffness)
Wagner et al. [48] 2016	Sweden	Prediabetes or diet-controlled T2D (67.3)	30,000 IU D3/week vs. placebo	44	2	No difference in insulin secretion/sensitivity, beta cell function and glucose tolerance
Tuomainen et al. [47] 2015	Finland	Prediabetes (65.7)	40 μg/day D3 or 80 μg/day D3 vs. placebo	68	5	No difference in glucose homeostasis indicators
Gagnon et al. [44] 2014	Australia	25(OH)D ≤ 22ng/ml at risk of T2D (54)	1200 mg calcium carbonate and 2000–6000 IU D3 day to target vs. placebo	95	6	No difference in insulin secretion/sensitivity and beta cell function. A post-hoc analysis (only prediabetes patients) showed a significant beneficial effect on insulin sensitivity
Sollid et al. [40] 2014	Norway	Prediabetes IFG or IGT (62.1)	20,000 IU D3/week vs. placebo	511	12	No difference in insulin secretion/sensitivity or glucose metabolism, blood pressure or lipid status
Oosterwerff et al. [15] 2014	Netherlands	Overweight, vitamin D deficient subjects with prediabetes (20–65)	Calcium carbonate 500 mg (all) and 1200 IU D3/day vs. placebo	130	4	No difference in insulin sensitivity or in beta cell function. A post hoc analysis (without diabetes patients at baseline) showed a significant increase in the insulinogenic index when 25(OH)D ≥ 60 nmol/L.
Salehpour et al. [46] 2013	Iran	Healthy, overweight/obese women (38)	25 μg D3/daily vs. placebo	77	4	No effect in glycemic indices (glucose, insulin, HbA1c and HOMA-IR)
Belenchia et al. [55] 2013	US	Obese adolescents (14.1)	4000 IU D3/day vs. placebo	35	6	Significant effect in fasting insulin, HOMA-IR and leptin-to-adiponectin ratio
Davidson et al. [43] 2013	US	Prediabetes and hypovitaminosis D (52)	D3 to target serum 25OHD level of 65–90 ng/mL vs. placebo	109	12	No difference on insulin secretion/sensitivity or the development of diabetes or returning to normal glucose tolerance
Mitri et al. [50] 2011	US	Prediabetes. At risk for T2D (57)	2000 IU D3/daily vs. calcium carbonate 800 mg/day	92	4	Significant effect in beta cell function and improvement in insulin secretion
von Hurst et al. [49] 2010	New Zealand	Insulin resistance. At risk for T2D 25(OH)D < 20 ng/mL (23–68)	4000 IU D3/day vs. placebo	81	6.5	No difference in FPG, HOMA2%B; C-peptide. Significant effect on HOMA IR and insulin
Jorde et al. [56] 2010	Norway	Overweight/Obese; At risk for T2D (21–70)	500 mg calcium/day plus D3, 40,000 IU/week or D3 20,000 IU/week	438	48	No difference in HbA1c, FPG, 2hs PG and HOMA-IR

BMI, body mass index; FPG, fasting plasma glucose; 2hs PG, 2 h plasma glucose; HbA1c, glycated hemoglobin; HOMA-IR, homeostatic model assessment of insulin resistance; IFG, impaired fasting glucose; IGT, impaired glucose tolerance; NAFLD, nonalcoholic fatty liver disease; T2D, type 2 diabetes.

Recently, the design of a new randomized clinical trial has been published and its results can be a determinant in clarifying many of the uncertainties that exist today. The D2d is a large randomized clinical trial (including participants from 22 sites across the U.S.) hypothesizing that supplementation with vitamin D_3 daily lowers risk of diabetes in adults with prediabetes [54]. This trial meets people with a large spectrum of diabetes risk, more convenient for testing the underlying hypothesis. D2d trial results are expected to answer two important questions: whether vitamin D supplementation is useful to prevent T2D and how the 2010 expanded American Diabetes Association (ADA) criteria for prediabetes would impact the natural history of this state previous to diabetes.

3.4. New Thresholds for the Relationship between Vitamin D and T2D

An important question that has arisen is what 25(OH)D levels are necessary to influence glycemic homeostasis and the risk of developing T2D. Three recent studies have addressed this issue. Von Horst et al. found that optimal 25OHD concentrations for reducing IR were around 50 ng/dL in a randomized controlled study with 81 Asian women [49]. Avila Rubio et al. [37], in a study conducted in women with postmenopausal osteoporosis, suggested that the established goal of reaching a level of 25(OH)D > 30 ng/mL was insufficient to improve glucose metabolism in these population. The data from this study indicates that 25(OH)D > 45 ng/mL are necessary to achieve this goal. These data are consistent with a cohort study of 903 adults of 12 years of duration in non-diabetic population where reaching values of 25(OH)D > 50 ng/mL contributed to reach the maximum benefits to reduce the risk of incident diabetes [36]. Therefore, it is important to establish what 25(OH)D values are necessary to achieve and, even more importantly, maintain all the potential benefits of vitamin D. The currently available studies do not allow us to answer this question with certainty.

4. Calcium Intake and T2D

4.1. Mechanistic Studies

To introduce and understand the underlying mechanisms that associates dairy products, and specifically dairy components to T2D prevention, mechanistic studies are essential. Further to the structural role it plays in the skeleton, calcium is an essential electrolyte necessary for many critical biological functions. Calcium may play a key role in a wide range of functions related to glucose homeostasis. Calcium regulates insulin-mediated intracellular processes in specific tissues that respond to insulin, participates in the secretory function of pancreatic beta cells and the phosphorylation of insulin receptors. Calcium also down-regulates specific regulatory genes encoding pro-inflammatory cytokines involved in insulin resistance [16,57,58].

Insulin secretion is a calcium-dependent process [59]. Calcium is vital for insulin-mediated intracellular processes in those tissues responding to insulin, such as muscle and fat [16,58]. There is a narrow range of intracellular calcium concentration needed for optimal insulin-mediated functions. When there are changes in intracellular calcium concentrations in insulin-responsive tissues there is a contribution to peripheral insulin resistance [17,60] through a dysregulated insulin signal transduction cascade that leads to a lower glucose transporter activity.

An appropriate range of intracellular calcium concentration is also required for some insulin-mediated activities in tissues such as liver, adipose and skeletal muscle [57]. It is important to maintain relatively low intracellular calcium concentrations in these target tissues to have a beneficial effect on the insulin signal transduction cascade [60] and peripheral insulin sensitivity. In addition, low intracellular calcium attenuates cytokine-induced inflammation, augments vascular relaxation and inhibits platelet aggregation. It is important to keep in mind that calcium intake should be considered in the context of dairy intake and dairy products, which provide other important nutrients besides calcium.

4.2. Dairy Intake and T2D Risk

Increased dairy consumption is linked to a lower risk of T2D, but the components responsible for this relation are not well established. The participation of specific dairy products needs to be further studied. Calcium, vitamin D, dairy fat, partially hydrogenated oils and specifically *trans*-palmitoleic acid (a natural *trans* fatty acid found in dairy) are key dairy components. They have been proposed to influence some metabolic pathways implicated in T2D prevention.

We have previously reported how vitamin D has a direct effect on insulin secretion by binding to VDR in pancreatic beta cells and an indirect effect via the regulation of extracellular calcium [13,57,61]. Moreover, vitamin D effects include suppression of inappropriately prolonged inflammation by modulating secretion of proinflammatory cytokines.

The role of dietary intake of *trans*-palmitoleic acid has been related to an improvement in metabolic regulation, hepatic and peripheral insulin resistance, and suppression of hepatic de novo lipogenesis and lower levels of fasting insulin, C-reactive protein, triglycerides and blood pressure [62,63]. In the Cardiovascular Health Study (CHS), a prospective cohort analysis about dietary intake of *trans*-palmitoleic acid, a significantly and considerably 62% risk reduction of incident T2D has been shown [62]. Moreover, the Multi-Ethnic Study of Atherosclerosis (MESA), a prospective cohort study, showed that dietary intake of *trans*-palmitoleic acid was associated with a 48% lower risk of incident T2D [63].

When we analyzed the fat content of dairy, the evidence finds relatively consistent results regarding a beneficial role of fatty dairy products in T2D prevention. But, to date, the differences between low, regular or high fat dairy are less known. Kratz et al. described in a systematic review including observational studies [64], that the majority of studies analyzed inversely associated high-fat dairy products with obesity, T2D and cardiometabolic disease, either significantly or insignificantly. However, the meta-analysis of cohort studies conducted by Alhazmi et al. showed that saturated fat ingestion was not associated with a risk of T2D [65].

Furthermore, the evidence regarding the role of specific types of dairy products (milk, yogurt, and cheese) is even more limited. Milk has generally been posted as part of total dairy consumption, and scarce evidence exists on milk particularly. It seems that milk consumption may be associated with a T2D risk reduction, with not well-established differences between regular-fat or whole fat milk and T2D [66–68]. The association between cheese consumption and a reduced risk of T2D still needs to be strongly supported because some findings are not statistically significant [68–71]. Finally, limited evidence suggested a protective role of fermented dairy products in general (including yogurt, cheese, buttermilk, and fermented milk), against T2D [69,71].

4.3. Observational Studies

More than twenty observational studies regarding calcium intake and T2D prevention were found. Different populations have investigated the association between calcium intake and T2D. The largest are four cohort studies. They were done in the United States ($n = 83,779$ [72], ($n = 41,186$) [73]), and the other two in Asian populations: China ($n = 64,191$) [74], and Japan ($n = 59,796$) [75]. They demonstrated an inverse association between dietary or total calcium intake and T2D risk among women but not in men, in the United States and in China. In the Japanese study, they found an inverse association in subjects with higher vitamin D intake.

In Korea, a smaller cohort study conducted in rural areas ($n = 8313$) also showed an inverse association between total and vegetable calcium intake and T2D risk among women, as previously reported [76]. Conversely, a relatively short study ($n = 5200$) in Australia did not find an association between dietary calcium and T2D [77]. Additionally, other studies provided mixed results when investigating the association between dairy products and the potential risk of T2D.

More recently, the Korean Genome study, a prospective cohort community-based trial followed for 10 years, explained the longitudinal associations between dietary calcium intake and the incidence of T2D [9]. The authors also associated dietary calcium intake and serum calcium levels at the baseline survey. They found that higher dietary calcium intake was associated with a lower risk of developing T2D. These results are important for public health and have implications for predicting and preventing T2D development. These findings can provide guidelines for calcium dietary and calcium supplementation.

At the same time, a Spanish study including more than 500 postmenopausal women without diabetes showed a decrease in fasting plasma glucose and glycated hemoglobin after the intervention. This supplementation consisted of a higher dose of vitamin D3 as part of an enriched milk, providing a daily intake of 600 IU of vitamin D3 and 900 mg of calcium [78].

Another population-based study using a prospective survey of 5582 adults, the Australian Diabetes Obesity and Lifestyle Study (AusDiab), showed a significant inverse association between the highest tertial of dairy intake and risk of diabetes in men after a following-up period of five years. They obtained these results after adjustment for confounding variables such as age, sex, energy intake, and other potential confounders (adjusted OR 0.53, 95% CI 0.29–0.96 [79]. This inverse association was non-significant in women (adjusted OR 0.71, 95% CI 0.48–1.05). When the authors analyzed different dairy products (low-fat milk, full-fat milk, yogurt, cheese), they only found significant inverse association with diabetes for low-fat milk (adjusted OR 0.65, 95% CI 0.44–0.94).

The Danish population-based lifestyle intervention study done by Struijk et al. called the Inter 99 Study, explained the association between specific types of dairy products and T2D incidence. They did not find a significant association between total dairy intake and T2D incidence (OR 0.95, 95% CI 0.86–1.06) and when they analyzed specific dairy products and T2D no association was reported. Particularly, cheese and other fermented dairy (including yogurt, and buttermilk) appeared to have a beneficial effect on glucose regulation markers, with an inverse association with fasting plasma glucose and glycated hemoglobin [69].

At the same time, the results of the Whitehall II prospective cohort study of working staff of Civil Service departments, were reported. They followed 4186 subjects for ten year and found that total dairy consumption was not significantly associated with T2D (hazard ratio (HR) 1.30, 95% CI 0.95–1.77). They analyzed all possible dairy (high-fat and low-fat dairy, total milk, yogurt, cheese and fermented products) and were not associated with T2D risk. But, nevertheless, fermented dairy products were significantly associated with an inverse risk of overall mortality [68].

In the French population, the Data from the Epidemiological Study on Insulin Resistance Syndrome (DESIR) study analyzed 3435 participants prospectively for nine years. This cohort study showed that global consumption of dairy products, but not cheese, was inversely associated with new impaired fasting glycemia diagnosis and T2D (adjusted OR 0.85, 95% CI 0.76–0.94). When analyzing cheese consumption, they did not find an association with T2D (adjusted OR 0.93, 95% CI 0.82–1.06). Curiously, they reported an inverse relationship between cheese and incident metabolic syndrome (adjusted OR 0.82, 95% CI 0.71–0.95) [70].

Moreover, data from the Nurses' Health Study II, including 37,038 women followed-up for seven years, evaluated the possible influence of dairy consumption during adolescence with the development of T2D later in adulthood. They adjusted for risk factors present in adolescence. Those women with the highest quintile intake of dairy during adolescence (two servings per day) had a 38% lower risk of T2D. They also adjusted for risk factors appearing in adulthood and still demonstrated a significant inverse association between adolescent dairy intake and T2D (RR 0.73, 95% CI 0.54–0.97). There was a 43% T2D risk reduction in women with high-dairy intakes for a long time (from adolescence to adulthood), highlighting the importance of persistence in dairy consumption. They also found a 25% risk reduction for the highest current dairy consumption (two servings per 1000 kcal), and a 26% and 28% risk reduction with low- and high-fat dairy consumption, respectively [80]. In contrast, the EPIC Study, including 16,835 participants in a nested case-cohort analysis including eight European countries, found no association between total dairy consumption and T2D (HR 1.01, 95% CI 0.83–1.34) [71]. There were an inverse association between the consumption of cheese and fermented dairy products (cheese, yogurt, and thick fermented milk) with T2D (HR 0.88, 95% CI 0.76–1.02 and HR 0.88, 95% CI 0.78–0.99, respectively).

Recently the PURE study was published [81]. It analyzes the association of dairy intake with cardiovascular disease and mortality in 21 countries from five continents. In this study, the dietary intake of dairy products of 136,384 individuals were recorded using country-specific validated food frequency questionnaires. During a follow-up period of 9.1 years, the incidence of cardiovascular events and mortality was evaluated. The authors concluded that higher consumption of dairy products is associated with lower risks of mortality and cardiovascular disease.

To date, there are no well-designed randomized controlled trials (RCTs) that have specifically studied the relationship between dairy products and the risk of incident T2D. However, there is a randomized crossover trial with 12 months follow up that need to be considered. It evaluated the consumption of low-fat dairy (four servings per day) and was associated with better insulin resistance, without negative effects on body weight and lipid profile [82].

4.4. Systematic Reviews and Meta-Analyses

Three meta-analyses of prospective cohort studies on dairy products and T2D are worth noting. In a meta-analysis conducted by Tong et al. the highest dairy consumption, compared to the lowest category, significantly reduced the risk of T2D by 14% [67]. They found a significant inverse association for low-fat dairy and yogurt with T2D. This association was not found for high-fat dairy and whole (regular-fat) milk. They described, in a dose-response analysis, how each additional daily serving of total dairy showed a decrease of 6% in T2D risk. Especially per each additional serving of low-fat dairy intake there was a 10% T2D risk reduction.

Elwood et al. have previously demonstrated in their meta-analysis including four prospective cohort studies on diabetes, that milk or dairy consumption played a protective role against T2D. Per each additional daily serving there was a 4%–9% risk reduction in diabetes incidence [66]. Pittas et al. found in their meta-analysis including mostly similar cohort studies that the highest versus lowest dairy intake (3–5 vs. 1.5 servings per day) was associated with a lower risk of incident T2D [57].

So, we can consider that, to date, there is some strong, consistent, and accumulating evidence about the influence of dairy intake on a reduced the risk of T2D [7].

However, it is important to notice possible confounding factors such as fat content in some dairy products, which can influence the protective effects of calcium [74,83]. Moreover, calcium intake may also depend on other products non-dairy foods (for example tofu, fish, rice, vegetables, and pulses). It is evident that the main source of dietary calcium differs between populations and different cultures.

5. Nutritional Recommendations for T2D Prevention

An important body of evidence has shown that dairy products can reduce the risk of T2D significantly and probably in a dose-response way.

The value of having an adequate intake of dairy products should be reinforced especially among those with prediabetes, obesity and metabolic syndrome.

In addition, cultural differences, nutritional habits, economic status and gender are related to the consumption of milk and dairy products. Unfortunately, a large percentage of the adult population, particularly older adults, do not to meet the international recommendations for optimal calcium intake and need to be encouraged to increase daily calcium intake.

Dairy products are largely under-consumed by all age groups and across populations. More than 80% Americans do not meet the minimum dairy requirements of the Dietary Guidelines for Americans (DGA) [84]. The same problems have been identified in other cultures, such as the Chinese population. Their milk intake is still quite low [85].

The amount of calcium needed daily varies by age. The recommendations given by the National Institutes of Health (NIH) proposed a daily intake of 1000 mg for men between 25 and 65 years [86]. This is the same recommendation for women between 25 and 50 years, with an exception for pregnant or lactating women or postmenopausal women not receiving estrogen replacement therapy. They should take 1500 mg/day [86]. For all subjects, men and women over 65 years, the NIH proposes a daily calcium intake of 1500 mg [86]. On the other hand, recently updated the US Institute of Medicine (IOM) recommendation of 1000 mg/day of calcium intake for all adults aged 19–50 years and for men until age 70 years. They recommend 1200 mg/day for women 51 years or older and both men and women aged >70 years [87]. They proposed in their guidelines that calcium-rich foods, especially milk and other dairy products, are the best source of calcium intake because they have showed a higher absorption efficiency. Alternatively, calcium supplementation may help reaching optimal intake for those subjects who cannot take adequate calcium through diet alone.

Although 25(OH)D blood concentration is the most commonly used biomarker to determine vitamin D status, there is no global consensus on what the 25(OH)D thresholds are for vitamin D deficiency or insufficiency. The main guidelines issued by the IOM and the Endocrine Society differ on their classification of vitamin D status. The differences can be explained because of the various populations recognized by the guidelines and the way evidence was described. The IOM guidelines focus on the general healthy population and emphasize on interventional studies. The IOM did not find appropriate evidence linking vitamin D and beneficial effects for non-skeletal outcomes, such as diabetes. Therefore, the IOM argued that a level of 25(OH)D >20 ng/mL is adequate and enough for skeletal outcomes, whereas only low evidence data ratify a higher level. Moreover, the IOM proposed that a level >50 ng/mL should be followed to avoid potential adverse events. In contrast, the Endocrine Society clinical practice guidelines focus on people at high risk for vitamin D deficiency and emphasize more on observational (epidemiological) studies. The latter guidelines determined that 25(OH)D concentrations >30 ng/mL are desirable for optimal skeletal outcomes without suggesting any upper limit to be concern for safety. However, the Endocrine Society guidelines have been criticized for the way they characterized several subgroups as a high-risk population and their wide recommendations for screening for vitamin D deficiency [88]. There is agreement between both guidelines about the requirement to reconsider current recommendations in the future when ongoing randomized trials become available. Thus, two important questions are raised. First, the existence of different thresholds for different beneficial effects. Second, the harmonization of techniques to determine circulating 25(OH)D concentrations to achieve comparable results [89].

6. Unsolved Questions

In this review, a large body of evidence has been discussed about the intake of calcium and vitamin D and its association with the incidence of T2D, although the results are inconsistent. To date, several observational studies and randomized trials have been performed including very heterogeneous subject populations. They differ in design and duration, and in which range of vitamin D types and calcium products and various dosing regimens used. Therefore, it seems necessary to clarify what vitamin D levels are needed to obtain a real benefit, if any, on glycemic status, and this concentration is probably higher than recommendations currently focused on obtaining a benefit on bone metabolism. Supplementation with vitamin D at doses around 4000 IU/day may be an option to increase 25(OH)D levels close to 50 ng/mL and improve homeostasis rates of glucose and insulin among non-diabetic subjects. Therefore, no consensus regarding whether the general population needs further supplementation of vitamin D to improve health outcomes has been found.

Furthermore, more research is needed to better understand the role of calcium intake from milk and specific types of dairy products (regular fat, skimmed, fermented, non-fermented) on the incidence of T2D and indices of glucose metabolism.

Establishing if specific populations such as those with prediabetes, the overweight or obese, could obtain significant benefits with nutritional recommendations regarding the intake of calcium and vitamin D has become a matter of special interest.

7. Conclusions and Perspectives

We conclude that the current literature is inadequate for drawing firm conclusions about the association between calcium intake and incident T2D, although it appears that a higher consumption of dairy products may be beneficial for glucose metabolism. Moreover, an adequate level of vitamin D may also have a helpful effect on T2D prevention, and a potential dose-response effect is suggested.

Nevertheless, specific studies with a close control of calcium intakes and higher vitamin D supplementation are needed to better understand their effects on glucose and insulin homeostasis.

Author Contributions: A.M.-G.: carried out the bibliographic search and wrote the manuscript. B.G.-F.: reviewed the manuscript. M.M.-T.: designed and revised the manuscript. All authors approved the manuscript.

Funding: This work was supported in part by grants from Instituto de Salud Carlos III (PI15/01207). This study has been co-funded by FEDER funds. A.M.G. is the recipient of a postdoctoral grant (Juan Rodes JR 17/00023) from the Spanish Ministry of Economy and Competitiveness.

Acknowledgments: This work was supported in part by grants from Instituto de Salud Carlos III (PI15/01207). This study has been co-funded by FEDER funds. A.M.G. is the recipient of a postdoctoral grant (Juan Rodes JR 17/00023) from the Spanish Ministry of Economy and Competitiveness. We acknowledge Nutraceutical Translations for English language editing of this review. All sources of funding of the study should be disclosed. We acknowledge Nutraceutical Translations for English language editing of this manuscript.

Conflicts of Interest: The authors declare no conflict of interest.

References

1. International Diabetes Federation. *IDF Diabetes Atlas*, 8th ed.; International Diabetes Federation: Brussels, Belgium, 2017; ISBN 978-2-930229-81-2.
2. Pittas, A.G.; Nelson, J.; Mitri, J.; Hillmann, W.; Garganta, C.; Nathan, D.M.; Hu, F.B.; Dawson-Hughes, B.; Diabetes Prevention Program Research Group. Plasma 25-hydroxyvitamin D and progression to diabetes in patients at risk for diabetes: An ancillary analysis in the Diabetes Prevention Program. *Diabetes Care* **2012**, *35*, 565–573. [CrossRef] [PubMed]
3. Maddaloni, E.; Cavallari, I.; Napoli, N.; Conte, C. Vitamin D and Diabetes Mellitus. *Front. Horm. Res.* **2018**, *50*, 161–176. [PubMed]
4. Ford, E.S.; Ajani, U.A.; McGuire, L.C.; Liu, S. Concentrations of serum vitamin D and the metabolic syndrome among U.S. adults. *Diabetes Care* **2005**, *28*, 1228–1230. [CrossRef]
5. Chiu, K.C.; Chu, A.; Go, V.L.W.; Saad, M.F. Hypovitaminosis D is associated with insulin resistance and β cell dysfunction. *Am. J. Clin. Nutr.* **2004**, *79*, 820–825. [CrossRef] [PubMed]
6. Lips, P.; Eekhoff, M.; van Schoor, N.; Oosterwerff, M.; de Jongh, R.; Krul-Poel, Y.; Simsek, S. Vitamin D and type 2 diabetes. *J. Steroid Biochem. Mol. Biol.* **2017**, *173*, 280–285. [CrossRef]
7. Kalergis, M.; Leung Yinko, S.S.L.; Nedelcu, R. Dairy products and prevention of type 2 diabetes: Implications for research and practice. *Front. Endocrinol.* **2013**, *4*, 90. [CrossRef] [PubMed]
8. Talaei, M.; Pan, A.; Yuan, J.M.; Koh, W.P. Dairy intake and risk of type 2 diabetes. *Clin. Nutr.* **2018**, *37*, 712–718. [CrossRef]
9. Kim, K.N.; Oh, S.Y.; Hong, Y.C. Associations of serum calcium levels and dietary calcium intake with incident type 2 diabetes over 10 years: The Korean Genome and Epidemiology Study (KoGES). *Diabetol. Metab. Syndr.* **2018**, *10*, 50. [CrossRef]
10. Cade, C.; Norman, A.W. Rapid normalization/stimulation by 1,25- dihydroxyvitamin d3 of insulin secretion and glucose tolerance in the vitamin d-deficient rat. *Endocrinology* **1987**, *120*, 1490–1497. [CrossRef]
11. Zeitz, U.; Weber, K.; Soegiarto, D.W.; Wolf, E.; Balling, R.; Erben, R.G. Impaired insulin secretory capacity in mice lacking a functional vitamin D receptor. *FASEB J.* **2003**, *17*, 509–511. [CrossRef]
12. Bouillon, R.; Carmeliet, G.; Verlinden, L.; Van Etten, E.; Verstuyf, A.; Luderer, H.F.; Lieben, L.; Mathieu, C.; Demay, M. Vitamin D and human health: Lessons from vitamin D receptor null mice. *Endocr. Rev.* **2008**, *29*, 726–776. [CrossRef] [PubMed]
13. Bland, R.; Markovic, D.; Hills, C.E.; Hughes, S.V.; Chan, S.L.F.; Squires, P.E.; Hewison, M. Expression of 25-hydroxyvitamin D3-1alpha-hydroxylase in pancreatic islets. *J. Steroid Biochem. Mol. Biol.* **2004**, *89–90*, 121–125. [CrossRef] [PubMed]

14. Reusch, J.E.; Begum, N.; Sussman, K.E.; Draznin, B. Regulation of GLUT-4 phosphorylation by intracellular calcium in adipocytes. *Endocrinology* **1991**, *129*, 3269–3273. [CrossRef] [PubMed]
15. Leung, P.S. The Potential Protective Action of Vitamin D in Hepatic Insulin Resistance and Pancreatic Islet Dysfunction in Type 2 Diabetes Mellitus. *Nutrients* **2016**, *8*, 147. [CrossRef] [PubMed]
16. Wright, D.C.; Hucker, K.A.; Holloszy, J.O.; Han, D.H. Ca^{2+} and AMPK both mediate stimulation of glucose transport by muscle contractions. *Diabetes* **2004**, *53*, 330–335. [CrossRef]
17. Draznin, B. Cytosolic calcium and insulin resistance. *Am. J. Kidney Dis.* **1993**, *21*, 32–38. [CrossRef]
18. Nimitphong, H.; Holick, M.F.; Fried, S.K.; Lee, M.-J. 25-hydroxyvitamin D(3) and 1,25-dihydroxyvitamin D(3) promote the differentiation of human subcutaneous preadipocytes. *PLoS ONE* **2012**, *7*, e52171. [CrossRef]
19. Blum, M.; Dolnikowski, G.; Seyoum, E.; Harris, S.S.; Booth, S.L.; Peterson, J.; Saltzman, E.; Dawson-Hughes, B. Vitamin D(3) in fat tissue. *Endocrine* **2008**, *33*, 90–94. [CrossRef]
20. Wamberg, L.; Christiansen, T.; Paulsen, S.K.; Fisker, S.; Rask, P.; Rejnmark, L.; Richelsen, B.; Pedersen, S.B. Expression of vitamin D-metabolizing enzymes in human adipose tissue—The effect of obesity and diet-induced weight loss. *Int. J. Obes.* **2013**, *37*, 651–657. [CrossRef]
21. Hyppönen, E.; Boucher, B.J. Adiposity, vitamin D requirements, and clinical implications for obesity-related metabolic abnormalities. *Nutr. Rev.* **2018**, *76*, 678–692. [CrossRef]
22. Chun, R.F.; Liu, P.T.; Modlin, R.L.; Adams, J.S.; Hewison, M. Impact of vitamin D on immune function: lessons learned from genome-wide analysis. *Front. Physiol.* **2014**, *5*, 151. [CrossRef] [PubMed]
23. Christakos, S.; Liu, Y. Biological actions and mechanism of action of calbindin in the process of apoptosis. *J. Steroid Biochem. Mol. Biol.* **2004**, *89–90*, 401–404. [CrossRef] [PubMed]
24. Salum, E.; Kals, J.; Kampus, P.; Salum, T.; Zilmer, K.; Aunapuu, M.; Arend, A.; Eha, J.; Zilmer, M. Vitamin D reduces deposition of advanced glycation end-products in the aortic wall and systemic oxidative stress in diabetic rats. *Diabetes Res. Clin. Pract.* **2013**, *100*, 243–249. [CrossRef] [PubMed]
25. Forouhi, N.G.; Luan, J.; Cooper, A.; Boucher, B.J.; Wareham, N.J. Baseline serum 25-hydroxy vitamin d is predictive of future glycemic status and insulin resistance: The Medical Research Council Ely Prospective Study 1990-2000. *Diabetes* **2008**, *57*, 2619–2625. [CrossRef] [PubMed]
26. Kayaniyil, S.; Vieth, R.; Retnakaran, R.; Knight, J.A.; Qi, Y.; Gerstein, H.C.; Perkins, B.A.; Harris, S.B.; Zinman, B.; Hanley, A.J. Association of vitamin D with insulin resistance and beta-cell dysfunction in subjects at risk for type 2 diabetes. *Diabetes Care* **2010**, *33*, 1379–1381. [CrossRef] [PubMed]
27. Maki, K.C.; Fulgoni, V.L., 3rd; Keast, D.R.; Rains, T.M.; Park, K.M.; Rubin, M.R. Vitamin D intake and status are associated with lower prevalence of metabolic syndrome in U.S. adults: National Health and Nutrition Examination Surveys 2003–2006. *Metab. Syndr. Relat. Disord.* **2012**, *10*, 363–372. [CrossRef]
28. Gannage-Yared, M.-H.; Chedid, R.; Khalife, S.; Azzi, E.; Zoghbi, F.; Halaby, G. Vitamin D in relation to metabolic risk factors, insulin sensitivity and adiponectin in a young Middle-Eastern population. *Eur. J. Endocrinol.* **2009**, *160*, 965–971. [CrossRef]
29. Scragg, R.; Holdaway, I.; Singh, V.; Metcalf, P.; Baker, J.; Dryson, E. Serum 25-hydroxyvitamin D3 levels decreased in impaired glucose tolerance and diabetes mellitus. *Diabetes Res. Clin. Pract.* **1995**, *27*, 181–188. [CrossRef]
30. Olson, M.L.; Maalouf, N.M.; Oden, J.D.; White, P.C.; Hutchison, M.R. Vitamin D deficiency in obese children and its relationship to glucose homeostasis. *J. Clin. Endocrinol. Metab.* **2012**, *97*, 279–285. [CrossRef]
31. Parikh, S.; Guo, D.-H.; Pollock, N.K.; Petty, K.; Bhagatwala, J.; Gutin, B.; Houk, C.; Zhu, H.; Dong, Y. Circulating 25-hydroxyvitamin D concentrations are correlated with cardiometabolic risk among American black and white adolescents living in a year-round sunny climate. *Diabetes Care* **2012**, *35*, 1133–1138. [CrossRef]
32. Kayaniyil, S.; Retnakaran, R.; Harris, S.B.; Vieth, R.; Knight, J.A.; Gerstein, H.C.; Perkins, B.A.; Zinman, B.; Hanley, A.J. Prospective associations of vitamin D with beta-cell function and glycemia: The PROspective Metabolism and ISlet cell Evaluation (PROMISE) cohort study. *Diabetes* **2011**, *60*, 2947–2953. [CrossRef] [PubMed]
33. Forouhi, N.G.; Ye, Z.; Rickard, A.P.; Khaw, K.T.; Luben, R.; Langenberg, C.; Wareham, N.J. Circulating 25-hydroxyvitamin D concentration and the risk of type 2 diabetes: Results from the European Prospective Investigation into Cancer (EPIC)-Norfolk cohort and updated meta-analysis of prospective studies. *Diabetologia* **2012**, *55*, 2173–2182. [CrossRef] [PubMed]

34. Afzal, S.; Bojesen, S.E.; Nordestgaard, B.G. Low 25-hydroxyvitamin D and risk of type 2 diabetes: A prospective cohort study and metaanalysis. *Clin. Chem.* **2013**, *59*, 381–391. [CrossRef]

35. Song, Y.; Wang, L.; Pittas, A.G.; Del Gobbo, L.C.; Zhang, C.; Manson, J.E.; Hu, F.B. Blood 25-hydroxy vitamin D levels and incident type 2 diabetes: A meta-analysis of prospective studies. *Diabetes Care* **2013**, *36*, 1422–1428. [CrossRef]

36. Park, S.K.; Garland, C.F.; Gorham, E.D.; BuDoff, L.; Barrett-Connor, E. Plasma 25-hydroxyvitamin D concentration and risk of type 2 diabetes and pre-diabetes: 12-year cohort study. *PLoS ONE* **2018**, *13*, e0193070. [CrossRef]

37. Avila-Rubio, V.; Garcia-Fontana, B.; Novo-Rodriguez, C.; Cantero-Hinojosa, J.; Reyes-Garcia, R.; Munoz-Torres, M. Higher Levels of Serum 25-Hydroxyvitamin D Are Related to Improved Glucose Homeostasis in Women with Postmenopausal Osteoporosis. *J. Women's Health* **2018**, *27*, 1007–1015. [CrossRef] [PubMed]

38. Zheng, J.-S.; Imamura, F.; Sharp, S.J.; van der Schouw, Y.T.; Sluijs, I.; Gundersen, T.E.; Ardanaz, E.; Boeing, H.; Bonet, C.; Gómez, J.H.; et al. Association of plasma vitamin D metabolites with incident type 2 diabetes: EPIC-InterAct case-cohort study. *J. Clin. Endocrinol. Metab.* **2019**, *104*, 1293–1303. [CrossRef]

39. Heath, A.K.; Williamson, E.J.; Hodge, A.M.; Ebeling, P.R.; Eyles, D.W.; Kvaskoff, D.; O'Dea, K.; Giles, G.G.; English, D.R. Vitamin D status and the risk of type 2 diabetes: The Melbourne Collaborative Cohort Study. *Diabetes Res. Clin. Pract.* **2018**, *149*, 179–187. [CrossRef] [PubMed]

40. Sollid, S.T.; Hutchinson, M.Y.S.; Fuskevag, O.M.; Figenschau, Y.; Joakimsen, R.M.; Schirmer, H.; Njolstad, I.; Svartberg, J.; Kamycheva, E.; Jorde, R. No effect of high-dose vitamin D supplementation on glycemic status or cardiovascular risk factors in subjects with prediabetes. *Diabetes Care* **2014**, *37*, 2123–2131. [CrossRef]

41. Forouhi, N.G.; Menon, R.K.; Sharp, S.J.; Mannan, N.; Timms, P.M.; Martineau, A.R.; Rickard, A.P.; Boucher, B.J.; Chowdhury, T.A.; Griffiths, C.J.; et al. Effects of vitamin D2 or D3 supplementation on glycaemic control and cardiometabolic risk among people at risk of type 2 diabetes: Results of a randomized double-blind placebo-controlled trial. *Diabetes Obes. Metab.* **2016**, *18*, 392–400. [CrossRef]

42. Griffin, S.J.; Little, P.S.; Hales, C.N.; Kinmonth, A.L.; Wareham, N.J. Diabetes risk score: Towards earlier detection of type 2 diabetes in general practice. *Diabetes. Metab. Res. Rev.* **2000**, *16*, 164–171. [CrossRef]

43. Davidson, M.B.; Duran, P.; Lee, M.L.; Friedman, T.C. High-dose vitamin D supplementation in people with prediabetes and hypovitaminosis D. *Diabetes Care* **2013**, *36*, 260–266. [CrossRef] [PubMed]

44. Gagnon, C.; Daly, R.M.; Carpentier, A.; Lu, Z.X.; Shore-Lorenti, C.; Sikaris, K.; Jean, S.; Ebeling, P.R. Effects of combined calcium and vitamin D supplementation on insulin secretion, insulin sensitivity and beta-cell function in multi-ethnic vitamin D-deficient adults at risk for type 2 diabetes: A pilot randomized, placebo-controlled trial. *PLoS ONE* **2014**, *9*, e109607. [CrossRef] [PubMed]

45. Oosterwerff, M.M.; Eekhoff, E.M.; Van Schoor, N.M.; Boeke, A.J.P.; Nanayakkara, P.; Meijnen, R.; Knol, D.L.; Kramer, M.H.; Lips, P. Effect of moderate-dose vitamin D supplementation on insulin sensitivity in vitamin D-deficient non-Western immigrants in the Netherlands: A randomized placebo-controlled trial. *Am. J. Clin. Nutr.* **2014**, *100*, 152–160. [CrossRef] [PubMed]

46. Salehpour, A.; Shidfar, F.; Hosseinpanah, F.; Vafa, M.; Razaghi, M.; Amiri, F. Does vitamin D3 supplementation improve glucose homeostasis in overweight or obese women? A double-blind, randomized, placebo-controlled clinical trial. *Diabet. Med.* **2013**, *30*, 1477–1481. [CrossRef] [PubMed]

47. Tuomainen, T.-P.; Virtanen, J.K.; Voutilainen, S.; Nurmi, T.; Mursu, J.; de Mello, V.D.F.; Schwab, U.; Hakumaki, M.; Pulkki, K.; Uusitupa, M. Glucose Metabolism Effects of Vitamin D in Prediabetes: The VitDmet Randomized Placebo-Controlled Supplementation Study. *J. Diabetes Res.* **2015**, *2015*, 672653. [CrossRef] [PubMed]

48. Wagner, H.; Alvarsson, M.; Mannheimer, B.; Degerblad, M.; Ostenson, C.-G. No Effect of High-Dose Vitamin D Treatment on beta-Cell Function, Insulin Sensitivity, or Glucose Homeostasis in Subjects With Abnormal Glucose Tolerance: A Randomized Clinical Trial. *Diabetes Care* **2016**, *39*, 345–352. [CrossRef]

49. Von Hurst, P.R.; Stonehouse, W.; Coad, J. Vitamin D supplementation reduces insulin resistance in South Asian women living in New Zealand who are insulin resistant and vitamin D deficient—A randomised, placebo-controlled trial. *Br. J. Nutr.* **2010**, *103*, 549. [CrossRef]

50. Mitri, J.; Dawson-Hughes, B.; Hu, F.B.; Pittas, A.G. Effects of vitamin D and calcium supplementation on pancreatic beta cell function, insulin sensitivity, and glycemia in adults at high risk of diabetes: The Calcium and Vitamin D for Diabetes Mellitus (CaDDM) randomized controlled trial. *Am. J. Clin. Nutr.* **2011**, *94*, 486–494. [CrossRef]

51. Manson, J.E.; Cook, N.R.; Lee, I.-M.; Christen, W.; Bassuk, S.S.; Mora, S.; Gibson, H.; Gordon, D.; Copeland, T.; D'Agostino, D.; et al. Vitamin D Supplements and Prevention of Cancer and Cardiovascular Disease. *N. Engl. J. Med.* **2018**, *380*, 33–44. [CrossRef]

52. Rafiq, S.; Jeppesen, P.B. Body mass index, vitamin d, and type 2 diabetes: A systematic review and meta-analysis. *Nutrients* **2018**, *10*, 1182. [CrossRef]

53. Tang, H.; Li, D.; Li, Y.; Zhang, X.; Song, Y.; Li, X. Effects of Vitamin D Supplementation on Glucose and Insulin Homeostasis and Incident Diabetes among Nondiabetic Adults: A Meta-Analysis of Randomized Controlled Trials. *Int. J. Endocrinol.* **2018**, *2018*, 7908764. [CrossRef] [PubMed]

54. LeBlanc, E.S.; Pratley, R.E.; Dawson-Hughes, B.; Staten, M.A.; Sheehan, P.R.; Lewis, M.R.; Peters, A.; Kim, S.H.; Chatterjee, R.; Aroda, V.R.; et al. Baseline Characteristics of the Vitamin D and Type 2 Diabetes (D2d) Study: A Contemporary Prediabetes Cohort That Will Inform Diabetes Prevention Efforts. *Diabetes Care* **2018**, *41*, 1590–1599. [CrossRef] [PubMed]

55. Belenchia, A.M.; Tosh, A.K.; Hillman, L.S.; Peterson, C.A. Correcting vitamin D insufficiency improves insulin sensitivity in obese adolescents: A randomized controlled trial. *Am. J. Clin. Nutr.* **2013**, *97*, 774–781. [CrossRef] [PubMed]

56. Jorde, R.; Sneve, M.; Torjesen, P.; Figenschau, Y. No improvement in cardiovascular risk factors in overweight and obese subjects after supplementation with vitamin D3 for 1 year. *J. Intern. Med.* **2010**, *267*, 462–472. [CrossRef] [PubMed]

57. Pittas, A.G.; Lau, J.; Hu, F.B.; Dawson-Hughes, B. The Role of Vitamin D and Calcium in Type 2 Diabetes. A Systematic Review and Meta-Analysis. *J. Clin. Endocrinol. Metab.* **2007**, *92*, 2017–2029. [CrossRef]

58. Ojuka, E.O. Role of calcium and AMP kinase in the regulation of mitochondrial biogenesis and GLUT4 levels in muscle. *Proc. Nutr. Soc.* **2004**, *63*, 275–278. [CrossRef] [PubMed]

59. Milner, R.D.G.; Hales, C.N. The role of calcium and magnesium in insulin secretion from rabbit pancreas studied in vitro. *Diabetologia* **1967**, *3*, 47–49. [CrossRef]

60. Zemel, M.B. Nutritional and endocrine modulation of intracellular calcium: Implications in obesity, insulin resistance and hypertension. *Mol. Cell. Biochem.* **1998**, *188*, 129–136. [CrossRef]

61. Dunlop, T.W.; Väisänen, S.; Frank, C.; Molnár, F.; Sinkkonen, L.; Carlberg, C. The Human Peroxisome Proliferator-activated Receptor δ Gene is a Primary Target of 1α,25-Dihydroxyvitamin D3 and its Nuclear Receptor. *J. Mol. Biol.* **2005**, *349*, 248–260. [CrossRef]

62. Mozaffarian, D.; Cao, H.; King, I.B.; Lemaitre, R.N.; Song, X.; Siscovick, D.S.; Hotamisligil, G.S. Trans-Palmitoleic Acid, Metabolic Risk Factors, and New-Onset Diabetes in U.S. Adults. *Ann. Intern. Med.* **2010**, *153*, 790. [CrossRef] [PubMed]

63. Mozaffarian, D.; de Oliveira Otto, M.C.; Lemaitre, R.N.; Fretts, A.M.; Hotamisligil, G.; Tsai, M.Y.; Siscovick, D.S.; Nettleton, J.A. trans-Palmitoleic acid, other dairy fat biomarkers, and incident diabetes: The Multi-Ethnic Study of Atherosclerosis (MESA). *Am. J. Clin. Nutr.* **2013**, *97*, 854–861. [CrossRef] [PubMed]

64. Kratz, M.; Baars, T.; Guyenet, S. The relationship between high-fat dairy consumption and obesity, cardiovascular, and metabolic disease. *Eur. J. Nutr.* **2013**, *52*, 1–24. [CrossRef] [PubMed]

65. Alhazmi, A.; Stojanovski, E.; McEvoy, M.; Garg, M.L. Macronutrient Intakes and Development of Type 2 Diabetes: A Systematic Review and Meta-Analysis of Cohort Studies. *J. Am. Coll. Nutr.* **2012**, *31*, 243–258. [CrossRef] [PubMed]

66. Givens, D.I.; Beswick, A.D.; Fehily, A.M.; Pickering, J.E.; Gallacher, J. The Survival Advantage of Milk and Dairy Consumption: An Overview of Evidence from Cohort Studies of Vascular Diseases, Diabetes and Cancer AU—Elwood, Peter C. *J. Am. Coll. Nutr.* **2008**, *27*, 723S–734S.

67. Tong, X.; Dong, J.-Y.; Wu, Z.-W.; Li, W.; Qin, L.-Q. Dairy consumption and risk of type 2 diabetes mellitus: A meta-analysis of cohort studies. *Eur. J. Clin. Nutr.* **2011**, *65*, 1027. [CrossRef]

68. Soedamah-Muthu, S.S.; Masset, G.; Verberne, L.; Geleijnse, J.M.; Brunner, E.J. Consumption of dairy products and associations with incident diabetes, CHD and mortality in the Whitehall II study. *Br. J. Nutr.* **2013**, *109*, 718–726. [CrossRef] [PubMed]

69. Struijk, E.A.; Heraclides, A.; Witte, D.R.; Soedamah-Muthu, S.S.; Geleijnse, J.M.; Toft, U.; Lau, C.J. Dairy product intake in relation to glucose regulation indices and risk of type 2 diabetes. *Nutr. Metab. Cardiovasc. Dis.* **2013**, *23*, 822–828. [CrossRef]

70. Fumeron, F.; Lamri, A.; Abi Khalil, C.; Jaziri, R.; Porchay-Baldérelli, I.; Lantieri, O.; Vol, S.; Balkau, B.; Marre, M. Dairy Consumption and the Incidence of Hyperglycemia and the Metabolic Syndrome. *Diabetes Care* **2011**, *34*, 813–817. [CrossRef] [PubMed]

71. Sluijs, I.; Forouhi, N.G.; Beulens, J.W.J.; van der Schouw, Y.T.; Agnoli, C.; Arriola, L.; Balkau, B.; Barricarte, A.; Boeing, H.; Bueno-de-Mesquita, H.B.; et al. The amount and type of dairy product intake and incident type 2 diabetes: Results from the EPIC-InterAct Study. *Am. J. Clin. Nutr.* **2012**, *96*, 382–390.

72. Pittas, A.G.; Dawson-Hughes, B.; Li, T.; Van Dam, R.M.; Willett, W.C.; Manson, J.E.; Hu, F.B. Vitamin D and calcium intake in relation to type 2 diabetes in women. *Diabetes Care* **2006**, *29*, 650–656. [CrossRef] [PubMed]

73. Van Dam, R.M.; Hu, F.B.; Rosenberg, L.; Krishnan, S.; Palmer, J.R. Dietary calcium and magnesium, major food sources, and risk of type 2 diabetes in U.S. black women. *Diabetes Care* **2006**, *29*, 2238–2243. [CrossRef] [PubMed]

74. Villegas, R.; Gao, Y.-T.; Dai, Q.; Yang, G.; Cai, H.; Li, H.; Zheng, W.; Shu, X.O. Dietary calcium and magnesium intakes and the risk of type 2 diabetes: The Shanghai Women's Health Study. *Am. J. Clin. Nutr.* **2009**, *89*, 1059–1067. [CrossRef]

75. Kirii, K.; Mizoue, T.; Iso, H.; Takahashi, Y.; Kato, M.; Inoue, M.; Noda, M.; Tsugane, S. Calcium, vitamin D and dairy intake in relation to type 2 diabetes risk in a Japanese cohort. *Diabetologia* **2009**, *52*, 2542–2550. [CrossRef] [PubMed]

76. Oh, J.M.; Woo, H.W.; Kim, M.K.; Lee, Y.-H.; Shin, D.H.; Shin, M.-H.; Choi, B.Y. Dietary total, animal, vegetable calcium and type 2 diabetes incidence among Korean adults: The Korean Multi-Rural Communities Cohort (MRCohort). *Nutr. Metab. Cardiovasc. Dis.* **2017**, *27*, 1152–1164. [CrossRef] [PubMed]

77. Gagnon, C.; Lu, Z.X.; Magliano, D.J.; Dunstan, D.W.; Shaw, J.E.; Zimmet, P.Z.; Sikaris, K.; Grantham, N.; Ebeling, P.R.; Daly, R.M. Serum 25-hydroxyvitamin D, calcium intake, and risk of type 2 diabetes after 5 years: Results from a national, population-based prospective study (the Australian diabetes, obesity and lifestyle study). *Diabetes Care* **2011**, *34*, 1133–1138. [CrossRef]

78. Reyes-Garcia, R.; Mendoza, N.; Palacios, S.; Salas, N.; Quesada-Charneco, M.; Garcia-Martin, A.; Fonolla, J.; Lara-Villoslada, F.; Muñoz-Torres, M. Effects of Daily Intake of Calcium and Vitamin D-Enriched Milk in Healthy Postmenopausal Women: A Randomized, Controlled, Double-Blind Nutritional Study. *J. Women's Heal.* **2018**, *27*, 561–568. [CrossRef]

79. Grantham, N.M.; Magliano, D.J.; Hodge, A.; Jowett, J.; Meikle, P.; Shaw, J.E. The association between dairy food intake and the incidence of diabetes in Australia: The Australian Diabetes Obesity and Lifestyle Study (AusDiab). *Public Health Nutr.* **2013**, *16*, 339–345. [CrossRef]

80. Malik, V.S.; Sun, Q.; van Dam, R.M.; Rimm, E.B.; Willett, W.C.; Rosner, B.; Hu, F.B. Adolescent dairy product consumption and risk of type 2 diabetes in middle-aged women1–3. *Am. J. Clin. Nutr.* **2011**, *94*, 854–861. [CrossRef]

81. Dehghan, M.; Mente, A.; Rangarajan, S.; Sheridan, P.; Mohan, V.; Iqbal, R.; Gupta, R.; Lear, S.; Wentzel-Viljoen, E.; Avezum, A.; et al. Association of dairy intake with cardiovascular disease and mortality in 21 countries from five continents (PURE): A prospective cohort study. *Lancet* **2018**, *392*, 2288–2297. [CrossRef]

82. Rideout, T.C.; Marinangeli, C.P.F.; Martin, H.; Browne, R.W.; Rempel, C.B. Consumption of low-fat dairy foods for 6 months improves insulin resistance without adversely affecting lipids or bodyweight in healthy adults: A randomized free-living cross-over study. *Nutr. J.* **2013**, *12*, 56. [CrossRef] [PubMed]

83. Aune, D.; Norat, T.; Romundstad, P.; Vatten, L.J. Dairy products and the risk of type 2 diabetes: A systematic review and dose-response meta-analysis of cohort studies. *Am. J. Clin. Nutr.* **2013**, *98*, 1066–1083. [CrossRef] [PubMed]

84. Krebs-Smith, S.M.; Guenther, P.M.; Subar, A.F.; Kirkpatrick, S.I.; Dodd, K.W. Americans do not meet federal dietary recommendations. *J. Nutr.* **2010**, *140*, 1832–1838. [CrossRef]

85. Liu, A.-D.; Zhang, B.; DU, W.-W.; Wang, H.-J.; Su, C.; Zhai, F.-Y. Milk consumption and its changing trend of Chinese adult aged 18–44 in nine provinces (autonomous region) from 1991 to 2006. *Zhonghua Yu Fang Yi Xue Za Zhi* **2011**, *45*, 304–309. [PubMed]

86. NIH Consensus conference. Optimal calcium intake. NIH Consensus Development Panel on Optimal Calcium Intake. *JAMA* **1994**, *272*, 1942–1948. [CrossRef]

87. Ross, A.C.; Taylor, C.L.; Yaktine, A.L.; Del Valle, H.B. (Eds.) *Dietary Reference Intakes for Calcium and Vitamin D*; National Academies Press: Washington, DC, USA, 2012; Volume 130, ISBN 978-0-309-16394-1.

88. Rosen, C.J.; Abrams, S.A.; Aloia, J.F.; Brannon, P.M.; Clinton, S.K.; Durazo-Arvizu, R.A.; Gallagher, J.C.; Gallo, R.L.; Jones, G.; Kovacs, C.S.; et al. IOM Committee Members Respond to Endocrine Society Vitamin D Guideline. *J. Clin. Endocrinol. Metab.* **2012**, *97*, 1146–1152. [CrossRef] [PubMed]

89. Scragg, R. Emerging Evidence of Thresholds for Beneficial Effects from Vitamin D Supplementation. *Nutrients* **2018**, *10*, 561. [CrossRef] [PubMed]

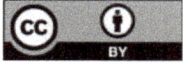

nutrients

Article

Cardiovascular Risk Factors and Their Association with Vitamin D Deficiency in Mexican Women of Reproductive Age

Alejandra Contreras-Manzano⬡, Salvador Villalpando *⬡, Claudia García-Díaz and Mario Flores-Aldana⬡

Center for Nutrition and Health Research, National Institute of Public Health, Cuernavaca 62100, Mexico; alejandra.contreras@insp.mx (A.C.-M.); clauw.g.diaz@gmail.com (C.G.-D.); mario.flores@insp.mx (M.F.-A.)
* Correspondence: svillalp@insp.mx; Tel.: +52-777-329-3000

Received: 13 March 2019; Accepted: 8 May 2019; Published: 28 May 2019

Abstract: Based on a nationally representative sample of young Mexican women aged 20 to 49 years (n = 3260), we sought to explore whether cardiovascular risk factors and acute myocardial infarction (AMI) were associated with vitamin D deficiency (VDD, defined as 25-OH-D <50 nmol/L). To this end, we obtained sociodemographic, serum and anthropometric data from the 2012 National Health and Nutrition Survey (ENSANUT 2012). Analyses were developed through logistic regression models adjusted for potential confounders. The prevalence of VDD was significantly higher in obese women (42.5%, 95% CI; 37.3–47.9) compared to women with a normal body mass index (29.9%, 95% CI; 23.5–37.1, p = 0.05), in those with high total cholesterol (TC) (45.6% 95% CI; 39.4–51.9) compared to those with normal TC levels (33.9%, 95% CI 30–38.1, p = 0.03), and in those with insulin resistance (IR) (44%, 95% CI; 36.9–51.7) or type 2 diabetes mellitus (T2DM) (58.6%, 95% CI 46.9–69.4) compared to those with normal glycemia (no insulin resistance: 34.7%, 95% CI; 30.9–38.8, p = 0.04 and no T2DM: 34.9%, 95% CI 31.4–38.6, p < 0.001). Utilizing individual models to estimate cardiovascular risk according to VDD, we found that the odds of being obese (odds ratio, OR: 1.53, 95% CI 1.02–2.32, p = 0.05), or having high TC levels (OR: 1.43, 95% CI; 1.05–2.01, p = 0.03), T2DM (OR: 2.64, 95% CI; 1.65–4.03, p < 0.001), or IR (OR: 1.48, 95% CI 1.04–2.10, p = 0.026) were significantly higher in women with VDD (p < 0.05). Odds were not statistically significant for overweight, high blood pressure, sedentarism, AMI, high serum concentration of triglycerides, homocysteine, or C-reactive protein models. In conclusion, our results indicate that young Mexican women with VDD show a higher prevalence of cardiovascular risk factors.

Keywords: vitamin D deficiency; 25-OH-D; women; cardiovascular risk factors; T2DM; obesity

---

1. Introduction

Receptors for vitamin D (VD) and VD activity have been found in many body tissues, suggesting non-calcemic effects of VD related to the regulation of cell proliferation and differentiation, immune response, insulin production, and insulin sensitivity [1–3]. These recognized actions of VD suggest that VD plays a role in the prevention of many chronic diseases such as cancer and cardiovascular disease (CVD) [4], but observational studies have not consistently found any association between VD deficiency (VDD) and chronic conditions such as type 2 diabetes mellitus (T2DM), metabolic syndrome, high blood pressure (HBP), and other cardiovascular risk factors [5–9]. Moreover, several supplementation experiments aimed at preventing pathologies associated with VDD have been carried out, but they have yielded contradictory results as regards to the association of VDD with obesity, insulin sensitivity, and insulin secretion, casting doubt on the association of these conditions with VDD [10–12].

In 2013, the three leading causes of disability-adjusted life years (DALYs) in Mexico were diabetes, ischemic heart disease, and chronic kidney disease, with fasting plasma glucose, high body-mass index (BMI), and HBP being the main risk factors [13]. It is crucial to understand the role of VDD in the occurrence of cardiovascular disease, particularly among young women, in order to help prevent negative health consequences not only for these women in the form of osteoporosis, preeclampsia, or chronic diseases [14,15], but also for their infants, whose bone health and neurological development are influenced by the VD status of their mothers [16,17].

Although little research has been performed concerning VDD in women of reproductive age [18], it is well known that long lactation periods and the use of sunscreen constitute risk factors for middle-aged and elderly women [19,20]. Studies in Mexico have revealed high rates of VDD among children and women of reproductive age (≈36%), with an even higher prevalence observed in the presence of obesity, in urban areas and in subjects with low dietary intake of VD [21,22].

A recent cohort study in Mexico documented an inverse association between VD intake and cardiovascular risk factors among adults; however, the sample was not nationally representative and 25-OH-D levels were not measured [23]. In addition, most international reports on the relationship between VDD and cardiovascular risks have not addressed several cardiovascular risks together, and few research efforts have focused on young and/or non-pregnant women [6]. Therefore, the objective of this study, conducted among a probabilistic national sample of Mexican women of reproductive age (20 to 49 years old), was to explore whether VDD was associated with sedentarism, overweight, obesity, T2DM, insulin resistance (IR), HBP, high total cholesterol (TC), low high-density lipoprotein cholesterol (HDL-C), high triglycerides (TGs), high homocysteine (Hcy) or C-reactive protein (CRP), and acute myocardial infarction (AMI).

2. Materials and Methods

Study population: This analysis was performed among a sample of 3260 women participating in the 2012 National Health and Nutrition Survey (ENSANUT 2012). The ENSANUT 2012 was a probabilistic population-based survey stratified by cluster and representative at the national, regional and urban/rural levels [24]. A detailed description of its sampling method has been published previously [25]. We analyzed the VD data of 3260 women aged 20–49 years with complete information on T2DM, serum concentrations of TC, HDL-C, TG, CRP, IR, and high levels of Hcy.

2.1. Sociodemographic Information

Sociodemographic information was collected using validated questionnaires. A Well-Being Index (WBI) was constructed according to the characteristics of and the property owned by households in a principal component analysis. The first component, representing 40% of total variability with a lambda of 3.4, was divided into tertiles in order to classify the WBI as low, medium, and high [26]. Localities with fewer than 2500 inhabitants were defined as rural and otherwise as urban. As in previous ENSANUTs, the country was divided into three regions: north, center (including Mexico City), and south. An individual was defined as indigenous where one of the members of the household spoke an indigenous language as his/her mother tongue.

2.2. Anthropometry

Body weight was measured using an electronic scale with a precision of 100 g, (Tanita Co., Tokyo, Japan), and height using a stadiometer with a precision of 1 mm (Dynatop, Mexico City). These measurements were performed by specialized personnel utilizing the Lohman method [27], and were standardized according to the Habitch method [28].

2.3. Blood Samples

Eight-hour-fasting blood samples were drawn from the winter of 2011 to the spring of 2012, between the latitudes of 14° 54' and 32° 31' N. Blood samples were drawn from an antecubital vein and collected in evacuated tubes. Serum was separated by in situ spinning-down at 3000 g. Serum samples were immediately stored in codified cryovials and preserved in liquid nitrogen until delivery to the Central Nutrition Laboratory at the National Institute of Public Health (INSP), in Cuernavaca, Morelos, Mexico. Thereafter, the samples were preserved at −70°C in a deep freezer until chemical analysis.

A chemiluminescence microparticle immunoassay was used to measure serum 25-OH-D, with intra- and inter-assay coefficient-of-variation (CV) results of 1.34 and 3.69%, respectively. This method has proved acceptable compared to LC/MS/MS ($r = 0.73$) [29]. Quality control was performed according to the reference standard serum NIST 968E of the National Institute of Standards & Technology. The serum concentrations of TC were measured using an enzymatic and oxidation method, glucose by the glucose oxidase technique, HDL-C by direct enzymatic assay after eliminating chylomicrons from the sample, TG by lipase hydrolysis, and Hcy and CRP using ultrasensitive monoclonal antibodies in an Architect CI8200 automatic analyzer (Abbott Lab, Michigan, MI, USA). The intra- and inter-assay CV results were 1.05 and 1.97% for glucose, 2.2% and 5.7% for TC, 3.5% and 5.02% for TG, 5.3 and 7.4% for HDL-C, 3.7% and 4.6% for Hcy, and 0% and 1.2% for CRP, respectively. For insulin, the intra-assay CV was 1.28 uU/mL.

2.4. Vitamin D Deficiency

VDD was defined as a serum level of 25-OH-D <50 nmol/L (<20 ng/mL), as in most studies in Latin America [3,30].

2.5. Definitions of Outcome Variables

T2DM was defined as diabetes previously diagnosed by a physician or a fasting blood glucose level of ≥126 mg/dL [31].

Serum biomarkers. The following were considered abnormal serum concentrations: TC >200 mg/dL, TG >150 mg/dL, and HDL-C ≤50 mg/dL [32]. Hcy >10.4 nmol/L was considered abnormal [33]. Inflammation was determined where CRP was >5 mg/dL [34], and IR was defined when homeostatic model assessment of IR (HOMA-IR) was ≥3.8 [35].

Overweight and obesity were based on the body mass index (BMI) as classified by the WHO guidelines (normal BMI ≤24.9 kg/m², overweight 25–29.9 kg/m², and obesity >30 kg/m²) [36].

HBP was defined as a previous diagnosis by a physician of hypertension or a systolic blood pressure >140 mmHg and/or a diastolic blood pressure >90 mmHg [37].

AMI was defined when acute myocardial infarction was self-reported by the subject.

Sedentarism. A lifestyle was defined as sedentary where a woman was classified as having low physical activity according to a validated International Physical Activity Questionnaires (IPAQ) [38].

2.6. Statistical Analysis

VDD prevalence rates were reported as proportions with a confidence interval (CI) of 95%; risks were expressed as odds ratios (ORs) with a CI of 95%. The significance level was established at an alpha <0.05, and regression models were adjusted by age, BMI, dwelling (urban/rural), geographical region, ethnicity, WBI, and sedentarism, as well as by the survey design, using the module SVY of STATA SE v14 (College Station, TX, USA, 2013).

Ethical aspects. The ENSANUT 2012 protocol was reviewed and approved by the Research, Ethics and Biosecurity Committees of the National Institute of Public Health in Mexico. Prior informed consent letters were signed by all participants.

3. Results

3.1. Characteristics of the Sample

Serum 25-OH-D levels were estimated for 3260 women representing 19 million Mexican women, aged 20–49 years. In this subsample, 33.4% suffered from overweight, 36.4% from obesity and 25% were sedentary. The prevalence rates for T2DM and HPB were 7.6% and 19.5%, respectively. The overall prevalence of cardiovascular risk factors was 48.3%, and within this group, 80.9% had a low HDL-C, 37.1% high TC, 37.1% high TG, 11.8% high Hcy, and 21.6% high CRP (Table 1).

Table 1. Characteristics and distribution of the sample.

Variable	Subgroup	% (95% CI) *
Age (years)	20–29	36.2 (33, 39.6)
	30–39	37.1 (33.8, 40.5)
	40–49	26.8 (24.2, 29.6)
Dwelling	Rural	21.5 (19.7, 23.4)
	Urban	78.6 (76.7, 80.4)
Region of the country	North	22.4 (20.7, 24.2)
	Center	47.7 (45.2, 50.2)
	South	30.1 (27.9, 32.3)
Well-Being Index	Tertile 1 (lower)	25.5 (23.2, 27.9)
	Tertile 2	31.6 (28.8, 34.6)
	Tertile 3 (higher)	43.1 (39.7, 46.6)
Ethnicity	No	94.7 (93.4, 95.7)
	Yes	5.3 (4.3, 6.6)
BMI category	Normal	30.3 (27.2, 33.5)
	Overweight	33.4 (30.4, 36.6)
	Obesity	36.4 (33.4, 39.6)
Sedentarism	No	70.4 (67.2, 73.3)
	Yes	29.6 (26.7, 32.8)
T2DM	No	92.4 (90.4, 94.0)
	Yes	7.6 (6.0, 9.7)
HBP	No	87.9 (85.3, 90.0)
	Yes	19.5 (17.0, 22.3)
TC	<200 mg/dL	75.8 (72.8, 78.6)
	≥200 mg/dL	24.2 (21.5, 27.2)
HDL-C	≥50 mg/dL	19.1 (16.3, 22.2)
	<50 mg/dL	80.9 (77.7, 83.7)
TG	<150 mg/dL	62.9 (59.8, 66.0)
	≥150 mg/dL	37.1 (34.0, 40.3)
AMI	No	98.7 (98.2, 99.1)
	Yes	1.20 (0.81, 1.76)
Hcy	<10.4 nmol/L	87.9 (85.3, 90.0)
	≥10.4 nmol/L	12.1 (9.9, 14.6)
IR	<3.8 HOMA-IR	79.4 (76.2, 82.3)
	≥3.8 HOMA-IR	20.6 (17.7, 23.8)
CRP	<5 g/L	78.4 (75.8, 80.9)
	≥ 5 g/L	21.6 (19.1, 24.2)

N sample = 3260, n expanded = 19,336,909. CI: Confidence Interval; BMI: body mass index; T2DM: type 2 diabetes mellitus; HBP: high blood pressure; TC: total cholesterol; HDL-C: high-density lipoprotein; TG: triglycerides; AMI: acute myocardial infarction; Hcy: homocysteine; IR: insulin resistance; CRP: C-reactive protein * Expanded % and 95% CI.

3.2. Prevalence of VDD

The overall prevalence of VDD was 37.2%, significantly higher among women with T2DM compared to women without it (58.6% vs. 34.5%, $p < 0.05$). VDD was also higher among women with obesity (42.5%) vs. normal BMI (29.9%, $p < 0.05$), and with high TC (45.6 vs. 33.9%, $p < 0.05$) and high TG (41.7 vs. 33.8%, $p < 0.09$). No differences emerged regarding the relationships between VDD prevalence and the other cardiovascular risk factors evaluated independently (Figure 1).

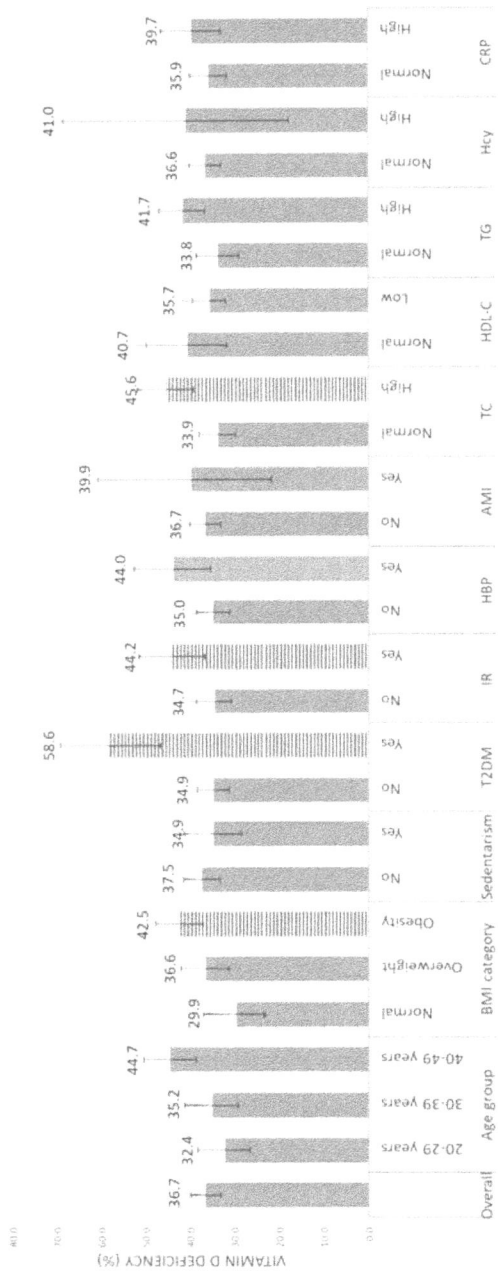

Figure 1. Adjusted prevalence (and 95% confidence interval) of vitamin D deficiency by age group and cardiovascular risk factor among Mexican women aged 20–49 years. BMI: body mass index; T2DM: type 2 diabetes mellitus; IR: insulin resistance; HBP: high blood pressure; TC: total cholesterol; HDL-C: high density lipoprotein; TG: triglycerides; AMI: acute myocardial infarction; Hcy: homocysteine; CRP: C-reactive protein. Horizontal bars indicate a statistical difference (p value < 0.05) among vitamin-D-deficiency prevalence rates in the subcategories. Reference subcategories are 20–29 years for age group; "Normal" for BMI, TC, HDL-C, TG, Hcy, and CRP; and "No" for sedentarism, T2DM, IR, HBP, and AMI. Logistic regression model was adjusted by area (urban/rurality), region of the country, Wellbeing index tertiles, ethnicity and all cardiovascular risk factors.

3.3. Cardiovascular Risk Factors and VDD

We analyzed adjusted logistic models introducing each chronic non-communicable disease and cardiovascular risk factor as dependent variables together with VDD as the independent variable (Figure 2 and Table S1). We found that the risk of obesity was significantly higher in women with VDD (OR: 1.53, $p < 0.05$) than in women without. The risk was also higher when IR (OR: 1.48, $p < 0.05$), T2DM (OR: 2.58, $p < 0.05$) or high TC (OR: 1.45, $p < 0.05$) was present. These models were adjusted by other cardiovascular risk factors as confounding variables. No association was significant between VDD and the rest of the cardiovascular risk factors.

In estimating the prevalence of severe VDD (<20 nmol/L), we found that it was notably low (2.3%, 95% CI 1.3–3.9) and had no significant relationship with cardiovascular outcomes (data not shown). We also tested interactions between VDD and age, BMI and sedentarism, and stratified analysis by oral use of hypoglycemic ($n = 154$), antihypertensive ($n = 129$), and hypolipemic drugs ($n = 210$), as well as by menstrual cycle status, and no impact was observed; therefore, the results were not presented.

4. Discussion

Our study found that VDD was associated with a higher risk for T2DM, obesity, and high TC concentrations in young Mexican women. The major finding of our analysis was the strong association between VDD and a greater risk of T2DM, a result also yielded by other cross-sectional studies [39–42]. On the other hand, some published clinical trials have reported an association between VDD and increased insulin resistance, metabolic syndrome hyperglycemia [43–45], while others have not [12,46].

Several researchers have found an association between intake of VD and calcium and the prevention of T2DM [11]. Other researchers have administered cholecalciferol weekly for six months and found no difference in insulin response or insulin sensitivity in adults at risk of diabetes mellitus [12]. However, for those with prediabetes, VD supplementation has been shown to improve insulin sensitivity [12,47]. Such an effect could be the result of the interaction of calcium fluxes with the VD receptors in the β-cells, needed for the optimal secretion of insulin [48,49]. 25-OH-D induces synchronous Ca^{2+} oscillations with a pattern of pulsatile insulin secretion from the β-cells [50,51]. This may explain the lower level of insulin sensitivity and secretion, as well as all levels of glucose intolerance. Our study showed that IR was significantly associated with VDD and T2DM.

An association between VDD and increased adiposity among Mexican women has previously been demonstrated [22]. Our analysis revealed that VDD was 12.6 percentage points higher in obese women than in those with a normal BMI. We hypothesized that such an association could increase the risk for high rates of TSDM, metabolic syndrome, hypertension, and dyslipidemias found in the Mexican population [52,53]. However, it is not yet known if VDD is a cause or a consequence of obesity in humans, and an ample review of the literature provides evidence for both arguments [54].

Although subjects with a higher BMI had greater skin exposure for VD conversion, an experimental exposure to UV rays produced half the amount of serum VD in women with a high as opposed to a normal BMI [55]. Thus, it is possible that the amount of VD previously contained in the body fat of obese women was large enough to interfere with the conversion or incorporation of 25-OH-D into the serum pool. In a clinical trial involving calcium and VD supplements among overweight and obese individuals, was observed a significant reduction of visceral fat [56]. Obese subjects have greater adipose stores of VD. This enlarged adipose mass in obese individuals serves as a VD reservoir, and the increased amount of VD required to saturate this depot may predispose obese individuals to have an inadequate level of 25-OH-D [57].

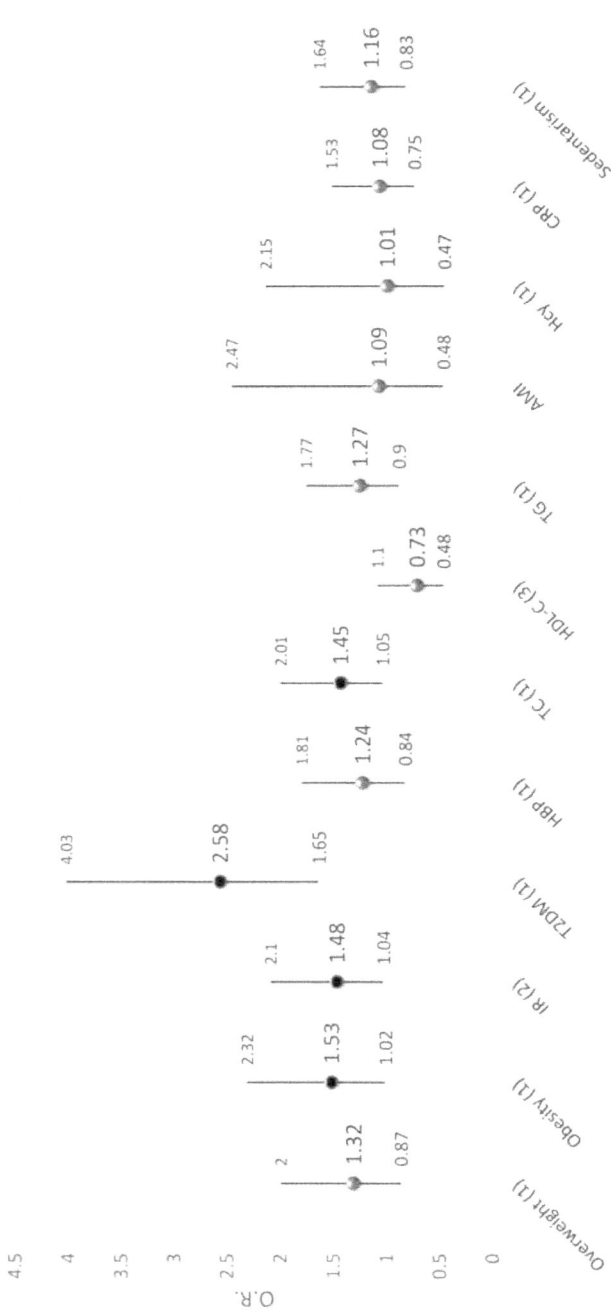

Figure 2. Odds ratios (OR) and 95% confidence interval adjusted for cardiovascular risk factors by vitamin D deficiency in Mexican women aged 20–49 years. BMI: body mass index; PA: physical activity; T2DM: type 2 diabetes mellitus; IR: insulin resistance; HBP: high blood pressure; TC: total cholesterol; HDL-C: high-density lipoprotein; TG: triglycerides; AMI: acute myocardial infarction; Hcy: homocysteine; CRP: C-reactive protein. (1) All models were adjusted by area (urban/rurality), region of the country, Wellbeing index tertiles, ethnicity and the following risk factor variables: HDL-C (<50 mg/dL), TG (<150 mg/dL), TC (<200 mg/dL), HBP, T2DM, CRP (<5 mg/dL), Hcy (<10 umol/L), sedentarism, overweight–obesity, IR, and AMI, except by the risk factor studied in the particular model. (2) Adjusted by all variables in model 1 excluding T2DM. (3) Adjusted by all variables in model 1 excluding TC. Black circle indicate a statistical difference (*p* value < 0.05).

Our study found that women with VDD had a 1.43 times greater risk (95% CI 1.03–1.99) for high levels of TC compared to women with sufficient VD concentrations ($p = 0.04$). This may be a result of the suppressive effect of VD on the parathyroid hormone (PTH), which reduces lipolysis. Similarly, it has been suggested that VD increases calcium concentrations, reducing the synthesis de novo and releasing hepatic TG [58]. Observational studies have reported that women with VDD have a higher risk of lipid concentration as compared to women with adequate VD status [59–61]. However, in a meta-analysis involving 12 clinical trials with 1346 subjects, VD supplementation was associated with improved LDL-C concentrations, but not with improved TG, HDL-C or TC levels [62]. Meanwhile, a recent randomized controlled trial in postmenopausal women showed positive effects in VD status, bone mineral density, glucose, TC, LDL-C, and apolipoprotein B100 after 24 months of intake of vitamin D-enriched milk [63].

Our study found no association between HBP and VDD, reflecting the findings of other studies [64,65]. However, some observational and randomized clinical trials have found a negative correlation between the two variables [66,67].

The cross-sectional nature of the 2012 ENSANUT makes it difficult to establish causality. However, our results are representative for the entire population of Mexican women aged 20–49 years and for countries with similar socioeconomic characteristics. Another limitation was that data for some variables were collected by means of self-reporting, potentially introducing a degree of measurement bias. Nonetheless, data for all variables were collected in a similar manner; thus, the bias will not affect results for the target population, and the results might even underestimate a potential association. In our analyses, we adjusted results by menstrual cycle status with no significant alteration in the associations, but we were unable to adjust by the current use of estrogen-containing contraception that has been associated with increases in 25-OH-D levels in other populations [19,68]. Nevertheless, in our sample 88% of women had been pregnant and 28% had been sterilized after childbirth. According to the National Survey Report, in 2012 the rate of use of hormonal contraceptives among Mexican women was 12.5% for those aged 20–29 years old, 7.3% among 30–39 year-olds, and 4.6 among 35–49 year-olds, while 42% to 53% reported not using any contraceptive method [69]. Among the strengths of this study is its population-based sample, that allows for representativeness for Mexican women 20–49 years, and the fact that the study includes information on VD serum levels and CVD risk factors.

5. Conclusions

The prevalence of VDD among women 20 to 49 years old is a public health problem in Mexico. Obesity, T2DM, IR, and high TC were found to be associated with VDD. Further research is necessary to assess the biological mechanisms underlying all of these factors and their association with VDD. Also, this study provides scientific evidence supporting the need for public health and nutrition interventions aimed at improving the vitamin D status of Mexican women.

Supplementary Materials: The following are available online at http://www.mdpi.com/2072-6643/11/6/1211/s1, Table S1: Multivariate logistic regression models for cardiovascular risk factors by Vitamin D Deficiency in Mexican women 20–49 years.

Author Contributions: A.C.-M. and S.V. designed and conducted research; A.C.-M. and C.G.-D. analyzed data; and A.C.-M., S.V., and M.F.-A. wrote the paper. S.V. had primary responsibility for the final content. All authors read and approved the final manuscript.

Funding: This research was supported by DSM Nutritional Products México S.A. de C.V. through a non-binding grant. DSM had no role in the planning, analyzing or drafting of this article. All authors declare that they have no conflict of interest.

Conflicts of Interest: The authors declare no conflict of interest.

References

1. Vieth, R. Vitamin D supplementation, 25 hydroxyvitamin D concentrations and safety. *Am. J. Clin. Nutr.* **1999**, *69*, 842–856. [CrossRef] [PubMed]
2. Marwaha, R.K.; Tandon, N.; Reddy, D.R.; Aggarwal, R.; Singh, R.; Sawhney, R.C.; Saluja, B.; Ganie, M.A.; Singh, S. Vitamin D and bone mineral density status of healthy school children in northern India. *Am. J. Clin. Nutr.* **2005**, *82*, 477–482. [CrossRef]
3. Holick, M.F.; Chen, T.C. Vitamin D deficiency: A worldwide problem with health consequences. *N. Engl. J. Med.* **2007**, *357*, 266–281. [CrossRef]
4. Rahmadhani, R.; Zaharan, N.L.; Mohamed, Z.; Moy, F.M.; Jalaludin, M.Y. The associations between VDR BsmI polymorphisms and risk of vitamin D deficiency, obesity and insulin resistance in adolescents residing in a tropical country. *PLoS ONE* **2017**, *12*, e0178695. [CrossRef]
5. Mirhosseini, N.; Vatanparast, H.; Mazidi, M.; Kimball, S.M. The Effect of Improved Serum 25-Hydroxyvitamin D Status on Glycemic Control in Diabetic Patients: A Meta-Analysis. *J. Clin. Endocrinol. Metab.* **2017**, *102*, 3097–3110. [CrossRef] [PubMed]
6. Judd, S.E.; Tangpricha, V. Vitamin D Deficiency and Risk for Cardiovascular Disease. *Am. J. Med. Sci.* **2009**, *338*, 40–44. [CrossRef]
7. Chiu, K.C.; Chu, A.; Go, V.L.; Saad, M.F. Hypovitaminosis D is associated with insulin resistance and B cell disfunction. *Am. J. Clin. Nutr.* **2004**, *79*, 820–825. [CrossRef] [PubMed]
8. Lind, L.; Hanni, A.; Lithell, H.; Hvarfner, A.; Sorensen, O.H.; Ljunghal, S. Vitamin D is related with blood pressure and other cardiovascular risk factors in middle aged men. *Am. J. Hypertens.* **1995**, *8*, 894–901. [CrossRef]
9. Witham, M.D.; Nadir, M.A.; Struthers, A.D. Effect of vitamin D on blood pressure: A systematic review and metaanalysis. *J. Hypertens.* **2009**, *27*, 1948–1954. [CrossRef]
10. Mai, S.; Walker, G.E.; Vietti, R.; Cattaldo, S.; Mele, C.; Priano, L.; Mauro, A.; Bona, G.; Aimaretti, G.; Scacchi, M.; et al. Acute Vitamin D_3 Supplementation in Severe Obesity: Evaluation of Multimeric Adiponectin. *Nutrients* **2017**, *9*, 459. [CrossRef]
11. Pittas, A.G.; Lau, J.; Hue, F.B.; Dowson-Hughs, B. The role of vitamin D and calcium on type 2 diabetes. A systematic review and meta-analyis. *J. Clin. Endocr. Metab.* **2007**, *92*, 2017–2029. [CrossRef]
12. Mousa, A.; Naderpoor, N.; de Courten, M.P.; Teede, H.; Kellow, N.; Walker, K.; Scragg, R.; de Courten, B. Vitamin D supplementation has no effect on insulin sensitivity or secretion in vitamin D-deficient, overweight or obese adults: A randomized placebo-controlled trial. *Am. J. Clin. Nutr.* **2017**, *105*, 1372–1381. [CrossRef]
13. Gómez-Dantés, H.; Fullman, N.; Lamadrid-Figueroa, H.; Cahuana-Hurtado, L.; Darney, B.; Avila-Burgos, L.; Correa-Rotter, R.; Rivera, J.A.; Barquera, S.; González-Pier, E. Dissonant health transition in the states of Mexico, 1990-2013: A systematic analysis for the Global Burden of Disease Study 2013. *Lancet* **2016**, *388*, 2386–2402. [CrossRef]
14. Bodnar, L.M.; Catov, J.M.; Simhan, H.N.; Holick, M.F.; Powers, R.W.; Roberts, J.M. Maternal vitamin D deficiency increases the risk of preeclampsia. *J. Clin. Endocrinol. Metab.* **2007**, *92*, 3517–3522. [CrossRef]
15. Krieger, J.; Cabaset, S.; Canonica, C.; Christoffel, L.; Richard, A.; Schröder, T.; von Wattenwyl, B.L.; Rohrmann, S.; Lötscher, K.Q. Prevalence and determinants of vitamin D deficiency in the third trimester of pregnancy: A multicentre study in Switzerland. *Br. J. Nutr.* **2018**, *119*, 299–309. [CrossRef]
16. Pet, M.A.; Brouwer-Brolsma, E.M. The Impact of Maternal Vitamin D Status on Offspring Brain Development and Function: A Systematic Review. *Adv. Nutr.* **2016**, *7*, 665–678. [CrossRef] [PubMed]
17. Agarwal, S.; Kovilam, O.; Agrawal, D.K. Vitamin D and its impact on maternal-fetal outcomes in pregnancy: A critical review. *Crit Rev. Food Sci. Nutr.* **2018**, *58*, 755–769. [CrossRef]
18. Callegari, E.T.; Garland, S.M.; Gorelik, A.; Reavley, N.; Wark, J.D. Predictors and correlates of serum 25-hydroxyvitamin D concentrations in young women: Results from the Safe-D study. *Br. J. Nutr.* **2017**, *118*, 263–272. [CrossRef]
19. Wagner, C.L.; Taylor, S.N.; Johnson, D.D.; Hollis, B.W. The role of vitamin D in pregnancy and lactation: Emerging concepts. *Women's Health (Lond. Engl.)* **2012**, *8*, 323–340. [CrossRef] [PubMed]
20. Kung, A.W.; Lee, K.K. Knowledge of vitamin D and perceptions and attitudes toward sunlight among Chinese middle-aged and elderly women: A population survey in Hong Kong. *BMC Public Health* **2006**, *6*, 226. [CrossRef] [PubMed]

21. Flores, A.; Flores, M.; Macias, N.; Hernández-Barrera, L.; Rivera, M.; Contreras, A.; Villalpando, S. In Mexican children aged 1–11 years Vitamin D deficiency is common and is associated with overweight. *Public Health Nutr.* **2017**, *28*, 1–9. [CrossRef]

22. Contreras-Manzano, A.; Villalpando, S.; Robledo-Perez, R. Estado de Vitamina D por factores sociodemograficos e índice de masa corporal en mujeres mexicanas en edad reproductiva. *Salud Pública Méx.* **2017**, *59*, 518–525. [CrossRef]

23. Muñoz-Aguirre, P.; Denova-Gutierrez, E.; Flores, M.; Salazar-Martinez, E.; Salmeron, J. High Vitamin D Consumption Is Inversely Associated with Cardiovascular Disease Risk in an Urban Mexican Population. *PLoS ONE* **2016**, *11*, e0166869. [CrossRef]

24. Gutierrez, J.P.; Rivera-Dommarco, J.A.; Shamah-Levy, T.; Villalpando, S.; Franco, A.; Cuevas-Nasu, L. *Encuesta Nacional de Salud y Nutrición 2012 Resultados Nacionales*; Instituto Nacional de Salud Pública: Cuernavaca, Mexico; Available online: https://ensanut.insp.mx/informes/ENSANUT2012ResultadosNacionales.pdf (accessed on 1 April 2019).

25. Romero-Martínez, M.; Shamah-Levy, T.; Franco-Núñez, A.; Villalpando, S.; Cuevas-Nasu, L.; Gutiérrez, J.P.; Rivera-Dommarco, J.A. Encuesta Nacional de Salud y Nutrición 2012: Diseño y cobertura. *Salud Pública Méx.* **2013**, *55* (Suppl. 2), S332–S340. [CrossRef]

26. Gutierrez, J.P. Household socioeconomic classification in the National Health and Nutrition Survey 2012. *Salud Pública Méx.* **2013**, *55* (Suppl. 2), s341–s346.

27. Lohman, T.; Martorell, R.; Roche, A.F. *Anthropometric Reference Standardization Manual*; Human Kinetics: Champaine, IL, USA, 1988.

28. Habicht, J.P. Standardization of quantitative epidemiological methods in the field. *Bol. Oficina. Sanit. Panam* **1974**, *76*, 375–384.

29. National Institute of Standards & Technology. Certificate of Analysis. *Standard Reference Material 968e. Fat-Soluble Vitamins, Carotenoids, and Cholesterol in Human Serum (internet document)*. Available online: https://www.aacb.asn.au/documents/item/1233 (accessed on 4 April 2017).

30. Brito, A.; Cori, H.; Ordóñez Pizarro, F.; Mujica, M.; Cediel, G. López de Romaña D. Less than adequate vitamin D status and intake in Latin America and the Caribbean: A problem of unknown magnitude. *Food Nutr. Bull.* **2013**, *34*, 52–64. [CrossRef]

31. American Diabetes Association. Diagnosis and Classification of Diabetes Mellitus. *Diabetes Care* **2013**, *36* (Suppl. 1), 67–74. [CrossRef] [PubMed]

32. Expert panel report on detection evaluation and treatment of high blood cholesterol in adults. Executive summary of the Third report of the national cholesterol education program (NCEP) expert panel on evaluation detection and treatment of high blood cholesterol in adults (adult treatment panel III). *JAMA* **2001**, *285*, 2483–2497.

33. Selhub, J.; Jacqus, P.F.; Rosenberg, I.H.; Rogers, G.; Bowman, B.A.; Gunter, E.W.; Wright, J.D.; Johnson, C.L. Serum total homocysteine concentrations in the third National Health and Nutrition Examination Survey (1991–1994); population reference ranges and contribution of vitamin status to high serum concentrations. *Ann. Intern. Med.* **1999**, *131*, 331–339. [PubMed]

34. Thurnham, D.; McCabe, L.D.; Haldar, S.; Wieringa, F.T.; Northrop-Clewes, C.A.; McCabe, G.P. Adjusting ferritin concentration to remove the effects of subclinical inflammation in the assessment of iron deficiency: A metaanalysis. *Am. J. Clin. Nutr.* **2010**, *92*, 546–555. [CrossRef]

35. Ascaso, J.F.; Romero, P.; Real, J.T.; Priego, A.; Valdecabres, C.; Carmena, R. Insulin resistance quantification by fasting insulin plasma values and HOMA index in a non-diabetic population. *Med. Clin.* **2001**, *117*, 530–533. [CrossRef]

36. WHO. Physical status: The use and interpretation of anthropometry. Report of a WHO Experts Committee. *WHO Tech. Rep. Ser.* **1995**, *854*, 1–452.

37. Chobanian, A.; Bakris, G.; Black, H. The Seventh Report of the Joint National Committee on Prevention, Detection and Evaluation and treatment of High Blood Pressure: The 7 JNC report. *JAMA* **2003**, *289*, 2560–2572. [CrossRef] [PubMed]

38. Medina, C.; Barquera, S.; Janssen, I. Validity and reliability of the International Physical Activity Questionnaire among adults in Mexico. *Rev. Panam Salud Publica* **2013**, *34*, 21–28.

39. Scragg, R.; Holdaway, I.; Metcalf, P.; Baker, J.; Dryson, E. Serum 25-hydroxivitamin D3 decreased impaired glucose tolerance and diabetes mellitus. *Diab. Res. Clin. Pract.* **1985**, *27*, 181–188. [CrossRef]

40. Isaia, G.; Giorgino, R.; Adami, S. High prevalence of hipovitaminosis D in females type 2 diabetic population (letter). *Diabetes Care* **2001**, *24*, 1496. [CrossRef] [PubMed]
41. Scragg, R.; Sower, M.; Bell, C. Serum 25 hydroxyvitamin D, diabetes and ethnicity in the Third National Health and Nutrition Examination Survey. *Diabetes Care* **2004**, *27*, 2813–2818. [CrossRef]
42. Hypönnen, E.; Boucher, E.J.; Berry, D.J.; Power, C. Vitamin D, IFG-1 and metabolic syndrome at 45 years. A cross sectional study in the 1958 British cohort study. *Diabetes* **2008**, *57*, 298–305. [CrossRef]
43. Abbasi, F.; Blasey, B.; Feldman, D.; Cauldfield, M.P.; Hantash, F.M.; Reaven, G.M. Low circulating 25 OH vitamin D concentrations are associated with defects of insulin action and insulin secretion in persons with prediabetes. *J. Nutr.* **2015**, *145*, 714–719. [CrossRef]
44. Kayaniyil, S.; Retnakaran, R.; Harris, S.B.; Vieth, R.; Knight, J.A.; Gerstein, H.C.; Perkins, B.A.; Zinman, B. Prospective Association of vitamin D and β-cell function and glycemia. The PROspective metabolism and Islet cell Evaluation. (PROMISE) cohort study. *Diabetes* **2011**, *60*, 2947–2953. [CrossRef]
45. Dutta, D.; Ali Mondal, S.; Choudhuri, S.; Maisnam, I.; Hasanoor Reza, A.; Bhattacharya, B.; Chowdhury, S.; Mukhopadhyay, S. Vitamin-D supplementation in prediabetes reduced progression to type 2 diabetes and was associated with decreased insulin resistance and systemic inflammation: An open label randomized prospective study from Eastern India. *Diabetes Res. Clin. Pract.* **2014**, *103*, e18–e23. [CrossRef]
46. Mitchell, D.M.; Leder, B.Z.; Cagliero, E.; Mendoza, N.; Henao, M.P.; Hayden, D.L.; Finkelstein, J.S.; Burnett-Bowie, S.M. Insulin secretion and sensitivity in healthy adults with low vitamin D are not affected by high-dose ergocalciferol administration: A randomized controlled trial. *Am. J. Clin. Nutr.* **2015**, *102*, 385–392. [CrossRef]
47. Gagnon, C.; Daly, R.M.; Carpentier, A.; Lu, Z.X.; Shore-Lorenti, C.; Sicaris, K.; Jean, S.; Eveling, P.R. Effect of combined with vitamin D and calcium supplementation on insulin secretion and insulin sensitivity and β-cell function in multiethnic vitamin-D deficient adults at risk of type 2 diabetes: A pilot randomized, placebo controlled trial. *PLoS ONE* **2014**, *9*, e109607. [CrossRef] [PubMed]
48. Zeitz, U.; Weber, K.; Soegiarto, D.W.; Wolf, E.; Balling, R.; Erben, R.G. Impaired insulin secretory capacity in mice lacking a functional vitamin D receptor. *FASEB J.* **2003**, *17*, 509–511. [CrossRef]
49. Sooy, K.; Schermerhorn, T.; Noda, M.; Surana, M.; Rhoten, W.B.; Meyer, M.; Fleischer, N.; Sharp, G.W.; Christakos, S. Calbindin-D(28k) controls [Ca(2+)](i) and insulin release. Evidence obtained from calbindin-d(28k) knockout mice and beta cell lines. *J. Biol. Chem.* **1999**, *274*, 34343–34349. [CrossRef] [PubMed]
50. Sergeev, I.N. Vitamin D-Cellular Ca2+ link to obesity and diabetes. *J. Steroid. Biochem. Mol. Biol.* **2016**, *164*, 326–330. [CrossRef]
51. Sergeev, I.N. 1,25-Dihydroxyvitamin D3 induces Ca^{2+}-mediated apoptosis in adipocytes via activation of calpain and caspase-12. *Biochem. Biophys. Res. Commun.* **2009**, *384*, 18–21. [CrossRef] [PubMed]
52. Barquera, S.; Campos-Nonato, I.; Hernandez-Barrera, L.; Pedroza-Tobias, A.; Rivera Dommarco, J.A. Prevalencia de obesidad en adultos Mexicanos. *Salud Pública Méx.* **2013**, *55* (Suppl. 2), s151–s160. [CrossRef] [PubMed]
53. Villalpando, S.; Shamah-Levy, T.; Rojas, R.; Aguilar-Salinas, C.A. Trends for type 2 diabetes and other cardiovascular risk factors in Mexico from 1993–2006. *Salud Publica Mex.* **2010**, *52* (Suppl. 1), S72–S79. [CrossRef]
54. Dix, C.F.; Barcley, J.L.; Wright, O.R.L. The role of vitamin D in adipogenesis. *Nutr. Rev.* **2018**, *76*, 47–59. [CrossRef]
55. Wortsman, J.; Matsuoka, L.Y.; Chen, T.C.; Lu, Z.; Holick, M.F. Decreased bioavailability of vitamin D in obesity. *Am. J. Clin. Nutr.* **2000**, *72*, 690–693. [CrossRef] [PubMed]
56. Rosenblum, J.L.; Castro, V.M.; Moore, C.E.; Kaplan, L.M. Calcium and vitamin D supplementation is associated with decreased abdominal visceral adipose tissue in overweight and obese adults. *Am. J. Clin. Nutr.* **2012**, *95*, 101–108. [CrossRef]
57. Carrelli, A.; Bucovsky, M.; Horst, R.; Cremers, S.; Zhang, C.; Bessler, M.; Schrope, B.; Evanko, J.; Blanco, J.; Silverberg, S.J.; et al. Vitamin D Storage in Adipose Tissue of Obese and Normal Weight Women. *J. Bone Miner. Res.* **2017**, *32*, 237–242. [CrossRef] [PubMed]
58. Mumford, S.L.; Schisterman, E.F.; Siega-Riz, A.M.; Browne, R.W.; Gaskins, A.J.; Trevisan, M.; Steiner, A.Z.; Daniels, J.L.; Zhang, C.; Perkins, N.J. A Longitudinal Study of Serum Lipoproteins in Relation to Endogenous Reproductive Hormones during the Menstrual Cycle: Findings from the BioCycle Study. *J. Clin. Endocrinol. Metab.* **2010**, *95*, E80–E85. [CrossRef]

59. Tosunbayraktar, G.; Bas, M.; Kut, A.; Buyukkaragoz, A.H. Low serum 25(OH)D levels are associated to higher BMI and metabolic syndrome parameters in adults subjects in Turkey. *Afri. Health Sci.* **2015**, *15*, 1161–1169. [CrossRef] [PubMed]

60. Boteon, E.; Nahas-Neto, J.; Bueloni-Dias, F.; Poloni, P.F.; Orsatti, C.L.; Petri Nahas, E.A. Vitamin D deficiency is associated with metabolic syndrome in postmenopausal women. *Maturitas* **2018**, *107*, 97–102.

61. Jorde, R.; Grimnes, G. Exploring the association between serum 25-hydroxyvitamin D and serum lipids-more than confounding? *Eur. J. Clin. Nutr.* **2018**, *72*, 526–533. [CrossRef] [PubMed]

62. Wang, H.; Xia, N.; Yang, Y.; Peng, D.Q. Influence of vitamin D supplementation on plasma lipids profiles: A metaanalysis of randomized controlled trials. *Lipid Health Dis.* **2012**, *11*, 42. [CrossRef]

63. Reyes-Garcia, R.; Mendoza, N.; Palacios, S.; Salas, N.; Quesada-Charneco, M.; Garcia-Martin, A.; Fonolla, J.; Lara-Villoslada, F.; Muñoz-Torres, M. Effects of Daily Intake of Calcium and Vitamin D-Enriched Milk in Healthy Postmenopausal Women: A Randomized, Controlled, Double-Blind Nutritional Study. *J. Womens Health (Larchmt)* **2018**, *27*, 561–568. [CrossRef] [PubMed]

64. Grübler, M.R.; Gaksch, M.; Kienreich, K.; Verheyen, N.D.; Schmid, J.; Müllner, C.; Richtig, G.; Scharnagl, H.; Trummer, C.; Schwetz, V.; et al. Effects of Vitamin D3 on asymmetric- and symmetric dimethylarginine in arterial hypertension. *J. Steroid. Biochem. Mol. Biol.* **2018**, *175*, 157–163. [CrossRef] [PubMed]

65. Golzarand, M.; Shab-Bidar, S.; Koochakpoor, G.; Speakman, J.R.; Djafarian, K. Effect of vitamin D3 supplementation on blood pressure in adults: An updated meta-analysis. *Nutr. Metab. Cardiovasc. Dis.* **2016**, *26*, 663–673. [CrossRef] [PubMed]

66. Mirhosseini, N.; Vatanparast, H.; Kimball, S.M. The Association between Serum 25(OH)D Status and Blood Pressure in Participants of a Community-Based Program Taking Vitamin D Supplements. *Nutrients* **2017**, *9*, 1244. [CrossRef]

67. Anderesen, L.B.; Pryzybil, L.; Haase, N.; von Bersen-Hoinck, F.; Qadri, F.; Jørgensen, J.S.; Sorensen, G.L.; Fruekilde, P.; Poglitsch, M.; Szijarto, I. Vitamin D depletion aggravates hypertension and target-organ damage. *J. Am. Hearth Assocc.* **2015**, *4*, e001417. [CrossRef]

68. Harmon, Q.E.; Umbach, D.M.; Baird, D.D. Use of Estrogen-Containing Contraception Is Associated With Increased Concentrations of 25-Hydroxy Vitamin D. *J. Clin. Endocrinol Metab.* **2016**, *101*, 3370–3377. [CrossRef]

69. Villalobos, A.; Allen, B.; Serrato, M.; Suárez, L.; De La Vara, E.; Castro, F. Uso de Anticonceptivos y Planificación Familiar Entre Mujeres Adolescentes y Adultas: Cerrando la Breca Entre Metas y Realidades. Available online: https://ensanut.insp.mx/doctos/seminario/M0203.pdf (accessed on 1 April 2019).

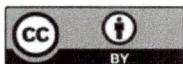

nutrients

MDPI

Review

Zinc Intake and Status and Risk of Type 2 Diabetes Mellitus: A Systematic Review and Meta-Analysis

José C. Fernández-Cao [1,2,*], Marisol Warthon-Medina [3,4], Victoria H. Moran [5], Victoria Arija [6], Carlos Doepking [1], Lluis Serra-Majem [7,8] and Nicola M. Lowe [4]

[1] Department of Nutrition and Dietetics, Faculty of Heath Sciences, University of Atacama, Av. Copayapu 2862, Copiapó, 1530000 Atacama Region, Chile; carlos.doepking@uda.cl

[2] Nutrition and Public Health, Universitat Rovira i Virgili, C/ Sant Llorenç 21, Reus, 43201 Tarragona, Spain

[3] Food Databanks National Capability, Quadram Institute Bioscience, Norwich Research Park, Norwich, Norfolk NR4 7UA, UK; marisol@warthon-medina.com

[4] International Institute of Nutritional Sciences and Food Safety Studies, University of Central Lancashire, Darwin Building c/o Psychology Scholl Office, Preston, Lancashire PR1 2HE, UK; NMLowe@uclan.ac.uk

[5] Maternal and Infant Nutrition and Nurture Unit, University of Central Lancashire, Preston, Lancashire PR 1 2HE, UK; VLMoran@uclan.ac.uk

[6] Research Group in Nutrition and Mental Health (NUTRISAM), Institut d'Investigació Sanitària Pere Virgili (IISPV), Rovira i Virgili University, Reus, 43201 Tarragona, Spain; victoria.arija@urv.cat

[7] Research Institute of Biomedical and Health Sciences, University of Las Palmas de Gran Canaria and CHUIMI, Canarian Health Service, 35016 Las Palmas de Gran Canaria, Spain; lluis.serra@ulpgc.es

[8] Consorcio CIBER, M.P. Fisiopatología de la Obesidad y Nutrición (CIBERObn), Instituto de Salud Carlos III (ISCIII), 28029 Madrid, Spain

* Correspondence: jose.fernandez.cao@uda.cl

Received: 26 March 2019; Accepted: 25 April 2019; Published: 8 May 2019

Abstract: Zinc could have a protective role against type 2 diabetes mellitus (T2DM). This systematic review and meta-analysis aimed to evaluate the association between dietary, supplementary, and total zinc intake, as well as serum/plasma and whole blood zinc concentration, and risk of T2DM. Observational studies, conducted on cases of incident diabetes or T2DM patients and healthy subjects that reported a measure of association between zinc exposure and T2DM, were selected. Random effects meta-analyses were applied to obtain combined results. Stratified meta-analyses and meta-regressions were executed to assess sources of heterogeneity, as well as the impact of covariates on the findings. From 12,136 publications, 16 studies were selected. The odds ratio (OR) for T2DM comparing the highest versus lowest zinc intake from diet was 0.87 (95% CI: 0.78–0.98). Nevertheless, no association between supplementary or total zinc intake from both diet and supplementation, and T2DM was observed. A direct relationship was found between serum/plasma zinc levels and T2DM (OR = 1.64, 95% CI: 1.25–2.14). A moderately high dietary zinc intake, in relation to the Dietary Reference Intake, could reduce by 13% the risk of T2DM, and up to 41% in rural areas. Conversely, elevated serum/plasma zinc concentration was associated with an increased risk of T2DM by 64%, suggesting disturbances in zinc homeostasis.

Keywords: zinc intake; zinc status; trace elements; type 2 diabetes mellitus; systematic review; meta-analysis; epidemiology

---

1. Introduction

Diabetes mellitus is a major public health challenge worldwide, and is a key contributor to morbidity and mortality. In 2016, diabetes mellitus was listed as the seventh leading cause of death globally [1]. According to the International Diabetes Federation (IDF) Diabetes ATLAS, the global prevalence of diabetes among individuals aged 20–79 years in 2017 was 8.8% (95% confidence interval

(CI): 7.2–11.3), i.e., 424.9 million people, with a total healthcare expenditure estimated at just under USD 727 billion [2]. The number of people suffering from diabetes is expected to increase to 628.6 million in 2045, a prevalence of over 9.9% (95% CI: 7.5–12.7). Around 90% of cases of diabetes are type 2 diabetes (T2DM) [2]. This disease results from the body's ineffective use of insulin [1], and is the result of the interaction of multiple genetic and environmental factors [3].

The role of zinc in the etiology of T2DM has been widely reported in recent decades. Longitudinal large prospective cohort studies, such as the Nurses' Health Study (NHS) cohort [4] in the USA; the Australian Longitudinal Study on Women's Health cohort study [5]; the Malmö Diet and Cancer Study cohort [6] in Sweden; and the Japan Collaborative Cohort study [7], among others, have investigated the effect of dietary, supplementary, and/or total zinc intake on the risk of developing T2DM. The NHS cohort was the first to prospectively analyze these relationships, and it reported that the higher the total and/or dietary zinc intake, the lower the risk of T2DM over subsequent years [4]. Although a non-significant association was observed between supplementary zinc intake and risk of T2DM in the overall sample, an inverse relationship was seen in those participants with low dietary zinc intake [4]. There is currently no evidence that supports the use of zinc supplements in the prevention of T2DM [8]. Nevertheless, a recent clinical trial based on zinc supplementation has found a reduction in the progression to diabetes in prediabetic subjects [9]. Some subsequent prospective cohort studies, however, have failed to confirm some of the results reported in the NHS cohort [6,10–12]. A systematic review of prospective studies that aimed to examine the role of zinc intake and status on the risk of T2DM revealed inconsistencies between studies, and suggested the possible influence of confounding factors on these relationships [13].

Similarly, findings on the relationship between serum/plasma zinc concentration and T2DM are contradictory [14–16]. The prospective Kuopio Ischaemic Heart Disease Risk Factor (KIHD) cohort study of 2220 Finnish men followed over twenty years showed that higher serum zinc levels were associated with an increased risk of T2DM [14]. Conversely, a cross-sectional study of 128 Russian postmenopausal women found an inverse relationship between serum zinc and T2DM [17]. The relationship between whole blood zinc concentration and T2DM has been investigated by two studies carried out within the same population-based Nord-Trøndelag Health Study (HUNT3), but their results were inconclusive [18,19]. The study conducted on newly diagnosed T2DM patients found a positive association between whole blood zinc concentration and T2DM [18], while the study performed in previously diagnosed T2DM patients showed no association [19]. In our previous systematic review and meta-analysis, which aimed to compare whole blood zinc concentration between T2DM patients and non-diabetic subjects, we observed a lower whole blood zinc concentration in T2DM patients [20]. It should be noted that diabetic subjects had, at least, 10.2 ± 8.6 years of duration of diabetes. Therefore, the duration of diabetes may have an impact on this association, and it is important to clarify this relationship.

The mechanism whereby zinc could have an impact on the risk of T2DM has not been completely elucidated, however zinc is an essential trace element that is involved in the physiology of carbohydrate metabolism in many ways. Zinc participates in the adequate insulin synthesis, storage, crystallization, and secretion in the pancreatic β-cell, as well as action and translocation of insulin into the cells [21–24]. In addition, zinc seems to play a role in insulin sensitivity through the activation of the phosphoinositol-3-kinase/protein kinase B cascade [25]. Due to its insulin–mimetic action, zinc also stimulates glucose uptake in insulin-dependent tissues [26]. Moreover, zinc is implicated in the suppression of proinflammatory cytokines, such as interleukin-1β [27] and nuclear factor kβ [28], avoiding β-cells' death and protecting insulin. All of these functions of zinc could support its potential protective role against diabetes mellitus.

Much remains uncertain concerning the effect of zinc on the risk of developing T2DM. Therefore, the purpose of this comprehensive systematic review and meta-analysis of observational studies was to evaluate the association between dietary, supplementary, and total zinc intake, as well as serum/plasma zinc and whole blood concentration and risk of T2DM in the adult population. A secondary objective was to examine potential confounding factors that may impact on these relationships.

2. Materials and Methods

The protocol for this systematic review and meta-analysis of observational studies was registered in PROSPERO (2015: CRD42015020178) and can be accessed here: (http://www.crd.york.ac.uk/ PROSPERO/display_record.php?ID=CRD42015020178). The study was conducted in accordance with the Meta-Analyses of Observational Studies in Epidemiology (MOOSE) criteria statement [29]. The MOOSE checklist is shown in Supplementary Materials Table S1.

2.1. Search Strategy

This systematic review and meta-analysis were carried out by six investigators within the framework of the EURopean micronutrient RECommendations Aligned (EURRECA) Network of Excellence, one aim of which was to undertake a series of systematic search for studies assessing the effect of zinc on different health outcomes. A comprehensive search was developed in MEDLINE (Ovid), Embase (Ovid), and The Cochrane Library (CENTRAL) up to January 2019, using search terms for ("study designs in humans") AND (Zinc) AND (intake OR status). Additional articles were identified through manual searching and citation tracking (Figure 1).

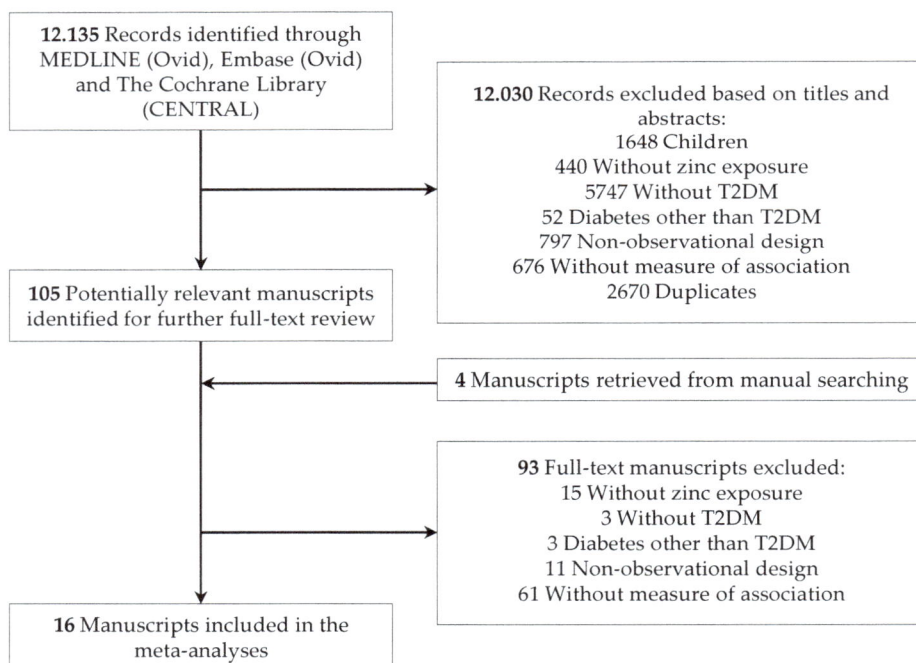

| **12.135** Records identified through MEDLINE (Ovid), Embase (Ovid) and The Cochrane Library (CENTRAL) | **12.030** Records excluded based on titles and abstracts: 1648 Children 440 Without zinc exposure 5747 Without T2DM 52 Diabetes other than T2DM 797 Non-observational design 676 Without measure of association 2670 Duplicates |

| **105** Potentially relevant manuscripts identified for further full-text review |

| **4** Manuscripts retrieved from manual searching |

| **93** Full-text manuscripts excluded: 15 Without zinc exposure 3 Without T2DM 3 Diabetes other than T2DM 11 Non-observational design 61 Without measure of association |

| **16** Manuscripts included in the meta-analyses |

Figure 1. Flowchart of the selection process.

2.2. Study Eligibility Criteria

Studies were selected according to the following inclusion criteria: (1) studies of observational design, including prospective cohort, case-control, and cross-sectional; (2) studies conducted on human adults, with type 2 diabetes mellitus (T2DM) or cases of incident diabetes and healthy control individuals or controls of non-incident diabetes; (3) publications reported in English, Spanish or other

European languages; (4) studies that reported a measure of association, such as relative risk (RR), odds ratio (OD) or hazard ratio (HR), between dietary, supplementary, and/or total zinc intake and/or serum/plasma and/or whole blood zinc concentration and T2DM, through a multivariable adjusted analysis that compared the highest quantile of zinc exposure versus the lowest. Studies that compared user versus non-user of zinc supplements in relation to T2DM were also selected. Other kinds of observational study designs, such as case reports, case series or ecological studies; reviews; and experimental or quasi-experimental studies, as well as those with participants diagnosed with diabetes mellitus other than T2DM, were excluded.

2.3. Study Selection

Titles and abstracts of studies identified through the literature search were independently screened for eligibility. Subsequently, the full text of relevant studies was retrieved and examined further against the inclusion and exclusion criteria. Reasons for excluding studies were recorded. The selection process was independently completed by members of the research team (JCFC, MWM, VHM, CD, and NL). A 10% sample was cross-checked by another investigator (MWM) to ensure consistency between reviewers, and any discrepancy or disagreement was resolved by discussion until consensus was reached among the reviewers.

2.4. Data Extraction and Study Quality Assessment

One reviewer (JCFC) carried out the data extraction process using a data-extraction spreadsheet. Two other reviewers (VHM and NL) independently screened the accuracy of the extracted data. In order to avoid the inclusion of duplicate data in the meta-analyses, some strategies were applied: first, the name of the project was recorded for all studies that met the inclusion criteria, as well as the geographic location where the studies had been conducted; second, the lists of authors were compared among them. Complementary data from the same project was included for a qualitative summary.

From each manuscript selected for inclusion, the following data were extracted into an excel spreadsheet: study identification (first author's name, year of publication, and name of the project), study characteristics (study design, period of follow-up, measure of association, adjustment variables, quality score, country, geographic regions, geographic area, sample base, matched design, sample size for each group and total, zinc assessment method, zinc quantiles adjusted for energy, ascertainment of T2DM, percentage of T2DM subjects, effect size, and 95% confidence interval (CI) for the most adjusted model), and study population (age, gender, ethnicity, area of residence—dietary, supplementary and total zinc intake, as well as serum, plasma, and whole blood zinc concentration—BMI, fasting glucose levels, stage of diabetes). To incorporate relevant data in forms other than the mean and standard deviation, such as median and the interquartile range, estimation methods proposed by Wan et al., [24] were applied, which are valid for both normal and skewed data. When covariates of interest were expressed as a range, the midpoint of the range was assumed. If any of the data were missing, the authors were contacted for additional data.

The quality of studies selected was evaluated by one research investigator (JCFC) using the Strengthening the Reporting of Observational Studies in Epidemiology (STROBE) Statement [25]. The STROBE checklist is shown in Supplementary Materials Table S2. The quality score was used to assess its possible influence on results.

2.5. Statistical Analysis

Meta-analyses comparing the highest versus the lowest quantile of exposure to zinc intake and/or status were performed when at least two studies with a common exposure in relation to T2DM were available. For all meta-analyses, effect size and 95% CIs were log-transformed. Estimated standard errors were calculated from log 95% CIs by subtracting the lower bound of the CI from the upper bound and subsequently dividing by two times 1.96. The method of a random-effects model and the generic inverse variance method were used to calculate the pooled effect sizes, reported as OR and 95% CI. Relative risks and hazard ratios were deemed equivalent to ORs [30]. The most adjusted model of the multivariable analysis in the selected studies was used to estimate the effect size in all meta-analyses. Forest plots were created to visualize individual and global estimates. As the studies included in the meta-analysis on supplementary zinc intake and T2DM reported exposure either in quantiles or as dichotomous variable (user versus no user), a stratified meta-analysis was performed based on these criteria.

Univariate and multivariate meta-regressions with Knapp–Hartung modification [31] were conducted to examine the potential impact of certain covariates on effect size. To display relevant results of a single continuous covariate in univariate meta-regressions, bubble plots were created. This graph represents the fitted regression line together with circles representing the estimates from each study, sized according to the precision of each estimate (the inverse of its within-study variance). Multivariate meta-regressions models were executed adding the covariate with the strongest association in univariate analysis first and then adding the next one in turn. Covariates showing collinearity were removed from the final multivariate model. Finally, a meta-regression equation was generated using the intercept (a), as well as the regression coefficient (b) of a specific covariate, to know how the effect size (OR for T2DM) changes with a unit increase in the exploratory covariate (Ln (OR_{T2DM}) = (a) + b × (covariate)).

Heterogeneity was assessed by the Cochran Q-statistic and the I^2 statistic to quantify the percentage of variation attributable to between-study heterogeneity [32]. I^2 values of 25%, 50%, and 75% were considered as low, medium, and high heterogeneity, respectively [33,34]. Potential sources of heterogeneity were explored through stratified analyses and univariate meta-regressions, even if an initial heterogeneity was non-significant [35], using different variables. Thus, categorical variables were: study design, study design and area of residence, measures of association, quality score, geographic regions, location, sample base, matched design, sample size, zinc intake assessment method, zinc serum/plasma assessment method, ascertainment of T2DM, diagnostic pattern, percentage of T2DM, gender, ethnicity, area of residence, group with higher serum/plasma zinc levels, zinc quantiles adjusted for energy. In addition, continuous variables were also used, such as sample size for each group and total, period of follow-up (years), quality score (%), percentage of T2DM subjects (%), age in cases and controls (years), age difference and ratio between cases and controls (years), serum/plasma zinc levels in cases and controls (μg/dL), serum/plasma zinc difference and ratio between cases and controls (μg/dL), BMI in cases and controls (kg/m^2), BMI difference and ratio between cases and controls (kg/m^2), fasting glucose levels in cases and controls (mmol/L), and fasting glucose difference and ratio between cases and controls (mmol/L). Multivariate meta-regressions were also utilized to examine further the covariates that had a significant influence on heterogeneity in univariate analysis. In addition, the proportion of between-study variance explained by one or more covariates was estimated through the adjusted R^2 (R_A^2). Likewise, the percentage of residual variation due to heterogeneity which remains unexplained by one or more covariates (I_r^2) was obtained.

To assess the power of each study on the overall pooled estimates, sensitivity analysis was performed using the leave-one-out method [36], where one study was excluded at a time, evaluating the impact of removing each of the studies on the summary results and the between-study heterogeneity. Furthermore, publication bias was investigated by visual inspection of funnel plots and quantitatively assessed using Egger's [37] and Begg's [38] tests. All analyses were performed with STATA statistical software, version 15.0. (STATA Corp., College Station, Texas, USA).

3. Results

The literature search strategy generated 12,136 publications, and 16 studies were finally selected for this systematic review and meta-analysis of observational studies [4–7,10–12,14–19,39–41]. There were no studies that were excluded for reasons of language. The details of the selection process and the reasons for exclusion are shown in the flowchart (Figure 1). The quality of selected publications, according to the Strengthening the Reporting of Observational Studies in Epidemiology (STROBE)

Statement [42], was high. The compliance percentages of the STROBE items were between 69 and 100%, 14 of the 16 selected studies above 80% [4–7,10–12,14–19,39,41]. The characteristics of the included studies for meta-analyses are summarized in Tables 1–3.

3.1. Dietary Zinc Intake and T2DM

Seven prospective cohort studies [4–7,10,11] and one cross-sectional study [39] were included in the meta-analysis of the association between dietary zinc intake and T2DM (Table 1). Five studies were carried out in the western countries (USA, the Nurses' Health Study (NHS) cohort [4], the Multi-Ethnic Study of Atherosclerosis (MESA) cohort [10], and the Coronary Artery Risk Development in Young Adults (CARDIA) cohort [11]; Australia, the Australian Longitudinal Study on Women's Health (ALSWH) cohort [5]; and Sweden, the Malmö Diet and Cancer Study (MDCS) cohort [6]), and two in the eastern countries (India [39], and Japan, the Japan Collaborative Cohort (JACC) [7]). This meta-analysis comprised 146,027 participants aged between 18 and 84 years, and of both genders, belonging to different ethnic groups (Hispanic, Caucasian, African American, Chinese or South Asian, among others), and areas of residence (rural or urban). During the follow-up of participants, between 4.8 years on average in the MESA cohort [10] and 24 years in the NHS cohort [4], 11,511 cases of T2DM were detected (7.8%). The percentage of T2DM cases was highly variable between the studies, from 2.5% in the JACC study [7] to 14.1% in the Swedish MDCS cohort [6].

Dietary zinc intake was collected using validated food frequency questionnaires (VFFQs) [4,5,7,10], validated diet history questionnaires (VDHQ) [6,11], or a 7-day dietary record [39]. The mean of dietary zinc intake ranged from 5.6 ± 1.6 mg/day in urban women from India [39] to 16.7 mg/day in urban subjects from the USA [11]. Ascertainment of T2DM was carried out through different criteria (fasting plasma glucose (FPG) and/or oral glucose tolerance test (OGTT), and/or self-reported, and/or using registries from different institutions, and/or use of antidiabetic drugs).

To evaluate the association between the dietary zinc intake and the T2DM, a meta-analysis was conducted (Figure 2). The pooled effect size for T2DM comparing the highest versus lowest dietary zinc intakes was 0.87 (95% CI: 0.78–0.98), with moderate to high heterogeneity (I^2 = 64.5%, p = 0.003).

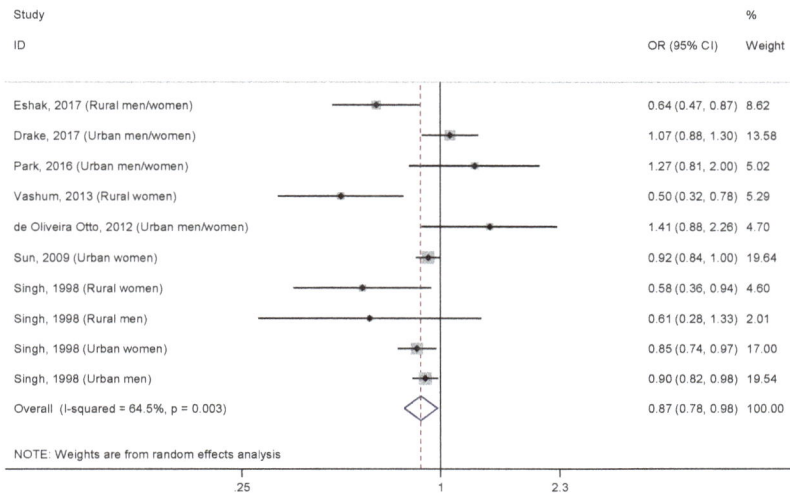

Study ID		OR (95% CI)	% Weight
Eshak, 2017 (Rural men/women)		0.64 (0.47, 0.87)	8.62
Drake, 2017 (Urban men/women)		1.07 (0.88, 1.30)	13.58
Park, 2016 (Urban men/women)		1.27 (0.81, 2.00)	5.02
Vashum, 2013 (Rural women)		0.50 (0.32, 0.78)	5.29
de Oliveira Otto, 2012 (Urban men/women)		1.41 (0.88, 2.26)	4.70
Sun, 2009 (Urban women)		0.92 (0.84, 1.00)	19.64
Singh, 1998 (Rural women)		0.58 (0.36, 0.94)	4.60
Singh, 1998 (Rural men)		0.61 (0.28, 1.33)	2.01
Singh, 1998 (Urban women)		0.85 (0.74, 0.97)	17.00
Singh, 1998 (Urban men)		0.90 (0.82, 0.98)	19.54
Overall (I-squared = 64.5%, p = 0.003)		0.87 (0.78, 0.98)	100.00

NOTE: Weights are from random effects analysis

.25   1   2.3

Figure 2. Forest plot of pooled effect size of the highest versus lowest dietary zinc intake for T2DM. Squares represent odds ratios (OR) for each study, and the size of the square is the study-specific statistical weight. Horizontal lines indicate the 95% CI of each study. Diamond represents the combined OR estimate with corresponding 95% CI.

Table 1. Characteristics of studies reporting the association between dietary zinc intake and risk of type 2 diabetes.

Author, Year (Study)	Location (Area)	Study Design	Follow-Up (Years)	Ethnicity	Gender	Age (Years) in Cases at Baseline (mean ± SD)	Age (Years) in Controls at Baseline (mean ± SD)	Sample Size (T2DM)	T2DM (%)	Ascertainment of T2DM	Zinc Assessment Method	Zinc Intake (mg/day) in Cases (mean ± SD)	Zinc Intake (mg/day) in Controls (mean ± SD)	Effect Size (95% CI)
Drake, 2017 (MDCS)	Sweden (urban)	Prospective cohort	Median: 19	White	Men/Women	58.0 ± 7.0	57.8 ± 7.7	26,132 (3676)	14.1	FPG ≥ 7.0 mmol/L (twice), or registries	VDHQ	11.6 ± 3.6	11.1 ± 3.3	HR: 1.07 (0.88–1.30)
Eshak, 2017 (JACC)	Japan (rural, mostly)	Prospective cohort	5	Japanese	Men/Women	Range: 40–65		16,160 (396)	2.5	Self-report	VFFQ	7.3 ± 0.8		OR: 0.64 (0.54–1.00)
Park, 2016 (CARDIA)	USA (urban)	Prospective cohort	23	African American, Caucasian	Men/Women	Range: 18–30; 27.03 ± 3.61		3960 (418)	10.6	FPG ≥ 7.0 mmol/L, or 2-h 75-g OGTT ≥ 11.1 mmol/L, or HbA1c ≥ 6.5%, or drugs	VDHQ	16.7	16.7	HR: 1.27 (0.81–2.01)
Vashum, 2013 (ALSWH)	Australia (rural, mostly)	Prospective cohort	6	Australian	Women	Range: 45–50		8921 (333)	3.7	Self-report	VFFQ	10.7	10.7	OR: 0.50 (0.32–0.77)
de Oliveira Otto, 2012 (MESA)	USA (urban)	Prospective cohort	Mean: 4.8	White, Asian, African American, Hispanic	Men/Women	Range: 45–84 61.8 ± 10.3		4982 (499)	10.0	FPG ≥ 6.99 mmol/L, or self-reported, or drugs	VFFQ	Median (standard error) 8.3 (4.4)		HR: 1.41 (0.88–2.27)
Sun, 2009 (NHS)	USA (urban)	Prospective cohort	24	White	Women	Range: 33–60		82,297 (6030)	7.3	Self-report	VFFQ	N/A	N/A	RR: 0.92 (0.84–1.00)
Singh, 1998	India (rural)	Cross-sectional study	N/A	South Asian	Men	25–64		894 (27)	3.0	FPG > 7.7 mmol/L, or 2-h 75-g OGTT > 11.1 mmol/L	7-day dietary record	8.8 ± 2.2		OR: 0.61 (0.35–1.66)
					Women			875 (24)	2.7			8.1 ± 2.1		OR: 0.58 (0.44–1.15)
	India (urban)				Men			904 (63)	7.0			7.0 ± 2.0		OR: 0.90 (0.82–0.98)
					Women			902 (45)	5.0			5.6 ± 1.6		OR: 0.85 (0.71–0.93)

Abbreviations: SD, Standard Deviation; T2DM, Type 2 Diabetes Mellitus; MDCS, Malmö Diet and Cancer Study; FPG, Fasting Plasma Glucose; VDHQ, Validated Diet History Questionnaire; HR, Hazard Ratio; CI, Confidence Interval; JACC, Japan Collaborative Cohort; VFFQ, Validated Food Frequency Questionnaire; OR, Odds Ratio; CARDIA, Coronary Artery Risk Development in Young Adults; OGTT, Oral Glucose Tolerance Test; HbA1c, Glycosylated Hemoglobin; ALSWH, Australian Longitudinal Study on Women's Health; MESA, Multi-Ethnic Study of Atherosclerosis; NHS, Nurses' Health Study; N/A, Not Applicable or Not Available; RR, Relative Risk.

Table 2. Characteristics of studies reporting the association between supplementary and total zinc intake and risk of type 2 diabetes.

Author, Year (Study)	Location (Area)	Study Design	Follow-Up (Years)	Ethnicity	Gender	Age (Years) in Cases at Baseline (mean ± SD)	Age (Years) in Controls at Baseline (mean ± SD)	Sample Size (T2DM)	T2DM (%)	Ascertainment of T2DM	Zinc Assessment Method	Zinc Intake (mg/day) in Cases (mean ± SD)	Zinc Intake (mg/day) in Controls (mean ± SD)	Effect Size (95% CI)
Supplementary zinc intake														
Drake, 2017 (MDCS)	Sweden (urban)	Prospective cohort	Median: 19	White	Men/Women	58.0 ± 7.0	57.8 ± 7.7	26,132 (3676)	14.1	FPG ≥ 7.0 mmol/L (twice), or registries	VDHQ	12.3% user	17.7% user	HR: 0.83 (0.71–0.98)
Song, 2011 (NIH-AARP)	USA (urban)	Prospective cohort	10	White, mostly	Men/Women	Range: 50–71	Range: 50–71	232,007 (14,130)	6.1	Self-report	Dietary survey	12.5% user	5.7% user	OR: 1.05 (0.98–1.13)
Sun, 2009 (NHS)	USA (urban)	Prospective cohort	24	White	Women with low dietary zinc intake	Range: 33–60	Range: 33–60	27,432 (2002)	7.3	Self-report	VFFQ	6.3% user in 1980–48.6% user in 2004		RR: 0.86 (0.74–0.99)
		Prospective cohort			Women with high dietary zinc intake			27,432 (2002)						RR: 1.05 (0.92–1.19)
Total zinc intake														
Drake, 2017 (MDCS)	Sweden (urban)	Prospective cohort	Median: 19	White	Men/Women	58.0 ± 7.0	57.8 ± 7.7	26,132 (3676)	14.1	FPG ≥ 7.0 mmol/L (twice), or registries	VDHQ	12.9 ± 5.4	13.0 ± 6.2	HR: 1.05 (0.88–1.25)
Sun, 2009 (NHS)	USA (urban)	Prospective cohort	24	White	Women	Range: 33–60	N/A	82,297 (6030)	7.3	Self-report	VFFQ	Median range: 4.9–18.0	N/A	RR: 0.90 (0.82–0.99)

Abbreviations: SD, Standard Deviation; T2DM, Type 2 Diabetes Mellitus; MDCS, Malmö Diet and Cancer Study; FPG, Fasting Plasma Glucose; VDHQ, Validated Diet History Questionnaire; HR, Hazard Ratio; NIH-AARP, National Institutes of Health-American Association of Retired Persons Diet and Health Study; OR, Odds Ratio; NHS, Nurses' Health Study; N/A, Not Applicable or Not Available; VFFQ, Validated Food Frequency Questionnaire; RR, Relative Risk.

Table 3. Characteristics of studies reporting the association between serum/plasma and whole blood zinc concentration and risk of type 2 diabetes.

Author, Year	Location	Study Design	Follow-Up (Years)	Ethnicity	Gender	Age (Years) in Cases at Baseline (mean ± SD)	Age (Years) in Controls at Baseline (mean ± SD)	Sample Size (T2DM)	T2DM (%)	Ascertainment of T2DM	Zinc Assessment Method	Zinc Levels (µg/dL) in Diabetic Subjects (mean ± SD)	Zinc Levels (µg/dL) in Controls (mean ± SD)	Effect Size (95% CI)
Serum/plasma zinc concentration														
Yuan, 2018 (DFTJ)	China (urban)	Nested case-control	4.6	Chinese	Men/Women	62.8 ± 7.2	62.9 ± 7.3	2078 (1039)	N/A	FPG ≥ 7.0 mmol/L, or HbA1c ≥ 6.5%, or self-reported, or drugs RPG ≥ 11.1 mmol/L and symptoms,	ICP-MS	169.6 ± 142.4	156.1 ± 126.5	OR: 1.09 (0.81–1.48)
Li, 2017	China (urban)	Cross-sectional	N/A	Chinese Han	Men/Women	Range: 40–92, mean: 66.3	Range: 40–92, mean: 66.5	551 (122)	N/A	2-h OGTT ≥ 11.1 mmol/L, or FPG ≥ 7.0 mmol/L, or HbA1c ≥ 6.5%	ICP-MS	Median: 63.4	Median: 57.5	OR: 2.26 (1.29–3.98)
Zhang, 2017 (REACTION)	China (urban)	Cross-sectional	N/A	Chinese	Men/Women	57.7 ± 7.4	55.2 ± 7.9	1837 (510)	N/A	Self-reported, or FPG > 7.0 mmol/L, or 2-h 75-g OGTT > 11.1 mmol/L	ICP-MS	109.0 ± 26.0	105.0 ± 25.0	OR: 1.79 (1.13–2.84)
Yary, 2016 (KIHD)	Finland (rural / urban)	Prospective cohort	20	N/A	Men	Range: 42–60		2220 (416)	18.7	Self-reported, or FPG ≥ 7.0 mmol/L or 2-h OGTT ≥ 11.1 mmol/L	AAS	95.0 ± 10.0	93.0 ± 12.0	HR: 1.39 (1.04–1.85)
Skalnaya, 2016	Russia (urban)	Cross-sectional	N/A	N/A	Women	55.8 ± 5.3	56.7 ± 6.1	128 (64)	N/A	HbA1c≥6.5%	ICP-MS	96.0 ± 0.2	105.0 ± 0.2	OR: 0.33 (0.14–0.76)
Shan, 2014	China (urban)	Cross-sectional	N/A	Chinese Han	Men/Women	51.0 ± 10.8	42.5 ± 11.6	1578 (785)	N/A	WHO 1999 criteria	ICP-MS	115.0 ± 45.0	172.5 ± 73.0	OR: 0.09 (0.06–0.13)
Whole blood zinc concentration														
Simic, 2017 (HUNT3)	Norway (rural, mostly)	Cross-sectional	N/A	Caucasian, mostly	Men/Women	65.4 ± 10.6	59.2 ± 12.2	876 (267)	N/A	Self-reported	ICP-MS	Median: 764.3 Range (10–90%): 643.6–893.3	Median: 751.2 Range (10–90%): 623.5–878.2	OR: 1.08 (0.59–1.97)
Hansen, 2017 (HUNT3)	Norway (rural, mostly)	Cross-sectional	N/A	Caucasian, mostly	Men/Women	65.2 ± 10.3	61.4 ± 14.1	883 (128)	N/A	FPG ≥ 7.0 mmol/L and/or 2-h OGTT ≥ 11.1 mmol/L	ICP-MS	Median: 799.0 Range (10–90%): 675.0–881.0	Median: 754.0 Range (10–90%): 628.0–885.0	OR: 2.19 (1.05–4.59)

Abbreviations: SD, Standard Deviation; T2DM, Type 2 Diabetes Mellitus; DFTJ, Dongfeng–Tongji; FPG, Fasting Plasma Glucose; N/A, Not Applicable or Not Available; HbA1c, Glycosylated Hemoglobin; ICP-MS, Inductively Coupled Plasma Mass Spectrometry; OR, Odds Ratio; RPG, Random Plasma Glucose; OGTT, Oral Glucose Tolerance Test; REACTION, Risk Evaluation of cAncers in Chinese diabeTic Individuals: a lONgitudinal; KIHD, Kuopio IschaemicHeart Disease Risk Factor Study; AAS, Atomic Absorption Spectrophotometry; HR, Hazard Ratio; WHO, World Health Organization; HUNT, North-TrØndelag Health.

Through a stratified analysis based on the area of residence of participants, rural versus urban, (Figure 3) we observed a higher and significant effect size in rural areas (OR = 0.59, 95% CI: 0.48–0.73), and undetectable heterogeneity (I^2 = 0.0%, p = 0.843), meanwhile in urban areas the effect became non-significant (OR = 0.94, 95% CI: 0.86–1.02; I^2 = 43.9%, p = 0.113). Subsequently, we used the adjusted R^2 to examine how much of the heterogeneity was accounted for by the area of residence (Table 4), and we found that the heterogeneity was explained to a great extent (R_A^2 = 100.0%; I_r^2 = 17.8%). Interestingly, through a stratified analysis by the covariate "study design and area of residence", we observed that this protective effect of dietary zinc intake in rural areas was found in both cross-sectional and prospective studies (Figure 4). In this analysis, results were statistically significant, and heterogeneity was reduced (I^2 = 0.0%, p > 0.050) for all subgroups, except for prospective studies conducted in urban areas (OR = 1.04, 95% CI: 0.88–1.24; I^2 = 50.7%, p = 0.107).

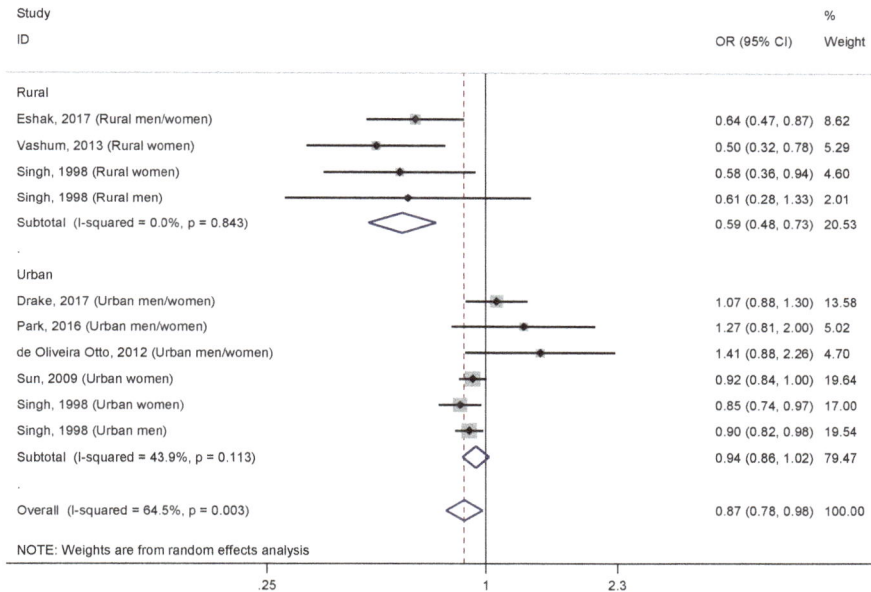

Figure 3. Forest plot of pooled effect size of the highest vs. lowest dietary zinc intake for T2DM according to area of residence (rural vs. urban). Squares represent ORs for each study, and the size of the square is the study-specific statistical weight. Horizontal lines indicate the 95% CI of each study. Diamond represents the combined OR estimate with corresponding 95% CI.

The corresponding adjusted R^2 for this covariate was 90.47%. However, the covariate that showed the greatest impact on the relationship studied was the percentage of T2DM, both as continuous and categorized variable. Thus, the stratified analysis (Figure 5) by this covariate categorized (<5/5–9.9/≥10) revealed a significant protective effect of dietary zinc intake in those studies with <5% of T2DM (OR = 0.59, 95% CI: 0.48–0.73; I^2 = 0.0%, p = 0.843), and those between 5–9.9% (OR = 0.90, 95% CI: 0.85–0.95; I^2 = 0.0%, p = 0.627), but not when it was higher than 10% (OR = 1.13, 95% CI: 0.96–1.34; I^2 = 0.0%, p = 0.499). It should be noted that the level of heterogeneity was reduced to 0.0% in all these subgroups. The importance of this covariate in the assessed relationship was supported by the large proportion of the between-study variance was explained (R_A^2 = 100.0%), as well as the undetectable percentage of the residual variation that was attributable to the between-study heterogeneity, after entering this covariate into a univariate meta-regression model (I_r^2 = 0.0%).

Table 4. Stratified meta-analyses and meta-regressions on the association between dietary zinc intake and risk of type 2 diabetes mellitus.

| Subgroup | Studies (n) | Effect Size (95% CI) | Heterogeneity | | Meta-Regressions | | | | | |
			I² (%)	p-Value	Regression Coefficients (95% CI)	Standard Error	p-Value	Tau²	I² Residual (%)	Adjusted R² (%)
Geographic area										
Western (1)	5	0.97 (0.77–1.22)	72.1%	0.006	−0.25 (−0.66; 0.17)	0.18	0.208	0.04	64.05%	6.68%
Eastern (2)	5	0.80 (0.70–0.92)	49.3%	0.096						
Geographic regions										
Oceania (1)	1	0.50 (0.32–0.78)	-	-						
Asia (2)	5	0.80 (0.70–0.92)	49.3%	0.096	0.22 (0.04–0.39)	0.08	0.022	0.02	50.38%	67.68%
America (3)	3	1.10 (0.82–1.47)	57.7%	0.094						
Europe (4)	1	1.07 (0.88–1.30)	-	-						
Area of residence										
Rural (1)	4	0.59 (0.48–0.73)	0.0%	0.843	0.45 (0.16; 0.73)	0.13	0.007	0.00	17.82%	100.0%
Urban (2)	6	0.94 (0.86–1.02)	43.9%	0.113						
Gender										
Men (1)	2	0.90 (0.82–0.98)	0.0%	0.331	0.14 (−0.17; 0.45)	0.13	0.330	0.06	67.67%	−30.54%
Women (2)	4	0.78 (0.65–0.95)	71.4%	0.015						
Men/Women (3)	4	1.02 (0.73–1.42)	74.1%	0.009						
Ethnicity										
White (1)	3	0.86 (0.66–1.12)	79.4%	0.008	0.10 (−0.06; 0.26)	0.07	0.194	0.06	68.30%	−17.63%
South Asian (2)	4	0.86 (0.77–0.95)	28.5%	0.241						
Japanese (3)	1	0.64 (0.47–0.87)	-	-						
Several ethnic groups (4)	2	1.34 (0.96–1.85)	0.0%	0.755						
Study design										
Prospective Cohort (1)	6	0.90 (0.73–1.12)	75.1%	0.001	−0.07 (−0.31; 0.16)	0.10	0.495	0.06	67.06%	−33.29%
Cross-sectional (2)	4	0.86 (0.77–0.95)	28.5%	0.241						
Study design and area of residence										
Prospective/Rural (1)	2	0.59 (0.46–0.76)	0.0%	0.367	0.18 (0.08; 0.29)	0.05	0.004	0.004	22.03%	90.47%
Cross-sectional/Rural (2)	2	0.58 (0.39–0.89)	0.0%	0.914						
Cross-sectional/Urban (3)	2	0.88 (0.82–0.95)	0.0%	0.489						
Prospective/Urban (4)	4	1.04 (0.88–1.24)	50.7%	0.107						
Measure of association										
Odds ratio (1)	5	0.75 (0.63–0.88)	63.2%	0.019	0.21 (0.05; 0.39)	0.07	0.016	0.02	49.76%	63.13%
Relative risk (2)	1	0.92 (0.84–1.00)	-	-						
Hazard ratio (3)	4	1.13 (0.96–1.34)	0.0%	0.499						

Table 4. Cont.

Subgroup	Studies (n)	Effect Size (95% CI)	Heterogeneity		Meta-Regressions					
			I² (%)	p-Value	Regression Coefficients (95% CI)	Standard Error	p-Value	Tau²	I² Residual (%)	Adjusted R² (%)
Sample size										
<1000	4	0.86 (0.77–0.95)	28.5%	0.241	0.03 (−0.09; 0.14)	0.05	0.578	0.06	66.27%	−29.83%
1000–4999	2	1.34 (0.96–1.85)	0.0%	0.755						
5000–9999	2	0.59 (0.46–0.76)	0.0%	0.367						
≥10,000	2	0.97 (0.84–1.11)	47.9%	0.166						
Percentage of T2DM										
<5%	4	0.59 (0.48–0.73)	0.0%	0.843	0.31 (0.15; 0.46)	0.07	0.002	0.00	0.00%	100.0%
5–9.9%	3	0.90 (0.85–0.95)	0.0%	0.627						
≥10%	3	1.13 (0.96–1.34)	0.0%	0.499						
Zinc intake assessment method										
VFFQ (1)	4	0.80 (0.57–1.12)	80.3%	0.002	−0.01 (−0.28; 0.26)	0.12	0.906	0.07	68.24%	−40.61%
VDHQ (2)	2	1.10 (0.92–1.31)	0.0%	0.497						
7-day dietary record (3)	4	0.86 (0.77–0.95)	28.5%	0.241						
Zinc quantiles adjusted for energy										
Adjusted (1)	9	0.86 (0.76–0.96)	65.3%	0.003	0.42 (−0.40; 1.25)	0.36	0.271	0.04	65.34%	6.11%
Not adjusted (2)	1	1.27 (0.81–2.00)	-	-						
Ascertainment of T2DM										
FPG/OGTT (1)	4	0.86 (0.77–0.95)	28.5%	0.241	0.19 (−0.05; 0.43)	0.10	0.112	0.04	62.01%	11.25%
Self-reported (2)	3	0.70 (0.48–1.01)	82.6%	0.003						
Several criteria (3)	3	1.13 (0.96–1.34)	0.0%	0.499						
Diagnostic pattern										
One diagnostic pattern	7	0.81 (0.72–0.91)	61.7%	0.016	0.41 (0.06; 0.77)	0.15	0.027	0.02	53.12%	51.60%
Several diagnostic pattern	3	1.13 (0.96–1.34)	0.0%	0.499						
Study quality										
80–89	6	0.83 (0.71–0.97)	58.4%	0.035	−0.11 (−0.36; 0.58)	0.21	0.598	0.06	65.99%	−23.10%
≥90	4	0.92 (0.73–1.16)	74.0%	0.009						

Abbreviations: CI, Confidence Interval; VDHQ, Validated Diet History Questionnaire; VFFQ, Validated Food Frequency Questionnaire; T2DM, Type 2 Diabetes Mellitus; FPG, Fasting Plasma Glucose; OGTT, Oral Glucose Tolerance Test.

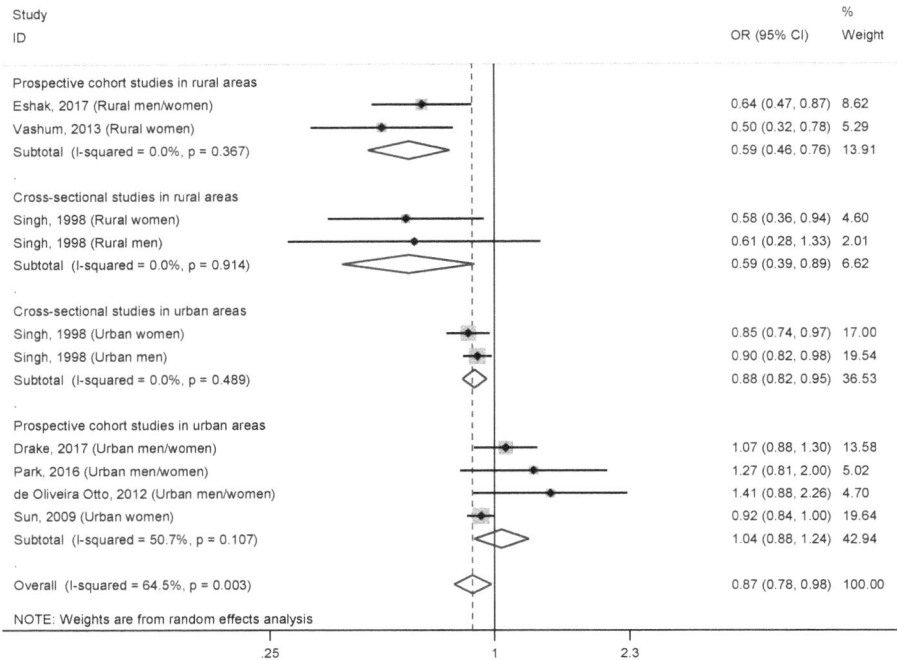

Figure 4. Forest plot of pooled effect size of the highest vs. lowest dietary zinc intake for T2DM according to study design and area of residence (prospective cohort studies in rural areas, cross-sectional studies in rural areas, cross-sectional studies in urban areas, and prospective cohort studies in urban areas). Squares represent ORs for each study, and the size of the square is the study-specific statistical weight. Horizontal lines indicate the 95% CI of each study. Diamond represents the combined OR estimate with corresponding 95% CI.

A multivariate meta-regression model adding the three covariates with a significantly higher impact on the association, showed that only a "percentage of T2DM" continued being significant (0.23, 95% CI: 0.02, 0.45, $p = 0.037$). Once the fourth covariate was introduced, none remained significant. When we analyzed the percentage of T2DM as a continuous variable, similar results were observed ($R_A^2 = 100.0\%$, $I_r^2 = 23.6\%$). A bubble plot was used to represent this covariate (Figure 6), and it was found that, as the percentage of T2DM increased, the protective effect of a moderately high dietary zinc intake was reduced in a relationship defined by the equation of the regression line: $(\text{Ln}(\text{OR}_{\text{T2DM}}) = (-0.4217314) + 0.0437897 \times (\text{percentage of T2DM}))$.

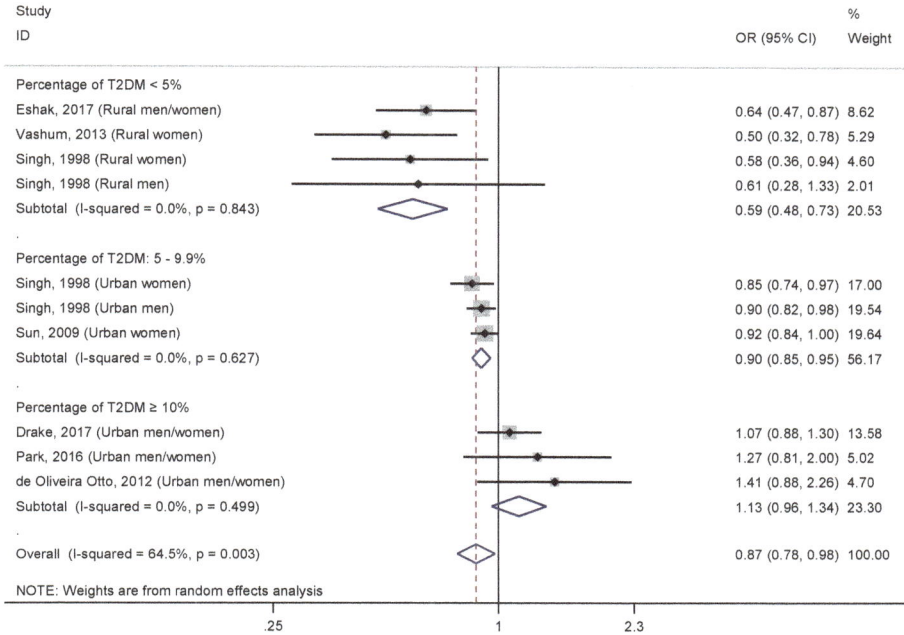

Figure 5. Forest plot of pooled effect size of the highest vs. lowest dietary zinc intake for T2DM according to the percentage of T2DM (<5%/5–9.9%/≥10%). Squares represent ORs for each study, and the size of the square is the study-specific statistical weight. Horizontal lines indicate the 95% CI of each study. Diamond represents the combined OR estimate with corresponding 95% CI.

The effect size ranged between (OR = 0.84, 95% CI: 0.75–0.96) after excluding the study carried out by Drake et al. [6], and (OR = 0.90, 95% CI: 0.81–0.99), after excluding the study conducted by Vashum et al. [5]. However, the combined overall effect size remained on the verge of statistical significance after removing the data obtained by Singh et al. [39] in urban Indian women (OR = 0.87, 95% CI: 0.76–1.00), or that of Eshak et al. [7] in Japanese subjects (OR = 0.90, 95% CI: 0.80–1.01). Finally, for this meta-analysis, an overall symmetry of the funnel plots was observed by visual inspection (Supplementary Materials Figure S1). This was confirmed by the Egger's (p = 0.429) and Begg's (p = 0.721) tests, indicating the absence of publication bias.

3.2. Supplementary Zinc Intake and T2DM

Three studies of 313,003 individuals assessed the association between supplementary zinc intake and T2DM (NHS cohort [4], National Institutes of Health-American Association of Retired Persons (NIH-AARP) Diet and Health Study [12], MDCS cohort [6]) (Table 2). The follow-up period of these prospective cohort studies ranged between 10 [12] to 24 years [4]. Participants were white (mostly) women [4] or subjects of both genders [6,12], aged between 33 and 71 years, and from urban areas. In total, 17,806 patients with incident diabetes (between 6.1 and 14.1%) were identified according to different diagnostic criteria (self-reported [4,12], or through an FPG ≥ 7.0 mmol/L measured twice, and institutional registries [6]).

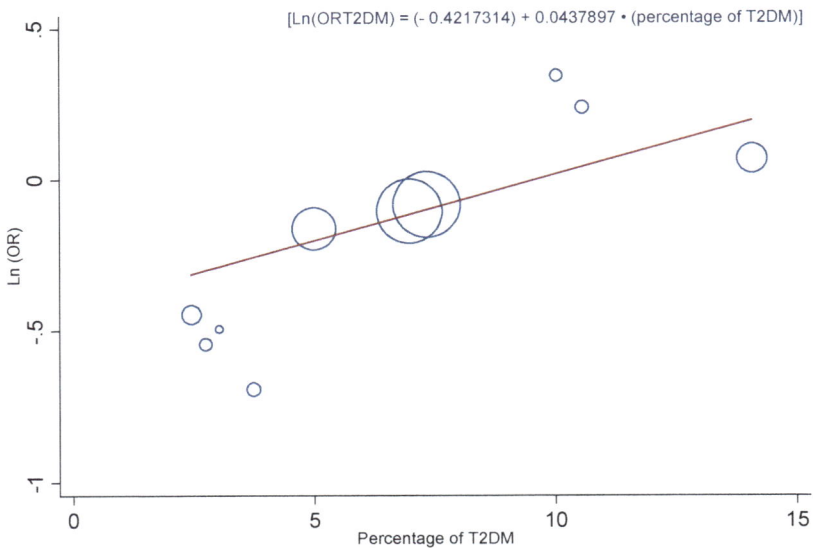

Figure 6. Bubble plot with a fitted meta-regression line of the relationship between the Ln(OR) and the percentage of T2DM. Circles are sized according to the precision of each estimate (the inverse of its within-study variance).

Supplementary zinc intake was determined using different food intake instruments, such as VFFQ [4], VDHQ [6], or dietary survey, including an FFQ and a short survey [12]. The percentage of patients with incident diabetes supplemented with zinc was around 12.5% [6,12], meanwhile in controls of non-incident diabetes, zinc supplementation ranged between 5.7% in the NIH-AARP Diet and Health Study [12], to 17.7%, in the MDCS cohort [6]. The NHS cohort reported a large increase in the proportion of women who were supplemented with zinc in 2004 (48.6%) compared with 1980 (6.3%) [4].

The association between supplementary zinc intake and the risk of T2DM was evaluated through a meta-analysis stratified by whether the analysis had been done comparing zinc supplement users versus non-users or comparing the highest versus lowest quantile of supplementary zinc intake, in order not to introduce bias in the analysis (Figure 7). Results revealed a non-significant association between zinc supplement users versus non-users and T2DM (OR = 0.94, 95% CI: 0.75–1.19; I^2 = 85.4%, p = 0.009), and between higher supplementary zinc intake versus lower and T2DM (OR = 0.95, 95% CI: 0.78–1.16; I^2 = 75.3%, p = 0.044), and an elevated heterogeneity in both cases.

Publication bias was unlikely in this meta-analysis, according to Egger's (p = 0.186), and Begg's (p = 0.089) tests (Figure S2).

3.3. Total Zinc Intake and T2DM

The final data set for the meta-analysis of total zinc intake and risk of T2DM included only two large prospective cohort studies [4,6] (Table 2). Nevertheless, both studies comprised 108,429 individuals, 9706 patients with incident diabetes and 98,723 controls of non-incident diabetes. Incidence of T2DM was 14.1% in the middle-aged Swedish cohort of urban men and women (MDCS) [6], and 7.3% in the American cohort of urban women (NHS) [4]. A VFFQ [4] and a VDHQ [6] were used to determine the total zinc intake, that ranged from 4.9 to 18.0 mg/day in the NHS cohort [4], and around 12.9 ± 5.4 mg/day in controls of non-incident diabetes and 13.0 ± 6.2 mg/day in patients with incident diabetes from the MDCS cohort [6].

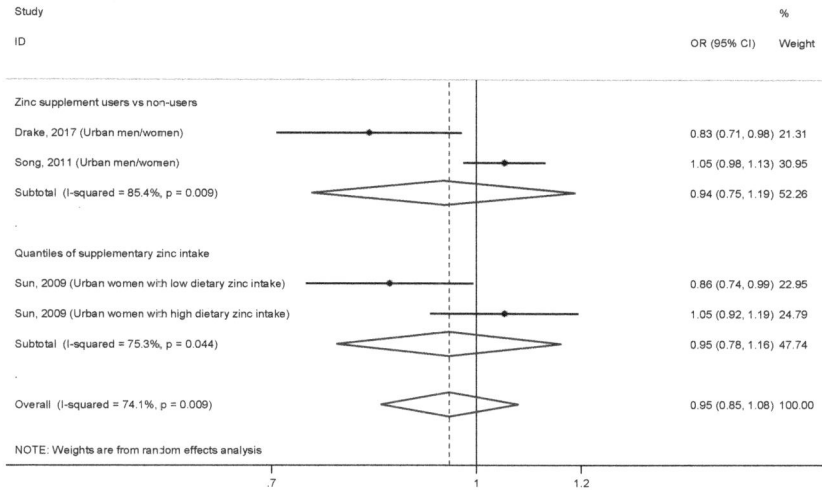

Figure 7. Forest plot of the pooled effect size of the highest versus lowest supplementary zinc intake for T2DM according to the analysis (zinc supplement users/non-users versus quantiles of supplementary zinc intake). Squares represent ORs for each study, and the size of the square is the study-specific statistical weight. Horizontal lines indicate the 95% CI of each study. Diamond represents the combined OR estimate with corresponding 95% CI.

After pooling data from both studies (Figure 8), we found that total zinc intake was not significantly associated with the incidence of T2DM (OR = 0.95, 95% CI: 0.82–1.11). There was moderate heterogeneity between the studies (I^2 = 56.5%, *p* = 0.129). Moreover, no evidence of publication bias was found (*p* = 1.000) (Supplementary Materials Figure S3).

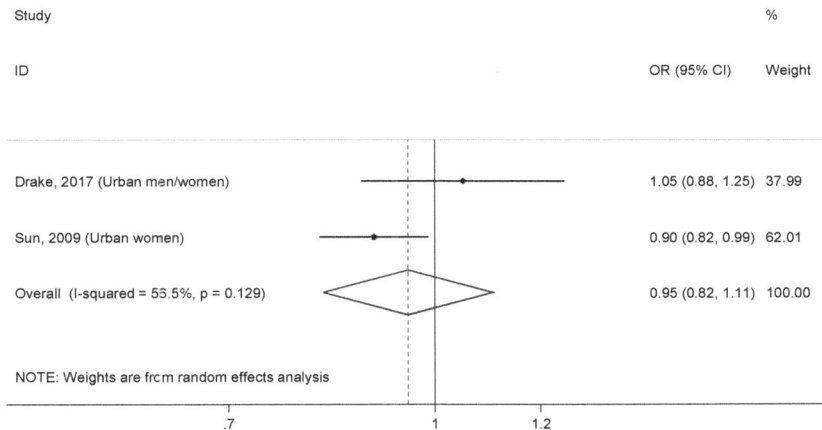

Figure 8. Forest plot of pooled effect size of the highest vs. lowest total zinc intake for T2DM. Squares represent ORs for each study, and the size of the square is the study-specific statistical weight. Horizontal lines indicate the 95% CI of each study. Diamond represents the combined OR estimate with corresponding 95% CI.

3.4. Whole Blood Zinc Concentration and T2DM

Only two cross-sectional studies carried out within the third survey of the population-based Nord-Trøndelag Health Study (HUNT3 Survey) were identified to assess the relationship between concentration of zinc in whole blood and T2DM [18,19]. The fact that both studies shared part of the same study sample prevented the execution of a meta-analysis to obtain a pooled result. Nevertheless, a qualitative summary was conducted to present the findings of these two studies (Table 3). Participants in both studies were men and women, mainly Caucasian, and aged around 61.5 ± 8.7 years old, who lived mainly in rural areas from Norway. The main difference between these two studies was the sampling strategy. Hansen et al. [18] selected 876 subjects at high risk for T2DM, but without previously known diabetes. In this study, 128 previously undiagnosed cases of T2DM, were detected by screening [18]. In contrast, Simic et al. [19] included 883 subjects, of which 267 had self-reported T2DM, i.e., they were patients in a more advanced stage of the disease. Curiously, while Hansen et al. [18] found a significant and positive association between a higher whole blood zinc concentration and the onset of T2DM (OR = 2.19, 95% CI: 1.05–4.59), Simic et al. [19] did not observe any significant relationship (OR = 1.08, 95% CI: 0.59–1.97). Differences in concentrations of zinc in whole blood between cases and controls, measured in both studies through inductively coupled plasma mass spectrometry (ICP-MS), were more evident in the study conducted by Hansen et al. [18] (median in cases: 799.0 µg/dL; median in controls: 754.0 µg/dL) compared to the one carried out by Simic et al. [19] (median in cases: 764.3 µg/dL; median in controls: 751.2 µg/dL). It is worth noting that the median whole blood zinc concentration in the control subjects in both studies was very similar, but not in those of the diabetic subjects.

3.5. Serum/Plasma Zinc Concentration and T2DM

Six observational studies (one prospective cohort study [14], one nested case-control study [15], and four cross-sectional studies [16,17,40,41]) were included in the meta-analysis of serum/plasma zinc concentration and T2DM (Table 3). Four studies were carried out on Chinese urban men and women between the ages of 40 and 90 years [15,16,40,41], one in Russian women with an average age of 56.3 ± 5.7 years [17], and one in Finnish men aged between 42 and 60 years [14]. The total number of cases of T2DM was 2936, among 8392 participants. The period of follow-up was between 4.6 years in the nested case control within the Dongfeng–Tongji (DFTJ) cohort [15], and 20 years in the KIHD study [14]. Serum/plasma zinc concentration was determined mainly by ICP-MS [15–17,40,41], meanwhile the KIHD used atomic absorption spectrophotometry (AAS) [14]. The levels of serum/plasma zinc in controls ranged from a median of 57.5 µg/dL to a mean of 172.5 ± 73.0 µg/dL; and in cases from a median of 63.4 µg/dL to a mean of 169.6 ± 142.4 µg/dL.

The combined effect size of T2DM for the highest versus lowest quantile of serum/plasma zinc concentration was 0.76 (95% CI: 0.29–2.01). However, a high level of heterogeneity was found ($I^2 = 97.1\%$, $p < 0.001$). Sensitivity analysis omitting one study at a time and calculating the heterogeneity for the remainder of the studies showed that the study conducted by Shan et al. [16] substantially influenced the overall heterogeneity, resulting in a reduction around 31% of this when it was excluded. In addition, the elimination of this study and the one carried out by Skalnaya et al. [17], decreased the level of heterogeneity by 44.5%, showing their impact on results (OR = 1.47, 95% CI: 1.11–1.95; $I^2 = 53.9\%$, $p = 0.090$). Nevertheless, the exclusion of any other study had a negligible effect on heterogeneity. When performing stratified analysis for "sample base" (Figure 9), a significant and positive association was found in the subgroup of "population or community-based studies" (OR = 1.64, 95% CI: 1.25–2.14), and a low heterogeneity ($I^2 > 22.5\%$, $p = 0.275$). On the other hand, "non-population or community-based studies" showed a very high level of heterogeneity ($I^2 > 98.0\%$, $p < 0.001$). Likewise, when it was stratified by the covariate "group with higher zinc levels", a relationship between serum/plasma zinc levels and T2DM (OR = 1.47, 95% CI: 1.11–1.95; $I^2 = 53.9\%$, $p = 0.090$) was observed in the subgroup of studies with higher zinc levels in the case group compared to controls (Table S3). Meanwhile, a significant negative relationship was found in the subgroup in which controls had higher serum/plasma concentration (OR = 0.16, 95% CI: 0.05–0.54), but with a high heterogeneity (I^2 = 86.4%, p = 0.007). Finally, the difference in mean serum/plasma zinc concentration between cases and controls, as well its ratio, also explained, to a large extent, the heterogeneity observed (R_A^2 = 85.2%, for mean difference; and R_A^2 = 92.6%, for mean ratio), as expected.

Although the funnel plot showed some degree of asymmetry (Figure S3), we did not detect any risk of publication bias according to the Egger's (p = 0.815) or Begg's tests (p = 0.707).

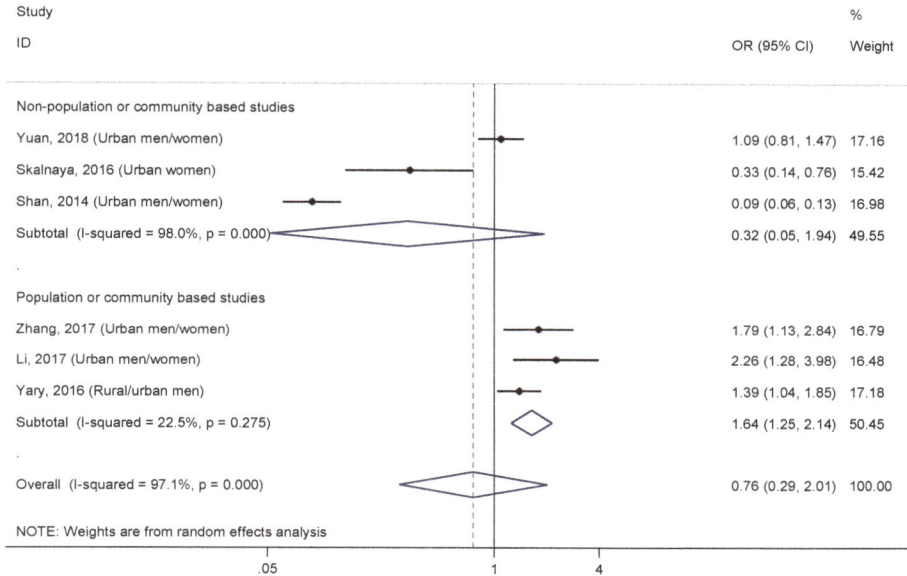

Figure 9. Forest plot of pooled effect size of the highest vs. lowest serum/plasma zinc concentration for T2DM according to the sample base (population/community-based studies vs. non-population/community-based studies). Squares represent ORs for each study, and the size of the square is the study-specific statistical weight. Horizontal lines indicate the 95% CI of each study. Diamond represents the combined OR estimate with corresponding 95% CI.

4. Discussion

This systematic review and meta-analysis of observational studies found an inverse association between dietary zinc intake and T2DM. This could suggest a potential beneficial role of zinc from diet to prevent the risk of this disease. In addition, the relationship seemed to be more evident in rural areas, and when the proportion of T2DM cases in the population was low or moderate. Conversely, a non-significant association between total or supplementary zinc intake and T2DM was observed, although data are limited. Whole blood zinc concentration could be directly related to T2DM only at an early phase of the diabetes disease, as suggested by results from the same cohort study. This hypothesis could not be examined for serum/plasma zinc concentration. Nevertheless, a positive relationship was found between this biomarker of zinc status and T2DM in population-based studies.

Our results suggest that a diet moderately elevated in zinc could help to prevent the development of T2DM. We tried to determine the cut-off point or range of dietary zinc intake with a protective effect against type 2 diabetes mellitus (T2DM); however, data were imprecise, heterogeneous, and not reported in all the studies. Despite these limitations in the data of the selected studies, it was notable that when the lowest quantiles (reference) did not reach the dietary reference intakes (DRI) according to the Institute Of Medicine (IOM) for adult men (11 mg/day) and women (8 mg/day) [43], those quantiles of dietary zinc intake that reached or moderately exceeded the DRI showed a protective effect, even in the intermediate quantiles [4,5]. Furthermore, when the highest quantiles of dietary zinc intake did not reach the DRI, no significant association was observed [10]. Interestingly, when the lowest quantiles of dietary zinc intake reached the DRI, the highest quantiles (>23.34 mg/day) did not show a protective effect on T2DM, and could even have a harmful impact on the risk of T2DM as observed in a model not fully adjusted [11]. These data seem to suggest that a dietary zinc intake within or slightly above the DRI could have a protective role on the risk of T2DM, but not when intake is very high. Consistent with our findings, several observational studies have shown a protective effect of a moderately high dietary zinc intake on cardiometabolic conditions, such as metabolic syndrome [44,45] and gestational hyperglycemia [46], and mortality by cardiovascular disease [47] and all causes [48]. Conversely, other studies have found no significant [10,49], or even direct associations [50,51] between dietary zinc intake and some of these cardiometabolic events. The first systematic review of prospective cohort studies on the association between zinc status, including dietary zinc intake, and risk of cardiovascular disease and T2DM [13] revealed a limited number of studies on this topic, as well as the inconsistency of their results. As the authors themselves suggested, the effect of confounding factors may have played an important role in the observed findings. In our meta-analysis we have evaluated a large number of confounding factors in order to identify and quantify those that could impact on the relationship between dietary zinc intake and T2DM. Gender is one of the confounding factors most reported in the above mentioned studies on the relationship between dietary zinc intake and metabolic syndrome [44,45], cardiovascular disease [13], and mortality [47]. Our results showed a similar significant inverse association between dietary zinc intake and T2DM in both men and women, suggesting that gender does not seem to have a relevant role in this relationship.

Interestingly, we observed that the covariate "area of residence" of participants (rural versus urban) had a key effect on our findings. While a strong inverse association was observed in studies conducted on participants living in rural areas, a null relationship was observed in those studies carried out on urban subjects (Figure 3). Interestingly, when we addressed these findings also taking into account the design of the studies, we observed a 41% reduction in the risk of T2DM in both cross-sectional and prospective studies conducted in rural areas (Figure 4). Conversely, the effect size was reduced to 12% in cross-sectional studies performed in urban areas, and in prospective cohort studies, the association was not significant. These observations support the hypothesis that living in urban areas may counteract the beneficial effect of an elevated dietary zinc intake on risk of T2DM. Accumulating evidence strongly suggests that the change from rural to urban environments may have a marked impact on lifestyle [52,53], resulting in the increase of certain risk factors, such as unhealthy diets, sedentary behavior, and smoking, among others, that account for a large contribution to global burden of major disease [54,55]. Thus, it has been revealed that T2DM risk factors are more common in urban than in rural areas [56]. The greater exposure to risk factors in urban environments could explain the small or null protective effect of the intake of zinc from diet against the risk of T2DM. Indeed, it is known that there is higher prevalence of T2DM in urban compared to rural areas [2,56]. According to the International Diabetes Federation (IDF) Diabetes ATLAS edition 2017, the global prevalence of diabetes in urban areas was 10.2%, i.e., 279.2 million people aged between 20–79 years, meanwhile in rural areas was notably lower, 6.9% (145.7 million) [2]. In addition, the number of people living with diabetes in urban areas is expected to increase to 472.6 million in 2045, due mainly to global urbanization [2].

It is interesting that the covariate which had the greatest impact on the association between dietary zinc intake and T2DM was the proportion of T2DM cases identified in each study, both as a continuous and categorized variable. When we conducted a meta-regression introducing the percentage of T2DM as a continuous variable, we found that for each percentage point that increased this covariate, the protective effect of a moderately high dietary zinc intake, relative to the DRI, against T2DM decreased 0.04 (95% CI: 0.01, 0.07, $p = 0.010$). Through a meta-regression equation represented in a bubble plot, we observed that when the proportion of T2DM subjects reached 10%, the protective effect from dietary zinc intake was nullified (Figure 6). Consistently, the three studies with a proportion of T2DM subjects of 10% or more, did not find a significant association between dietary zinc intake and T2DM [6,10,11]. In addition, stratified analysis based on the percentage of T2DM in each study (<5%, 5%–9.9%, and ≥10%) showed an undetectable heterogeneity in all the three subgroups (I^2 = 0.0%, p > 0.100), which provides high reliability to the results. Furthermore, a significant inverse association was found between intake of zinc from diet and T2DM when the percentage of T2DM was lower than 10%, and with the highest effect size when that was less than 5% (Figure 5). It should be noted that the studies with less proportion of T2DM subjects (<5%) were those carried out in rural areas, while those with the highest percentage of diabetics (5%–9.9%, and ≥10%) were the studies conducted in urban areas. In addition, among studies of urban areas, those with a moderate proportion of T2DM (5%–9.9%) retained a significant association between dietary zinc intake and T2DM, although it was more attenuated than those in rural areas. Nevertheless, the studies with higher percentage of T2DM did not find any significant relationship (Figure 5). These results suggest that in rural areas, with less T2DM risk factors, and consequently, less T2DM prevalence, the association between dietary zinc intake and T2DM is significant and the effect size is strong; meanwhile, in urban areas, with a greater exposure to T2DM risk factors and a higher T2DM prevalence, the association is still significant but with a low effect size when T2DM prevalence is moderate, and not significant when the T2DM prevalence is high.

Only two studies have evaluated the effect of a high total zinc intake on the risk of T2DM [4,6], and the overall pooled estimates showed no significant association (Figure 8). The NHS cohort showed a moderate protective effect of total zinc intake, while the MDCS cohort did not find a relationship. Consistent with results from the meta-analysis of the dietary zinc intake, the NHS cohort [4] had a moderate proportion of T2DM (7.3%), meanwhile the MDCS cohort [6] presented the highest percentage of T2DM of all included studies in this systematic review (14.1%). This supports the hypothesis previously raised regarding the impact of the T2DM prevalence on the association between zinc intake and risk of T2DM.

Although, there is currently some evidence of the beneficial effect of zinc supplementation on glycemic control in T2DM patients [9,57], scarce studies support the use of zinc supplements in the prevention of this disease [8]. A recent clinical trial based on zinc supplementation has found a reduction in the progression to T2DM in prediabetic subjects, in addition to an improvement in blood glucose and insulin levels, insulin resistance, and β–cell function [9]. Observational studies that have assessed the association between supplementary zinc intake and risk of T2DM are also scarce [4,6,12]. The overall pooled estimates did not show any significant relationship, neither comparing zinc supplement users versus non-users, nor comparing the highest versus lowest quantile of supplementary zinc intake (Figure 7). Those studies that compared zinc supplement users versus non-users against the risk of T2DM, failed to differentiate between participants who obtained zinc from multivitamin/mineral supplements from those taking individual zinc supplements [6,12]. Thus, a synergistic effect or an interaction between minerals and vitamins supplemented, along with zinc, could have affected the relationship between supplementary zinc intake and the risk of T2DM. Interestingly, the NHS cohort reported a significant inverse association in participants with low dietary zinc intake, but not in those with high dietary zinc intake [4]. In addition, dietary zinc intake was more strongly associated with a lower risk of T2DM among those participants with low zinc intakes from supplements. This seems to suggest that only when the zinc intake is insufficient, zinc supplementation may have benefits. However, when dietary intake is adequate, additional zinc intake from supplementation may not confer further benefit.

To the best of our knowledge, only two cross-sectional studies, conducted within the same population-based HUNT3 study, have evaluated the association between whole blood zinc concentration and T2DM [18,19]. However, the results were dissimilar, likely due to characteristics of participants selected during the sampling. Interestingly, Hansen et al. [18] reported a significant and positive association between whole blood zinc concentration and T2DM, in previously undiagnosed diabetic patients and control subjects [18]. Meanwhile, Simic et al. [19], did not find a significant relationship in previously diagnosed T2DM patients and control subjects. These results seem to suggest that when T2DM is in the early stages, i.e., newly diagnosed, zinc levels are more elevated than non-diabetic subjects, and progressively they are reduced as the disease progresses, which is consistent with our previous systematic review and meta-analysis [20]. That meta-analysis which aimed to compare whole blood zinc concentration between T2DM patients and non-diabetic subjects, showed that duration of T2DM had a relevant influence on concentration of zinc in whole blood [20]. In addition, we found a lower whole blood zinc concentration in T2DM patients; however, this group had, at least, 10.2 ± 8.6 years of duration of diabetes, and differences between cases and controls in that study were not observed [58], in concordance with the study of Simic et al. [19], among previously diagnosed T2DM participants [19].

Since the use of whole blood zinc concentration may be not representative of the total zinc body burden [56], we also assessed the association between zinc and T2DM, through a more reliable biomarker of zinc status, the serum/plasma zinc concentration [59]. We wanted to contrast the hypothesis regarding the impact of the T2DM phases on serum/plasma zinc concentration; however, data were limited to carry out that analysis. Only six studies evaluated this relationship, and results were inconsistent [14–17,40,41], which was highlighted by high heterogeneity observed after the results were combined. Two of the included studies were responsible for 44.5% of the heterogeneity detected [16,17]. After both studies were excluded, the combined result was more reliable (OR = 1.47, 95% CI: 1.11–1.95; $I^2 = 53.9\%$, $p = 0.090$). Curiously, these two studies, together with the third that contributed more to the global heterogeneity, were conducted on non-population or community-based studies, i.e., hospital-based settings [16], retired employees of a motor company [15] and postmenopausal women on a voluntary basis [17], so the results could not be extrapolated to the general population. However, the other three studies were carried out on population [14] or community-based [40,41] studies. Stratified analysis according to the "sample base" (Figure 9) showed a high heterogeneity in the "non-population or community-based studies" group ($I^2 = 98.0\%$, $p < 0.001$), and a low heterogeneity in the "population or community-based studies" group ($I^2 = 22.5\%$, $p = 0.275$). The pooled estimates for this last subgroup revealed a direct and significant association between serum/plasma zinc concentration and T2DM (OR = 1.64, 95% CI: 1.25–2.14). This finding is not consistent with a previous meta-analysis that compared serum/plasma zinc levels between T2DM patients and healthy controls [60]. Results of this previous meta-analysis showed significantly lower serum/plasma zinc concentration in diabetic subjects compared to healthy controls, but with high heterogeneity. The high heterogeneity suggests that results were influenced by confounding factors, but its source was not analyzed in that meta-analysis. Finally, a recent cross-sectional study reported that urinary zinc levels were positively associated with T2DM [61]. These findings suggest this is a response mechanism against zinc excess in serum/plasma in diabetic patients, and it seems to be in concordance with the direct relationship between serum/plasma and T2DM that we observed in our meta-analysis.

Several limitations in the present systematic review and meta-analysis should be considered. First, the number of results and studies included in meta-analyses was small, and stratified analyses might have insufficient power to identify potential confounding factors, as well as to detect potential sources of heterogeneity. To correct this weakness, random effects meta-regressions were carried out. Furthermore, our findings were likely to be influenced by imprecise measurement of zinc intake. However, VFFQ and VDHQ were used to assess dietary, supplementary, and/or total zinc intake, in all but two studies. In addition, differences in diagnostic criteria for the ascertainment of T2DM over the years could have introduced misclassification bias and could affect results. Finally, meta-analyses were based on observational studies, which are prone to confounding and reverse causation. Nevertheless, for meta-analyses of dietary, supplementary and/or total zinc intake, all but one of the included studies were prospective cohort studies, which allows stronger inferences than cross-sectional studies [62].

Our study has also several strengths. Firstly, the comprehensive and robust search strategy within the framework of the EURRECA Network of Excellence was designed to avoid the loss of relevant studies. Moreover, there were no studies that were excluded for reasons of language, avoiding language bias. In addition, standard tests and visual inspection of funnel plots did not show any evidence for risk of publication bias in any meta-analysis. Furthermore, included studies were of high quality, according to the STROBE Statement [42]. The meta-analyses included 575,851 subjects, had a wide geographical spread, and a diverse ethnicity, giving more validity to the results. Finally, heterogeneity was low or moderate in most of the meta-analyses, which also contributes to the study validity.

The important role of zinc on carbohydrate metabolism via several mechanisms is well established, and this could explain the protective effect of dietary zinc intake on risk of T2DM observed in our meta-analysis. Zinc is involved in synthesis, storage, crystallization, and secretion, as well as the action of insulin and translocation of insulin into the cells [21–24]. In addition, zinc seems to play a role in insulin sensitivity through the activation of the phosphoinositol-3-kinase/protein kinase B cascade [25]. It has also a role insulin–mimetic, being involved in the regulation process of glucose homeostasis [26]. Moreover, zinc may participate in the suppression of proinflammatory cytokines, such as interleukin-1β [27] and nuclear factor kβ [28], avoiding β-cells' death and protecting insulin. The underlying mechanism whereby higher serum/plasma and/or whole blood zinc concentration could be related to T2DM is unclear. However, strong evidence supports disturbances in zinc homeostasis associated with T2DM, that could not be linked to zinc status [63,64]. In recent years, it has been proposed that the cellular zinc transport system may play a key role in the pathophysiology of T2DM [65,66]. Thus, differences between diabetic patients and healthy controls in gene expressions for most zinc transporters has been observed [63]. This zinc dyshomeostasis may be caused in the early stages of T2DM, as observed in a trend of increased serum zinc levels from healthy to prediabetic and diabetic postmenopausal women [67].

5. Conclusions

Findings from this systematic review and meta-analysis revealed a potential protective effect of a moderately high dietary zinc intake, related to the DRI, on the risk of T2DM. The relationship seems to be stronger and more evident in rural compared to urban areas. In addition, T2DM prevalence may be also a confounding factor for this association, being stronger when the prevalence is low, weak when it is moderate, and disappearing with a high prevalence. Conversely, no associations were observed between total or supplementary zinc intake and T2DM. However, more data are required to explore this relationship more fully.

In addition, an elevated serum/plasma zinc concentration is associated with an increased risk of T2DM in the general population. Meanwhile, high whole blood zinc concentration could be associated with T2DM, likely only at an early phase of the diabetes disease. Additional studies are required to confirm these results, and determine the role of serum/plasma and whole blood zinc concentration in the pathophysiology of T2DM.

Supplementary Materials: The following are available online at http://www.mdpi.com/2072-6643/11/5/1027/s1, Figure S1: Funnel plot of publication biases of studies included in the meta-analysis of the association between dietary zinc intake and T2DM. Each dot stands for an individual study. Figure S2: Funnel plot of publication biases of studies included in the meta-analysis of the association between supplementary zinc intake and T2DM. Each dot stands for an individual study. Figure S3: Funnel plot of publication biases of studies included in the meta-analysis of the association between serum/plasma zinc concentration and T2DM. Each dot stands for an individual study. Table S1: MOOSE Checklist for Meta-analyses of Observational Studies. Table S2: STROBE Statement Checklist. Table S3: Stratified meta-analyses and meta-regressions on the association between serum/plasma zinc concentration and risk of type 2 diabetes mellitus.

Author Contributions: Conceptualization, N.M.L. and V.H.M.; methodology, N.M.L., V.H.M., M.W.-M., and J.C.F.-C.; formal analysis, J.C.F.-C.; investigation, J.C.F.-C., M.W.-M., V.H.M., V.A., C.D., L.S.-M., and N.M.L.; writing—original draft preparation, J.C.F.-C.; writing—review and editing, J.C.F.-C., M.W.-M., V.H.M., V.A., C.D., L.S.-M., and N.M.L.; supervision, N.M.L.

Funding: This research received no external funding.

Acknowledgments: JCFC thanks the support from the University Staff Training (FPU) grant by the Ministry of Education, Spain; and the mobility aid for university staff in training by the Ministry of Education, Spain. JCFC also thanks the support from the project ATA 1756 of the Ministry of Education of Chile.

Conflicts of Interest: The authors declare no conflict of interest.

References

1. World Health Organization Noncommunicable Diseases: Key Facts. Available online: http://www.who.int/news-room/fact-sheets/detail/noncommunicable-diseases (accessed on 7 February 2019).
2. International Diabetes Federation (IDF) IDF Diabetes Atlas 8th Edition. Available online: http://www.diabetesatlas.org/ (accessed on 7 February 2019).
3. Qi, L.; Hu, F.B.; Hu, G. Genes, environment, and interactions in prevention of type 2 diabetes: A focus on physical activity and lifestyle changes. *Curr. Mol. Med.* **2008**, *8*, 519–532. [CrossRef] [PubMed]
4. Sun, Q.; Van Dam, R.M.; Willett, W.C.; Hu, F.B. Prospective study of zinc intake and risk of type 2 diabetes in women. *Diabetes Care* **2009**, *32*, 629–634. [CrossRef]
5. Vashum, K.P.; McEvoy, M.; Shi, Z.; Milton, A.H.; Islam, M.R.; Sibbritt, D.; Patterson, A.; Byles, J.; Loxton, D.; Attia, J. Is dietary zinc protective for type 2 diabetes? Results from the Australian longitudinal study on women's health. *BMC Endocr. Disord.* **2013**, *13*, 40. [CrossRef] [PubMed]
6. Drake, I.; Hindy, G.; Ericson, U.; Orho-Melander, M. A prospective study of dietary and supplemental zinc intake and risk of type 2 diabetes depending on genetic variation in SLC30A8. *Genes Nutr.* **2017**, *12*, 30. [CrossRef] [PubMed]
7. Eshak, E.S.; Iso, H.; Maruyama, K.; Muraki, I.; Tamakoshi, A. Associations between dietary intakes of iron, copper and zinc with risk of type 2 diabetes mellitus: A large population-based prospective cohort study. *Clin. Nutr.* **2018**, *37*, 667–674. [CrossRef]
8. El Dib, R.; Gameiro, O.L.F.; Ogata, M.S.P.; Módolo, N.S.P.; Braz, L.G.; Jorge, E.C.; do Nascimento, P.; Beletate, V. Zinc supplementation for the prevention of type 2 diabetes mellitus in adults with insulin resistance. *Cochrane Database Syst. Rev.* **2015**, CD005525. [CrossRef]
9. Ranasinghe, P.; Wathurapatha, W.S.; Galappatthy, P.; Katulanda, P.; Jayawardena, R.; Constantine, G.R. Zinc supplementation in prediabetes: A randomized double-blind placebo-controlled clinical trial. *J. Diabetes* **2018**, *10*, 386–397. [CrossRef] [PubMed]
10. De Oliveira Otto, M.C.; Alonso, A.; Lee, D.-H.; Delclos, G.L.; Bertoni, A.G.; Jiang, R.; Lima, J.A.; Symanski, E.; Jacobs, D.R.; Nettleton, J.A. Dietary Intakes of Zinc and Heme Iron from Red Meat, but Not from Other Sources, Are Associated with Greater Risk of Metabolic Syndrome and Cardiovascular Disease. *J. Nutr.* **2012**, *142*, 526–533. [CrossRef]
11. Park, J.S.; Xun, P.; Li, J.; Morris, S.J.; Jacobs, D.R.; Liu, K.; He, K. Longitudinal association between toenail zinc levels and the incidence of diabetes among American young adults: The CARDIA Trace Element Study. *Sci. Rep.* **2016**, *6*, 23155. [CrossRef] [PubMed]
12. Song, Y.; Xu, Q.; Park, Y.; Hollenbeck, A.; Schatzkin, A.; Chen, H. Multivitamins, Individual Vitamin and Mineral Supplements, and Risk of Diabetes Among Older U.S. Adults. *Diabetes Care* **2011**, *34*, 108–114. [CrossRef]
13. Chu, A.; Foster, M.; Samman, S. Zinc status and risk of cardiovascular diseases and type 2 diabetes mellitus—A systematic review of prospective cohort studies. *Nutrients* **2016**, *8*, 707. [CrossRef]
14. Yary, T.; Virtanen, J.K.; Ruusunen, A.; Tuomainen, T.-P.; Voutilainen, S. Serum zinc and risk of type 2 diabetes incidence in men: The Kuopio Ischaemic Heart Disease Risk Factor Study. *J. Trace Elem. Med. Biol.* **2016**, *33*, 120–124. [CrossRef]
15. Yuan, Y.; Xiao, Y.; Yu, Y.; Liu, Y.; Feng, W.; Qiu, G.; Wang, H.; Liu, B.; Wang, J.; Zhou, L.; et al. Associations of multiple plasma metals with incident type 2 diabetes in Chinese adults: The Dongfeng-Tongji Cohort. *Environ. Pollut.* **2018**, *237*, 917–925. [CrossRef]
16. Shan, Z.; Bao, W.; Zhang, Y.; Rong, Y.; Wang, X.; Jin, Y.; Song, Y.; Yao, P.; Sun, C.; Hu, F.B.; et al. Interactions Between Zinc Transporter-8 Gene (SLC30A8) and Plasma Zinc Concentrations for Impaired Glucose Regulation and Type 2 Diabetes. *Diabetes* **2014**, *63*, 1796–1803. [CrossRef]

17. Skalnaya, M.G.; Skalny, A.V.; Yurasov, V.V.; Demidov, V.A.; Grabeklis, A.R.; Radysh, I.V.; Tinkov, A.A. Serum Trace Elements and Electrolytes Are Associated with Fasting Plasma Glucose and HbA1c in Postmenopausal Women with Type 2 Diabetes Mellitus. *Biol. Trace Elem. Res.* **2017**, *177*, 25–32. [CrossRef]

18. Hansen, A.F.; Simić, A.; Åsvold, B.O.; Romundstad, P.R.; Midthjell, K.; Syversen, T.; Flaten, T.P. Trace elements in early phase type 2 diabetes mellitus—A population-based study. The HUNT study in Norway. *J. Trace Elem. Med. Biol.* **2017**, *40*, 46–53. [CrossRef] [PubMed]

19. Simić, A.; Hansen, A.F.; Åsvold, B.O.; Romundstad, P.R.; Midthjell, K.; Syversen, T.; Flaten, T.P. Trace element status in patients with type 2 diabetes in Norway: The HUNT3 Survey. *J. Trace Elem. Med. Biol.* **2017**, *41*, 91–98. [CrossRef]

20. Fernández-Cao, J.C.; Warthon-Medina, M.; Hall Moran, V.; Arija, V.; Doepking, C.; Lowe, N.M. Dietary zinc intake and whole blood zinc concentration in subjects with type 2 diabetes versus healthy subjects: A systematic review, meta-analysis and meta-regression. *J. Trace Elem. Med. Biol.* **2018**. [CrossRef] [PubMed]

21. Coffman, F.D.; Dunn, M.F. Insulin-metal ion interactions: The binding of divalent cations to insulin hexamers and tetramers and the assembly of insulin hexamers. *Biochemistry* **1988**, *27*, 6179–6187. [CrossRef]

22. Keller, S.R. Role of the insulin-regulated aminopeptidase IRAP in insulin action and diabetes. *Biol. Pharm. Bull.* **2004**, *27*, 761–764. [CrossRef]

23. Meyer, J.A.; Spence, D.M. A perspective on the role of metals in diabetes: Past findings and possible future directions. *Metallomics* **2009**, *1*, 32–41. [CrossRef]

24. Moore, W.T.; Bowser, S.M.; Fausnacht, D.W.; Staley, L.L.; Suh, K.-S.; Liu, D. Beta Cell Function and the Nutritional State: Dietary Factors that Influence Insulin Secretion. *Curr. Diabetes Rep.* **2015**, *15*, 76. [CrossRef]

25. Tang, X.; Shay, N.F. Zinc has an insulin-like effect on glucose transport mediated by phosphoinositol-3-kinase and Akt in 3T3-L1 fibroblasts and adipocytes. *J. Nutr.* **2001**, *131*, 1414–1420. [CrossRef]

26. Chabosseau, P.; Rutter, G.A. Zinc and diabetes. *Arch. Biochem. Biophys.* **2016**, *611*, 79–85. [CrossRef]

27. Von Bülow, V.; Rink, L.; Haase, H. Zinc-mediated inhibition of cyclic nucleotide phosphodiesterase activity and expression suppresses TNF-alpha and IL-1 beta production in monocytes by elevation of guanosine 3′,5′-cyclic monophosphate. *J. Immunol.* **2005**, *175*, 4697–4705. [CrossRef]

28. Prasad, A.S.; Bao, B.; Beck, F.W.J.; Kucuk, O.; Sarkar, F.H. Antioxidant effect of zinc in humans. *Free Radic. Biol. Med.* **2004**, *37*, 1182–1190. [CrossRef]

29. Stroup, D.F.; Berlin, J.A.; Morton, S.C.; Olkin, I.; Williamson, G.D.; Rennie, D.; Moher, D.; Becker, B.J.; Sipe, T.A.; Thacker, S.B. Meta-analysis of observational studies in epidemiology: A proposal for reporting. Meta-analysis Of Observational Studies in Epidemiology (MOOSE) group. *JAMA* **2000**, *283*, 2008–2012. [CrossRef]

30. Greenland, S. Quantitative methods in the review of epidemiologic literature. *Epidemiol. Rev.* **1987**, *9*, 1–30. [CrossRef]

31. Knapp, G.; Hartung, J. Improved tests for a random effects meta-regression with a single covariate. *Stat. Med.* **2003**. [CrossRef]

32. Huedo-Medina, T.B.; Sánchez-Meca, J.; Marín-Martínez, F.; Botella, J. Assessing heterogeneity in meta-analysis: Q statistic or I^2 index? *Psychol. Methods* **2006**, *11*, 193–206. [CrossRef]

33. Higgins, J.P.T.; Thompson, S.G. Quantifying heterogeneity in a meta-analysis. *Stat. Med.* **2002**, *21*, 1539–1558. [CrossRef]

34. Higgins, J.P.T. Measuring inconsistency in meta-analyses. *BMJ* **2003**, *327*, 557–560. [CrossRef]

35. Thompson, S.G.; Higgins, J.P.T. How should meta-regression analyses be undertaken and interpreted? *Stat. Med.* **2002**, *21*, 1559–1573. [CrossRef]

36. Patsopoulos, N.A.; Evangelou, E.; Ioannidis, J.P.A. Sensitivity of between-study heterogeneity in meta-analysis: Proposed metrics and empirical evaluation. *Int. J. Epidemiol.* **2008**, *37*, 1148–1157. [CrossRef]

37. Egger, M.; Davey Smith, G.; Schneider, M.; Minder, C. Bias in meta-analysis detected by a simple, graphical test. *BMJ* **1997**, *315*, 629–634. [CrossRef]

38. Begg, C.B.; Mazumdar, M. Operating Characteristics of a Rank Correlation Test for Publication Bias. *Biometrics* **1994**, *50*, 1088. [CrossRef]

39. Singh, R.B.; Niaz, M.A.; Rastogi, S.S.; Bajaj, S.; Gaoli, Z.; Shoumin, Z. Current Zinc Intake and Risk of Diabetes and Coronary Artery Disease and Factors Associated with Insulin Resistance in Rural and Urban Populations of North India. *J. Am. Coll. Nutr.* **1998**, *17*, 564–570. [CrossRef]

40. Li, X.T.; Yu, P.F.; Gao, Y.; Guo, W.H.; Wang, J.; Liu, X.; Gu, A.H.; Ji, G.X.; Dong, Q.; Wang, B.S.; et al. Association between Plasma Metal Levels and Diabetes Risk: A Case-control Study in China. *Biomed. Environ. Sci.* **2017**, *30*, 482–491. [CrossRef]

41. Zhang, H.; Yan, C.; Yang, Z.; Zhang, W.; Niu, Y.; Li, X.; Qin, L.; Su, Q. Alterations of serum trace elements in patients with type 2 diabetes. *J. Trace Elem. Med. Biol.* **2017**, *40*, 91–96. [CrossRef]

42. Von Elm, E.; Altman, D.G.; Egger, M.; Pocock, S.J.; Gøtzsche, P.C.; Vandenbroucke, J.P. The Strengthening the Reporting of Observational Studies in Epidemiology (STROBE) statement: Guidelines for reporting of observational studies. *Der Internist* **2008**, *49*, 688–693. [CrossRef]

43. Panel on Micronutrients: Subcommittee on Upper Reference Levels of Nutrients; Subcommittee on Interpretation and Uses of Dietary Reference Intakes; Standing Committee on the Scientific Evaluation of Dietary Reference Intakes; Food and Nutrition Board, Institute of Medicine. *Dietary Reference Intakes for Vitamin A, Vitamin K, Arsenic, Boron, Chromium, Copper, Iodine, Iron, Manganese, Molybdenum, Nickel, Silicon, Vanadium, and Zinc*; National Academies Press: Washington, DC, USA, 2001.

44. Suarez-Ortegón, M.F.; Ordoñez-Betancourth, J.E.; Aguilar-de Plata, C. Dietary zinc intake is inversely associated to metabolic syndrome in male but not in female urban adolescents. *Am. J. Hum. Biol.* **2013**, *25*, 550–554. [CrossRef]

45. Al-Daghri, N.; Khan, N.; Alkharfy, K.; Al-Attas, O.; Alokail, M.; Alfawaz, H.; Alothman, A.; Vanhoutte, P. Selected Dietary Nutrients and the Prevalence of Metabolic Syndrome in Adult Males and Females in Saudi Arabia: A Pilot Study. *Nutrients* **2013**, *5*, 4587–4604. [CrossRef]

46. Bo, S.; Lezo, A.; Menato, G.; Gallo, M.-L.; Bardelli, C.; Signorile, A.; Berutti, C.; Massobrio, M.; Pagano, G.F. Gestational hyperglycemia, zinc, selenium, and antioxidant vitamins. *Nutrition* **2005**, *21*, 186–191. [CrossRef]

47. Eshak, E.S.; Iso, H.; Yamagishi, K.; Maruyama, K.; Umesawa, M.; Tamakoshi, A. Associations between copper and zinc intakes from diet and mortality from cardiovascular disease in a large population-based prospective cohort study. *J. Nutr. Biochem.* **2018**, *56*, 126–132. [CrossRef]

48. Bates, C.J.; Hamer, M.; Mishra, G.D. Redox-modulatory vitamins and minerals that prospectively predict mortality in older British people: The National Diet and Nutrition Survey of people aged 65 years and over. *Br. J. Nutr.* **2011**, *105*, 123–132. [CrossRef]

49. Shi, Z.; Yuan, B.; Qi, L.; Dai, Y.; Zuo, H.; Zhou, M. Zinc intake and the risk of hyperglycemia among Chinese adults: The prospective Jiangsu Nutrition Study (JIN). *J. Nutr. Health Aging* **2010**, *14*, 332–335. [CrossRef]

50. Milton, A.H.; Vashum, K.P.; McEvoy, M.; Hussain, S.; McElduff, P.; Byles, J.; Attia, J. Prospective Study of Dietary Zinc Intake and Risk of Cardiovascular Disease in Women. *Nutrients* **2018**, *10*, 38. [CrossRef]

51. Shi, Z.; Chu, A.; Zhen, S.; Taylor, A.W.; Dai, Y.; Riley, M.; Samman, S. Association between dietary zinc intake and mortality among Chinese adults: Findings from 10-year follow-up in the Jiangsu Nutrition Study. *Eur. J. Nutr.* **2018**, *57*, 2839–2846. [CrossRef]

52. McDade, T.W.; Adair, L.S. Defining the "urban" in urbanization and health: A factor analysis approach. *Soc. Sci. Med.* **2001**, *53*, 55–70. [CrossRef]

53. Pretorius, S.; Sliwa, K. Perspectives and perceptions on the consumption of a healthy diet in Soweto, an urban African community in South Africa. *SA Hear.* **2017**, *8*, 178–183. [CrossRef]

54. Lopez, A.D.; Mathers, C.D.; Ezzati, M.; Jamison, D.T.; Murray, C.J.L. Global and regional burden of disease and risk factors, 2001: Systematic analysis of population health data. *Lancet (London, England)* **2006**, *367*, 1747–1757. [CrossRef]

55. Ezzati, M.; Lopez, A.D.; Rodgers, A.; Vander Hoorn, S.; Murray, C.J.L. Comparative Risk Assessment Collaborating Group Selected major risk factors and global and regional burden of disease. *Lancet (London, England)* **2002**, *360*, 1347–1360. [CrossRef]

56. Al-Moosa, S.; Allin, S.; Jemiai, N.; Al-Lawati, J.; Mossialos, E. Diabetes and urbanization in the Omani population: An analysis of national survey data. *Popul. Health Metr.* **2006**, *4*, 5. [CrossRef]

57. Jayawardena, R.; Ranasinghe, P.; Galappatthy, P.; Malkanthi, R.; Constantine, G.; Katulanda, P. Effects of zinc supplementation on diabetes mellitus: A systematic review and meta-analysis. *Diabetol. Metab. Syndr.* **2012**, *4*, 13. [CrossRef]

58. Forte, G.; Bocca, B.; Peruzzu, A.; Tolu, F.; Asara, Y.; Farace, C.; Oggiano, R.; Madeddu, R. Blood metals concentration in type 1 and type 2 diabetics. *Biol. Trace Elem. Res.* **2013**, *156*, 79–90. [CrossRef]

59. Lowe, N.M.; Fekete, K.; Decsi, T. Methods of assessment of zinc status in humans: A systematic review. *Am. J. Clin. Nutr.* **2009**, *89*, 2040S–2051S. [CrossRef]

60. Sanjeevi, N.; Freeland-Graves, J.; Beretvas, S.N.; Sachdev, P.K. Trace element status in type 2 diabetes: A meta-analysis. *J. Clin. Diagn. Res.* **2018**, *12*, OE01–OE08. [CrossRef]

61. Liu, B.; Feng, W.; Wang, J.; Li, Y.; Han, X.; Hu, H.; Guo, H.; Zhang, X.; He, M. Association of urinary metals levels with type 2 diabetes risk in coke oven workers. *Environ. Pollut.* **2016**, *210*, 1–8. [CrossRef]

62. Carlson, M.D.A.; Morrison, R.S. Study design, precision, and validity in observational studies. *J. Palliat. Med.* **2009**, *12*, 77–82. [CrossRef]

63. Chu, A.; Foster, M.; Hancock, D.; Petocz, P.; Samman, S. Interrelationships among mediators of cellular zinc homeostasis in healthy and type 2 diabetes mellitus populations. *Mol. Nutr. Food Res.* **2017**, *61*. [CrossRef]

64. Ranasinghe, P.; Pigera, S.; Galappatthy, P.; Katulanda, P.; Constantine, G.R. Zinc and diabetes mellitus: Understanding molecular mechanisms and clinical implications. *Daru* **2015**, *23*, 44. [CrossRef]

65. Tamaki, M.; Fujitani, Y.; Hara, A.; Uchida, T.; Tamura, Y.; Takeno, K.; Kawaguchi, M.; Watanabe, T.; Ogihara, T.; Fukunaka, A.; et al. The diabetes-susceptible gene SLC30A8/ZnT8 regulates hepatic insulin clearance. *J. Clin. Investig.* **2013**, *123*, 4513–4524. [CrossRef]

66. Myers, S.A.; Nield, A.; Chew, G.-S.; Myers, M.A. The Zinc Transporter, Slc39a7 (Zip7) Is Implicated in Glycaemic Control in Skeletal Muscle Cells. *PLoS ONE* **2013**, *8*, e79316. [CrossRef]

67. Skalnaya, M.G.; Skalny, A.V.; Tinkov, A.A. Serum copper, zinc, and iron levels, and markers of carbohydrate metabolism in postmenopausal women with prediabetes and type 2 diabetes mellitus. *J. Trace Elem. Med. Biol.* **2017**, *43*, 46–51. [CrossRef]

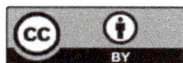

nutrients

MDPI

Article

Intakes of Zinc, Potassium, Calcium, and Magnesium of Individuals with Type 2 Diabetes Mellitus and the Relationship with Glycemic Control

Paula Nascimento Brandão-Lima [1] [iD], Gabrielli Barbosa de Carvalho [2],
Ramara Kadija Fonseca Santos [2], Beatriz da Cruz Santos [3], Natalia Lohayne Dias-Vasconcelos [3],
Vivianne de Sousa Rocha [4], Kiriaque Barra Ferreira Barbosa [1,2,3] and Liliane Viana Pires [2,3,*] [iD]

[1]   Health Sciences Postgraduate Program, Department of Medicine, Federal University of Sergipe, Rua Cláudio
      Batista, S/N, Cidade Nova, Aracaju, 49060-108 Sergipe, Brazil; paulanblima@gmail.com (P.N.B.-L.);
      kiribarra@yahoo.com.br (K.B.F.B.)
[2]   Nutrition Sciences Postgraduate Program, Department of Nutrition, Federal University of Sergipe,
      Avenida Marechal Rondon, S/N, Jardim Rosa Elze, São Cristovão, 49100-000 Sergipe, Brazil;
      gabicarvalho_31@hotmail.com (G.B.d.C.); rkadijanutri@gmail.com (R.K.F.S.)
[3]   Undergraduate Nutrition Program, Department of Nutrition, Federal University of Sergipe,
      Avenida Marechal Rondon, S/N, Jardim Rosa Elze, São Cristovão, 49100-000 Sergipe, Brazil;
      cruz14_bia@outlook.com (B.d.C.S.); diaslohayne@gmail.com (N.L.D.-V.)
[4]   Department of Nutrition, Federal University of Sergipe, Avenida Governador Marcelo Déda, 13, Centro,
      Lagarto, 49400-000 Sergipe, Brazil; viviannesrocha@gmail.com
*   Correspondence: lvianapires@gmail.com or lvpires@usp.br; Tel.: +55-79-31947498

Received: 9 November 2018; Accepted: 6 December 2018; Published: 8 December 2018

Abstract: The role of the concomitant intake of zinc, potassium, calcium, and magnesium in the glycemic control of individuals with type 2 diabetes mellitus (T2DM) has not been extensively discussed. We evaluated the relationship between the dietary intake of these micronutrients and glycemic markers in 95 individuals with T2DM (mean age 48.6 ± 8.4 years). Hierarchical grouping analysis was used to divide the individuals into two clusters according to their micronutrient intake, and differences between clusters were statistically assessed. Effects of individual and combination intake of micronutrients on glycated hemoglobin percentage (%HbA1c) were assessed using multiple linear regression and binary logistic regression analysis. We observed a high likelihood of inadequate intake of the four micronutrients. The group with lower micronutrient intake (cluster 1) displayed higher %HbA1c ($p = 0.006$) and triglyceride ($p = 0.010$) levels. High %HbA1c showed an association with cluster 1 (odds ratio (OR) = 3.041, 95% confidence interval (CI) = 1.131; 8.175) and time of T2DM diagnosis (OR = 1.155, 95% CI = 1.043; 1.278). Potassium ($\beta = -0.001$, $p = 0.017$) and magnesium ($\beta = -0.007$, $p = 0.015$) intakes were inversely associated with %HbA1c. Reduced concomitant intake of the four micronutrients studied proved to be associated with risk of increased %HbA1c in individuals with T2DM, which was particularly predicted by magnesium and potassium intakes.

Keywords: micronutrients; trace elements; food: glycated hemoglobin A; hyperglycemia

---

1. Introduction

Type 2 diabetes mellitus (T2DM) is characterized by failures in blood glucose homeostasis and is considered a global public health problem [1]. Chronic hyperglycemia leads to increased oxidative stress and production of proinflammatory cytokines, disrupting insulin signaling pathways, lipid metabolism, protein synthesis, and cell differentiation, and may alter body concentrations of micronutrients [2–5]. The maintenance of the glycemic control in individuals with T2DM involves strategies for lifestyle changes, drug therapy, and adoption of healthy eating habits [1,2]. A balanced diet with adequate nutrient content can reduce the glycated hemoglobin percentage (%HbA1c) in subjects with T2DM by 0.3–2% [6]. Over the last few years, studies have verified the participation of minerals in the synthesis, secretion, and action of insulin. Among them, the minerals zinc, potassium, calcium, and magnesium are considered essential for the homeostasis of glucose metabolism [5,7,8].

Zinc plays a key role in the insulin biosynthesis as part of the hexameric structure of this hormone, and in the sensitivity to insulin in target tissues through stimulation of insulin receptors [9,10]. Calcium and potassium regulate voltage-dependent channels in pancreatic β-cells, which are essential for insulin exocytosis [11,12]. Magnesium is important for β-cell functioning and acts as a cofactor of many enzymes involved in the glucose metabolism, like tyrosine kinase enzymes, which phosphorylate insulin receptors and trigger the signaling cascade [4,12,13].

Thus, an inadequate intake of these micronutrients may impair the insulin synthesis, secretion, and signaling pathways [4,11,14]. It is possible to observe in the literature studies that associate the low intake and serum concentration of these minerals with risk of T2DM development [2,13,15–18]. Nevertheless, studies that evaluate the relationship between the dietary intake of these minerals in glycemic control in subjects with established disease are not widely found. In addition, no studies have assessed the relationship of the concomitant intake of these four micronutrients with the glycemic control, insulin biosynthesis, and insulin sensitivity of individuals with T2DM. In this scenario, the present study aimed to evaluate the relationship of the dietary intake of zinc, potassium, calcium, and magnesium with glycemic markers in individuals with T2DM in order to expand the understanding of these relationships in glycemic control.

2. Materials and Methods

2.1. Study Design and Participants

In this cross-sectional study, to be eligible for enrollment, individuals had to be 19–59 years old and have diagnosis of T2DM. Thus, 102 individuals with T2DM who visited the Family Health Units in the state of Sergipe, Brazil, were evaluated. Exclusion criteria adopted were the use of vitamin–mineral supplements, pregnancy, status as a current smoker, and the presence of the following diseases: rheumatoid arthritis, cancer, chronic renal failure, thyroid dysfunction, and acute infections or inflammatory processes such as influenza and urinary tract infection. The study followed the guidelines of the Declaration of Helsinki and all participants provided written informed consent. The study was approved by the Ethical Committee of the Federal University of Sergipe (Approval number 1.370.831).

Venous blood samples were obtained, after an overnight fast for at least 10 hours, in ethylenediamine tetra-acetic acid (EDTA) tubes for estimation of concentration of glycated hemoglobin (HbA1c) in whole blood, and in gel tubes for the determination of fasting glucose, lipid profile, insulin, and C-peptide in serum. Measurements of anthropometric parameters, body fat percentage, and blood pressure were performed. All the measurements were realized by trained technicians, and the individuals were instructed to avoid physical activity or effort one day before the tests. In combination, dietary intake assessments of macro and micronutrients was performed. Information about socioeconomic conditions, medical history, and lifestyle were obtained using a questionnaire.

2.2. Anthropometric Parameters, Bioelectric Impedance and Blood Pressure Measurements

Weight and height measurements were performed to calculate the body mass index (BMI). The BMI was calculated by dividing the body weight value (in kilograms) by the square value of the body height (in meters). The participants were classified as malnourished (BMI < 18.5 kg/m^2), normal weight (BMI 18.5–24.9 kg/m^2) or overweight/obese (BMI ≥ 25 kg/m^2), assessed according to the cut-off values proposed by the World Health Organization [19]. Waist circumference was measured with a non-extendable tape positioned at the midpoint between the last floating rib and the top of the iliac crest. The cut-off point used for waist circumference was ≥80 cm for women and ≥94 cm for men [20].

Measurement of body fat percentage was performed using the BIA 310 Bioimpedance Analyzer (Biodynamics Corporation, Shoreline, WA, USA), following the manufacturer's instructions. Blood pressure was measured using aneroid sphygmomanometers and a stethoscope according to the recommendations of the Brazilian Society of Cardiology [21] at rest in a sitting position.

2.3. Biochemical Analyses

Serum concentrations of glucose, triglycerides, total cholesterol, and high-density lipoprotein cholesterol (HDL-c) were measured by an enzymatic colorimetric method using commercial kits (Labtest®, Lagoa Santa/MG, Brazil). The HbA1c was measured by immunoturbidimetric inhibition. All biochemical tests were performed using an automatic biochemical analyzer CMD 800i (Wiener Lab Group®, Rosario, Argentina). Serum insulin and C-peptide concentrations were measured by chemiluminescence using commercial kits (Abbott®, Abbott Park, IL, USA) and the automatic immunoassay analyzer Architect i1000SR (Abbott®, Abbott Park, IL, USA). The homeostasis model assessment (HOMA) was used to assess insulin sensitivity, based on C-peptide and glucose levels. Calculations were made using the HOMA calculator (University of Oxford, United Kingdom).

2.4. Food Intake

The 24-h dietary recalls over three days (including two weekdays and one weekend day) were obtained by Multiple-Pass method [22], and analyzed using the NutWin software (Department of Informatics, Paulista School of Medicine/UNIFESP, São Paulo/SP, Brazil), which includes the updated versions of the Brazilian Table of Food Composition (TACO), the Table of Nutritional Composition of Food Consumed in Brazil, the United States Department of Agriculture (USDA) Food Composition Databases, and food labels. The adequacy of usual dietary intake of nutrients by each group was evaluated according to the estimated average requirement (EAR) and adequate intake (AI) for potassium values proposed by the dietary reference intakes [23,24]. The probability of inadequate food intake by group was evaluated by z-score, which was calculated from the difference between the EAR corresponding to each nutrient and the mean ingestion of the group divided by the standard deviation of the intake. Potassium intake values were compared with AI values [24].

2.5. Statistical Analyses

The Kolmogorov–Smirnov test was used to evaluate data homogeneity. Non-homogeneous data were subjected to logarithmic transformation. The identification of individuals with inaccurate report of energy intake was performed using the methodology proposed by Mccrory et al. [25], based on the ratio between the reported energy intake and the total energy expenditure predicted, calculated by the equation of Vinken et al. [26] and considering the cut-off value of ± one standard deviation. The usual dietary intake was calculated using the Multiple Sources Method (MSM) (https://msm.dife.de/) [27]. Micronutrient intake values were adjusted for total energy intake according to residual method proposed by Willett et al. [28].

To verify associations between response variables, and to characterize individuals according to dietary intake of zinc, magnesium, calcium, and potassium, a hierarchical cluster analysis was used. From this analysis, the mean values corresponding to the energy-adjusted dietary intake of the four minerals were auto-scaled, and the similarities between the individuals calculated according to the Euclidean squared distance, while the Ward's method was used for the formation of clusters. Differences between the two clusters formed was assessed using the Student's *t*-test (for normal data distribution) or the Mann–Whitney test (for non-normal data distribution).

Regression models were used to assess the effect of the micronutrient intake on the glycemic control. Independent variables with $p \leq 0.20$ in the bivariate analyses were included in the models using the enter method. $p \leq 0.20$ was adopted according to the criterion of Wang et al. [29], established for the testing of a greater number of predictor variables in the model. Thus, a binary logistic regression model was applied using %HbA1c values above 7.0 [30] and cluster 1 (lower micronutrient intake) as risk variables. In addition, multiple regression models were applied to assess the effect of each micronutrient intake on %HbA1c separately. Multicollinearity was assessed by variance inflation factors (VIF) and no correlation was identified between the independent variables (VIF <10). Both regression models used sex, age, and time of T2DM diagnosis as adjustment variables.

The results were expressed as means and standard deviations, and as absolute and relative frequencies. A significance level of 5% was adopted for all tests. All statistical analyses were performed using SPSS for Windows Version 17.0 (SPSS Inc., Chicago, IL, USA).

3. Results

After exclusion of participants with missing dietary information, 95 individuals with T2DM were finally evaluated; 69.5% of them were female and mean age was 48.6 ± 8.4 years. Most individuals were overweight or obese (81.0%), and mean BMI and body fat percentage values were 30.22 ± 6.78 kg/m^2 and 34.98 ± 7.94%, respectively. Waist circumference measurement showed 85.3% of the participants at increased risk of obesity-associated metabolic diseases (Table 1).

Deficient glycemic control was observed, as indicated by values of fasting glucose and %HbA1c above the cut-off point for disease control (fasting glucose < 154 mg/dL; %HbA1c < 7.0) [30]. Regarding lipid profile, 73.7% of the participants presented low HDL-c levels, and 37.9%, 10.5%, and 3.1% presented hypertriglyceridemia, mixed hyperlipidemia, and hypercholesterolemia, respectively.

Table 1. Clinical, biochemical and nutrient intake variables of individuals with type 2 diabetes mellitus (T2DM).

Variables	T2DM (n = 95)
Age, years	48.6 ± 8.4
Sex	
Men, n (%)	29 (30.5)
Women, n (%)	66 (69.5)
Time of T2DM diagnosis [1], years	7.3 ± 6.2
Insulin therapy [2], n (%)	21 (22.1)
Oral antidiabetic agents [2], n (%)	70 (73.7)
Lipid-lowering agents [2], n (%)	24 (25.3)
Antihypertensive agents [2], n (%)	46 (48.4)
Weight, kg	78.9 ± 19.3
BMI, kg/m^2	30.2 ± 6.8
Fat mass [2], %	35.0 ± 7.9
Waist circumference, cm	99.8 ± 14.3
Men, n (%)	
<94 cm	8 (27.6)
≥94 cm	21 (72.4)
Women, n (%)	
<80 cm	6 (9.1)
≥80 cm	60 (90.9)
SBP [3], mmHg	129.2 ± 17.0
DBP [3], mmHg	83.5 ± 15.3
Fasting glucose, mg/dL	180.1 ± 84.1
%Hb1Ac	8.1 ± 2.1
Insulin, μU/mL	13.8 ± 13.5
C-peptide, ng/mL	2.7 ± 0.8
HOMA2-%B	77.0 ± 56.2
HOMA2-%S	42.8 ± 20.9
HOMA2-IR	3.3 ± 2.9
Total cholesterol, mg/dL	193.4 ± 47.3
HDL-c, mg/dL	41.1 ± 10.4
LDL-c, mg/dL	117.4 ± 39.8
Triglycerides, mg/dL	174.3 ± 117.1

Table 1. *Cont.*

Variables	T2DM (*n* = 95)
Energy intake, kcal/day	1469.4 ± 478.5
Protein intake, g/day	80.0 ± 20.2
Carbohydrate intake, g/day	210.1 ± 73.6
Lipid intake, g/day	37.1 ± 15.6
Zinc intake, mg/day	5.2 ± 1.5
Potassium intake, mg/day	1848.5 ± 543.4
Calcium intake, mg/day	469.0 ± 195.3
Magnesium intake mg/day	218.4 ± 68.1

Results presented in mean ± standard deviation and absolute frequency; [1] *n* = 91; [2] *n* = 93; [3] *n* = 89. %HbA1c: glycated hemoglobin percentage; BMI: body mass index; DBP: diastolic blood pressure; HDL-c: high-density lipoprotein cholesterol; HOMA: Homeostasis Assessment Model; LDL-c: low-density lipoprotein cholesterol; T2DM: type 2 diabetes mellitus; SBP: systolic blood pressure. Micronutrients adjusted for total energy intake using the residual method [28].

Energy intake was found to be underreported by 84.2% of the individuals. A prevalence of inadequacy in energy-adjusted zinc intake of 99.9% in males and 82.6% in females was observed. The prevalence of inadequate energy-adjusted magnesium intake for males and females was 96.4% and 74.9%, respectively. The energy-adjusted calcium intake showed a prevalence of inadequacy of 95.5%. All the individuals evaluated had energy-adjusted potassium intake below the AI values (Figure 1).

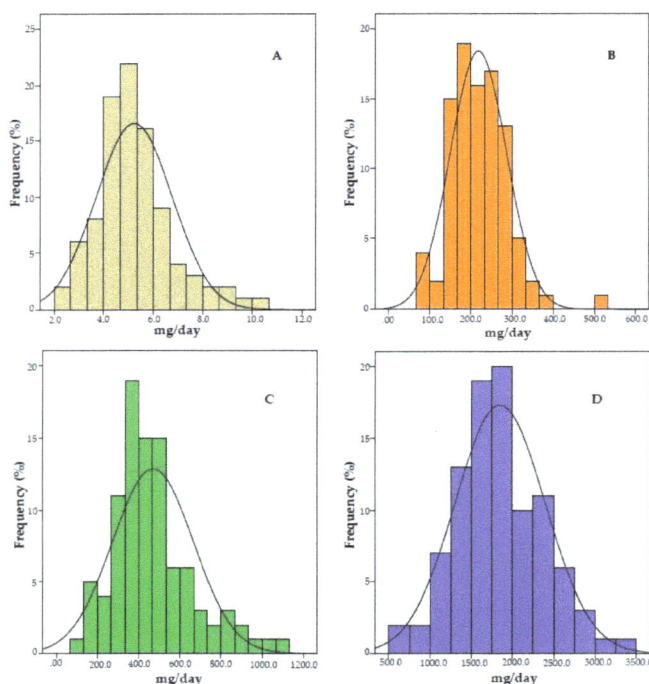

Figure 1. Histogram of energy-adjusted intake of zinc (**A**), magnesium (**B**), calcium (**C**), and potassium (**D**), and prevalence of inadequate intake in individuals with type 2 diabetes mellitus (T2DM) (*n* = 95). (**A**) Group intake (mean ± SD): 5.23 ± 1.53 mg/day; Z-score: 3.06 (men) and 0.94 (women). (**B**) Group intake (mean ± SD): 218.36 ± 68.13 mg/day; Z-score: 1.80 (men) and 0.67 (women). (**C**) Group intake (mean ± SD): 468.95 ± 195.3 mg/day; Z-score: 1.96 (group). (**D**) Group intake (mean ± SD): 1848.45 ± 543.43 mg/day. SD: Standard deviation.

When energy-adjusted micronutrient (zinc, potassium, calcium, and magnesium) intake was compared between clusters, the group with lower micronutrient intake (cluster 1) showed significantly higher %HbA1c ($p = 0.006$) and serum triglyceride concentration ($p = 0.01$) in comparison with the group with higher intake (cluster 2). No statistical differences were seen with regard to the other variables studied (Table 2).

Table 2. Clinical, biochemical and nutrient intake variables of individuals with type 2 diabetes mellitus (T2DM).

Variables	*Cluster 1 (n = 65)*	*Cluster 2 (n = 30)*	*p*-value
Age, years	48.6 ± 8.6	48.9 ± 7.9	0.866 [¥]
Time of T2DM diagnosis, years	7.2 ± 6.4	7.4 ± 6.0	0.909
BMI, kg/m^2	30.4 ± 6.9	29.9 ± 6.7	0.762 [¥]
Waist circumference, cm	100.8 ± 13.7	97.7 ± 15.5	0.332
Fat mass, %	34.6 ± 8.0	35.8 ± 7.8	0.483
Total cholesterol, mg/dL	198.8 ± 49.7	181.5 ± 40.0	0.097
HDL-c, mg/dL	41.9 ± 10.5	39.2 ± 10.3	0.247
LDL-c, mg/dL	117.9 ± 42.2	116.4 ± 34.5	0.867
Triglycerides, mg/dL	194.9 ± 131.1	129.6 ± 58.5	0.010
%Hb1Ac	8.3 ± 2.1	7.2 ± 1.7	0.006
C-peptide, ng/mL	2.7 ± 0.9	2.7 ± 0.7	0.963
Fasting glucose, mg/dL	190.3 ± 88.2	158.1 ± 70.7	0.082 [¥]
Insulin, µU/mL	13.2 ± 11.7	15.1 ± 16.8	0.525
HOMA2-%B	73.7 ± 59.4	84.0 ± 48.8	0.407 [¥]
Energy intake, kcal/day	1452.3 ± 471.4	1506.3 ± 499.7	0.611
Lipid intake, g/day	37.4 ± 15.1	36.5 ± 16.8	0.796
Protein intake, g/day	80.2 ± 19.7	79.4 ± 21.4	0.856
Carbohydrate intake, g/day	203.6 ± 74.1	224.2 ± 71.7	0.207
Zinc intake, mg/day	4.8 ± 1.4	6.1 ± 1.5	<0.001
Potassium intake, mg/day	1556.5 ± 344.3	2480.9 ± 301.4	<0.001
Calcium intake, mg/day	400.6 ± 136.4	616.9 ± 222.4	<0.001
Magnesium intake mg/day	191.5 ± 54.2	276.6 ± 58.5	<0.001

Results presented in mean ± standard deviation. *p*-value <0.05 was considered statistically significant. Student's *t*-test for independent samples and [¥] Mann–Whitney test. %HbA1c: glycated hemoglobin percentage; BMI: body mass index; HDL-c: high-density lipoprotein cholesterol; HOMA: Homeostasis Assessment Model; LDL-c: low-density lipoprotein cholesterol; T2DM: type 2 diabetes mellitus. Micronutrients adjusted for total energy intake using the residual method [28].

Considering the significant difference in %HbA1c between clusters, a binary logistic regression model was applied in order to investigate the risk factors for increased %HbA1c (Table 3). We found that alterations in the %HbA1c were dependent of the time (in years) taken to diagnose T2DM ($p = 0.005$) and lower micronutrient intake (cluster 1) ($p = 0.028$).

Table 3. Binary logistic regression model of glycated hemoglobin percentage (%HbA1c) and clusters formed from energy-adjusted mineral intake by individuals with type 2 diabetes mellitus (T2DM).

Dependent Variable	Covariables	OR (95% CI)	*p*-value
	Age (years) [£]	0.987 (0.931; 1.046)	0.661
%Hb1Ac [§]	Sex [§]	1.598 (0.580; 4.405)	0.365
	Time of T2DM diagnosis (years) [£]	1.155 (1.043; 1.278)	0.005
	Cluster 1 [§]	3.041 (1.131; 8.175)	0.028

p-value <0.05 was considered significant. *p*-value of model: 0.003 and r^2: 0.221. Hosmer and Lemeshow test: 0.591. [§] Variables included in the model in the dichotomous format. [£] Variables included in the model in continuous format. Model adjusted by sex, age, and time of T2DM diagnosis. %HbA1c: glycated hemoglobin percentage; CI: confidence interval; OR: odds ratio; T2DM: type 2 diabetes mellitus. Risk classification used %HbA1c >7% [30] and cluster 1 with lower combined intake of zinc, potassium, calcium, and magnesium.

Multiple regression analyses showed that, for every 1 g of potassium and 100 mg of magnesium ingested, there was 1% and 0.7% reduction in %HbA1c, respectively. These results were influenced by sex and time taken to diagnose T2DM (Table 4).

Table 4. Multiple linear regression models of glycated hemoglobin percentage (%HbA1c; dependent variable) and energy-adjusted mineral intake by individuals with type 2 diabetes mellitus (T2DM).

	Independent Variables	β (95%CI)	*p*-value	r^2 Adjusted
Model 1 [1]	Age (years)	−0.032 (−0.082; 0.019)	0.216	
	Sex [§]	1.069 (0.209; 1.930)	0.015	
	Time of T2DM diagnosis (years)	0.117 (0.051; 0.183)	0.001	0.143
	Zinc intake (mg/day)	−0.017 (−0.283; 0.250)	0.902	
Model 2 [2]	Age (years)	−0.028 (−0.077; 0.021)	0.259	
	Sex [§]	0.925 (0.086; 1.765)	0.031	
	Time of T2DM diagnosis (years)	1.118 (0.054; 0.182)	<0.001	0.198
	Potassium intake (mg/day)	−0.001 (−0.002; 0.000)	0.017	
Model 3 [2]	Age (years)	−0.029 (−0.079; 0.021)	0.253	
	Sex [§]	1.025 (0.163; 1.887)	0.020	
	Time of T2DM diagnosis (years)	0.119 (0.053; 0.184)	0.001	0.151
	Calcium intake (mg/day)	−0.001 (−0.003; 0.001)	0.377	
Model 4 [2]	Age (years)	−0.031 (0.080; 0.017)	0.206	
	Sex [§]	1.009 (0.177; 1.840)	0.018	
	Time of T2DM diagnosis (years)	0.117 (0.053; 0.181)	<0.001	0.201
	Magnesium intake (mg/day)	−0.007 (−0.012; −0.001)	0.015	

[1] *p*-value of model: 0.002. [2] *p*-value of model: <0.001. β non-standardized. Variables included in the models in the continuous format and in the [§] dichotomous format. All models adjusted by sex, age and time of T2DM diagnosis. %HbA1c: glycated hemoglobin percentage; CI: confidence interval; T2DM: type 2 diabetes mellitus.

4. Discussion

After assessing the effect of the energy-adjusted dietary intake of zinc, potassium, calcium, and magnesium on the glycemic control of individuals with T2DM, we found a three-fold increased risk of high %HbA1c when dietary intake was reduced. In addition, potassium and magnesium intakes were predictive of %HbA1c decrease. It is noteworthy that most evaluated individuals were likely to have inadequate ingestion of these micronutrients.

The association between low micronutrient intake and deficient glycemic control is well known and poor intake of these micronutrients is widely documented in T2DM [2,3,12,31]. However, most studies looked at the intake of each micronutrient individually, and studies evaluating the concomitant intake thereof are scarce.

Epidemiological studies have shown a significant association between low daily zinc intake and risk of T2DM [10,18,32], and the risk can be reduced by 20% upon daily intake of more than 13 mg of zinc [33]. Kanoni et al. [34] found a significant correlation between zinc intake and fasting glucose values, where the daily intake of every 1 mg of zinc was able to reduce the glucose concentration by 0.02 mg/dL. The same study was included in a recent systematic review, which reported that the serum zinc concentration has been negatively correlated with %HbA1c and fasting glucose values in T2DM [16].

The role of zinc in the functioning and maintenance of pancreatic β-cell mass, insulin biosynthesis, and maturation of secretory granules is well documented [9,10]. In addition, zinc inhibits tyrosine phosphatases by stimulating auto phosphorylation of insulin receptors [14,16]. Moreover, it is essential in the redox mechanisms as a component of the superoxide dismutase enzyme, thus being helpful against the oxidative stress generated by hyperglycemia [10,14].

The role of magnesium in the glycemic control has been shown in experimental studies on rats with induced T2DM. Magnesium supplementation improved insulin secretion and sensitivity, lipid profile, and inflammatory status [35,36]. Morakinyo et al. [36] also showed that rats supplemented with magnesium improved GLUT4 translocation and, consequently, the metabolic control.

Previous evidence also points to an inverse association between magnesium intake and T2DM risk [13,37]. Hypomagnesemia and low magnesium intake are very prevalent in individuals diagnosed with T2DM, especially in those with poor glycemic control [12,31,38]. In addition, reduced plasma concentration of magnesium may lead to changes in the glycemic control, since the body distribution of this micronutrient has an impact on insulin secretion and action [12].

However, studies addressing the effect of magnesium supplementation on glycemic control are controversial. Some studies have shown positive effects of magnesium supplementation on blood glucose and %HbA1c lowering, and on the increased insulin sensitivity [8,39–41]. However, other studies did not observe such effects, which may be explained by the presence of normomagnesemia, time of supplementation, and reduced number of individuals assessed [42–47]. Two meta-analyses studies showed reduction of 0.56 mmol/L (95% confidence interval (CI) = −1.10; −0.01) [48] and 0.37 mmol/L (95% CI = −0.74; −0.00) [4], respectively, in the fasting glucose levels upon magnesium supplementation.

Magnesium is an important cofactor of enzymes involved in the glucose metabolism, in which it binds to an ATP molecule, yielding the Mg–ATP complex that acts in phosphate transfer reactions [4,12,37]. Thus, magnesium participates in the autophosphorylation of the β-subunit of insulin receptors, proliferation and maintenance of pancreatic β-cells, activity of tyrosine kinases, and stimulation of proteins and substrates of the insulin signaling cascade [12,13].

Enhanced intakes of calcium and potassium are also associated with reduced risk of T2DM [5,15], due to the combined action of these minerals in the process of insulin release [7]. Within the pancreatic β-cells, the intracellular ATP/ADP ratio that follows the glucose metabolism leads to the closure of ATP-sensitive potassium channels, and subsequent depolarization of the plasma membrane. Calcium channels are then opened, allowing the calcium influx to the cells and subsequent activation of exocytosis of the insulin granules [7,11].

The fundamental role of calcium in body weight control and, consequently, in the maintenance of insulin sensitivity in the adipose tissue, is observed in animal models. Dietary calcium induces suppression of calcitriol, thus reducing lipogenesis and increasing lipolysis. In addition, it increases the uncoupling protein-2 (UCP2) expression in the adipose tissue. UCP2 is responsible for the transport and oxidation of mitochondrial fatty acids, which reduces lipid storage and adiposity [49].

Few studies have assessed the effect of calcium intake on the glycemic control. In an eight-week study, calcium supplementation (1500 mg per day) improved the insulin sensitivity in individuals with T2DM [50]. However, insulin sensitivity was not changed after non-diabetic obese individuals underwent 24 weeks of supplementation with 1000 mg of calcium per day [49].

Furthermore, magnesium intake is likely to be a confounding factor as it is highly correlated with calcium metabolism as observed in studies addressing the association between intake of both minerals and the risk of T2DM [51,52]. A relationship between calcium and vitamin D intakes was also observed as the interaction of these nutrients leads to reduced fasting insulin and %HbA1c levels in individuals with T2DM [53].

The relation between potassium intake and variables of glycemic control in individuals with T2DM is not widely addressed in the literature. Both low potassium intake and reduced potassium concentration in serum were shown to be significantly associated with reduced insulin sensitivity and with a compensatory increase in insulin secretion [5], as well as with risk of T2DM [17,54].

Considering that the adoption of healthy dietary and body weight control patterns is fundamental for the T2DM management [1,6], a high rate of underreported energy intake is observed among individuals with T2DM in this study, and this can be the main reason for the high prevalence of overweight and obesity here documented. Underreporting is a commonly observed practice among obese individuals and can affect the estimation of nutrient intake, consequently impairing nutritional and disease assessments [55,56]. In addition, the analysis of food intake that relies on 24-hour recalls may have limitations, since this method is susceptible to inaccurate reports about both

Nutrients **2018**, *10*, 1948

the food consumed and the size of its portions [25]. However, these limitations were mitigated after calculation of intra and interindividual variability, in combination with the adjustment for energy intake of nutrients.

Furthermore, food evaluation involves data of tables of food composition, and such tables can be different depending on where the food is produced. Therefore, similar to the present study, the use of region or country-specific food composition tables may help to correct this confounding factor.

5. Conclusions

Overall, studies evaluating the effect of the concomitant intake of micronutrients on variables of glycemic metabolism in individuals with T2DM are scarce, especially when it comes to zinc, potassium, calcium, and magnesium. This highlights the importance of our results for a better evaluation of usual food intake in this population, which is a simple and low-cost procedure, as %HbA1c is routinely measured in individuals with T2DM and it is the gold standard for glycemic control evaluation.

Therefore, inadequate concomitant intake of zinc, potassium, calcium, and magnesium is related to poor glycemic control in individuals with T2DM, and the intakes of magnesium and potassium are predictors of %HbA1c reduction. Further studies on dietary intake of individuals with T2DM and their relation with glucose metabolism are needed.

Author Contributions: P.N.B.-L. and L.V.P. designed the study; All authors performed the analysis and contributed to the writing of the manuscript. All authors approved the final version of the manuscript.

Funding: This research was funded by the National Council for Scientific and Technological Development (CNPq), grant number 455117/2014-4.

Acknowledgments: The authors would like to thank the research volunteers, Alan Santos Oliveira for the support in data collection, the National Council for Scientific and Technological Development (CNPq) for the financial support, the Foundation for Research and Technological Innovation Support of the State of Sergipe (Fapitec/SE), and the Coordination of Improvement of Higher Education Personnel (CAPES).

Conflicts of Interest: The authors declare no conflict of interest.

References

1. International Diabetes Federation. *IDF Diabetes Atlas*, 8th ed.; IDF: Brussels, Belgium, 2017.
2. Shah, M.; Vasandani, C.; Adams-Huet, B.; Garg, A. Comparison of nutrient intakes in South Asians with type 2 diabetes mellitus and controls living in the United States. *Diabetes Res. Clin. Pract.* **2018**, *138*, 47–56. [CrossRef] [PubMed]
3. Perez, A.; Rojas, P.; Carrasco, F.; Basfi-fer, K.; Perez-Bravo, F.; Codoceo, J.; Inostroza, J.; Galgani, J.E.; Gilmore, L.A.; Ruz, M. Association between zinc nutritional status and glycemic control in individuals with well-controlled type-2 diabetes. *J. Trace Elem. Med. Biol.* **2018**, *50*, 560–565. [CrossRef] [PubMed]
4. Veronese, N.; Watutantrige-Fernando, S.; Luchini, C.; Solmi, M.; Sartore, G.; Sergi, G.; Manzato, E.; Barbagallo, M.; Maggi, S.; Stubbs, B. Effect of magnesium supplementation on glucose metabolism in people with or at risk of diabetes: A systematic review and meta-analysis of double-blind randomized controlled trials. *Eur. J. Clin. Nutr.* **2016**, *70*, 1354–1359. [CrossRef] [PubMed]
5. Chatterjee, R.; Biggs, M.L.; de Boer, I.H.; Brancati, F.L.; Svetkey, L.P.; Barzilay, J.; Djoussé, L.; Ix, J.H.; Kizer, J.R.; Siscovick, D.S.; et al. Potassium and Glucose Measures in Older Adults: The Cardiovascular Health Study. *J. Gerontol. A Biol. Sci. Med. Sci.* **2015**, *70*, 255–261. [CrossRef] [PubMed]
6. American Diabetes Association. Lifestyle Management: Standards of Medical Care in Diabetes-2018. *Diabetes Care* **2018**, *41*, S38–S50. [CrossRef] [PubMed]
7. Fu, Z.; Gilbert, E.R.; Liu, D. Regulation of insulin synthesis and secretion and pancreatic Beta-cell dysfunction in diabetes. *Curr. Diabetes Rev.* **2013**, *9*, 25–53. [CrossRef]
8. Solati, M.; Ouspid, E.; Hosseini, S.; Soltani, N.; Keshavarz, M.; Dehghani, M. Oral magnesium supplementation in type II diabetic patients. *Med. J. Islam. Repub. Iran* **2014**, *28*, 67.
9. Wijesekara, N.; Chimienti, F.; Wheeler, M.B. Zinc, a regulator of islet function and glucose homeostasis. *Diabetes Obes. Metab.* **2009**, *11*, 202–214. [CrossRef]

10. Sun, Q.; Van Dam, R.M.; Willett, W.C.; Hu, F.B. Prospective Study of Zinc Intake and Risk of Type 2 Diabetes in Women. *Diabetes Care* **2009**, *32*, 629–634. [CrossRef]

11. Bonfanti, D.H.; Alcazar, L.P.; Arakaki, P.A.; Martins, L.T.; Agustini, B.C.; de Moraes Rego, F.G.; Frigeri, H.R. ATP-dependent potassium channels and type 2 diabetes mellitus. *Clin. Biochem.* **2015**, *48*, 476–482. [CrossRef]

12. Sales, C.H.; Pedrosa, L.F.; Lima, J.G.; Lemos, T.M.; Colli, C. Influence of magnesium status and magnesium intake on the blood glucose control in patients with type 2 diabetes. *Clin. Nutr.* **2011**, *30*, 359–364. [CrossRef] [PubMed]

13. Hruby, A.; Meigs, J.B.; O'Donnell, C.J.; Jacques, P.F.; McKeown, N.M. Higher magnesium intake reduces risk of impaired glucose and insulin metabolism and progression from prediabetes to diabetes in middle-aged americans. *Diabetes Care* **2014**, *37*, 419–427. [CrossRef] [PubMed]

14. Chabosseau, P.; Rutter, G.A. Zinc and Diabetes. *Arch. Biochem. Biophys.* **2016**, *611*, 79–85. [CrossRef] [PubMed]

15. Villegas, R.; Gao, Y.T.; Dai, Q.; Yang, G.; Cai, H.; Li, H.; Zheng, W.; Shu, X.O. Dietary calcium and magnesium intakes and the risk of type 2 diabetes: The Shanghai Women's Health Study. *Am. J. Clin. Nutr.* **2009**, *89*, 1059–1067. [CrossRef] [PubMed]

16. de Carvalho, G.B.; Brandão-Lima, P.N.; Maia, C.S.; Barbosa, K.B.F.; Pires, L.V. Zinc's role in the glycemic control of patients with type 2 diabetes: A systematic review. *BioMetals* **2017**, *30*, 151–162. [CrossRef] [PubMed]

17. Chatterjee, R.; Colangelo, L.A.; Yeh, H.C.; Anderson, C.A.; Daviglus, M.L.; Liu, K.; Brancati, F.L. Potassium intake and risk of incident type 2 diabetes mellitus: The Coronary Artery Risk Development in Young Adults (CARDIA) Study. *Diabetologia* **2012**, *55*, 1295–1303. [CrossRef] [PubMed]

18. Drake, I.; Hindy, G.; Ericson, U.; Orho-Melander, M. A prospective study of dietary and supplemental zinc intake and risk of type 2 diabetes depending on genetic variation in SLC30A8. *Genes Nutr.* **2017**, *12*, 30. [CrossRef] [PubMed]

19. World Health Organization. *Obesity: Preventing and Managing the Global Epidemic*; WHO Technical Report Series 894; WHO: Geneva, Switzerland, 2000; ISBN 92 4 120894 5.

20. World Health Organization. *Waist Circumference and Waist-Hip Ratio: Report of a WHO Expert Consultation*; World Health Organization: Geneva, Switzerland, 2011; ISBN 978 92 4 150149 1.

21. Brazilian Society of Cardiology. *7ª Diretriz Brasileira de Hipertensão Arterial*; Arq Bras Cardiol: Rio de janeiro, Brazil, 2016; ISSN 0066-782X.

22. Guenther, P.M.; DeMaio, T.J.; Ingwersen, L.A.; Berlin, M. The multiple-pass approach for the 24 hour recall in the Continuing Survey of food intakes by individuals (CSFII) 1994–1996. In Proceedings of the 2nd International Conference on Dietary Assessment Methods, Boston, MA, USA, 22–24 January 1995.

23. Institute of Medicine. *Dietary Reference Intakes for Calcium and Vitamin D*; National Academy of Sciences: Washington, DC, USA, 2011; ISBN 978-0-309-16394-1.

24. Institute of Medicine. *Dietary Reference Intakes: The Essential Guide to Nutrient Requirements*; National Academy of Sciences: Washington, DC, USA, 2006; ISBN 978-0-309-10091-5.

25. Mccrory, M.A.; Hajduk, C.L.; Roberts, S.B. Procedures for screening out inaccurate reports of dietary energy intake. *Public Health Nutr.* **2002**, *5*, 873–882. [CrossRef] [PubMed]

26. Vinken, A.G.; Bathalon, G.P.; Sawaya, A.L.; Dallal, G.E.; Tucker, K.L.; Roberts, S.B. Equations for predicting the energy requirements of healthy adults aged 18–81 y. *Am. J. Clin. Nutr.* **1999**, *69*, 920–926. [CrossRef]

27. German Institute of Human Nutrition Potsdam-Rehbrücke (DIfE). *The Multiple Source Method (MSM)*; DIfE: Nuthetal, Germany, 2012; Available online: https://msm.dife.de (accessed on 25 April 2018).

28. Willett, W.C.; Howe, G.R.; Kushi, L.H. Adjustment for total energy intake in epidemiologic studies. *Am. J. Clin. Nutr.* **1997**, *65*, 1220S–1231S. [CrossRef] [PubMed]

29. Wang, Q.; Koval, J.J.; Mills, C.A.; Lee, K.-I.D. Determination of the Selection Statistics and Best Significance Level in Backward Stepwise Logistic Regression. *Commun. Stat. Simul. C* **2007**, *37*, 62–72. [CrossRef]

30. American Diabetes Association. Glycemic Targets: Standards of Medical Care in Diabetes-2018. *Diabetes Care* **2018**, *41*, S55–S64. [CrossRef]

31. Sampaio, F.A.; Feitosa, M.M.; Sales, C.H.; Silva, D.M.C.; Cruz, K.J.C.; Oliveira, F.E.; Colli, C.; Marreiro, D.N. Influence of magnesium on biochemical parameters of iron and oxidative stress in patients with type 2 diabetes. *Nutr. Hosp.* **2014**, *30*, 570–576. [CrossRef]

32. Eshak, E.S.; Iso, H.; Maruyama, K.; Muraki, I.; Tamakoshi, A. Associations between dietary intakes of iron, copper and zinc with risk of type 2 diabetes mellitus: A large population-based prospective cohort study. *Clin. Nutr.* **2018**, *37*, 667–674. [CrossRef] [PubMed]

33. Vashum, K.P.; McEvoy, M.; Shi, Z.; Milton, A.H.; Islam, M.R.; Sibbritt, D.; Patterson, A.; Byles, J.; Loxton, D.; Attia, J. Is dietary zinc protective for type 2 diabetes? Results from the Australian longitudinal study on women's health. *BMC Endocr. Disord.* **2013**, *13*, 40. [CrossRef] [PubMed]

34. Kanoni, S.; Nettleton, J.A.; Hivert, M.F.; Ye, Z.; van Rooij, F.J.; Shungin, D.; Sonestedt, E.; Ngwa, J.S.; Wojczynski, M.K.; Lemaitre, R.N.; et al. Total Zinc Intake May Modify the Glucose-Raising Effect of a Zinc Transporter (SLC30A8) Variant: A 14-Cohort Meta-analysis. *Diabetes* **2011**, *60*, 2407–2416. [CrossRef] [PubMed]

35. Ige, A.O.; Ajayi, O.A.; Adewoye, E.O. Anti-inflammatory and insulin secretory activity in experimental type-2 diabetic rats treated orally with magnesium. *J. Basic Clin. Physiol. Pharmacol.* **2018**, *29*, 507–514. [CrossRef] [PubMed]

36. Morakinyo, A.O.; Samuel, T.A.; Adekunbi, D.A. Magnesium upregulates insulin receptor and glucose transporter-4 in streptozotocin-nicotinamide-induced type-2 diabetic rats. *Endocr. Regul.* **2018**, *52*, 6–16. [CrossRef]

37. Dong, J.Y.; Xun, P.; He, K.; Qin, L.Q. Magnesium Intake and Risk of Type 2 Diabetes: Meta-analysis of prospective cohort studies. *Diabetes Care* **2011**, *34*, 2116–2122. [CrossRef]

38. Barbagallo, M.; Dominguez, L.J. Magnesium and type 2 diabetes. *World J. Diabetes* **2015**, *6*, 1152–1157. [CrossRef]

39. Rodríguez-Morán, M.; Guerrero-Romero, F. Oral magnesium supplementation improves insulin sensitivity and metabolic control in type 2 diabetic subjects: A randomized double-blind controlled trial. *Diabetes Care* **2003**, *26*, 1147–1152. [CrossRef]

40. Paolisso, G.; Sgambato, S.; Pizza, G.; Passariello, N.; Varricchio, M.; D'Onofrio, F. Improved insulin response and action by chronic magnesium administration in aged NIDDM subjects. *Diabetes Care* **1989**, *12*, 265–269. [CrossRef]

41. Paolisso, G.; Scheen, A.; Cozzolino, D.; Di Maro, G.; Varricchio, M.; D'Onofrio, F.; Lefebvre, P.J. Changes in glucose turnover parameters and improvement of glucose oxidation after 4-week magnesium administration in elderly noninsulin-dependent (type II) diabetic patients. *J. Clin. Endocrinol. Metab.* **1994**, *78*, 1510–1514. [CrossRef] [PubMed]

42. Navarrete-Cortes, A.; Ble-Castillo, J.L.; Guerrero-Romero, F.; Cordova-Uscanga, R.; Juárez-Rojop, I.E.; Aguilar-Mariscal, H.; Tovilla-Zarate, C.A.; Lopez-Guevara Mdel, R. No effect of magnesium supplementation on metabolic control and insulin sensitivity in type 2 diabetic patients with normomagnesemia. *Magnes. Res.* **2014**, *27*, 48–56. [CrossRef] [PubMed]

43. Lima, M.L.; Cruz, T.; Pousada, J.C.; Rodrigues, L.E.; Barbosa, K.; Cangucu, V. The Effect of Magnesium Supplementation in Increasing Doses on the Control of Type 2 Diabetes. *Diabetes Care* **1998**, *21*, 682–686. [CrossRef]

44. de Valk, H.W.; Verkaaik, R.; van Rijn, H.J.; Geerdink, R.; Struyvenberg, A. Oral magnesium supplementation in insulin-requiring Type 2 diabetic patients. *Diabet. Med.* **1998**, *15*, 503–507. [CrossRef]

45. Gullestad, L.; Jacobsen, T.; Dolva, L. Effect of Magnesium Treatment on Glycemic Control and Metabolic Parameters in NIDDM Patients. *Diabetes Care* **1994**, *17*, 460–461. [CrossRef] [PubMed]

46. Purvis, J.R.; Cummings, D.M.; Landsman, P.; Carroll, R.; Barakat, H.; Bray, J.; Whitley, C.; Horner, R.D. Effect of oral magnesium supplementation on selected cardiovascular risk factors in non-insulin-dependent diabetics. *Arch. Fam. Med.* **1994**, *3*, 503–508. [CrossRef] [PubMed]

47. Eibl, N.L.; Kopp, H.P.; Nowak, H.R.; Schnack, C.J.; Hopmeier, P.G.; Schernthaner, G. Hypomagnesemia in Type II Diabetes: Effect of a 3-month replacement therapy. *Diabetes Care* **1995**, *18*, 188–192. [CrossRef]

48. Song, Y.; He, K.; Levitan, E.B.; Manson, J.E.; Liu, S. Effects of oral magnesium supplementation on glycaemic control in Type 2 diabetes: A meta-analysis of randomized double-blind controlled trials. *Diabet. Med.* **2006**, *23*, 1050–1056. [CrossRef]

49. Shalileh, M.; Shidfar, F.; Haghani, H.; Eghtesadi, S.; Heydari, I. The influence of calcium supplement on body composition, weight loss and insulin resistance in obese adults receiving low calorie diet. *J. Res. Med. Sci.* **2010**, *15*, 191–201.

50. Pikilidou, M.I.; Lasaridis, A.N.; Sarafidis, P.A.; Befani, C.D.; Koliakos, G.G.; Tziolas, I.M.; Kazakos, K.A.; Yovos, J.G.; Nilsson, P.M. Insulin sensitivity increase after calcium supplementation and change in intraplatelet calcium and sodium-hydrogen exchange in hypertensive patients with Type 2 diabetes. *Diabet. Med.* **2009**, *26*, 211–219. [CrossRef] [PubMed]

51. Dong, J.Y.; Qin, L.Q. Dietary calcium intake and risk of type 2 diabetes: Possible confounding by magnesium. *Eur. J. Clin. Nutr.* **2012**, *66*, 408–410. [CrossRef] [PubMed]

52. Van Dam, R.M.; Hu, F.B.; Rosenberg, L.; Krishnan, S.; Palmer, J.R. Dietary Calcium and Magnesium, Major Food Sources, and Risk of Type 2 Diabetes in U.S. Black Women. *Diabetes Care* **2006**, *29*, 2238–2243. [CrossRef] [PubMed]

53. Santos, R.K.F.; Brandão-Lima, P.N.; Tete, R.M.D.D.; Freire, A.R.S.; Pires, L.V. Vitamin D ratio and glycaemic control in individuals with type 2 diabetes mellitus: A systematic review. *Diabetes Metab. Res. Rev.* **2018**, *34*, 1–11. [CrossRef] [PubMed]

54. Chatterjee, R.; Yeh, H.C.; Shafi, T.; Selvin, E.; Anderson, C.; Pankow, J.S.; Miller, E.; Brancati, F. Serum and dietary potassium and risk of incident type 2 diabetes mellitus: The Atherosclerosis Risk in Communities (ARIC) study. *Arch. Intern. Med.* **2010**, *170*, 1745–1751. [CrossRef] [PubMed]

55. Becker, W.; Welten, D. Under-reporting in dietary surveys—Implications for development of food-based dietary guidelines. *Public Health Nutr.* **2001**, *4*, 683–687. [CrossRef] [PubMed]

56. Mirmiran, P.; Esmaillzadeh, A.; Azizi, F. Under-reporting of energy intake affects estimates of nutrient intakes. *Asia Pac. J. Clin. Nutr.* **2006**, *15*, 459–464. [PubMed]

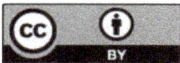

nutrients

MDPI

Article

Dietary Patterns Related to Triglyceride and High-Density Lipoprotein Cholesterol and the Incidence of Type 2 Diabetes in Korean Men and Women

Sihan Song [1] and Jung Eun Lee [1,2,*]

1 Department of Food and Nutrition, College of Human Ecology, Seoul National University, 1 Gwanak-ro, Gwanak-gu, Seoul 08826, Korea; songsihan@snu.ac.kr
2 Research Institute of Human Ecology, Seoul National University, 1 Gwanak-ro, Gwanak-gu, Seoul 08826, Korea
* Correspondence: jungelee@snu.ac.kr; Tel.: +82-2880-6834

Received: 20 November 2018; Accepted: 17 December 2018; Published: 20 December 2018

Abstract: We aimed to examine whether dietary patterns that explain the variation of triglyceride (TG) to high-density lipoprotein cholesterol (HDL-C) ratio were associated with the incidence of type 2 diabetes in Korean adults. We included a total of 5097 adults without diabetes at baseline with a mean follow-up of 11.54 years. Usual diet was assessed by a validated food frequency questionnaire, and serum levels of TG and HDL-C were measured at baseline. We derived dietary pattern scores using 41 food groups as predictors and the TG/HDL-C ratio as a response variable in a stepwise linear regression. We calculated the odds ratio (OR) with the 95% confidence interval (CI) of type 2 diabetes according to pattern scores using multivariate logistic regression. A total of 1069 incident cases of type 2 diabetes were identified. A list of foods characterizing the dietary pattern differed by sex. Higher dietary pattern scores were associated with an increased risk of type 2 diabetes; ORs (95% CIs) comparing extreme quintiles were 1.53 (1.12–2.09; *p* for trend = 0.008) for men and 1.33 (0.95–1.86; *p* for trend = 0.011) for women. Our study suggests the evidence that dietary patterns associated with low levels of TG/HDL-C ratio may have the potential to reduce the burden of type 2 diabetes.

Keywords: dietary pattern; triglyceride; high-density lipoprotein cholesterol; type 2 diabetes

---

1. Introduction

The estimated global prevalence of diabetes mellitus has increased about 50% over the last decade, increased from 5.9% in 2007 to 8.8% in 2017 according to the International Diabetes Foundation [1,2] Over 90% of diabetes cases are of type 2 [2], and the rapid increase is largely attributed to changes in lifestyle factors, such as being overweight or obese, physical inactivity, unhealthy diet, and smoking [3,4]. To reduce the burden of diabetes and its complications, the early detection and treatment of diabetes and evidence-based guideline for diabetes prevention or management are important [5]. The World Health Organization (WHO) and the Food and Agriculture Organization (FAO) provide dietary recommendations for type 2 diabetes prevention, which include limiting saturated fat and obtaining an adequate fiber intake [6]. In addition, WHO recommends reducing the free sugar intake to prevent non-communicable diseases (NCDs), including type 2 diabetes [7].

Because nutrients and foods are consumed in combination, dietary pattern analysis can provide more practical evidence than single-nutrient analysis [8,9]. In addition, the consumption of dietary factors associated with the risk of type 2 diabetes may correlate with each other; therefore, dietary pattern analysis that reflects the complexity of diets may provide scientific insight and practical strategies for disease prevention. Approaches to assess the effects of dietary patterns on the risk of diabetes have been implemented in epidemiologic studies [10,11]. Several previous studies have found significant associations between the risk of type 2 diabetes and posteriori-derived dietary patterns that explain the variation in diabetes-related biomarkers, such as blood glucose, lipids, or inflammatory markers [12–21].

Insulin resistance, a phenomenon involving the resistance to insulin-stimulated glucose uptake, is involved in the pathogenesis of type 2 diabetes, hypertension, and coronary heart disease [22,23]. Indices derived from fasting glucose and insulin including homoeostasis model assessment-insulin resistance (HOMA-IR) and quantitative insulin-sensitivity check index (QUICKI) are widely used to quantify insulin resistance [24]. In addition, the triglyceride (TG) to high-density lipoprotein cholesterol (HDL-C) ratio has been suggested as a simple measure of insulin resistance [25–28]. Vega et al. [29] found that a high TG/HDL-C ratio was associated with an increased risk of type 2 diabetes and cardiovascular disease (CVD) mortality among men participating in the Cooper Center Longitudinal Study (CCLS). In the Korean population, the TG/HDL-C ratio was also significantly associated with insulin resistance [30,31], and the risk of type 2 diabetes [32].

The aim of our study was to identify posteriori-dietary patterns that explain variation in the TG/HDL-C ratio and to examine their association with the risk of type 2 diabetes in Korean adults. Given the sex-differences in TG and HDL-C levels [33] and dietary behavior [34], we identified the dietary patterns among men and women separately.

2. Materials and Methods

2.1. Study Population

The Ansan and Ansung study is part of the Korean Genome and Epidemiology Study (KoGES), which was designed to prospectively investigate the genetic and environmental influences on chronic disease in Korean adults [35]. The Ansan and Ansung study included 10,030 adults (4758 men and 5272 women) aged 40–69 years from the general population of urban (Ansan) and rural (Ansung) areas in 2001–2002. Clinical examination and interviewer-administered questionnaires were conducted at baseline and at biennial follow up. The follow-up rate was 62.8% at the 6th follow-up in 2013–2014 from baseline [35]. All participants provided informed consent. This study was approved by the Seoul National University Institutional Review Board (IRB No. E1811/001-009).

Of 10,030 participants at baseline, we excluded participants who had been diagnosed with or treated for diabetes ($n = 683$), cancer ($n = 247$), CVD ($n = 408$) or had missing data on relevant information ($n = 7$); those who had used insulin treatment ($n = 93$), an oral hypoglycemic drug ($n = 360$) or stroke medication ($n = 21$). We further excluded participants who did not have baseline fasting plasma glucose, 2-h plasma glucose after a 75 g oral glucose tolerance test (OGTT), or hemoglobin A1c (HbA1c) measurements ($n = 67$) as well as undiagnosed diabetes cases who met the American Diabetes Association (ADA) criteria for the diagnosis of diabetes ($n = 692$). We also excluded participants who did not have serum TG or HDL measurements ($n = 1$) or had outlier values for TG or HDL-C levels as determined by a box-plot method (greater than 3*interquartile range; $n = 4$).

KoGES provided food frequency questionnaires (FFQs) data after excluding individuals who: 1) did not answer any questions on the FFQs, 2) left more than 12 blanks for frequency questions, 3) did not answer any questions about rice intake, or 4) had extremely low (<100 kcal/day) or high (≥10,000 kcal/day) energy intake [36], resulting in exclusion of 255 participants. Furthermore, we excluded individuals who reported implausible energy intake (<500 or >3500 kcal/day for women and <800 or >4200 kcal/day for men; $n = 230$) or did not have data on alcohol consumption ($n = 247$). Among those participants who met the inclusion criteria at baseline ($n = 7338$), we excluded those who were not followed at the 5th (2011–2012) or 6th (2013–2014) follow up ($n = 2228$) as well as for those whose information on the ascertainment of type 2 diabetes during the follow-up ($n = 754$) was not available. As a result, a total of 5097 participants (2410 men and 2687 women) were included in the current study. Flow diagram of inclusion for study participants is presented in Figure S1.

2.2. Dietary Assessment

Usual dietary intake was assessed using an interviewer-administered semi-quantitative 103 item FFQ at baseline. The questionnaire was previously validated using 12-day dietary records among 124 participants of KoGES; Pearson's correlation coefficients for energy-adjusted nutrient intakes ranged from 0.23 (vitamin A) to 0.64 (carbohydrate) [37]. Daily energy and nutrient intake were estimated based on the seventh edition of the Food Composition Tables of the Korean Nutrition Society [38]. Participants were asked to report the frequency and portion size of each food item during the previous year. Nine frequency categories ranging from "never or seldom" to "three times or more a day" and three portion sizes (small, medium, or large) were given as options. Alcoholic beverage consumption was assessed separately at baseline and at each biennial follow up. Alcohol drinking status was defined as nondrinker, past drinker, or current drinker. Current alcohol drinkers were asked to report the amount and frequency of alcohol beverage consumption in the previous month, and total alcohol consumption (g/day) was calculated based on the alcohol content of one standard drink.

2.3. Ascertainment of Type 2 Diabetes and Biomarker Assessment

A diagnostic test for diabetes and interviewer-administered questionnaires on diabetes diagnosis or treatment were repeated at biennial follow up. We defined incident type 2 diabetes cases as those who had: 1) a diagnosis of diabetes according to the ADA criteria including HbA1c $\geq$ 6.5% or fasting plasma glucose $\geq$ 126 mg/dl or 2-h plasma glucose $\geq$ 200 mg/dl after a 75 g OGTT [39]; or 2) a diagnosis of type 2 diabetes by physicians or treatment with insulin or oral hypoglycemic medication. Participants who developed type 2 diabetes after baseline were classified as diabetes cases and were otherwise categorized as non-cases.

Blood samples were collected after an overnight fast (at least 8 h) at baseline and at each biennial follow-up examination. Fasting plasma glucose, 1-h and 2-h plasma glucose after a 75 g OGTT were measured enzymatically using an automatic analyzer (ADIVA 1650; Siemens, USA). Whole blood HbA1c level was measured by high-performance liquid chromatography (BIO-RAD Variant II—Turbo; BIORAD, Japan). Serum TG and HDL-C were measured enzymatically using an automatic analyzer (ADIVA 1650; Siemens, USA). The TG/HDL-C ratio was calculated as the ratio of TG to HDL-C.

2.4. Covariate Assessment

Trained interviewers administered a questionnaire regarding sociodemographic factors, lifestyle factors, disease history or current treatment, medication history, family disease history, and reproductive factors. Smoking status was categorized into nonsmoker, past smoker, or current smoker. Pack-years of smoking were calculated using detailed information on smoking history among past or current smokers. When information regarding age at menopause was missing ($n = 326$), we considered the participant postmenopausal if they had been diagnosed after the age of 50, which was the median age of menopause in Korean postmenopausal women aged 40–69 years in 2001 [40]. Participants were asked to report: 1) the hours per day spent on four-intensity physical activity levels (sedentary, light, moderate, and vigorous activity) and 2) the frequency of leisure time spent on physical activity per week and the hours spent on each activity (aerobic, jogging, walking, swimming, tennis, golf, bowling, health club exercise, and mountain climbing). Physical activity was expressed as metabolic equivalents (METs) hours per week by multiplying the hours per week engaged in that activity by the activity's corresponding MET value [41,42]. Anthropometric factors of body weight, height, waist circumference, hip circumference, and blood pressure were obtained by trained examiners. Body mass index (BMI) was calculated as weight (kg) divided by height-squared (m^2).

2.5. Statistical Analysis

We derived dietary patterns that explained the variation in TG/HDL-C ratio using reduced rank regression (RRR) [43]. RRR is a posteriori method used to derive linear combinations of predictor variables (food groups) that explain as much as possible of the variation of response variables (disease-related markers) [43]. When using only one response variable, RRR is identical to multiple linear regression [12,44].

When we derived the dietary patterns of the participants at baseline, we included participants who had never been diagnosed with dyslipidemia and used hyperlipidemia drugs, and participants who had normal HbA1c and plasma glucose levels according to the ADA criteria to avoid the effect of these symptoms on their diet. As a result, 3630 participants (1716 men and 1914 women) were included in the study to derive dietary patterns.

We grouped 103 food items from FFQ and alcohol consumption into 41 groups (g/day) on the basis of similarities in food composition or nutrient content, and these were used as predictor variables to derive dietary patterns. As a response variable, the TG/HDL-C ratio was log-transformed for normality and adjusted for age using a residual method. We then derived dietary patterns that explained as much as possible of the variation of age-adjusted TG/HDL-C using a stepwise linear regression model in men and women separately. A significance level of 0.05 was used for entry and retention in the model. We calculated dietary pattern scores by summing the intakes of selected food groups that were weighted by the regression coefficients for all the study participants.

We used Spearman's correlation coefficients to assess the correlations of dietary pattern and selected foods with the TG/HDL-C ratio. We divided the study participants according to the quintiles of dietary pattern scores and identified the intakes of selected food groups as well as demographic, lifestyle, and clinical characteristics. We used multivariate logistic regression models to calculate the odds ratio (OR) and 95% confidence interval (CI) of type 2 diabetes in each quintile of dietary pattern scores using the lowest quintile as the reference group. In multivariate models, we adjusted for age (continuous, years), living area (Ansan and Ansung), energy intake (continuous, kcal/day), menopausal status (pre and postmenopausal status for women), smoking status (0, >0 and <15, 15–<30, and 30≤ pack-years for men; ever and never smoking for women), alcohol consumption (0, >0 and <5, 5–<15, 15–<30, and 30≤ g/day for men; ever and never drinking for women), family history of diabetes (yes, no), chronic disease status at baseline (yes, no; diagnosis or use of medication for hypertension or hyperlipidemia), and physical activity (continuous, METs-hours/week). We further adjusted for BMI (kg/m^2), which may be an intermediate factor in the causal pathway between dietary patterns related to TG/HDL-C ratio and the risk of type 2 diabetes. We calculated the p value for the trend across quintiles by assigning the median value of each quintile to corresponding participants and treating this value as a continuous variable in the model. We tested for effect modification by age, menopausal status, and BMI at baseline by performing stratified analyses and the likelihood ratio test (LRT) for each variable. We also conducted a sensitivity analysis by excluding incident cases of type 2 diabetes during 2 years of follow up when we examined the association between dietary pattern scores and the risk of type 2 diabetes. All statistical analyses were performed using SAS statistical software version 9.4 (SAS Institute Inc., Cary, NC). All hypothesis tests were evaluated using two-tailed tests of significance at $p < 0.05$.

3. Results

When we derived dietary patterns associated with TG/HDL-C ratio, the list of selected food items differed by sex (Table 1). A high dietary pattern score was characterized in men by higher intakes of noodles, fruits, fermented salted seafood and lower intakes of candy and chocolate, nuts, and pork, whereas that in women was characterized by higher intakes of organ and other meats and lower intakes of dairy products and nuts. The calculated dietary pattern scores were positively associated with TG/HDL-C ratio; the Spearman's correlation coefficients were 0.15 for men and 0.13 for women.

Table 1. Spearman correlation coefficients between dietary pattern scores, selected foods, and the TG/HDL-C ratio, and the mean intake of selected food groups (g/day) according to the quintile of dietary pattern scores.

	Spearman's Correlation with Dietary Pattern Scores		Quintile of TG/HDL-C Ratio-Related Dietary Pattern Scores		
	Dietary Pattern Scores	TG/HDL-C Ratio	Quintile1	Quintile3	Quintile5
Men (*n* = 2410)					
Diet pattern scores	1.00	0.15 [a]			
Positive associations				Mean ± SD	
Noodles	0.37 [a]	0.07 [a]	63.24 ± 54.12	68.18 ± 47.97	152.57 ± 120.93
Fruits	0.33 [a]	0.03	156.68 ± 150.35	154.63 ± 145.63	426.23 ± 382.61
Fermented salted seafood	0.23 [a]	0.03	1.26 ± 2.66	0.88 ± 1.58	4.91 ± 8.12
Inverse associations					
Candy and chocolate	−0.30 [a]	−0.06 [a]	5.02 ± 8.62	0.68 ± 1.42	0.69 ± 1.90
Nuts	−0.29 [a]	−0.06 [a]	2.46 ± 4.40	0.39 ± 1.02	0.36 ± 1.08
Pork	−0.26 [a]	−0.03	69.70 ± 55.90	32.44 ± 29.14	37.11 ± 34.88
Women (*n* = 2687)					
Diet pattern scores	1.00	0.13 [a]			
Positive associations				Mean ± SD	
Organ and other meats	0.10 [a]	−0.01	0.94 ± 3.11	0.97 ± 2.44	3.62 ± 16.72
Inverse associations					
Dairy products	−0.88 [a]	−0.12 [a]	292.40 ± 173.30	75.75 ± 40.48	9.51 ± 32.10
Nuts	−0.42 [a]	−0.09 [a]	2.50 ± 5.02	0.33 ± 0.57	0.04 ± 0.17

Abbreviations: TG, triglyceride; HDL-C, high-density lipoprotein cholesterol. [a] Spearman's correlation coefficient was statistically significant (*p* < 0.05).

The baseline characteristics of men and women are presented in Table 2 according to the quintiles of sex-specific dietary pattern associated with TG/HDL-C ratio. Men who had higher dietary pattern scores were more likely to live in a rural area, have a higher energy intake, and be a current smoker. Women who had higher dietary pattern scores were more likely to be older and postmenopausal, live in a rural area, and have a lower energy intake and physical activity. Participants who had higher dietary pattern scores were more likely to have a higher TG/HDL-C ratio, higher TG levels and lower HDL-C levels than those who had lower dietary pattern scores.

Table 2. Baseline characteristics of the study participants according to the quintiles for TG/HDL-C ratio-related dietary pattern scores.

	Quintile of TG/HDL-C Ratio-Related Dietary Pattern Scores		
	Quintile1	Quintile3	Quintile5
Men (*n* = 2410)	482	482	482
Age (years), mean ± SD	50.38 ± 8.08	50.50 ± 7.99	51.10 ± 8.19
Residential area, *n* (%)			
Rural (Ansung)	148 (30.71)	209 (43.36)	260 (53.94)
Urban (Ansan)	334 (69.29)	273 (56.64)	222 (46.06)
Energy intake (kcal/day), mean ± SD	2095.97 ± 527.68	1802.31 ± 437.21	2289.32 ± 603.02
BMI (kg/m²), mean ± SD [a]	24.02 ± 2.88	24.27 ± 2.77	24.37 ± 2.90
Physical activity (METs h/week), mean ± SD	9.65 ± 14.83	8.06 ± 12.29	8.76 ± 12.05
Smoking status, *n* (%) [a]			
Non-smoker	116 (24.07)	97 (20.12)	99 (20.54)
Past smoker	175 (36.31)	165 (34.23)	130 (26.97)
Current smoker	191 (39.63)	220 (45.64)	253 (52.49)
Alcohol consumption status, *n* (%)			
Non-drinker	94 (19.50)	101 (20.95)	80 (16.60)
Past drinker	48 (9.96)	32 (6.64)	51 (10.58)
Current drinker	340 (70.54)	349 (72.41)	351 (72.82)
Family history of diabetes, *n* (%)			
No	434 (90.04)	433 (89.83)	437 (90.66)
Yes	48 (9.96)	49 (10.17)	45 (9.34)
TG/HDL-C ratio, mean ± SD	3.66 ± 2.79	4.14 ± 2.95	4.97 ± 4.06
TG (mg/dL), mean ± SD	150.52 ± 92.96	166.22 ± 92.86	191.56 ± 123.95
HDL-C (mg/dL), mean ± SD	44.88 ± 9.96	43.69 ± 9.27	42.73 ± 10.10

Table 2. *Cont.*

	Quintile of TG/HDL-C Ratio-Related Dietary Pattern Scores		
	Quintile1	Quintile3	Quintile5
Women (*n* = 2687)	538	531	512
Age (years), mean ± SD	50.02 ± 8.06	50.24 ± 8.26	54.41 ± 8.97
Menopausal status, *n* (%) [a]			
Pre-menopause	243 (52.83)	263 (55.96)	165 (35.71)
Post-menopause	217 (47.17)	207 (44.04)	297 (64.29)
Residential area, *n* (%)			
Rural (Ansung)	199 (36.99)	236 (44.44)	358 (69.92)
Urban (Ansan)	339 (63.01)	295 (55.56)	154 (30.08)
Energy intake (kcal/day), mean ± SD	2081.36 ± 513.71	1818.15 ± 480.73	1679.94 ± 517.76
BMI (kg/m^2), mean ± SD [a]	24.21 ± 2.97	24.72 ± 2.97	25.13 ± 3.23
Physical activity (METs h/week), mean ± SD	11.72 ± 16.47	9.46 ± 14.56	6.69 ± 10.16
Smoking status, *n* (%) [a]			
Non-smoker	510 (96.05)	511 (96.78)	481 (95.06)
Past smoker	4 (0.75)	5 (0.95)	10 (1.98)
Current smoker	17 (3.20)	12 (2.27)	15 (2.96)
Alcohol consumption status, *n* (%)			
Non-drinker	368 (68.40)	378 (71.19)	371 (72.46)
Past drinker	10 (1.86)	14 (2.64)	18 (3.52)
Current drinker	160 (29.74)	139 (26.18)	123 (24.02)
Family history of diabetes, *n* (%)			
No	467 (86.80)	469 (88.32)	461 (90.04)
Yes	71 (13.20)	62 (11.68)	51 (9.96)
TG/HDL-C ratio, mean ± SD	3.08 ± 2.24	3.27 ± 2.64	3.74 ± 2.59
TG (mg/dL), mean ± SD	133.63 ± 74.45	136.19 ± 81.17	153.49 ± 82.92
HDL-C (mg/dL), mean ± SD	47.72 ± 10.1	45.59 ± 9.76	45.11 ± 9.95

Abbreviations: BMI, body mass index; METs, metabolic equivalents; TG, triglyceride; HDL-C, high-density lipoprotein cholesterol. [a] Some participants did not provide relevant information (among men, 1 missing for BMI; and among women, 326 missing for menopausal status and 27 missing for smoking status).

A total of 1069 (560 men and 509 women) cases of type 2 diabetes were identified over a mean follow up of 11.54 years. Multivariate adjusted OR (95% CIs) comparing extreme quintiles was 1.53 (1.12–2.09; *p* for trend = 0.008) among men and 1.33 (0.95–1.86; *p* for trend = 0.011) among women (Table 3). For women, OR (95% CI) comparing the 3rd versus the 1st quintile was 1.45 (1.06–1.99). After further adjustment for BMI, the association was slightly attenuated in both men and women. We examined whether the associations between dietary pattern scores and incident type 2 diabetes varied by age (≤median, >median), menopausal status, and BMI (<25, ≥25 kg/m^2) at baseline regarding the risk of type 2 diabetes (Table 4). The associations appeared to be stronger among older or postmenopausal women than among younger or premenopausal women; the ORs (95% CI) comparing the extreme quintiles were 1.10 (0.65–1.86) for younger women and 1.61 (1.03–2.54) for older women. For BMI, the association appeared to be stronger among men with lower BMI than among those with higher BMI; the ORs (95% CI) comparing the extreme quintiles were 1.82 (1.19–2.80) for men with lower BMI and 1.17 (0.74–1.85) for men with higher BMI. However, there were no significant interactions by these factors.

In the sensitivity analysis, we excluded incident cases that were identified during 2 years of follow-up (*n* = 193), and the estimates of the association between the dietary pattern scores and the incidence of type 2 diabetes were similar to those found in the main analysis (Table S1).

Table 3. Odds ratios (ORs) and 95% confidence intervals (CIs) of incident type 2 diabetes according to the quintiles of TG/HDL-C ratio-related dietary pattern scores.

	Quintiles of TG/HDL-C Ratio-Related Dietary Pattern Scores					p for Trend
	Quintile1	Quintile2	Quintile3	Quintile4	Quintile5	
Men (n = 2410)						
Case/non-case	99/383	110/372	106/376	112/370	133/349	
Unadjusted model	Reference	1.14 (0.84–1.56)	1.09 (0.80–1.49)	1.17 (0.86–1.59)	1.47 (1.10–1.99)	0.010
Age-adjusted model	Reference	1.15 (0.85–1.57)	1.09 (0.80–1.48)	1.17 (0.86–1.60)	1.46 (1.08–1.97)	0.013
Multivariate adjusted model1 [a]	Reference	1.17 (0.85–1.61)	1.12 (0.81–1.54)	1.19 (0.87–1.63)	1.53 (1.12–2.09)	0.008
Multivariate adjusted model2 [b]	Reference	1.16 (0.84–1.59)	1.08 (0.78–1.49)	1.12 (0.82–1.53)	1.48 (1.09–2.03)	0.019
Women (n = 2687)						
Case/non-case	89/449	76/461	118/413	114/455	112/400	
Unadjusted model	Reference	0.83 (0.60–1.16)	1.44 (1.06–1.96)	1.26 (0.93–1.72)	1.41 (1.04–1.92)	0.002
Age-adjusted model	Reference	0.83 (0.59–1.15)	1.44 (1.06–1.95)	1.20 (0.88–1.64)	1.27 (0.93–1.74)	0.014
Multivariate adjusted model1 [c]	Reference	0.83 (0.59–1.16)	1.45 (1.06–1.99)	1.23 (0.88–1.71)	1.33 (0.95–1.86)	0.011
Multivariate adjusted model2 [b]	Reference	0.80 (0.57–1.13)	1.37 (1.00–1.89)	1.14 (0.81–1.59)	1.21 (0.86–1.70)	0.053

Abbreviations: TG, triglyceride; HDL-C, high-density lipoprotein cholesterol. [a] Adjusted for age (continuous, years), living area (Ansan and Ansung), energy intake (continuous, kcal/day), pack-years of smoking (0, >0 and <15, 15–<30, and 30≤ pack-years), alcohol consumption (0, >0 and <5, 5–<15, 15–<30, and 30≤ g/day), family history of diabetes (yes, no), hypertension or hyperlipidemia at baseline (yes, no), and physical activity (continuous, metabolic equivalents-hours/week). [b] Further adjusted for body mass index (continuous, kg/m²) in addition to the variables included in Model 1. [c] Adjusted for age (years), living area (Ansan and Ansung), energy intake (continuous, kcal/day), menopausal status (pre and postmenopausal status), smoking status (ever and never), alcohol consumption (ever and never), family history of diabetes (yes, no), hypertension or hyperlipidemia at baseline (yes, no), and physical activity (continuous, metabolic equivalents-hours/week).

Table 4. Odds ratios (ORs) and 95% confidence intervals (CIs) of incident type 2 diabetes according to the quintiles of dietary pattern scores by age, menopausal status, and BMI at baseline.

	Quintiles of TG/HDL-C Ratio-Related Dietary Pattern Scores					p for Trend	p for Interaction
	Quintile1	Quintile2	Quintile3	Quintile4	Quintile5		
Men [a]							
≤48 years, median (n = 1229)	Reference	1.26 (0.80–1.98)	1.02 (0.63–1.64)	1.12 (0.71–1.77)	1.65 (1.05–2.61)	0.052	0.788
>48 years (n = 1181)	Reference	1.09 (0.70–1.70)	1.21 (0.79–1.88)	1.26 (0.82–1.94)	1.46 (0.96–2.23)	0.063	
Women [b]							
≤49 years, median (n = 1376)	Reference	0.73 (0.45–1.18)	1.20 (0.76–1.90)	1.02 (0.63–1.66)	1.10 (0.65–1.86)	0.407	0.319
>49 years (n = 1311)	Reference	0.90 (0.55–1.46)	1.75 (1.12–2.73)	1.49 (0.94–2.38)	1.61 (1.03–2.54)	0.004	
Menopausal-status at baseline [c]							
Pre-menopause (n = 1143)	Reference	0.83 (0.49–1.41)	1.47 (0.90–2.41)	1.17 (0.68–2.01)	1.15 (0.64–2.07)	0.236	0.324
Post-menopause (n = 1218)	Reference	0.84 (0.50–1.41)	1.57 (0.97–2.55)	1.43 (0.87–2.33)	1.55 (0.96–2.50)	0.013	
Men [a]							
<25 kg/m² (n = 1441)	Reference	1.20 (0.78–1.85)	1.21 (0.78–1.89)	1.20 (0.76–1.89)	1.82 (1.19–2.80)	0.007	0.238
≥25 kg/m² (n = 968)	Reference	1.12 (0.69–1.80)	0.92 (0.57–1.50)	0.98 (0.63–1.53)	1.17 (0.74–1.85)	0.593	
Women [b]							
<25 kg/m² (n = 1543)	Reference	0.63 (0.38–1.05)	1.53 (0.98–2.39)	1.04 (0.64–1.69)	1.17 (0.71–1.93)	0.138	0.625
≥25 kg/m² (n = 1144)	Reference	1.00 (0.62–1.61)	1.31 (0.83–2.07)	1.31 (0.82–2.08)	1.29 (0.81–2.05)	0.133	

Abbreviations: TG, triglyceride; HDL-C, high-density lipoprotein cholesterol; BMI, body mass index. [a] Adjusted for age (continuous, years), living area (Ansan and Ansung), energy intake (continuous, kcal/day), pack-years of smoking (0, >0 and <15, 15–<30, and 30≤ pack-years), alcohol consumption (0, >0 and <5, 5–<15, 15–<30, and 30≤ g/day), family history of diabetes (yes, no), hypertension or hyperlipidemia at baseline (yes, no), and physical activity (continuous, metabolic equivalents-hours/week). [b] Adjusted for age (continuous, years), living area (Ansan and Ansung), energy intake (continuous, kcal/day), menopausal status (pre and postmenopausal status), smoking status (ever and never), alcohol consumption status (ever and never), family history of diabetes (yes, no), hypertension or hyperlipidemia at baseline (yes, no), and physical activity (continuous, metabolic equivalents-hours/week). [c] Adjusted for age (years), living area (Ansan and Ansung), energy intake (kcal/day), smoking status (ever and never), alcohol consumption status (ever and never), family history of diabetes (yes, no), hypertension or hyperlipidemia at baseline (yes, no), and physical activity (continuous, metabolic equivalents-hours/week).

4. Discussion

We derived dietary patterns that explain the variation in the diabetes-related biomarker, the TG/HDL-C ratio, in men and women separately. The dietary pattern was characterized by high intakes of noodles, fruits, fermented salted seafood and low intakes of candy and chocolate, nuts, and pork among men and by high intakes of organ and other meats and low intakes of dairy products and nuts among women. Dietary pattern scores were positively associated with the TG/HDL-C ratio. High dietary pattern score was associated with an increased risk of type 2 diabetes. The associations appeared to be stronger among older or postmenopausal women, albeit without statistical significance.

Insulin resistance is a major risk factor for the development of type 2 diabetes [22,23, 45]. The consequences of insulin resistance and its compensatory hyperinsulinemia include glucose intolerance, dyslipidemia (increased TG and/or decreased HDL-C), high blood pressure, hyperuricemia, and increased plasminogen activator inhibitor (PAI)-1 activity [23]. Several studies have examined the association between risk of type 2 diabetes and dietary patterns that explain the variation of biomarkers that are linked to diabetes [12–21]. Biomarkers linked to diabetes that have been used to derive dietary patterns include inflammatory markers (e.g., PAI-1, tumor necrosis factor-α receptor 2, C-reactive protein (CRP), and Interleukin 6) [12,13,19,21], glucose (e.g., HbA1c, HOMA-IR, and fasting glucose) [12,14,16,20], lipid-related metabolites (e.g., TG, HDL-C, adiponectin, and leptin) [12,16,18,21], and uric acids [17]. Food groups that have been frequently reported to be associated with an increased risk of type 2 diabetes have been characterized by high intakes of sugar-sweetened beverages or soft drinks [12–14,16,17,21], processed meats [12,13,16,21], red meats [12,15,16,21], refined grains [13,16], white rice [21] or bread [14,19] and low intakes of wine [13,15,16], whole grains [16,21], and yellow [13,16,21] and green [16,21] vegetables. In our study, noodles positively contributed to the dietary pattern scores among men. Batis et al. [20] also identified a positive association of wheat noodles with dietary pattern scores that explained variations of HbA1c, HOMA-IR, and fasting glucose levels among Chinese men and women. Additionally, consistent with previous studies that identified a positive contribution of red meats to diabetes-related dietary pattern scores [12,15,16,21], we found a positive contribution of organ and other meats to dietary pattern scores among women.

The estimates of the association between dietary pattern scores and the risk of type 2 diabetes are comparable to those found in previous studies. Jannasch et al. [11] conducted meta-analyses of the association between posteriori-dietary patterns associated with diabetes-related biomarkers and risk of type 2 diabetes [12–14,16,46]; combined relative risks (95% CIs) were 0.51 (0.27–0.98) for dietary pattern related to HbA1c, HDL-C, CRP, and adiponectin [12,16,46], 2.53 (1.56–4.10) for dietary pattern related to inflammatory markers [13,16,46] and 1.39 (1.25–1.54) for dietary patterns associated with HOMA-IR [14,16,46].

Previous studies have identified the TG/HDL-C ratio as a clinically useful surrogate estimate of insulin resistance [25–28]. Methods for estimating TG and HDL-C concentrations are well standardized [26], and the ratio of the two values provides information on the atherogenic lipoprotein profile associated with the risk of CVD [47] as well as insulin resistance. A high TG/HDL-C ratio is associated with an increased risk of type 2 diabetes [29,32,48,49] and with CHD and/or CVD events [50,51] and mortality [29,52]. Tabung et al. [53] developed an empirical dietary index for insulin resistance using the TG/HDL-C ratio as a response variable and food groups as explanatory variables in a stepwise linear regression model in a female cohort, the Nurses' Health Study (NHS). An empirical dietary index for insulin resistance was characterized by high intakes of low-calorie beverages, margarine, red meat, refined grains, processed meats, tomatoes, other vegetables, other fish, fruit juice, and creamy soups and low intakes of coffee, wine, liquor, beer, green leafy vegetables, high-fat dairy products, dark yellow vegetables, and nuts [53]. Consistent with a previous study that developed a dietary index for insulin resistance, our study also found that dietary pattern was positively associated with organ and other meats and negatively associated with dairy products and nuts among women. According to the meta-analysis of prospective cohort studies for individual food groups, a higher consumption of red meats was associated with an increased risk of type 2 diabetes [54], whereas higher consumption of dairy products [55,56] and nuts [57] were associated with a reduced risk of type 2 diabetes.

There were unexpected inverse associations of dietary pattern scores with pork and candy/chocolate among men. Even though we used an age-adjusted TG/HDL-C ratio, a difference in pork by age may exist. Low consumption of pork among older men may explain our finding; mean intake of pork among men aged 40s, 50s, and 60s was 47.19 g/day, 42.25 g/day, and 37.65 g/day, respectively. Further study is needed to examine dietary patterns associated with various biomarkers that have been linked to diabetes and their prediction of type 2 diabetes risk in different study populations.

This study has several limitations. We did not use person-years of follow-up to analyze the association because we did not have information on type 2 diabetes incidence for more than 20% of the original study participants. Therefore, we included participants whose fasting plasma glucose, 2-h plasma glucose after a 75 g OGTT, and HbA1c were available during the follow-up. This may limit the generalizability of our findings; however, we tried to remove the potential bias that could occur from loss to follow-up. We also cannot rule out the possibility of the presence of measurement error in the dietary assessment or residual or unknown confounding factors.

The strengths of our study include the measurement of biomarkers to detect the incidence of type 2 diabetes. Fasting plasma glucose, 2-h plasma glucose after a 75 g OGTT, and HbA1c were measured at baseline and at every biannual follow up. This is the first cohort study in Korea to examine the association between biomarker-related dietary pattern and type 2 diabetes incidence. We were able to examine a temporal relationship between dietary patterns and the risk of type 2 diabetes, given a cohort study design. Information on sociodemographic and lifestyle factors as well as medical status allowed us to adjust for potential confounders. Last, we additionally derived the dietary patterns of men and women separately. Providing sex-specific findings is important because of the sex difference in biological and behavioral characteristics and sex-specific results may provide appropriate evidence on modifiable factors that contributing to disease prevention in men and women [58]. We found that the components of dietary patterns differed by sex, and the results were consistent with previous studies that examined the association in a sex-specific way.

5. Conclusions

The present study derived posteriori-dietary patterns using the TG/HDL-C ratio as a biomarker that is linked to type 2 diabetes, and examined the associations between the dietary pattern scores and the risk of type 2 diabetes among Korean men and women. Among men, dietary pattern was characterized by higher intakes of noodles, fruits, fermented salted seafood and lower intakes of candy and chocolate, nuts, and pork; and the dietary pattern for women was characterized by higher intakes of organ and other meats and lower intakes of dairy products and nuts. Higher dietary pattern scores were associated with an increased risk of type 2 diabetes. Our study provides sex-specific evidence on dietary patterns associated with the risk of type 2 diabetes, which may partly be mediated by the TG/HDL-C ratio. Consideration of TG/HDL-C ratio related dietary patterns to reduce the burden of type 2 diabetes may be needed and our study warrants further replication.

Supplementary Materials: The following are available online at http://www.mdpi.com/2072-6643/11/1/8/s1, Figure S1: Flow diagram of inclusion for study participants, Table S1: Odds ratios (ORs) and 95% confidence intervals (CIs) of incident 2 diabetes according to the quintiles of TG/HDLC-related dietary pattern after excluding incident cases during 2 years of follow up.

Author Contributions: Conceptualization, J.E.L. and S.S.; Formal Analysis, S.S.; Writing—Original Draft Preparation, S.S.; Writing—Review & Editing, J.E.L.; Funding Acquisition, J.E.L.

Funding: This research was supported by the Support Program for Women in Science, Engineering and Technology through the National Research Foundation of Korea (NRF) funded by the Ministry of Science and ICT (No. 2016H1C3A1903202).

Acknowledgments: Data in this study were from the Korean Genome and Epidemiology Study (KoGES; 4851-302), National Research Institute of Health, Centers for Disease Control and Prevention, Ministry for Health and Welfare, Republic of Korea.

Conflicts of Interest: The authors declare no conflict of interest. The funders had no role in the design of the study; in the collection, analyses, or interpretation of data; in the writing of the manuscript, or in the decision to publish the results.

References

1. International Diabetes Foundation. *IDF Diabetes Atlas*, 3rd ed.; International Diabetes Foundation: Brussels, Belgium, 2006.
2. International Diabetes Federation. *IDF Diabetes Atlas*, 8th ed.; International Diabetes Foundation: Brussels, Belgium, 2017.
3. Zimmet, P.; Alberti, K.; Shaw, J. Global and societal implications of the diabetes epidemic. *Nature* **2001**, *414*, 782. [CrossRef]
4. Chen, L.; Magliano, D.J.; Zimmet, P.Z. The worldwide epidemiology of type 2 diabetes mellitus—Present and future perspectives. *Nat. Rev. Endocrinol.* **2012**, *8*, 228. [CrossRef] [PubMed]
5. World Health Organization. *Global Report on Diabetes*; World Health Organization: Geneva, Switzerland, 2016.
6. World Health Organization. *Diet, Nutrition, and the Prevention of Chronic Diseases: Report of a Joint Who/Fao Expert Consultation*; World Health Organization: Geneva, Switzerland, 2003.
7. World Health Organization. *Guideline: Sugars Intake for Adults and Children*; World Health Organization: Geneva, Switzerland, 2015.
8. National Research Council. *Diet and Health: Implications for Reducing Chronic Disease Risk*; National Academies Press: Washington, DC, USA, 1989.
9. Hu, F.B. Dietary pattern analysis: A new direction in nutritional epidemiology. *Curr. Opin. Lipidol.* **2002**, *13*, 3–9. [CrossRef] [PubMed]
10. Ley, S.H.; Hamdy, O.; Mohan, V.; Hu, F.B. Prevention and management of type 2 diabetes: Dietary components and nutritional strategies. *The Lancet* **2014**, *383*, 1999–2007. [CrossRef]
11. Jannasch, F.; Kroger, J.; Schulze, M.B. Dietary Patterns and Type 2 Diabetes: A Systematic Literature Review and Meta-Analysis of Prospective Studies. *J. Nutr.* **2017**, *147*, 1174–1182. [CrossRef]
12. Heidemann, C.; Hoffmann, K.; Spranger, J.; Klipstein-Grobusch, K.; Mohlig, M.; Pfeiffer, A.F.; Boeing, H. A dietary pattern protective against type 2 diabetes in the European Prospective Investigation into Cancer and Nutrition (EPIC)–Potsdam Study cohort. *Diabetologia* **2005**, *48*, 1126–1134. [CrossRef]
13. Schulze, M.B.; Hoffmann, K.; Manson, J.E.; Willett, W.C.; Meigs, J.B.; Weikert, C.; Heidemann, C.; Colditz, G.A.; Hu, F.B. Dietary pattern, inflammation, and incidence of type 2 diabetes in women. *Am. J. Clin. Nutr.* **2005**, *82*, 675–684. [CrossRef]
14. McNaughton, S.A.; Mishra, G.D.; Brunner, E.J. Dietary patterns, insulin resistance, and incidence of type 2 diabetes in the whitehall II study. *Diabetes Care* **2008**, *31*, 1343–1348. [CrossRef]
15. Liese, A.D.; Weis, K.E.; Schulz, M.; Tooze, J.A. Food intake patterns associated with incident type 2 diabetes: The insulin resistance atherosclerosis study. *Diabetes Care* **2009**, *32*, 263–268. [CrossRef]
16. Imamura, F.; Lichtenstein, A.H.; Dallal, G.E.; Meigs, J.B.; Jacques, P.F. Generalizability of dietary patterns associated with incidence of type 2 diabetes mellitus. *Am. J. Clin. Nutr.* **2009**, *90*, 1075–1083. [CrossRef]
17. Sluijs, I.; Beulens, J.W.; van der, A.D.; Spijkerman, A.M.; Schulze, M.B.; van der Schouw, Y.T. Plasma uric acid is associated with increased risk of type 2 diabetes independent of diet and metabolic risk factors. *Am. J. Clin. Nutr.* **2013**, *143*, 80–85. [CrossRef] [PubMed]
18. Frank, L.K.; Jannasch, F.; Kroger, J.; Bedu-Addo, G.; Mockenhaupt, F.P.; Schulze, M.B.; Danquah, I. A Dietary Pattern Derived by Reduced Rank Regression is Associated with Type 2 Diabetes in An Urban Ghanaian Population. *Nutrients* **2015**, *7*, 5497–5514. [CrossRef] [PubMed]
19. McGeoghegan, L.; Muirhead, C.R.; Almoosawi, S. Association between an anti-inflammatory and anti-oxidant dietary pattern and diabetes in British adults: Results from the national diet and nutrition survey rolling programme years 1–4. *Int. J. Food Sci. Nutr.* **2015**, *67*, 553–561. [CrossRef]

20. Batis, C.; Mendez, M.A.; Gordon-Larsen, P.; Sotres-Alvarez, D.; Adair, L.; Popkin, B. Using both principal component analysis and reduced rank regression to study dietary patterns and diabetes in Chinese adults. *Public Health Nutr.* **2016**, *19*, 195–203. [CrossRef]

21. Jacobs, S.; Kroeger, J.; Schulze, M.B.; Frank, L.K.; Franke, A.A.; Cheng, I.; Monroe, K.R.; Haiman, C.A.; Kolonel, L.N.; Wilkens, L.R.; et al. Dietary Patterns Derived by Reduced Rank Regression Are Inversely Associated with Type 2 Diabetes Risk across 5 Ethnic Groups in the Multiethnic Cohort. *Curr. Dev. Nutr.* **2017**, *1*, e000620. [CrossRef] [PubMed]

22. Reaven, G.M. Role of Insulin Resistance in Human Disease. *Diabetes* **1988**, *37*, 1595–1607. [CrossRef] [PubMed]

23. Reaven, G.M. Pathophysiology of insulin resistance in human disease. *Physiol. Rev.* **1995**, *75*, 473–486. [CrossRef]

24. Antuna-Puente, B.; Disse, E.; Rabasa-Lhoret, R.; Laville, M.; Capeau, J.; Bastard, J.-P. How can we measure insulin sensitivity/resistance? *Diabetes Metab.* **2011**, *37*, 179–188. [CrossRef]

25. McLaughlin, T.; Abbasi, F.; Cheal, K.; Chu, J.; Lamendola, C.; Reaven, G. Use of metabolic markers to identify overweight individuals who are insulin resistant. *Ann. Intern. Med.* **2003**, *139*, 802–809. [CrossRef]

26. McLaughlin, T.; Reaven, G.; Abbasi, F.; Lamendola, C.; Saad, M.; Waters, D.; Simon, J.; Krauss, R.M. Is there a simple way to identify insulin-resistant individuals at increased risk of cardiovascular disease? *Am. J. Cardiol.* **2005**, *96*, 399–404. [CrossRef]

27. Li, C.; Ford, E.S.; Meng, Y.-X.; Mokdad, A.H.; Reaven, G.M. Does the association of the triglyceride to high-density lipoprotein cholesterol ratio with fasting serum insulin differ by race/ethnicity? *Cardiovasc. Diabetol.* **2008**, *7*, 4. [CrossRef] [PubMed]

28. Salazar, M.R.; Carbajal, H.A.; Espeche, W.G.; Leiva Sisnieguez, C.E.; Balbín, E.; Dulbecco, C.A.; Aizpurúa, M.; Marillet, A.G.; Reaven, G.M. Relation Among the Plasma Triglyceride/High-Density Lipoprotein Cholesterol Concentration Ratio, Insulin Resistance, and Associated Cardio-Metabolic Risk Factors in Men and Women. *Am. J. Cardiol.* **2012**, *109*, 1749–1753. [CrossRef] [PubMed]

29. Vega, G.L.; Barlow, C.E.; Grundy, S.M.; Leonard, D.; DeFina, L.F. Triglyceride-to–high-density-lipoprotein-cholesterol ratio is an index of heart disease mortality and of incidence of type 2 diabetes mellitus in men. *J. Investig. Med.* **2014**, *62*, 345–349. [CrossRef] [PubMed]

30. Kang, H.-T.; Yoon, J.-H.; Kim, J.-Y.; Ahn, S.-K.; Linton, J.; Koh, S.-B.; Kim, J.-K. The association between the ratio of triglyceride to HDL-C and insulin resistance according to waist circumference in a rural Korean population. *Nutr. Metab. Cardiovasc. Dis.* **2012**, *22*, 1054–1060. [CrossRef] [PubMed]

31. Kim, J.-S.; Kang, H.-T.; Shim, J.-Y.; Lee, H.-R. The association between the triglyceride to high-density lipoprotein cholesterol ratio with insulin resistance (HOMA-IR) in the general Korean population: Based on the National Health and Nutrition Examination Survey in 2007–2009. *Diabetes Res. Clin. Pract.* **2012**, *97*, 132–138. [CrossRef] [PubMed]

32. Sung, K.-C.; Park, H.-Y.; Kim, M.-J.; Reaven, G. Metabolic markers associated with insulin resistance predict type 2 diabetes in Koreans with normal blood pressure or prehypertension. *Cardiovasc. Diabetol.* **2016**, *15*, 47. [CrossRef] [PubMed]

33. Wang, X.; Magkos, F.; Mittendorfer, B. Sex differences in lipid and lipoprotein metabolism: It's not just about sex hormones. *J. Clin. Endocrinol. Metab.* **2011**, *96*, 885–893. [CrossRef]

34. Arganini, C.; Saba, A.; Comitato, R.; Virgili, F.; Turrini, A. Gender differences in food choice and dietary intake in modern western societies. In *Public Health-Social and Behavioral Health*; InTech Open Access Publisher: Rijeka, Croatia, 2012.

35. Kim, Y.; Han, B.-G.; KoGES Group. Cohort Profile: The Korean Genome and Epidemiology Study (KoGES) Consortium. *Int. J. Epidemiol.* **2017**, *46*, e20. [CrossRef]

36. KCDC Center for Genome Sciences. FFQ guideline for Korean Genome and Epidemiology Study (KoGES). 2014. Available online: http://www.cdc.go.kr/NIH_NEW/contents/NihKrContentView.jsp?cid=141857&menuIds=HOME005-MNU2016-MNU1010-MNU1023#menu2_2_2 (accessed on 20 October 2018).

37. Ahn, Y.; Kwon, E.; Shim, J.; Park, M.; Joo, Y.; Kimm, K.; Park, C.; Kim, D. Validation and reproducibility of food frequency questionnaire for Korean genome epidemiologic study. *Eur. J. Clin. Nutr.* **2007**, *61*, 1435. [CrossRef]

38. Korean Nutrition Society. *Recommended Dietary Allowances for Koreans*, 7th ed.; Korean Nutrition Society: Seoul, Korea, 2000.

39. American Diabetes Association. 2. Classification and diagnosis of diabetes. *Diabetes Care* **2015**, *38*, S8–S16. [CrossRef]
40. Korea Centers for Disease Control and Prevention. *The Second Korea National Health and Nutrition Examination Survey (KNHANES II), 2001*; Korea Centers for Disease Control and Prevention: Seoul, Korea, 2002.
41. Ainsworth, B.E.; Haskell, W.L.; Whitt, M.C.; Irwin, M.L.; Swartz, A.M.; Strath, S.J.; O Brien, W.L.; Bassett, D.R.; Schmitz, K.H.; Emplaincourt, P.O. Compendium of physical activities: An update of activity codes and MET intensities. *Med. Sci. Sports Exerc.* **2000**, *32*, S498–S504. [CrossRef] [PubMed]
42. Ainsworth, B.E.; Haskell, W.L.; Herrmann, S.D.; Meckes, N.; Bassett, D.R., Jr.; Tudor-Locke, C.; Greer, J.L.; Vezina, J.; Whitt-Glover, M.C.; Leon, A.S. 2011 Compendium of Physical Activities: A second update of codes and MET values. *Med. Sci. Sports Exerc.* **2011**, *43*, 1575–1581. [CrossRef] [PubMed]
43. Hoffmann, K.; Schulze, M.B.; Schienkiewitz, A.; Nothlings, U.; Boeing, H. Application of a new statistical method to derive dietary patterns in nutritional epidemiology. *Am J. Epidemiol.* **2004**, *159*, 935–944. [CrossRef] [PubMed]
44. Fung, T.T.; Hu, F.B.; Schulze, M.; Pollak, M.; Wu, T.; Fuchs, C.S.; Giovannucci, E. A dietary pattern that is associated with C-peptide and risk of colorectal cancer in women. *Cancer Causes Control* **2012**, *23*, 959–965. [CrossRef]
45. Lillioja, S.; Mott, D.M.; Spraul, M.; Ferraro, R.; Foley, J.E.; Ravussin, E.; Knowler, W.C.; Bennett, P.H.; Bogardus, C. Insulin resistance and insulin secretory dysfunction as precursors of non-insulin-dependent diabetes mellitus: Prospective studies of Pima Indians. *N. Engl. J. Med.* **1993**, *329*, 1988–1992. [CrossRef] [PubMed]
46. InterAct Consortium. Adherence to predefined dietary patterns and incident type 2 diabetes in European populations: EPIC-InterAct Study. *Diabetologia* **2014**, *57*, 321–333. [CrossRef] [PubMed]
47. Dobiásová, M.; Frohlich, J. The plasma parameter log (TG/HDL-C) as an atherogenic index: Correlation with lipoprotein particle size and esterification rate inapob-lipoprotein-depleted plasma (FERHDL). *Clin. Biochem.* **2001**, *34*, 583–588. [CrossRef]
48. Zhang, M.; Zhou, J.; Liu, Y.; Sun, X.; Luo, X.; Han, C.; Zhang, L.; Wang, B.; Ren, Y.; Zhao, Y. Risk of type 2 diabetes mellitus associated with plasma lipid levels: The rural Chinese cohort study. *Diabetes Res. Clin. Pract.* **2018**, *135*, 150–157. [CrossRef]
49. He, S.; Wang, S.; Chen, X.; Jiang, L.; Peng, Y.; Li, L.; Wan, L.; Cui, K. Higher ratio of triglyceride to high-density lipoprotein cholesterol may predispose to diabetes mellitus: 15-year prospective study in a general population. *Metabolism* **2012**, *61*, 30–36. [CrossRef]
50. Hadaegh, F.; Khalili, D.; Ghasemi, A.; Tohidi, M.; Sheikholeslami, F.; Azizi, F. Triglyceride/HDL-cholesterol ratio is an independent predictor for coronary heart disease in a population of Iranian men. *Nutr. Metab. Cardiovasc. Dis.* **2009**, *19*, 401–408. [CrossRef]
51. Bittner, V.; Johnson, B.D.; Zineh, I.; Rogers, W.J.; Vido, D.; Marroquin, O.C.; Bairey-Merz, C.N.; Sopko, G. The triglyceride/high-density lipoprotein cholesterol ratio predicts all-cause mortality in women with suspected myocardial ischemia: A report from the Women's Ischemia Syndrome Evaluation (WISE). *Am. Heart J.* **2009**, *157*, 548–555. [CrossRef] [PubMed]
52. Asia Pacific Cohort Studies Collaboration. A Comparison of Lipid Variables as Predictors of Cardiovascular Disease in the Asia Pacific Region. *Ann. Epidemiol.* **2005**, *15*, 405–413. [CrossRef] [PubMed]
53. Tabung, F.K.; Wang, W.; Fung, T.T.; Hu, F.B.; Smith-Warner, S.A.; Chavarro, J.E.; Fuchs, C.S.; Willett, W.C.; Giovannucci, E.L. Development and validation of empirical indices to assess the insulinaemic potential of diet and lifestyle. *Br. J. Nutr.* **2016**, *116*, 1787–1798. [CrossRef] [PubMed]
54. Pan, A.; Sun, Q.; Bernstein, A.M.; Schulze, M.B.; Manson, J.E.; Willett, W.C.; Hu, F.B. Red meat consumption and risk of type 2 diabetes: 3 cohorts of US adults and an updated meta-analysis. *Am. J. Clin. Nutr.* **2011**, *94*, 1088–1096. [CrossRef] [PubMed]
55. Tong, X.; Dong, J.; Wu, Z.; Li, W.; Qin, L. Dairy consumption and risk of type 2 diabetes mellitus: A meta-analysis of cohort studies. *Eur. J. Clin. Nutr.* **2011**, *65*, 1027. [CrossRef] [PubMed]
56. Gijsbers, L.; Ding, E.L.; Malik, V.S.; de Goede, J.; Geleijnse, J.M.; Soedamah-Muthu, S.S. Consumption of dairy foods and diabetes incidence: A dose-response meta-analysis of observational studies. *Am. J. Clin. Nutr.* **2016**, *103*, 1111–1124. [CrossRef] [PubMed]

57. Afshin, A.; Micha, R.; Khatibzadeh, S.; Mozaffarian, D. Consumption of nuts and legumes and risk of incident ischemic heart disease, stroke, and diabetes: A systematic review and meta-analysis. *Am. J. Clin. Nutr.* **2014**, *100*, 278–288. [CrossRef] [PubMed]

58. Song, S.; Kim, S.; Lee, J.E. Sex consideration in diet–biomarker-related indices: A systematic review. *Public Health Nutr.* **2018**, 1–13. [CrossRef]

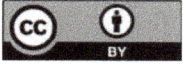

nutrients

MDPI

Article

A Randomized Controlled Trial to Compare the Effect of Peanuts and Almonds on the Cardio-Metabolic and Inflammatory Parameters in Patients with Type 2 Diabetes Mellitus

Yun-Ying Hou [1,†], Omorogieva Ojo [2,†], Li-Li Wang [1], Qi Wang [1], Qing Jiang [3], Xin-Yu Shao [3] and Xiao-Hua Wang [1,*]

[1] School of Nursing, Medical College, Soochow University, Suzhou 215006, China;
houyunying@suda.edu.cn (Y.-Y.H.); wanglili83476@suda.edu.cn (L.-L.W.); xuweipan@whu.edu.cn (Q.W.)
[2] Faculty of Education and Health, University of Greenwich, London SE9 2UG, UK; o.ojo@greenwich.ac.uk
[3] Medical College, Soochow University, Suzhou 215006, China; jiangqing2015@suda.edu.cn (Q.J.);
wudan@suda.edu.cn (X.-Y.S.)
* Correspondence: wangxiaohua@suda.edu.cn; Tel.: +86-138-1488-0208
† Yun-Ying Hou and Omorogieva Ojo are co-first authors.

Received: 24 August 2018; Accepted: 18 October 2018; Published: 23 October 2018

Abstract: A low carbohydrate diet (LCD), with some staple food being replaced with nuts, has been shown to reduce weight, improve blood glucose, and regulate blood lipid in patients with type 2 diabetes mellitus (T2DM). These nuts include tree nuts and ground nuts. Tree nut consumption is associated with improved cardio-vascular and inflammatory parameters. However, the consumption of tree nuts is difficult to promote in patients with diabetes because of their high cost. As the main ground nut, peanuts contain a large number of beneficial nutrients, are widely planted, and are affordable for most patients. However, whether peanuts and tree nuts in combination with LCD have similar benefits in patients with T2DM remains unknown; although almonds are the most consumed and studied tree nut. This study sought to compare the effect of peanuts and almonds, incorporated into a LCD, on cardio-metabolic and inflammatory measures in patients with T2DM. Of the 32 T2DM patients that were recruited, 17 were randomly allocated to the Peanut group ($n = 17$) and 15 to the Almond group ($n = 15$) in a parallel design. The patients consumed a LCD with part of the starchy staple food being replaced with peanuts (Peanut group) or almonds (Almond group). The follow-up duration was three months. The indicators for glycemic control, other cardio-metabolic, and inflammatory parameters were collected and compared between the two groups. Twenty-five patients completed the study. There were no significant differences in the self-reported dietary compliance between the two groups. Compared with the baseline, the fasting blood glucose (FBG) and postprandial 2-h blood glucose (PPG) decreased in both the Peanut and Almond groups ($p < 0.05$). After the intervention, no statistically significant differences were found between the Peanut group and the Almond group with respect to the FBG and PPG levels. A decrease in the glycated hemoglobin A1c (HbA1c) level from the baseline in the Almond group was found ($p < 0.05$). However, no significant difference was found between the two groups with respect to the HbA1c level at the third month. The peanut and almond consumption did not increase the body mass index (BMI) and had no effect on the blood lipid profile or interleukin-6 (IL-6). In conclusion, incorporated into a LCD, almonds and peanuts have a similar effect on improving fasting and postprandial blood glucose among patients with T2DM. However, more studies are required to fully establish the effect of almond on the improvement of HbA1c.

Keywords: type 2 diabetes mellitus; peanut; almond; glycemic control; body mass index; lipids; interleukin-6

1. Introduction

Type 2 diabetes mellitus (T2DM) is a chronic disease that involves a heterogeneous group of disorders of the intermediary metabolism, characterized by glucose intolerance [1]. The incidence and prevalence of T2DM have increased markedly worldwide, and its complications are the leading causes of morbidity and premature mortality [2]. The use of diet in the prevention, treatment, and control of T2DM has been recommended, and is one of the strategies for managing the condition. According to the American Diabetes Association (ADA), the nutritional goals for patients with T2DM are to achieve normoglycemia and a cardio protective lipid profile that reduces the risk for cardiovascular disease (CVD) [3].

In recent years, a low carbohydrate diet (LCD) has gained popularity [4], and its effectiveness in reducing weight, improving blood glucose, and regulating blood lipid in patients with T2DM has been confirmed by the American Diabetes Association and Diabetes UK [5,6]. ALCD combined with a low saturated fat intake may be best for patients [7].

Nuts are high in unsaturated fat and are a rich source of bioactive nutrients that have the potential to provide metabolic and cardiovascular benefits [8]. Bodies concerned with diabetes and CVD (e.g., the Canadian Cardiovascular Society and the European Atherosclerosis Society) are now advocating for an increase in nut consumption as part of their dietary recommendations [9–12].

Nuts include tree nuts (almond, walnut, hazelnut, pistachio, pine nut, cashew, pecan, macadamia, and Brazil nut) and ground nuts (mainly peanut). Almonds are the most studied tree nut. Clinical trials have shown that the consumption of almonds as well as other tree nuts is associated with improved glycemic control, insulin sensitivity, decreased inflammation, and reduced/sustained body weight [13–16]. However, tree nuts are difficult to promote in patients with diabetes because of their high cost, especially in developing and under-developed countries.

As the main ground nut, peanuts have a similar nutrient composition to tree nuts, thus being nutrient-dense and rich in monounsaturated fatty acid (MUFA) (40% of energy). They are also a good source of arginine, fiber, phytosterols, polyphenols, niacin, folic acid, and vitamin E [17]. In addition, peanuts are widely planted and are much cheaper than tree nuts, and they are affordable for most T2DM patients. Randomized controlled and cross-over trials have shown that peanut consumption helps to moderate glucose concentrations [18], improve the postprandial lipid response, and preserve endothelial function [19]. However, whether peanuts and tree nuts have similar benefits for T2DM patients remains unknown.

Almonds are the most consumed tree nut [20]. We aim to compare the effect of peanuts and almonds incorporated into LCD on cardio-metabolic and inflammatory measures in T2DM patients.

2. Materials and Methods

2.1. Subjects

The participants were recruited from a diabetes club and from the Endocrine Division of the First Affiliated Hospital of Soochow University. The inclusion criteria were as follows: The patients were diagnosed with T2DM, had glycated hemoglobin A1c (HbA1c) of less than 10%, had no change in oral antidiabetic drugs or in insulin half a month before the intervention, were between 40 to 80 years old [15,21], were able to communicate, had volunteered to participate in this study, and were willing to provide informed consent. Those that were excluded were the patients who ate nuts regularly ($\geq$four per day/week) [22]; were allergic to nuts or other food; had difficulty in chewing nuts as a result of fewer teeth or for other reasons; could not adhere to a LCD strategy; received other dietary interventions; had severe conditions including indigestion, hepatic failure, renal failure, severe gallbladder and pancreatic diseases, stroke, malignant tumors, or unstable cardiovascular diseases (such as myocardial infarction, ketosis, or hyperthyroidism); those who were taking glucocorticoid; and those whose fasting blood glucose (FBG) was more than 16.7 mmol/L [23] during the intervention.

2.2. Study Design

This study is a prospective, randomized controlled trial (RCT) that was performed between December 2015 and April 2016. The recruited patients were randomly allocated to the Peanut and Almond groups using a table of random numbers. The random numbers were generated by one researcher, and were concealed to the researcher who was responsible for the allocation, and the participants were blinded prior to assignment. Before the intervention, all of the subjects underwent a one-week washout period [23] to diminish the effect of background diets on the study. This study followed the Declaration of Helsinki and the Guidelines for Good Clinical Practice, and was approved by the ethics committee of the First Affiliated Hospital of Soochow University (no. 2015106). All of the enrolled participants signed a consent form.

2.3. Sample Size Calculation

Evidence from the literature showed that the mean difference of the changes in the HbA1c levels were 1.6% between the Peanut group and the Almond group [21,24]. Therefore, we calculated 13 participants for each group, with $\alpha = 0.05$ and power = 0.80. In light of the sample loss of 10%, the number for each group was calculated to be 16. Finally, we recruited 15 participants for the Peanut group and 17 participants for the Almond group in this study.

2.4. Intervention

We incorporated peanuts or almonds into a low-carbohydrate diet (LCD), which is a dietary strategy that refers to a carbohydrate intake of between 30–200 g/day or calories from carbohydrates/total calories <45%, being supplemented instead with fat or protein [24]. Our team developed a LCD education handbook [24] for patients with T2DM based on evidence from the literature, guidelines regarding T2DM dietary management, consultation with diabetes experts and nutritionists, and reviews by patients. The researcher and patients reviewed the LCD handbook, and the researcher trained the patients to restrict their intake of starchy staple food (such as potatoes and broad beans) to 50 g/meal per day during the one-on-one education session. The reduced staple food/meal was substituted by consuming 60 g/day peanuts for men and 50 g/day for women in the Peanut group [25], and 55 g/day almonds for men and 45 g/day for women in the Almond group [25,26]. The peanuts and almonds (without salt and with the skin intact, and free of charge) were prepared in vacuum packing, according to a daily amount. The patients were instructed to consume nuts between meals or with breakfast, or when hungry. For those whose fasting plasma glucose were higher than normal (>6.1 mmol/L), the nuts were required to be consumed before 10:00 a.m. in the morning [27]. The patients were instructed to consume 50% of the nuts before bedtime if there was a risk of a nocturnal hypoglycemic event. The intervention duration was three months for the two groups.

The follow-ups were conducted once a week in the first month of the intervention, and once every two weeks in the second and third months. The duration of each follow-up session was about 10 min. The patients' compliance to the dietary plan was reviewed and those with a poor compliance were supported in order to adhere to the plan. The data relating to modification of hypoglycemic agents and the occurrence of hypoglycemia were also collected. Those whose diets did not meet the requirements of the dietary program in the intervention period were excluded from the study.

2.5. Diet Record

The patients maintained a diet record, including details of the diet of any day over the weekend and two working days, as well as the time of nut consumption. The types and quantities of the food consumed were assessed to determine the patients' adherence to a LCD strategy. Among the patients who met the dietary requirements for a LCD, the number of bags of nuts consumed per week was assessed to determine the patients' dietary adherence.

2.6. Cardio-Metabolic and Anthropometric Parameters

The cardio-metabolic and anthropometric parameters included the FBG, postprandial 2-h blood glucose (PPG) levels, HbA1c, total cholesterol, low density lipoprotein cholesterol (LDL-C), high density lipoprotein cholesterol (HDL-C), triglycerides, and body mass index (BMI). The HbA1c, blood lipids, and BMI were measured at the baseline and at the end of the third month. Venous blood samples were collected at the School of Nursing of Soochow University after a 12 h overnight fast. The HbA1c was measured by high-performance liquid chromatography using Afinion AS100 Analyzer (Alere, Inc., Shanghai, China), and the total cholesterol, LDL-C, HDL-C, and triglycerides were measured using the spectrophotometry method in the molecular laboratory of the School of Nursing of Soochow University. The height and weight were measured using a calibrated stadiometer, and the patients were weighed wearing light clothing and without shoes. The BMI was calculated as the weight (in kilograms) divided by the square of the height (in meters). The FBG and PPG levels were measured by collecting the peripheral blood from the fingers using a rapid glycemic apparatus by patients once a week at home. The glycemic meters were checked by the research staff and the patients were educated to measure the FBG and PPG correctly so as to reduce the subject bias.

2.7. Hypoglycemic Episodes and Antidiabetic Medication Modification

Hypoglycemic episodes in this study were determined by the patients' self-reported hypoglycemic symptoms, with or without a measured plasma glucose concentration of $\leq$70 mg/dL ($\leq$3.9 mmol/L), according to the definition of hypoglycemia in diabetes, given by the American Diabetes Association [28]. To assess the modification of the hypoglycemic agents, the use and changes of the doses of oral antidiabetic drugs and insulin were recorded at the baseline and in the third month.

2.8. Interleukin-6

Interleukin-6 (IL-6) was measured to assess the impact of peanuts and almonds on inflammation. The fasting venous blood was collected and the serum was separated in the molecular laboratory of the School of Nursing of Soochow University. Human IL-6 ELISA kit (R&D Systems™, Emeryville, CA, USA) was used to determine the IL-6 levels in the Hematology Center of the Cyrus Tang Medical Institute at Soochow University.

2.9. Ratio of Urinary Albumin/Creatinine

In order to determine the safety of peanuts and almonds in patients with diabetes, a mid-stream specimen of random urine was collected, and the ratio of urinary albumin/creatinine (ACR) was measured using a dry immune marker scattering quantitative method [29].

2.10. Statistical Analysis

A statistical analysis was performed using SPSS 18.0 software (SPSS, Inc., Dhicago, IL, USA). For continuous variables, the results were presented as mean $\pm$ standard deviation (SD). Comparisons were performed using a *t*-test for the independent samples for general baseline demographic, and clinical characteristics, and one-way analysis of variance (ANOVA) for the outcomes of interest. To eliminate the problem of imbalance in the baseline characteristics, the comparisons of anthropometric and metabolic variables between the groups after the intervention were performed using a covariance analysis with the baseline measurements adjusted. The trends in the dietary adherence, FBG, and PPG in the two groups, which were assessed once a week during the intervention, were analyzed using repeated ANOVA, and have been presented as a fold line diagram. The intention-to-treat (ITT) of HbA1c was performed so as to ensure the reliability of the research results. For the categorical variables, the results were presented as numbers and percentages, and comparisons between the groups were performed using the Chi-squared test or the Fisher's exact test. A *p* value of <0.05 was considered statistically significant.

3. Results

3.1. Study Participants

On the basis of inclusion and exclusion criteria, 32 T2DM participants were recruited and randomly allocated to the Peanut group (*n* = 15) and the Almond group (*n* = 17). Four participants in the Peanut group and three participants in the Almond group withdrew from the study. In the Peanut group, one participant did not like peanuts, one showed abnormally elevated FPG after the first week, one's uric acid increased during the second week (with a history of increased uric acid), and one showed a poor adherence (<four per day/week). In the Almond group, one did not like almonds, one was lost to follow-up, and one could not adhere to the diet program because of toothache. Finally, the data of 11 patients in the Peanut group and 14 in the Almond group were analyzed (Figure 1). The mean age of the participants was 69.60 ± 7.25 years, and 15 (60.0%) were men. The general characteristics of the enrolled participants in each group are shown in Table 1. There were no statistically significant differences in any of the parameters between the two groups (*p* > 0.05, Table 1). The time of exercise per week in the two groups did not change significantly from the baseline, and there was no statistically significant difference found at the third month.

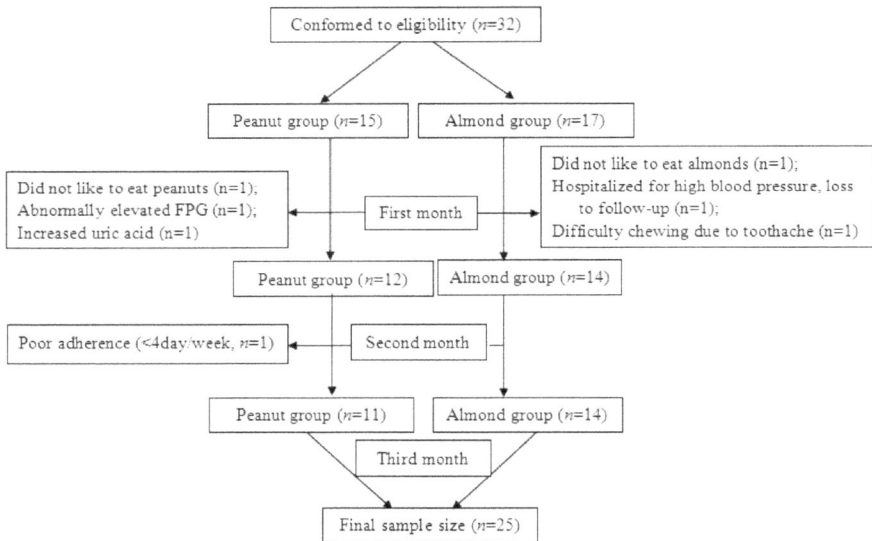

Figure 1. Flow diagram of the patients included in the study.

Table 1. Baseline characteristics.

Variables		Peanut (*n* = 11)	Almond (*n* = 14)	t/χ^2	*p*
		x̄ ± SD/*n* (%)	x̄ ± SD/*n* (%)		
Demographic data					
Age (years)		68.00 ± 5.80	70.86 ± 8.21	−0.977 [a]	NS
Gender—male		5 (45.5)	10 (71.4)	_ [b]	NS
Exercise (min/week)		430.9 ± 222.2	421.4 ± 318.5	0.084 [a]	NS
Exercise habits	Never regular exercise	4 (36.4)	10 (71.4)	_ [b]	NS
	Regular exercise	7 (63.6)	4 (28.6)		
Like sweets or rice or noodles—no		1 (9.1)	1 (7.1)	_ [b]	NS
The amount of staple food, liang/day (1 liang = 50 g)		3.77 ± 1.75	3.61 ± 2.02	0.215 [a]	NS
Consuming nuts—yes		9 (81.8)	13 (92.9)	_ [b]	NS
Clinical data					
Smoking—yes		2 (18.2)	0 (0)	_ [b]	NS
SBP (mmHg)		130.73 ± 7.56	128.00 ± 13.77	0.589 [a]	NS
DBP (mmHg)		79.55 ± 10.25	75.71 ± 8.89	1.000 [a]	NS
Family history of diabetes—yes		5 (45.5)	6 (42.9)	_ [b]	NS
Diabetes duration, years		11.27 ± 6.36	15.21 ± 8.82	−1.247 [a]	NS
Complications—yes		4 (36.4)	6 (42.9)	_ [b]	NS
Accompanying diseases—yes		9 (81.8)	7 (50.0)	_ [b]	NS

p-value for comparisons between the treatment diets by an independent samples *t*-test or Chi-square test. [a] *t*-test; [b] Fisher's exact test. SBP—systolic blood pressure; DBP—diastolic blood pressure; NS: Differences were not significant. SD—standard deviation. Complications included diabetic retinopathy, nephropathy, neuropathy, cardiopathy, foot ulcers, and cognitive impairment.

3.2. Dietary Adherence

The dietary adherence was assessed through the bags of nuts consumed by the participants per week. A fold line diagram was performed to compare the dietary compliance between the two groups (Peanut versus Almond). The results showed that there were no significant differences in the self-reported dietary compliance per week between the two groups ($p > 0.05$, Figure 2).

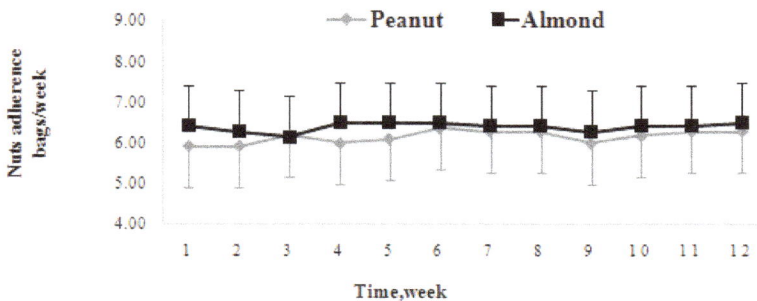

Figure 2. The changing trends of dietary adherence in the Peanut and Almond groups. Values are means, with their standard deviations represented by vertical bars.

3.3. Effect of Peanuts and Almonds on Glycemic Control

3.3.1. Fasting Blood Glucose

Changing Trends of Fasting Blood Glucose

The changing trends of FBG in the two groups during the intervention are described by the fold line diagram (Figure 3). The results show that, for the Peanut group, the levels of FBG were stable with a slight decline, down to the tenth week to the lowest level. For the Almond group, the levels of FBG decreased significantly for the first three weeks, and then fluctuated around the level of the third month.

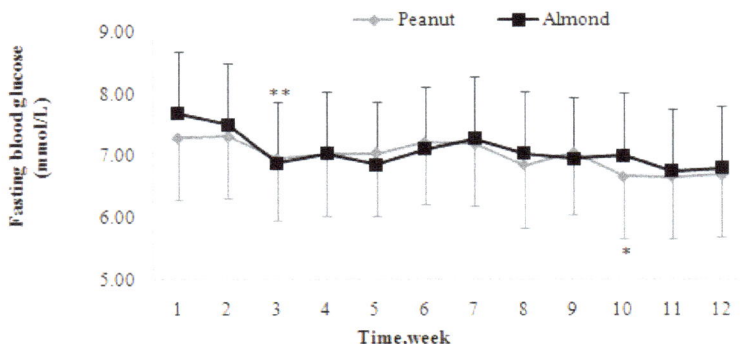

Figure 3. The changing trends of fasting blood glucose (FBG) in the Peanut and Almond groups. Values are means, with their standard deviations represented by vertical bars. For the Peanut group, * FBG was significantly lower at the tenth week than that at the sixth week ($p = 0.035$). For the Almond group, ** FBG was significantly lower at the third week than that at the first week ($p = 0.001$).

Comparison of Fasting Blood Glucose Levels

Compared to the baseline, the FBG levels of the two groups decreased significantly ($p < 0.05$). However, the differences between the two groups, with respect to FBG, were not statistically significant ($p > 0.05$) (Table 2).

Table 2. Comparison of fasting blood glucose (mmol/L) between the two groups.

Study Period	Peanut ($n = 11$)	Almond ($n = 14$)	F	p
Baseline	7.73 ± 1.19	8.28 ± 2.05	0.537	NS
Third month	6.69 ± 0.54 (adjusted: 6.77 ± 0.20)	6.79 ± 0.92 (adjusted: 6.73 ± 0.17)	0.016	NS
F	6.945	5.785	-	-
p	0.016 *	0.024 *	-	-

F-value and p-value for comparisons by one-way analysis of variance or covariance analysis for between-group differences at the third month, with adjusted data presented as mean ± standard error. * $p < 0.05$; NS: differences were not significant.

3.3.2. Postprandial Two-Hour Blood Glucose

Trends in Postprandial Two-Hour Blood Glucose

The changing trends of PPG in the two groups during the intervention are described by the fold line diagram (Figure 4). Both of the groups showed fluctuation, and the amplitude of the fluctuation of the Peanut group was significantly larger than that of the Almond group.

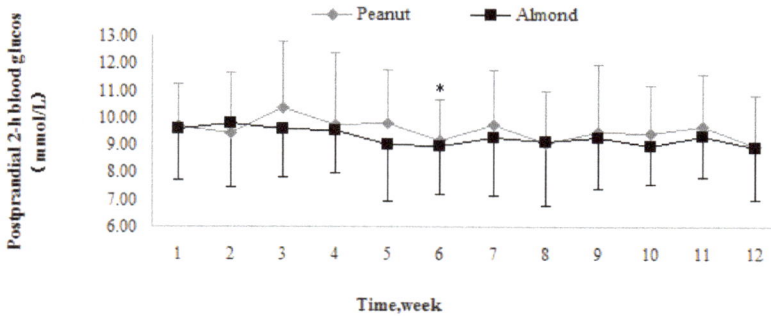

Figure 4. The changing trends of postprandial 2-h blood glucose in the Peanut and Almond groups. Values are means, with their standard deviations represented by vertical bars. For the Peanut group, * PPG was significantly lower at the sixth week than that at the third week ($p = 0.027$).

Comparison of Postprandial Two-Hour Blood Glucose

Compared to the baseline, the PPG in the two groups improved significantly ($p < 0.05$). However, there were no significant differences between the two groups at the third month ($p > 0.05$) (Table 3).

Table 3. Comparison of postprandial 2-h blood glucose (mmol/L) in the two groups.

Study Period	Peanut ($n = 11$)	Almond ($n = 14$)	F	p
Baseline	10.36 ± 1.40	10.61 ± 2.83	0.072	NS
Third month	8.94 ± 1.55 (adjusted: 9.03 ± 0.38)	8.91 ± 1.89 (adjusted: 8.85 ± 0.34)	0.115	NS
F	5.011	4.487	-	-
p	0.037 *	0.044 *	-	-

F-value and p-value for comparisons by one-way analysis of variance or covariance analysis for between-group differences at the third month, with adjusted data presented as mean ± standard error. * $p < 0.05$; NS: differences were not significant.

3.3.3. Glycated Hemoglobin

At the baseline, the HbA1c levels were not significantly different between the Peanut and Almond groups. Compared with the baseline, the HbA1c decreased significantly in the Almond group ($p < 0.05$, Table 4). However, there were no significant differences between the two groups by the third month. The intention-to-treat (ITT) in relation to the HbA1c levels were performed so as to ensure the stability of the above results. The ITT results were found to be in agreement with the earlier findings (Table 5).

Table 4. Comparison of glycated hemoglobin (%) between the two groups.

Study Period	Peanut ($n = 11$)	Almond ($n = 14$)	F	p
Baseline	6.81 ± 0.82	7.39 ± 1.16	0.072	NS
Third month	6.76 ± 0.91 (adjusted: 6.97 ± 0.15)	6.81 ± 0.73 (adjusted: 6.65 ± 0.13)	2.453	NS
F	0.015	4.541	-	-
p	NS	0.043 *	-	-

F-value and p-value for comparisons by one-way analysis of variance or covariance analysis for between-group differences at the third month, with adjusted data presented as mean ± standard error. * $p < 0.05$; NS: differences were not significant.

Table 5. Glycated hemoglobin (%) between the two groups in intention-to-treat (ITT).

Study Period	Peanut (*n* = 15)	Almond (*n* = 17)	*F*	*p*
Baseline	6.96 ± 0.89	7.36 ± 1.07	2.119	NS
Third month	6.93 ± 0.96 (adjusted: 6.90 ± 0.18)	6.88 ± 0.71 (adjusted: 6.65 ± 0.11)	2.361	NS
F	0.015	4.210	-	-
p	NS	0.048 *	-	-

F-value and *p*-value for comparisons by one-way analysis of variance or covariance analysis for between-group difference at the third month, with adjusted data presented as mean ± standard error. * $p < 0.05$; ITT—intention-to-treat; NS: differences were not significant.

3.4. Effect of Peanuts and Almonds on Other Cardio-Metabolic and Anthropometric Indicators

Compared with the baseline, the BMI, total cholesterol, LDL-C, HDL-C, and triglycerides in the two groups did not improve significantly by the third month. After the intervention, the cardio-metabolic and anthropometric indicators were not significantly different between the two groups (Table 6).

Table 6. Comparison of other cardio-metabolic indicators between the two groups.

Variables	Study Period	Peanut (*n* = 11)	Almond (*n* = 14)	*F*	*p*
BMI (Kg/m^2)	Baseline	22.84 ± 2.48	24.08 ± 3.15	1.141	NS
	Third month	22.67 ± 2.44 (adjusted: 23.30 ± 0.22)	23.43 ± 2.90 (adjusted: 22.94 ± 0.20)	1.482	NS
	F	0.025	1.141	-	-
	p	NS	NS	-	-
Total cholesterol (mmol/L)	Baseline	4.48 ± 0.77	4.90 ± 1.00	1.362	NS
	Third month	4.25 ± 0.93 (adjusted: 4.40 ± 0.21)	4.51 ± 0.86 (adjusted:4.39 ± 0.19)	0.002	NS
	F	0.398	1.260	-	-
	p	NS	NS	-	-
LDL-C (mmol/L)	Baseline	2.48 ± 0.72	2.97 ± 0.84	2.290	NS
	Third month	2.51 ± 0.84 (adjusted: 2.69 ± 0.15)	2.74 ± 0.63 (adjusted: 2.59 ± 0.14)	0.234	NS
	F	0.006	0.653	-	-
	p	NS	NS	-	-
HDL-C (mmol/L)	Baseline	1.49 ± 0.28	1.36 ± 0.30	1.219	NS
	Third month	1.53 ± 0.22 (adjusted: 1.49 ± 0.05)	1.34 ± 0.26 (adjusted: 1.38 ± 0.04)	3.123	NS
	F	0.197	0.029	-	-
	p	NS	NS	-	-
Triglycerides (mmol/L)	Baseline	1.05 ± 0.46	1.87 ± 1.19	2.184	NS
	Third month	0.96 ± 0.46 (adjusted: 0.98 ± 0.23)	1.26 ± 0.87 (adjusted: 1.25 ± 0.20)	0.777	NS
	F	0.207	1.317	-	-
	p	NS	NS	-	-

F-value and *p*-value for comparisons by one-way analysis of variance or covariance analysis for between-group differences at the third month, with adjusted data presented as mean ± standard error.BMI—body mass index; LDL-C—low density lipoprotein cholesterol; HDL-C—high density lipoprotein cholesterol; NS: differences were not significant.

3.5. Hypoglycemia and Medication Changes

3.5.1. Incidence of Hypoglycemia

The incidence of hypoglycemia in the two groups showed no significant differences during the three months before the intervention (baseline) and during the intervention period. One patient in the Almond group and none in the Peanut group sustained a hypoglycemic episode during the trial.

3.5.2. Antidiabetic Drugs Used

During the study, one subject in the Peanut group and two subjects in the Almond group had a decrease in the dose of oral hypoglycemic drugs, and one subject in the Almond group had an increase in the dose of oral hypoglycemic drugs, according to the recommendations of physicians. There were no significant differences in the antidiabetic drugs used between the two groups at baseline and by the third month (Table 7).

Table 7. Comparison of antidiabetic drugs between the two groups.

Study Period		Peanut (*n* = 11)	Almond (*n* = 14)	F/χ^2	*p*
		$\bar{x} \pm SD/n$ (%)	$\bar{x} \pm SD/n$ (%)		
Baseline	No	1 (9.1%)	2 (14.3%)	0.423 [a]	NS
	Oral antidiabetic drugs	7 (63.6%)	9 (64.3%)		
	Insulin	0 (0%)	0 (0%)		
	Both	3 (27.3)	3 (21.4%)		
Third month	No	1 (9.1%)	1 (7.1%)	0.581 [a]	NS
	Oral antidiabetic drugs	7 (63.6%)	10 (71.4%)		
	Insulin	0 (0%)	0 (0%)		
	Both	3 (27.3)	3 (21.4%)		
Insulin dose (IU)	Baseline	28.33 ± 11.59	36.00 ± 24.58	0.239 [b]	NS
	Third month	27.00 ± 10.82 (adjusted: 30.19 ± 1.18 [d])	33.33 ± 20.03 (adjusted: 30.14 ± 1.18 [d])	0.001 [c]	NS

[a] Fisher's exact test; [b] one-way analysis of variance; [c] covariance analysis; [d] standard error; NS: differences were not significant.

3.6. Effect of Peanuts and Almonds on Interleukins-6

Compared with the baseline, the IL-6 in the two groups did not improve significantly by the third month. After the intervention, the IL-6 was not significantly different between the two groups (Table 8).

Table 8. Comparison of interleukin-6 (IL-6) ($\bar{x} \pm s$, pg/mL) in the two groups.

Study Period	Peanut (*n* = 11)	Almond (*n* = 14)	*F*	*p*
Baseline	12.78 ± 30.62	2.18 ± 1.10	1.696	NS
Third month	10.65 ± 26.91 (adjusted: 5.44 ± 0.52)	2.70 ± 1.83 (adjusted: 6.79 ± 0.45)	3.761	NS
F	0.030	0.832	-	-
p	NS	NS	-	-

p-value for comparisons by one-way analysis of variance or covariance analysis for between-group differences at the third month, with adjusted data presented as mean ± standard error. NS: differences were not significant.

3.7. Effect of Peanuts and Almonds on Ratio of Urinary Albumin/Creatinine

There were no significant differences between the two groups at baseline and by the third month (Table 9).

Table 9. Comparison of albumin/creatinine (ACR) ($\bar{x} \pm s$, mg/g) in the two groups.

Study Period	Peanut (*n* = 11)	Almond (*n* = 14)	*F*	*p*
Baseline	25.58 ± 26.40	18.53 ± 16.19	0.679	NS
Third month	31.47 ± 48.70 (adjusted: 25.55 ± 5.26)	17.88 ± 21.87 (adjusted: 22.54 ± 4.65)	0.182	NS
F	0.124	0.008	-	-
p	NS	NS	-	-

p-value for comparisons by one-way analysis of variance or covariance analysis for between-group difference at the third month, with adjusted data presented as mean ± standard error. ACR—ratio of urinary albumin/creatinine; NS: differences were not significant.

4. Discussion

This is the first study that compared the effect of peanuts and almonds in patients with T2DM, when incorporated into a LCD diet in order to replace some staple food. The diet diaries revealed that the participants had a good adherence to the dietary intervention, and no significant difference with respect to nut adherence was found between the two groups. This RCT showed that, in combination with a LCD diet, peanuts yielded similar reductions in FBG and PPG compared to almonds.

4.1. Effect of Peanuts and Almonds on Glycemic Control

High levels of FBG, PPG, and HbA1c are some of the most difficult challenges faced by patients with T2DM, and these parameters could be used as the main indicators in order to establish a glycemic control [30]. This study showed that both peanuts and almonds incorporated into a LCD diet resulted in reductions in FBG and PPG after the intervention, which is consistent with previous research results [18,21,31]. The reason might lie in the fact that there is a decrease in the total amount of carbohydrate rich foods in a LCD. In addition, peanuts and almonds are rich in fat, they possess a low-glycemic index, and could alter the glycemic index of co-consumed foods [32]. What is more, the greater fat availability may reduce the gastric emptying rate, and may decrease the carbohydrate absorption rate [33].

However, the content of unsaturated fatty acids (UFAs) and soluble fiber in almonds is higher than that in peanuts [17]. UFAs could facilitate the movement of the glucose receptor to the cell surface, thus increasing the insulin sensitivity [34]. UFAs also act through the stimulation of GLP-1 secretion, which improves the efficacy of the β-cell function [35]. Soluble fiber increases the gastric distention, viscosity in the gastrointestinal tract, and the slower absorption of macronutrients [36]. In this way, it lowers the speed of carbohydrate absorption and the concentration of PPG [37]. Based on the above reasons, the glycemic effect of almonds may be more stable than that of peanuts. In our study, although peanuts and almonds yielded similar reductions in FBG and PPG by the end of the three-months intervention, the amplitude of the fluctuation of the PPG in the Peanut group was significantly larger than that of the Almond group.

The HbA1c level can reflect the mean blood glucose level over the last 8–12 weeks, and can be used to evaluate the long-term glycemic control of patients [30]. HbA1c has a closer association with PPG than FPG [38]. In the present study, the effect of peanuts on the HbA1c reduction was not significant. This might be due to the fluctuation of PPG in the Peanut group. The result of our study is in line with the RCT by Wien et al. [39], which did not find that incorporating peanuts into an American Diabetes Association meal plan had a significant effect in decreasing HbA1c in adults with T2DM. Although there was a 0.48% decrease in HbA1c from the baseline caused by almond consumption, the greater effect of almonds on the improvement of HbA1c was not found by the third month, compared to peanuts. The short-term duration of the follow-up may be one of the reasons for this. After a 24-week almond intervention, Gulati et al. [40] found a statistically significant improvement in the levels of HbA1c compared with the control diet.

4.2. Other Cardio-Metabolic Indicators

The consumption of peanuts and almonds has not been associated with increased body weight, despite their high lipid content. Human feeding trials have shown that nut ingestion moderates appetite postprandially [41]. The inclusion of peanuts and almonds increases a feeling of satiety and leads to a strong dietary compensation effect. In addition, because of the inefficiency in energy absorption, nut consumption does not promote a greater energy intake than other foods [41]. In a randomized cross-over study, after 12 weeks of incorporating high oleic peanuts into the diet, a less than predicted increase in the body weight was found, despite a large additional amount of energy being consumed from the peanuts [25]. Similarly, Li et al. [26] and Gulati et al. [40] also reported no changes in the body weight and BMI with the almond diet, however, a statistically significant improvement was seen in the body fat [26], waist circumference, and waist-to-height ratio [40]. Sato et al. [42] reported a significant improvement of BMI on a LCD diet on in T2DM patients with higher baseline levels of BMI (26.5 Kg/m^2). Among the subjects with a relative normal baseline BMI, this study did not find that peanuts or almonds incorporated into a LCD diet had a significant reduction on the BMI.

The total cholesterol, LDL-C, HDL-C, and triglyceride levels were not altered significantly with an almond or peanut diet in this study, contrary to many other studies [14]. However, the cholesterol lowering effects of nuts are shown to be the greatest in individuals with higher baseline lipids [43]. The subjects in this study had an average healthy baseline lipid level. Barbour et al. [25] and Wien et al. [39] also reported no differences in lipids with peanut consumption in subjects with healthy baseline lipid levels.

4.3. Hypoglycemia and Medication Changes

The antidiabetic drugs and insulin doses used in the Peanut and Almond groups were identical. There was no interference caused by the agents when comparing the glycemic control effects between peanuts and almonds in this study.

We used hypoglycemia as a safety indicator. Although there was no significant difference in the between-group comparison, the percentage of hypoglycemia was reduced from 18.2% to zero in the Peanut group. Nocturnal hypoglycemia occurred in two participants in the Peanut group before the intervention, and it was recommended that they consume 50% of their prescribed peanuts before bedtime. The occurrence of hypoglycemia in the morning causes the body to produce a large amount of glucocorticoids, namely the Somogyi effect, leading to increased blood glucose in the morning [44]. Peanuts and almonds, which are rich in healthy fat, can delay the speed of gastric emptying, and can continuously supply energy [27] to the body so as to prevent the occurrence of the Somogyi effect. During the intervention in the Almond group, daytime hypoglycemia occurred in one case because of strenuous exercise, and there was no nocturnal hypoglycemia found.

4.4. Effect of Peanuts and Almonds on Interleukin-6

IL-6 was chosen as an indicator of inflammation. Chronic low-level inflammation plays an important role in the occurrence and development of DM [17,45]. IL-6 is the source of the metabolic syndrome induced by inflammation, and plays a core regulatory role in the inflammatory response [46,47]. IL-6 can inhibit insulin signaling transduction and could therefore impede the action of insulin [47].

Peanuts are rich in folic acid, which can inhibit the cascade of a reaction in the process of inflammation in vessel wall, and this may reduce the release of vascular inflammatory factors [48]. Although the administration of folic acid can cause a decrease in the concentration of homocysteine, and, as a consequence, could influence the decrease in the concentration of the indicators of inflammation [49], a decrease of IL-6 caused by peanut consumption was not found in this study. As an indicator of inflammation, the C reactive protein (CRP) did not improve after 12-week of peanut consumption in the study by Barbour et al. [25]. Contrary to our study, in the study by Gulati et al. [40], a significant improvement in the CRP was found after 24-weeks of almond consumption. Whether the inconsistency in the improvement of inflammation between studies is correlated to the different intervention duration needs to be further verified.

4.5. Effect of Peanuts and Almonds on Kidney Burden

ACR is a sensitive indicator of early renal damage [50], which is used to assess the impact of peanuts and almonds incorporated into a LCD on renal function in this study. Our study found that peanut and almond consumption with a LCD did not increase the burden on the kidney. Díaz-López et al. also reported no change in ACR after a one-year Mediterranean diet supplemented with nuts [51].

5. Limitation

There are some limitations to this study. Firstly, the sample size was small. There was also an imbalance in the gender, diabetes duration, and baseline HbA1c level between groups, although there were no significant differences found. The prolonged effect of peanuts and almonds on the prognosis of T2DM was not observed because of the short follow-up duration. Finally, measurement differences might exist in the FBG and PPG levels, which were measured by the patients themselves, using different blood glucose meters at home.

6. Conclusions

Incorporated into a low-carbohydrate diet, both peanuts and almonds can improve the fasting blood glucose and postprandial 2-h blood glucose in patients with T2DM. The effect of almonds in promoting long-term glycemic control needs to be confirmed by more studies.

Author Contributions: Y.-Y.H., O.O., and X.-H.W. analyzed the data. Y.-Y.H. wrote the initial draft, which was revised by O.O., X.-H.W., and X.-Y.S. L.-L.W., Q.W., and Q.J. collected the data. X.-H.W. contributed most to the design of this research, and all of the other authors participated in the study design and quality control. Y.-Y.H. and O.O. contributed equally to this study. X.-H.W. was the corresponding author.

Funding: This research was funded by Suzhou Science and Technology Project, China (Grant number SYS201513) and the APC was funded by Yuhui Huang.

Acknowledgments: We thank the patients with DM who volunteered to participate in this study. We also thank all of the staff in the Endocrine Division of the First Affiliated Hospital of Soochow University—Huijuan Zhou, Xiaoyan Zhang, and Li Wang—who provided us with assistance so as to ensure that the study was conducted.

Conflicts of Interest: The authors declare no conflicts of interest.

References

1. Adeghate, E.; Schattner, P.; Dunn, E. An Update on the Etiology and Epidemiology of Diabetes Mellitus. *Ann. N. Y. Acad. Sci.* **2006**, *1084*, 1–29. [CrossRef] [PubMed]
2. World Health Organization. World Health Organization Global Report on Diabetes: Executive Summary. 2016. Available online: http://www.who.int/diabetes/global-report (accessed on 20 May 2018).
3. American Diabetes Association; Bantle, J.P.; Wylie-Rosett, J.; Albright, A.L.; Apovian, C.M.; Clark, N.G.; Franz, M.J.; Hoogwerf, B.J.; Lichtenstein, A.H.; Mayer-Davis, E.; et al. Nutrition recommendations and interventions for diabetes: A position statement of the American Diabetes Association. *Diabetes Care* **2010**, *33*, S61–S78.
4. Forouhi, N.G.; Misra, A.; Mohan, V.; Taylor, R.; Yancy, W. Dietary and nutritional approaches for prevention and management of type 2 diabetes. *BMJ* **2018**, *361*, k2234. [CrossRef] [PubMed]
5. Dyson, P.A.; Kelly, T.; Deakin, T.; Duncan, A.; Frost, G.; Harrison, Z.; Khatri, D.; Kunka, D.; McArdle, P.; Mellor, D. Diabetes UK evidence-based nutrition guidelines for the prevention and management of diabetes. *Diabet. Med.* **2011**, *28*, 1282–1288. [CrossRef] [PubMed]
6. Wheeler, M.L.; Dunbar, S.A.; Jaacks, L.M.; Wahida, K.; Mayer-Davis, E.J.; Judith, W.R., Jr.; William, S. Macronutrients, Food Groups, and Eating Patterns in the Management of Diabetes. *Diabetes Care* **2010**, *35*, 434–445. [CrossRef] [PubMed]
7. Tay, J.; Luscombe-Marsh, N.D.; Thompson, C.H.; Noakes, M.; Buckley, J.D.; Wittert, G.A.; Yancy, W.S., Jr.; Brinkworth, G.D. Comparison of low- and high-carbohydrate diets for type 2 diabetes management: A randomized trial. *Am. J. Clin. Nutr.* **2015**, *102*, 780–790. [CrossRef] [PubMed]
8. Souza, R.G.M.; Gomes, A.C.; Naves, M.M.V.; Mota, J.F. Nuts and legume seeds for cardiovascular risk reduction: Scientific evidence and mechanisms of action. *Nutr. Rev.* **2015**, *73*, 335–347. [CrossRef] [PubMed]
9. Cheng, A.Y.Y.; Barnes, T. Canadian Diabetes Association 2013 Clinical Practice Guidelines for the Prevention and Management of Diabetes in Canada. *Can. J. Diabetes* **2013**, *373*, S291–S360. [CrossRef]
10. Anderson, T.J.; Gregoire, J.; Hegele, R.A.; Couture, P.; Mancini, G.B.J.; McPherson, R.; Francis, G.A.; Poirier, P.; Lau, D.C.; Grover, S.; et al. 2012 Update of the Canadian Cardiovascular Society Guidelines for the Diagnosis and Treatment of Dyslipidemia for the Prevention of Cardiovascular Disease in the Adult. *Can. J. Cardiol.* **2013**, *29*, 151–167. [CrossRef] [PubMed]

11. Stroes, E.S.; Thompson, P.D.; Corsini, A.; Vladutiu, G.D.; Raal, F.J.; Ray, K.K.; Roden, M.; Stein, E.; Tokgozoglu, L.; Nordestgaard, B.G.; et al. Statin-associated muscle symptoms: Impact on statin therapy-European Atherosclerosis Society Consensus Panel Statement on Assessment, Aetiology and Management. *Eur. Heart J.* **2015**, *36*, 1012–1022. [CrossRef] [PubMed]

12. Mann, J.I.; De Leeuw, I.; Hermansen, K.; Karamanos, B.; Karlstrom, B.; Katsilambros, N.; Riccardi, G.; Rivellese, A.A.; Rizkalla, S.; Slama, G.; et al. Evidence-based nutritional approaches to the treatment and prevention of diabetes mellitus. *Nutr. Metab. Cardiovasc.* **2004**, *14*, 373–394. [CrossRef]

13. Viguiliouk, E.; Kendall, C.W.C.; Mejia, B.S.; Cozma, A.I.; Ha, V. Effect of Tree Nuts on Glycemic Control in Diabetes: A Systematic Review and Meta-Analysis of Randomized Controlled Dietary Trials. *PLoS ONE* **2014**, *9*, e103376. [CrossRef] [PubMed]

14. Musa-Veloso, K.; Paulionis, L.; Poon, T.; Lee, H.Y. The effects of almond consumption on fasting blood lipid levels: A systematic review and meta-analysis of randomised controlled trials. *J. Nutr. Sci.* **2016**, *5*, e34. [CrossRef] [PubMed]

15. Liu, J.; Liu, Y.; Chen, C.; Chang, W.; Chen, C.O. The effect of almonds on inflammation and oxidative stress in Chinese patients with type 2 diabetes mellitus: A randomized crossover controlled feeding trial. *Eur. J. Nutr.* **2013**, *52*, 927–935. [CrossRef] [PubMed]

16. Jenkins, D.J.A.; Hu, F.B.; Tapsell, L.C.; Josse, A.R.; Kendall, C.W.C. Possible benefit of nuts in type 2 diabetes. *J. Nutr.* **2008**, *138*, 1752S–1756S. [CrossRef] [PubMed]

17. Ros, E. Health Benefits of Nut Consumption. *Nutrients* **2010**, *2*, 652–682. [CrossRef] [PubMed]

18. Reis, C.E.G.; Ribeiro, D.N.; Costa, N.M.B.; Bressan, J.; Alfenas, R.C.G.; Mattes, R.D. Acute and second-meal effects of peanuts on glycaemic response and appetite in obese women with high type 2 diabetes risk: A randomised cross-over clinical trial. *Brit. J. Nutr.* **2013**, *109*, 2015–2023. [CrossRef] [PubMed]

19. Liu, X.; Hill, A.; West, S.; Gabauer, R.; McCrea, C.; Fleming, J.; Kris-Etherton, P. Acute Peanut Consumption Alters Postprandial Lipids and Vascular Responses in Healthy Overweight or Obese Men. *J. Nutr.* **2017**, *147*, 835–840. [CrossRef] [PubMed]

20. Buzby, J.; Pollack, S. Almonds lead increase in tree nut consumption. *Amber Waves* **2008**, *6*, 5.

21. Cohen, A.E.; Johnston, C.S. Almond ingestion at mealtime reduces postprandial glycemia and chronic ingestion reduces hemoglobin A(1c) in individuals with well-controlled type 2 diabetes mellitus. *Metabolism* **2011**, *60*, 1312–1317. [CrossRef] [PubMed]

22. Asghari, G.; Ghorbani, Z.; Mirmiran, P.; Azizi, F. Nut consumption is associated with lower incidence of type 2 diabetes: The Tehran Lipid and Glucose Study. *Diabetes Metab.* **2017**, *43*, 18–24. [CrossRef] [PubMed]

23. Chen, L. A brief discussion on the increase of fasting blood glucose. *Health Guide* **2014**, *20*, 34–35.

24. Wang, Q. Effect of Loose Low Carbohydrate Diet on Metabolism in Patients with Type 2 Diabetes Mellitus. Master's Thesis, Soochow University, Suzhou, China, 2015.

25. Barbour, J.A.; Howe, P.R.C.; Buckley, J.D.; Bryan, J.; Coates, A.M. Effect of 12 Weeks High Oleic Peanut Consumption on Cardio-Metabolic Risk Factors and Body Composition. *Nutrients* **2015**, *7*, 7381–7398. [CrossRef] [PubMed]

26. Li, S.; Liu, Y.; Liu, J.; Chang, W.; Chen, C.; Chen, C.O. Almond consumption improved glycemic control and lipid profiles in patients with type 2 diabetes mellitus. *Metabolism* **2011**, *60*, 474–479. [CrossRef] [PubMed]

27. Collier, G.; O'Dea, K. He effect of coingestion of fat on the glucose, insulin, and gastric inhibitory polypeptide responses to carbohydrate and protein. *Am. J. Clin. Nutr.* **1983**, *37*, 941–944. [CrossRef] [PubMed]

28. Childs, B.P.; Clark, N.G.; Cox, D.J.; Cryer, P.E.; Davis, S.N.; Dinardo, M.M.; Kahn, R.; Kovatchev, B.; Shamoon, H. Defining and reporting hypoglycemia in diabetes—A report from the American Diabetes Association Workgroup on Hypoglycemia. *Diabetes Care* **2005**, *28*, 1245–1249.

29. Shi, H. The Change of Urinary Albumin-to-Creatinine Ratio in Patients with Coronary Heart Disease and the Relationship between Urinary Albumin-to-Creatinine Ratio and the Severity of Coronary Stenosis. Master's Thesis, Fudan University, Shanghai, China, 2010.

30. Chinese Diabetes Society. Guidelines for the prevention and treatment of type 2 diabetes in China. *Chin. Med. J.* **2017**, 4–67.

31. Reis, C.E.G.; Bordalo, L.A.; Rocha, A.L.C.; Freitas, D.M.O.; Da Silva, M.V.L.; de Faria, V.C.; Martino, H.S.D.; Costa, N.M.B.; Alfenas, R.C. Ground roasted peanuts leads to a lower post-prandial glycemic response than raw peanuts. *Nutr. Hosp.* **2011**, *26*, 745–751. [PubMed]

32. Hernandez-Alonso, P.; Camacho-Barcia, L.; Bullo, M.; Salas-Salvado, J. Nuts and Dried Fruits: An Update of Their Beneficial Effects on Type 2 Diabetes. *Nutrients* **2017**, *9*, 673. [CrossRef] [PubMed]

33. Gentilcore, D.; Chaikomin, R.; Jones, K.L.; Russo, A.; Feinle-Bisset, C.; Wishart, J.M.; Rayner, C.K.; Horowitz, M. Effects of fat on gastric emptying of and the glycemic, insulin, and incretin responses to a carbohydrate meal in type 2 diabetes. *J. Clin. Endocrinol. Metab.* **2006**, *91*, 2062–2067. [CrossRef] [PubMed]

34. Kien, C.L. Dietary interventions for metabolic syndrome: Role of modifying dietary fats. *Curr. Diabetes Rep.* **2009**, *9*, 43–50. [CrossRef]

35. Riserus, U.; Willett, W.C.; Hu, F.B. Dietary fats and prevention of type 2 diabetes. *Prog. Lipid Res.* **2009**, *48*, 44–51. [CrossRef] [PubMed]

36. Chandalia, M.; Garg, A.; Lutjohann, D.; von Bergmann, K.; Grundy, S.M.; Brinkley, L.J. Beneficial effects of high dietary fiber intake in patients with type 2 diabetes mellitus. *N. Engl. J. Med.* **2000**, *342*, 1392–1398. [CrossRef] [PubMed]

37. Hopping, B.N.; Etber, E.; Grandinetti, A.; Verheus, M.; Kolonel, L.N.; Maskarinec, G. Dietary Fiber, Magnesium, and Glycemic Load Alter Risk of Type 2 Diabetes in a Multiethnic Cohort in Hawaii. *J. Nutr.* **2010**, *140*, 68–74. [CrossRef] [PubMed]

38. Ketema, E.B.; Kibret, K.T. Correlation of fasting and postprandial plasma glucose with HbA1c in assessing glycemic control; systematic review and meta-analysis. *Arch. Public Health* **2015**, *73*, 43. [CrossRef] [PubMed]

39. Wien, M.; Oda, K.; Sabate, J. A randomized controlled trial to evaluate the effect of incorporating peanuts into an American Diabetes Association meal plan on the nutrient profile of the total diet and cardiometabolic parameters of adults with type 2 diabetes. *Nutr. J.* **2014**, *13*, 10. [CrossRef] [PubMed]

40. Gulati, S.; Misra, A.; Pandey, R.M. Effect of Almond Supplementation on Glycemia and Cardiovascular Risk Factors in Asian Indians in North India with Type 2 Diabetes Mellitus: A 24-Week Study. *Metab. Syndr. Relat. Disord.* **2017**, *15*, 98–105. [CrossRef] [PubMed]

41. Tan, S.Y.; Dhillon, J.; Mattes, R.D. A review of the effects of nuts on appetite, food intake, metabolism, and body weight. *Am. J. Clin. Nutr.* **2014**, *100*, 412S–422S. [CrossRef] [PubMed]

42. Sato, J.; Kanazawa, A.; Hatae, C.; Makita, S.; Komiya, K.; Shimizu, T.; Ikeda, F.; Tamura, Y.; Ogihara, T.; Mita, T.; et al. One year follow-up after a randomized controlled trial of a 130 g/day low-carbohydrate diet in patients with type 2 diabetes mellitus and poor glycemic control. *PLoS ONE* **2017**, *12*, e0188892. [CrossRef] [PubMed]

43. Sabate, J.; Oda, K.; Ros, E. Nut Consumption and Blood Lipid Levels A Pooled Analysis of 25 Intervention Trials. *Arch. Intern. Med.* **2010**, *170*, 821–827. [CrossRef] [PubMed]

44. Rybicka, M.; Krysiak, R.; Okopien, B. The dawn phenomenon and the Somogyi effect-two phenomena of morning hyperglycaemia. *Endokrynol. Pol.* **2011**, *62*, 276–283. [PubMed]

45. Yu, Z.; Malik, V.S.; Keum, N.; Hu, F.B.; Giovannucci, E.L.; Stampfer, M.J.; Willett, W.C.; Fuchs, C.S.; Bao, Y. Associations between nut consumption and inflammatory biomarkers. *Am. J. Clin. Nutr.* **2016**, *104*, 722–728. [CrossRef] [PubMed]

46. Chen, Y.; Zheng, S.; Meng, C.; Hao, J. The role of IL-6 on liver insulin resistance in type 2 diabetes mellitus rats. *Chin. J. Lab. Diagn.* **2013**, *17*, 436–439.

47. When, H.J.; Yang, J.S.; Zhang, J.J. Effect of folic acid combined with pravastatin on inflammatory factors in patients with carotid artery stenosis. *Chin. J. Integr. Med. Cardio-Cerebrovasc. Dis.* **2013**, *11*, 111–112.

48. Scheurig, A.C.; Thorand, B.; Fischer, B.; Heier, M.; Koenig, W. Association between the intake of vitamins and trace elements from supplements and C-reactive protein: Results of the MONICA/KORA Augsburg study. *Eur. J. Clin. Nutr.* **2008**, *62*, 127–137. [CrossRef] [PubMed]

49. Baszczuk, A.; Kopczynski, Z.; Kopczynski, J.; Cymerys, M.; Thielemann, A.; Bielawska, L.; Banaszewska, A. Impact of administration of folic acid on selected indicators of inflammation in patients with primary arterial hypertension. *Postep. Hig. Med. Dosw.* **2015**, *69*, 429–435. [CrossRef]

50. Hasanato, R.M. Diagnostic efficacy of random albumin creatinine ratio for detection of micro and macro-albuminuria in type 2 diabetes mellitus. *Saudi Med. J.* **2016**, *37*, 268–273. [CrossRef] [PubMed]
51. Diaz-Lopez, A.; Bullo, M.; Angel Martinez-Gonzalez, M.; Guasch-Ferre, M.; Ros, E.; Basora, J.; Covas, M.; Del Carmen Lopez-Sabater, M.; Salas-Salvado, J. Effects of Mediterranean Diets on Kidney Function: A Report from the PREDIMED Trial. *Am. J. Kidney Dis.* **2012**, *60*, 380–389. [CrossRef] [PubMed]

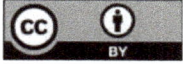

nutrients

MDPI

Article

Dietary Approaches for Japanese Patients with Diabetes: A Systematic Review

Satoru Yamada [1],*, Yusuke Kabeya [2] and Hiroshi Noto [3]

1   Diabetes Center, Kitasato Institute Hospital, 5-9-1 Shirokane, Minato-ku, Tokyo 108-8642, Japan
2   Department of Home Care Medicine, Saiyu Clinic, 3-217-1 Sagamicho, Koshigaya-shi,
    Saitama 343-0823, Japan; ykabeyan@yahoo.co.jp
3   Endocrinology Department, St. Luke's International Hospital, 9-1 Akashicho, Chuo-ku,
    Tokyo 104-8560, Japan; noto-tky@umin.net
*   Correspondence: yamada-s@insti.kitasato-u.ac.jp; Tel.: +81-3-3444-6161

Received: 6 July 2018; Accepted: 8 August 2018; Published: 13 August 2018

Abstract: This study aimed to elucidate the effect of an energy restricted and carbohydrate restricted diet on the management of Japanese diabetes patients. Several databases including MEDLINE, EMBASE, and the Japan Medical Abstracts Society were searched for relevant articles published prior to June 2017. The articles identified were systematically reviewed. We identified 286 articles on an energy restricted diet, assessed seven and included two studies in our review. On a carbohydrate restricted diet, 75 articles were extracted, seven articles assessed and three included in the review, of which two were the studies that were selected for the energy restricted diet group, since they compared energy restricted diets with carbohydrate restricted diets. All selected studies were on Japanese patients with type 2 diabetes. No studies for type 1 diabetes were found in our search. Two randomized controlled trials on an energy restricted diet were also included in the three studies for a carbohydrate restricted diet. All the three randomized controlled trials showed better glucose management with the carbohydrate restricted diet. Our study revealed that there is very little evidence on diets, particularly in Japanese patients with diabetes, and that the energy restricted diet, which has been recommended by the Japan Diabetes Society in the sole dietary management approach, is not supported by any scientific evidence. Our findings suggest that the carbohydrate restricted diet, but not the energy restricted diet, might have short term benefits for the management of diabetes in Japanese patients. However, since our analysis was based on a limited number of small randomized controlled trials, large scale and/or long term trials examining the dietary approaches in these patients are needed to confirm our findings.

Keywords: energy restricted diet; low energy diet; carbohydrate restricted diet; low carbohydrate diet; diabetes; Japanese

---

1. Introduction

Nutrition therapy plays an integral role in the management of diabetes [1]. Several dietary approaches such as the Mediterranean diet, dietary approaches to stop hypertension (DASH), a vegetarian diet, and a carbohydrate restricted diet have been recommended by the American Diabetes Association (ADA) and reviewed by Ley et al. in *The Lancet* [2,3]. On the other hand, the Japan Diabetes Society (JDS) has officially recommended only an energy restricted diet since 1965 [4], as it believes that the pathophysiology and food preferences of Japanese patients with diabetes are unique when compared to patients in Western countries [5]. As per the JDS guidelines, energy restriction was calculated based on the ideal body weight as follows: total energy intake (kcal) = ideal body weight (kg = height (m) × height (m) × 22) × physical activity index (obese, 20–25; non-obese sedentary, 25–30; non-obese normal intensity active, 30–35; non-obese high intensity active, 35 and above). In fact, a recent study of the trajectory of body mass index (BMI) in Japanese patients with diabetes has shown it to be continuously normal (approximately 24.4) and not obese [6]. The BMI of Japanese individuals is very different from that of Americans [7] and Europeans [8], suggesting that there must be differences in the pathophysiology as well. However, because the European Association for the Study of Diabetes (EASD) mentioned that energy restriction is not needed in patients whose BMI is lower than 25 [9], the discrepancy in the position of energy restriction between the JDS and the Western countries seems more problematic. Although the JDS guidelines [4] on the dietary recommendations are reportedly based on 86 studies, none of those references support the JDS recommended an energy restriction diet. Eighty-three of these papers were not studies on dietary approach for Japanese patients with type 2 diabetes. The remaining three references were on dietary approaches for Japanese diabetic patients, where one is the 'eating vegetables before carbohydrate' diet [10], one is the before-after study on exercise and energy restriction diet which instructed a deficit of 140 kcal/d from the baseline for subjects with metabolic syndrome [11], and the last is the carbohydrate restriction diet [12]. Thus, it is evident that the JDS guidelines are not based on any supportive evidence for energy restriction in diabetic patients with normal BMI, despite the fact that energy restriction is the basis of the consensus in preparing the guidelines by the writing committee [4]. However, since the JDS recognizes that an evaluation of the effectiveness and safety of dietary approaches is needed in their recommendation [5], in this study we have tried to evaluate the effectiveness of the energy restricted diet in Japanese patients with diabetes. Furthermore, in recent years, emerging evidence has suggested that a restricted carbohydrate diet improves glycemic control [13], although it is not yet conclusive, especially in long term follow-ups [1,14]. We have, therefore, evaluated the effectiveness of the carbohydrate restricted diet as well.

2. Materials and Methods

2.1. Study Search

Searches of MEDLINE, EMBASE, and Japan Medical Abstracts Society (JAMAS) databases from their inception (MEDLINE 1966, EMBASE 1947, AND JAMAS 1964) until 30 June 2017, were performed. To identify studies related to an energy restricted diet, we used a combination of the following keywords: "low-energy" or "energy-restriction" or "low-calorie" or "caloric-restriction" and "diabetes," and "Japanese" in the MEDLINE and EMBASE databases. Similarly, for articles related to a carbohydrate restricted diet, we used the terms "low-carbohydrate" or "carbohydrate-restriction," and "diabetes," and "Japanese" in the MEDLINE and EMBASE databases. In the JAMAS database, we used the same combination of keywords in Japanese. Other dietary approaches such as, the Mediterranean diet, DASH (dietary approaches to stop hypertension), fat restriction (low fat) diet, low glycemic index (low GI) diet, vegetarian diet, and high-protein diet were excluded because preliminary searches by one author (S.Y.) found no relevant study in Japanese (partly presented in 60th JDS annual meeting in 2017, Nagoya by S.Y.).

2.2. Study Selection

The following exclusion criteria were applied: (1) non-Japanese data, (2) non-diabetic patient data, (3) other dietary approaches, (4) unpublished data (including abstracts presented only in scientific meetings), and (5) studies not appropriate for our evaluation such as case series and case reports.

After each search, based on the title and abstract, two authors (S.Y. and Y.K.) extracted relevant reports independently. One author (S.Y.) collected the papers for a full-text evaluation by two independent authors (S.Y and Y.K). Disagreements were primarily resolved through discussions and by consulting a third author (H.N.). We did not perform any quantitative data analysis because our search found few studies that were not enough to perform a meta-analysis.

2.3. Validity and Quality Assessment

The risk of bias was assessed against the key criteria: random sequence generation; allocation concealment; blinding of participants, personnel, and assessors; incomplete outcome data; selective outcomes reporting; and other sources of bias, in accordance with the recommendations of the Medical Information Network Distribution Service (Minds) [15].

2.4. Data Abstraction

We reviewed each full-text report to determine its eligibility and extracted and tabulated all the relevant data independently. The extracted data included the characteristics of the subjects (including age, gender), the study design, publication year, follow-up period, and risk parameters. Any disagreement was resolved by consensus among the investigators.

3. Results

We identified a total of 286 articles related to an energy restricted diet, of which seven [16–22] were assessed for their eligibility for inclusion in our review (Figure 1). All were studies on patients with type 2 diabetes. No study was identified for type 1 diabetes. There were no articles outlining the adverse effects of energy restriction. Five articles were excluded from the systematic review because (a) counseling [16], (b) meal delivery [17], and (c) periodization [18] were evaluated under the same level of energy restriction in three studies; one study assessed the effects of very strict energy restriction under hospitalization (1000 kcal/day) [19]; while another did not evaluate an energy restricted diet [20]. After excluding these five studies, the remaining two randomized controlled trials (RCTs) were appraised in our systematic review [21,22]. The two selected articles were moderately homogeneous in terms of the level of energy restriction. Both studies adopted a carbohydrate restricted diet as the control group. The sample sizes in these two studies were 24 [21] and 66 [22].

Both studies were also selected in the carbohydrate restricted diet section. To avoid redundancy, we created a summary table that included the two studies each on a carbohydrate restricted diet and an energy restricted diet, and an energy restricted diet was used as the control group (Table 1). In both studies, the energy restricted diet (Table 1, control group) had inferior effects on HbA1c improvement when compared to the carbohydrate restriction group (Table 1, intervention group). However, a review of dietary energy in one study [21] revealed that the levels of energy intake were similar in both the energy and carbohydrate restriction groups. In the other study [22], the levels of energy intake were higher in the energy restriction group compared to those in the carbohydrate restriction group. Thus, we concluded that the net effect of energy restriction on glycemic control could not be assessed in both studies (Table 2).

We identified a total of 75 articles related to a carbohydrate restricted diet, of which seven were assessed for their eligibility to be included in our review (Figure 2) [19–25]. All were studies on patients with type 2 diabetes. No studies were identified for type 1 diabetes. There were no articles that showed adverse effects of carbohydrate restriction. Four articles were excluded from the study because the same levels of carbohydrate restriction were recommended for all participants, and a longitudinal change in glycemic control was observed in two studies [20,23]. One study evaluated the effect of very strict energy restriction under hospitalization (1000 kcal/day) [19]. In one study, carbohydrate restriction was prescribed only on a single day (admission day 8) [24]. After excluding these four studies, the remaining three RCTs were appraised in our systematic review [21,22,25]. The three selected articles were moderately homogeneous in terms of the level of carbohydrate restriction. Among these studies, two had an energy restricted diet as the control groups and were the same studies selected for the energy restricted diet analysis [21,22], while the third study had a carbohydrate-rich diet with similar energy intake [25]. The sample sizes in these three studies were 24 [21], 66 [22], and 15 [25].

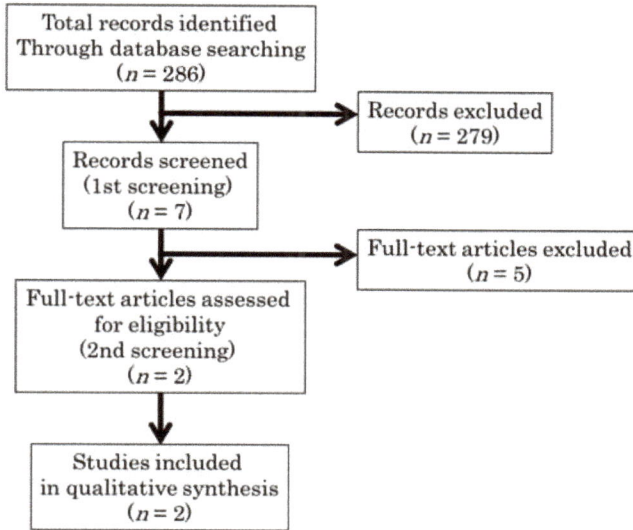

Figure 1. Flow diagram of selecting the energy restriction studies included in our study. Two randomized controlled trials were appraised in our systematic review.

Table 1 shows the summary of each study. A carbohydrate restricted diet had superior effects on improvement of HbA1c [21,22] or the postprandial glucose levels as determined by continuous glucose monitoring [25] compared to the control group in all three studies. However, in one study the energy intake was lower in the intervention (carbohydrate restriction) group than in the control (energy restriction) group [22] (Table 2). Thus, we concluded that a carbohydrate restriction diet was supported by limited evidence in Japanese patients with type 2 diabetes.

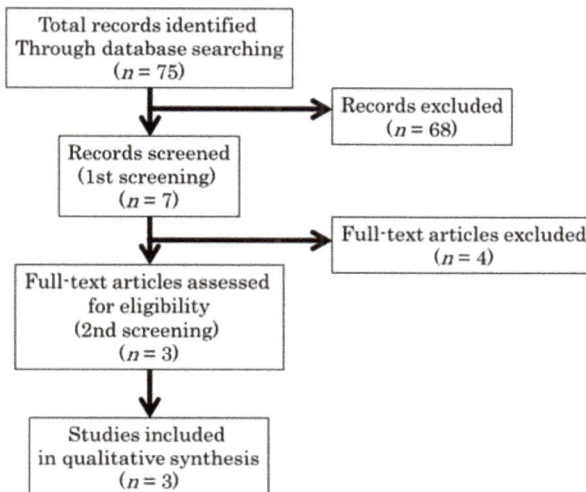

Figure 2. Flow diagram of selecting the carbohydrate studies included in our study. Three randomized controlled trials were appraised in our systematic review.

Table 1. Summary table of studies on carbohydrate restriction diet (including energy restriction studies as control group [21,22]).

Study ID (Reference Number)	Setting	Study Design	Number of Participants	Number of Dropouts	Sex (M/F)	Age	Duration of Diabetes (Years)	Intervention	Control	Primary Outcome	Results Intervention	Control	Median Difference
Yamada et al., 2014 [21]	Outpatient University Hospital	RCT	24	C:0 E:0	C:7/5 E:5/7	C:63.3 ± 13.5 E:63.2 ± 10.2	C:8.9 ± 3.6 E:9.5 ± 4.8	Carbohydrate: 70–130 g/day	IBW (kg) ×25 kcal/day	HbA1c change after 6 month	−0.6 ± 0.48	−0.2 ± 0.68	−0.40
Sato et al., 2017 [22]	Outpatient University Hospital	RCT	66	C:1 E:3	C:23/7 E:24/8	C:60.5 ± 10.5 E:58.4 ± 10.0	(median) C:14.0 E:13.0	Carbohydrate 130 g/day	IBW (kg) × 28 kcal/day	HbA1c change after 6 month	(median)−0.65	(median) 0.00	−0.65
Yabe et al., 2017 [25]	Meal test 2 Medical Institutions	RCT	15	C:0 H:0	C:7/0 E:5/3	C:56.9 ± 7.3 H:54.3 ± 5.2	C:7.6 ± 4.3 E:4.4 ± 3.3	Carbohydrate 180 g/day, Energy 1800 kcal/d	Carbohydrate 247.5 g/day, Energy 1800 kcal/day	CGM data during 5–7 days	130.32 ± 27.72	142.92 ± 39.6	n.a.

C: carbohydrate restriction group = intervention group. E: energy restriction group = control group [21,22]. H: high carbohydrate group=control group, RCT: randomized controlled trials. M = male, F = female. IBW: ideal body weight. n.a.; not available.

Table 2. Methodological quality and risk of bias of carbohydrate restriction studies (including energy restriction studies as control group [21,22]).

Study ID [Reference Number]	Sample Size Calculation	Random Sequence Generation	Allocation Concealment *	Blinding of Participants and Personnel *	Blinding of Outcome Assessment *	Incomplete Outcome Data	Selective Reporting	Other Source of Bias	Study free from total biases *	Indirectness Subjects	Intervention	Control	Outcome	Total Indirectness
Yamada et al., 2014 [21]	Yes	Yes	Low	Unclear	Unclear	Low	Low	Unclear	Unclear	No	No	No	No	No
Sato et al., 2017 [22]	Yes	Yes	Low	Unclear	Unclear	Low	Low	Unclear	Unclear	Yes **	Yes ***	No	No	No
Yabe et al., 2017 [25]	n.a.	Yes	Low	Unclear	Unclear	Low	Low	Unclear	Unclear	Yes **	Yes ****	Yes ****	No	Yes

* In dietary study, blinding and concealment are impossible. Thus, no dietary study is unbiased. ** In these studies [22,25], female/male ratio was different between intervention and control group. *** In this study [22], energy intake is strictly restricted to the intervention group. **** This study [25] used test meals supplied by Nichirei Foods Inc. (Tokyo, Japan).

4. Discussion

The present study was an attempt to elucidate the effects of an energy restricted diet and carbohydrate restricted diet on the management of diabetes in Japanese patients by reviewing previous studies from available databases. The first and most important finding of our study is that there is very little evidence on diets in Japanese patients with diabetes.

Our second finding was that an energy restricted diet, which has been recommended by the JDS as the sole dietary management approach, is not supported by any scientific evidence so far. The two studies in our review were not appropriate to judge the effects of an energy restricted diet on glycemic control because the levels of energy intake in the energy restriction group were not lower than those in the control group [21,22]. While in one study the energy restriction group showed a non-significant reduction of HbA1c (from 7.7 ± 0.6 to 7.5 ± 1.0%, p = 0.45) [18], no change was seen in HbA1c in another study [22], indicating that an energy restricted diet is not supported by scientific evidence in Japan. The available data on the effects of an energy restricted diet are very limited, which results in difficulties in the evaluation and recommendation of such a diet. Furthermore, the CALERIE (Comprehensive Assessment of Long term Effects of Reducing Intake of Energy) study revealed that energy restriction in non-obese subjects leads to loss of bone mineral density [26] and lean body mass [27] in a two year period. In light of these findings, a multi-faceted evaluation might be required for patients with diabetes in terms of examining the effects and safety of energy restriction. If the JDS continues to adopt dietary guidelines [4] different from those in Western countries, it should be backed by sufficient evidence that can be critically evaluated. Well-designed, multi-centered RCTs to establish dietary evidence should be actively encouraged.

The third finding of our study was that as a short-term management approach a carbohydrate restricted diet is more effective than an energy restricted diet. All three RCTs in our review were small but well-designed [21,22,25]. Although observational studies have presented safety concerns regarding the carbohydrate restricted diet in Western countries [28,29], a similar study in Japan was in favor of carbohydrate restriction [30]. Furthermore, recently the PURE (Prospective Urban and Rural Epidemiological) study, which was held in 18 countries, showed that carbohydrate intake was positively correlated with mortality [31], suggesting the safety of carbohydrate restriction.

Regarding the long-term effects of carbohydrate restriction, Sato et al. have recently reported that the statistical superiority of a carbohydrate restricted diet receded in an 18-month follow-up study. In their cohort, the median HbA1c level changed from 8.3% at baseline to 8.2% at 18 months in the energy restriction group and from 8.0% to 7.7% in the carbohydrate restriction group [32]. Hence, Sato et al. concluded that well-constructed nutrition therapy, including both energy and carbohydrate restricted diets, might be equally effective in improving HbA1c levels in the long term [32]. However, improvement in HbA1c have not yet been observed with energy restricted diets. Furthermore, although it was a non-RCT, Haimoto et al. [33] have previously shown that the carbohydrate restriction group had better HbA1c, BMI, and tapering of sulfonylureas during a 24-month period. Sanada et al. [34] have reported that a carbohydrate restriction diet was effective during a 36-month period. Thus, we cannot exclude the possibility that a carbohydrate restricted diet is effective in the long term. Unlike other carbohydrate restriction studies, the study by Sato et al. [22,32], showed that the carbohydrate restriction group consumed less energy than the energy restriction group. This reduced energy intake in the energy non-restricted group may explain the rebound in the carbohydrate restriction group in the study by Sato et al. [32]. Our findings therefore point towards the possibility that a carbohydrate restricted diet could potentially be an option as a first line dietary approach for Japanese patients with diabetes. However, longer-term and larger RCTs are needed to confirm this hypothesis.

Our study has some limitations. First, all three studies included in our review were small and short term. Second, the included studies all have a potential performance bias because the subjects and healthcare providers were not blinded. However, it might be difficult to solve this problem in studies evaluating dietary effects on glycemic control under actual clinical situations.

5. Conclusions

Our systematic review revealed that there are only a few dietary studies in Japanese patients with diabetes. Large-scale trials are needed to more fully evaluate the risks and benefits of an energy restricted diet, which is recommended by JDS. On the other hand, the effectiveness of a carbohydrate restricted diet is supported by limited evidence, at least in the short term. Well-designed and more sophisticated trials are needed to establish evidence-based dietary approaches specifically for these patients.

Author Contributions: Conceptualization, S.Y., Y.K. and H.N.; Methodology, S.Y., Y.K. and H.N.; Data curation, S.Y. and Y.K.; Formal Analysis, S.Y. and Y.K.; Writing-Original Draft Preparation, S.Y.; Supervision, H.N.

Funding: This research received no external funding.

Acknowledgments: Our study was supported by the Kitasato Institute Hospital Study Grant. The funders had no role in the design of the study; in the collection, analyses, or interpretation of data; in the writing of the manuscript, and in the decision to publish the results. We would like to thank Editage (https://www.editage.com/) for editing and reviewing this manuscript for English language.

Conflicts of Interest: S.Y. declares receiving lecture fees from Astellas Inc., Elly Lilly, MSD, Ono Pharmaceuticals, Sanofi, and Tanabe-Mitsubishi. Y.K. declares no conflict of interest. H.N. declares receiving lecture fees from Elly Lilly.

References

1. American Diabetes Association. Lifestyle management: Standards of Medical Care in Diabetes—2018. *Diabetes Care* **2018**, *41*, S38–S50. [CrossRef] [PubMed]
2. Evert, A.B.; Boucher, J.L.; Cypress, M.; Dunbar, S.A.; Franz, M.J.; Mayer-Davis, E.J.; Neumiller, J.J.; Nwankwo, R.; Verdi, C.L.; Urbanski, P.; et al. Nutrition therapy recommendations for the management of adults with diabetes. *Diabetes Care* **2013**, *36*, 3821–3824. [CrossRef] [PubMed]
3. Ley, S.H.; Hamdy, O.; Mohan, V.; Hu, F.B. Prevention and management of type 2 diabetes: Dietary components and nutritional strategies. *Lancet* **2014**, *383*, 1999–2007. [CrossRef]
4. The Japan Diabetes Society. Diet therapy. In *Practice Guideline for the Treatment for Diabetes in Japan*; Nankodo: Tokyo, Japan, 2016; pp. 37–66. (In Japanese)
5. The Japan Diabetes Society. Recommendation of Diet Therapy for Japanese Patients with Diabetes. Available online: http://www.jds.or.jp/modules/important/index.php?page=article&storyid=40 (accessed on 30 December 2017).
6. Heianza, Y.; Arase, Y.; Kodama, S.; Tsuji, H.; Tanaka, S.; Saito, K.; Hara, S.; Sone, H. Trajectory of body mass index before the development of type2 diabetes in japanese men: Toranomon hospital health management center study 15. *J. Diabetes Investig.* **2015**, *6*, 289–294. [CrossRef] [PubMed]
7. Looker, H.C.; Knowler, W.C.; Hanson, R.L. Changes in bmi and weight before and after the development of type 2 diabetes. *Diabetes Care* **2001**, *24*, 1917–1922. [CrossRef] [PubMed]
8. De Fine Olivarius, N.; Richelsen, B.; Siersma, V.; Andreasen, A.H.; Beck-Nielsen, H. Weight history of patients with newly diagnosed type 2 diabetes. *Diabet. Med.* **2008**, *25*, 933–941. [CrossRef] [PubMed]
9. Mann, J.I.; De Leeuw, I.; Hermansen, K.; Karamanos, B.; Karlström, B.; Katsilambros, N.; Riccardi, G.; Rivellese, A.A.; Rizkalla, S.; Slama, G.; et al. Diabetes and Nutrition Study Group (DNSG) of the European Association. Evidence-based nutritional approaches to the treatment and prevention of diabetes mellitus. *Nutr. Metab. Cardiovasc. Dis.* **2004**, *14*, 373–394. [CrossRef]
10. Imai, S.; Matsuda, M.; Hasegawa, G.; Fukui, M.; Obahashi, H.; Ozasa, N.; Kajiyama, S. A simple meal plan of 'eating vegetables before carbohydrate' was more effective for achieving glycemic control than an exchange-based meal plan in Japanese patients with type 2 diabetes. *Asia Pac. J. Clin. Nutr.* **2011**, *20*, 161–168. [PubMed]
11. Muramoto, A.; Yamamoto, N.; Nakamura, M.; Koike, J.; Numata, T.; Tamakoshi, A.; Tsushita, K. Effect of intensive lifestyle intervention programs on metabolic syndrome and obesity. *Himan Kenkyuu* **2010**, *16*, 182–187.

12.   Nanri, A.; Mizoue, T.; Kurotani, K.; Goto, A.; Oba, S.; Noda, M.; Sawada, N.; Tsugane, S. Low-carbohydrate diet and type 2 diabetes risk in japanese men and women: The japan public health center-based prospective study. *PLoS ONE* **2015**, *10*, e0118377. [CrossRef] [PubMed]

13.   Feinman, R.D.; Pogozelski, W.K.; Astrup, A.; Bernstein, R.K.; Fine, E.J.; Westman, E.C.; Accurso, A.; Frassetto, L.; Gower, B.A.; McFarlane, S.I.; et al. Dietary carbohydrate restriction as the first approach in diabetes management: Critical review and evidence base. *Nutrition* **2015**, *31*, 1–13. [CrossRef] [PubMed]

14.   Snorgaard, O.; Poulsen, G.M.; Andersen, H.K.; Astrup, A. Systematic review and meta-analysis of dietary carbohydrate restriction in patients with type 2 diabetes. *BMJ Open Diabetes Res. Care* **2017**, *5*, e000354. [CrossRef] [PubMed]

15.   Fukui, T.; Yamaguchi, N. Systematic Review. In *Minds Guide to Establish Clinical Guideline*; Igakushoin: Tokyo, Japan, 2014; pp. 29–50.

16.   Noda, K.; Zhang, B.; Iwata, A.; Nishikawa, H.; Ogawa, M.; Nomiyama, T.; Miura, S.; Sako, H.; Matsuo, K.; Yahiro, E.; et al. Lifestyle changes through the use of delivered meals and dietary counseling in a single-blind study. STYLIST study. *Circ. J.* **2012**, *76*, 1335–1344. [CrossRef] [PubMed]

17.   Yamanouchi, T.; Isobe, K.; Terashima, H.; Hayashi, T.; Hiroshima, Y.; Hosaka, A. Intervention with delivered meals changes lifestyle and improves weight and glycemic control in patients with impaired glucose tolerance. *J.J.C.L.A.* **2017**, *42*, 26–30. (In Japanese)

18.   Enosawa, N.; Inoue, M.; Sato, T.; Suzuki, S. New trial in diet therapy for weight reduction in obese type 2 diabetic patients. *J. Jap. Diab. Soc.* **2004**, *47*, 635–641. (In Japanese)

19.   Miyashita, Y.; Itoh, Y.; Hashiguchi, S.; Shirai, K. Effect of low carbohydrate content of low calorie diet for obese non-insulin-dependent diabetes mellitus patients on glucose and lipid metabolism. *J. Jap. Diab. Soc.* **1998**, *41*, 885–890. (In Japanese)

20.   Sato, A.; Ueno, K.; Sugimoto, I. Diet therapy in diabetes mellitus. *Nippon. Byouinkai Zasshi* **2012**, *59*, 314–316. (In Japanese)

21.   Yamada, Y.; Uchida, J.; Izumi, H.; Tsukamoto, Y.; Inoue, G.; Watanabe, Y.; Irie, J.; Yamada, S. A non-calorie-restricted low-carbohydrate diet is effective as an alternative therapy for patients with type 2 diabetes. *Intern. Med.* **2014**, *53*, 13–19. [CrossRef] [PubMed]

22.   Sato, J.; Kanazawa, A.; Makita, S.; Hatae, C.; Komiya, K.; Shimizu, T.; Ikeda, F.; Tamura, Y.; Ogihara, T.; Mita, T.; et al. A randomized controlled trial of 130 g/day low-carbohydrate diet in type 2 diabetes with poor glycemic control. *Clin. Nutr.* **2017**, *36*, 992–1000. [CrossRef] [PubMed]

23.   Okada, K.; Ito, Y.; Kitagawa, M.; Maeda, K.; Nakamura, R. The effect of low carbohydrate diet for type 2 diabetic patients. *Nippon Rinsho Eiyougakkai Zasshi* **2013**, *35*, 103–113. (In Japanese)

24.   Nishimura, R.; Omiya, H.; Sugio, K.; Ubukata, M.; Sakai, S.; Samukawa, Y. Sodium-glucose cotransporter 2 inhibitor luseogliflozin improves glycaemic control, assessed by continuous glucose monitoring, even on a low-carbohydrate diet. *Diabetes Obes. Metab.* **2016**, *18*, 702–706. [CrossRef] [PubMed]

25.   Yabe, D.; Iwasaki, M.; Kuwata, H.; Haraguchi, T.; Hamamoto, Y.; Kurose, T.; Sumita, K.; Yamazato, H.; Kanada, S.; Seino, Y. Sodium-glucose co-transporter-2 inhibitor use and dietary carbohydrate intake in japanese individuals with type 2 diabetes: A randomized, open-label, 3-arm parallel comparative, exploratory study. *Diabetes Obes. Metab.* **2017**, *19*, 739–743. [CrossRef] [PubMed]

26.   Villareal, D.T.; Fontana, L.; Das, S.K.; Redman, L.; Smith, S.R.; Saltzman, E.; Bales, C.; Rochon, J.; Pieper, C.; Huang, M.; et al. Effect of two-year caloric restriction on bone metabolism and bone mineral density in non-obese younger adults: A randomized clinical trial. *J. Bone Miner. Res.* **2016**, *31*, 40–51. [CrossRef] [PubMed]

27. Das, S.K.; Roberts, S.B.; Bhapkar, M.V.; Villareal, D.T.; Fontana, L.; Martin, C.K.; Racette, S.B.; Fuss, P.J.; Kraus, W.E.; Wong, W.W.; et al. Body-composition changes in the comprehensive assessment of long-term effects of reducing intake of energy (calerie)-2 study: A 2-y randomized controlled trial of calorie restriction in nonobese humans. *Am. J. Clin. Nutr.* **2017**, *105*, 913–927. [CrossRef] [PubMed]

28. Fung, T.T. Low-carbohydrate diets and all-cause and cause-specific mortality. *Ann. Intern. Med.* **2010**, *153*, 289. [CrossRef] [PubMed]

29. Noto, H.; Goto, A.; Tsujimoto, T.; Noda, M. Low-carbohydrate diets and all-cause mortality: A systematic review and meta-analysis of observational studies. *PLoS ONE* **2013**, *8*, e55030. [CrossRef] [PubMed]

30. Nakamura, Y.; Okuda, N.; Okamura, T.; Kadota, A.; Miyagawa, N.; Hayakawa, T.; Kita, Y.; Fujiyoshi, A.; Nagai, M.; Takashima, N.; et al. Low-carbohydrate diets and cardiovascular and total mortality in japanese: A 29-year follow-up of nippon data80. *Columbia J. Nutr.* **2014**, *112*, 916–924. [CrossRef] [PubMed]

31. Dehghan, M.; Mente, A.; Zhang, X.; Swaminathan, S.; Li, W.; Mohan, V.; Iqbal, R.; Kumar, R.; Wentzel-Viljoen, E.; Rosengren, A.; et al. Associations of fats and carbohydrate intake with cardiovascular disease and mortality in 18 countries from five continents (PURE): A prospective cohort study. *Lancet* **2017**, *390*, 2050–2062. [CrossRef]

32. Sato, J.; Kanazawa, A.; Hatae, C.; Makita, S.; Komiya, K.; Shimizu, T.; Ikeda, F.; Tamura, Y.; Ogihara, T.; Mita, T.; et al. One year follow-up after a randomized controlled trial of a 130g/day low-carbohydrate diet in patients with type 2 diabetes mellitus and poor glycemic control. *PLoS ONE* **2017**, *12*, e0188892. [CrossRef] [PubMed]

33. Haimoto, H.; Iwata, M.; Wakai, K.; Umegaki, H. Long-term effects of a diet loosely restricting carbohydrates on HbA1c levels, BMI and tapering of sulfonylureas in type 2 diabetes: A 2-year follow-up study. *Diabetes Res. Clin. Pract.* **2008**, *79*, 350–356. [CrossRef] [PubMed]

34. Sanada, M.; Kabe, C.; Hata, H.; Uchida, J.; Inoue, G.; Tsukamoto, Y.; Yamada, Y.; Irie, J.; Tabata, S.; Tabata, M.; et al. Efficacy of a moderate low carbohydrate diet in a 36-month observational study of Japanese patients with type 2 diabetes. *Nutrients* **2018**, *10*, 528. [CrossRef] [PubMed]

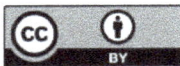

nutrients

MDPI

Protocol

How Does Diet Change with A Diagnosis of Diabetes? Protocol of the 3D Longitudinal Study

Emily Burch [1], Lauren T. Williams [1], Harriet Makepeace [1], Clair Alston-Knox [2] and Lauren Ball [1,*]

[1] Menzies Health Institute Queensland, Griffith University, Gold Coast 4215, Australia; emily.burch@griffithuni.edu.au (E.B.); lauren.williams@griffith.edu.au (L.T.W.); harriet.makepeace@griffithuni.edu.au (H.M.)

[2] Office of the Pro-Vice Chancellor, Arts, Education and Law, Griffith University, Mount Gravatt Campus, Brisbane 4222, Australia; c.alston-knox@griffith.edu.au

* Correspondence: l.ball@griffith.edu.au

Received: 8 December 2018; Accepted: 10 January 2019; Published: 12 January 2019

Abstract: Diet quality influences glycemic control in people with type 2 diabetes (T2D), impacting their risk of complications. While there are many cross-sectional studies of diet and diabetes, there is little understanding of the extent to which people with T2D change their diet after diagnosis and of the factors that impact those changes. This paper describes the rationale for and design of the 3D longitudinal Study which aims to: (i) describe diet quality changes in the 12 months following T2D diagnosis, (ii) identify the demographic, physical and psychosocial predictors of sustained improvements in diet quality and glycemic control, and (iii) identify associations between glycemic control and diet quality in the 12 months following diagnosis. This cohort study will recruit adults registered with the Australian National Diabetes Services Scheme who have been recently diagnosed with T2D. Participants will be involved in five purposefully developed telephone surveys, conducted at 3 monthly intervals over a 12-month period. Diet quality will be determined using a 24-h dietary recall at each data collection point and the data will be scored using the Dietary Approaches to Stop Hypertension (DASH) diet-quality tool. This study is the first dedicated to observing how people newly diagnosed with T2D change their diet quality over time and the predictors of sustained improvements in diet and glycemic control.

Keywords: type 2 diabetes mellitus; nutrition; DASH; diet quality; diabetes management; dietary intake; longitudinal analysis; lifestyle management

1. Introduction

Diet quality plays a vital role in helping people with type 2 diabetes (T2D) to achieve and maintain optimal glycemic control, thereby lowering their risk of developing diabetes-related complications [1]. Diet quality can be described as the extent to which food intake complies with national or international dietary guidelines or a priori diet quality score [2]. Investigating diet quality based on dietary patterns, defined as multiple dietary components operationalized as a single exposure [3], provides valuable information, beyond analyzing specific nutrients (e.g., protein) or food groups (e.g., dairy) [4]. This is because dietary patterns closely reflect actual dietary behavior and have a stronger influence on disease risk than specific nutrients or foods [5]. Findings from dietary pattern analyses may facilitate the translation of useful recommendations to health professionals and the general population [5,6]. A dietary pattern rich in whole-grains, fruits, vegetables, legumes, and nuts; moderate in alcohol; and low in refined grains, red or processed meats, and sugar-sweetened beverages has been shown to improve glycemic control in people with T2D [7]. Consequently, a key feature of international T2D management recommendations is to eat healthy foods that provide a high-quality diet [8–10].

However, evidence has shown that people with T2D have low-quality diets, despite these recommendations [10–15]. Our recent systematic review identified that internationally, people with T2D do not adhere to food group recommendations outlined in dietary guidelines [15]. Qualitative studies examining lived experiences report that people with T2D find it challenging to adopt and maintain healthy dietary behaviors after diagnosis [13,14]. Our previous qualitative study that investigated the experiences and perceptions of Australian adults newly diagnosed with T2D found that while participants reported making immediate, widespread changes to dietary behaviors that led to improvements in diet quality initially, they found it challenging to maintain dietary change [13]. Participants described feeling restricted in food choice, being uncertain of ideal dietary behaviors and felt unheard and rushed when speaking about their diet with health professionals [13]. Similar results were obtained in a qualitative study in Mexico where people reported making only short-term adherence to improvements in dietary intake due to difficulties with controlling appetite and eating with others [14]. While these qualitative findings of experiences raise concerns, it is important to also investigate quantitative aspects of diet quality change following diagnosis.

Cross-sectional research has assessed the diet quality of people with T2D at a single-point in time [15], however, no research has quantitatively explored changes in diet quality after diagnosis. Consequently, there is no evidence as to whether diet quality remains fixed once an individual is diagnosed with T2D, or whether there are periods of marked increases or decreases in diet quality. Prospective, observational studies are valuable as they measure events in temporal sequence and can distinguish causes from effects [16,17]. Many factors influence diet quality. These include non-modifiable factors such as age and sex, and modifiable factors such as self-efficacy, perception of current diet, environmental factors such as marketing and food availability, and relationships with health professionals [11,13]. There is currently no data on the demographic and health characteristics influencing diet quality change for people with T2D [13,18]. There is a clear need to investigate how diet changes over time so targeted strategies can be developed to facilitate improved glycemic control.

This paper describes the methodological protocol of the 3D Longitudinal Study, so named because seeing something in three dimensions adds clarity. In this case it refers to the 3D's of <u>D</u>iet, after <u>D</u>iagnosis with <u>D</u>iabetes. The study aims are to:

(i)   Describe diet quality changes in the 12 months following T2D diagnosis.
(ii)   Identify the demographic, physical and psychosocial predictors of improvements in diet quality and glycemic control.
(iii)   Identify associations between glycemic control and diet quality in the 12 months following diagnosis.

2. Theoretical Framework

The ability to predict and explain health-related behavior is important for developing strategies to change those behaviors [19]. The theory of planned behavior (TPB) is among the most influential and widely applied theories of the factors influencing health-related behavior [19]. According to the TPB, the single best predictor of a person's behavior is the intention to perform that behavior [20]. This is predicted by three constructs: attitude, subjective norm, and perceived behavioral control (PBC). The greater the PBC and more favorable the attitude and subjective norms, the stronger the intent will be to perform the behavior [20]. According to the TPB, people with T2D will intend to improve their diet quality to the extent that they believe the likely outcomes of consumption to be favorable, perceive social pressure from those who are important to them and feel capable of improving their diet quality without difficulty [21]. The constructs of the TPB are considered strong predictors of healthful eating and are commonly applied in the development of dietary behavior change interventions [21,22]. This study will integrate the TPB into its design in order to explore the factors that may serve as moderators in influencing the TPB constructs, thus affecting dietary behaviors and T2D management.

3. Materials and Methods

3.1. Study Design

The 3D Longitudinal Study is a prospective observational cohort study that will be conducted in Australia between 2018–2019. The study will recruit people newly diagnosed with T2D and monitor their dietary intake over 12 months. The Strengthening the Reporting of Observational Studies in Epidemiology (STROBE) checklist for cohort studies was used to guide the development of the research protocol [23]. The 3D Longitudinal Study is registered with the Australian New Zealand Clinical Trials Registry (ANZCTR) (ref: ACTRN12618000375257) and was approved by the Griffith University Human Research Ethics Committee (ref: 2017/951). Study results will be published in peer-reviewed journals and presented at scientific conferences.

3.2. Potential Participants

Eligible participants will be adults aged 18 years or older who have been recently diagnosed with T2D (<6 months prior to recruitment contact), are registered with the Australian National Diabetes Service Scheme (NDSS) and have indicated their willingness to be contacted for research purposes. The NDSS is an initiative of the Australian Government and is administered with the assistance of Diabetes Australia [24]. In 2017, there were approximately 1.1 million people registered with the NDSS [25]. Registration is part of usual care for people diagnosed with T2D, therefore this potential participant pool provides broad representation of the target population. People with T2D are authorized to register for free if they live in Australia or are visiting from a country with which Australia has a Reciprocal Health Care Agreement on an applicable visa [24]. Registering with the NDSS enables individuals to access a range of government approved diabetes-related products and information services [24]. All registrants have the option of consenting to being contacted for research purposes. Upon registration, patients are required to register their personal details on a form signed by a registered Australian medical practitioner, nurse practitioner or a credentialed diabetes educator [24]. The majority of T2D diagnoses in Australia are made by general practitioners (GPs), who are the usual coordinators of management [7]. A detailed participant inclusion and exclusion criteria is listed in Table 1.

Table 1. Inclusion and exclusion criteria for the 3D Longitudinal Study.

Inclusion Criteria	Exclusion Criteria
Adults aged >18 years	Individuals aged <18 years.
Diagnosed with T2D <6 months prior to recruitment contact	Diagnosed with LADA, T1D, gestational diabetes or pre-diabetes
Registered with the Australian NDSS and indicated their willingness to be contacted for research purposes.	Individuals who have been placed on a special diet due to a co-morbidity (e.g., renal disease)
Able to communicate in English	

LADA, Latent Autoimmune Diabetes in Adults; NDSS, National Diabetes Service Scheme; T1D, Type 1 diabetes; T2D, Type 2 diabetes.

3.3. Participant Recruitment and Screening

A convenience sample of all individuals registered with the NDSS with a new diagnosis of T2D over the previous 6-month period will be sent an initial invitation letter and a plain-language summary of the research project via email by Diabetes Australia. Interested individuals will be invited to contact the research team via email or telephone to confirm eligibility, provide informed consent and arrange data collection. Participants will be informed they can withdraw from the study at any stage. This recruitment method has been trialed in a feasibility study conducted in 2016–2017 (unpublished) which successfully recruited 22 participants from 1000 email invitees. Of these 22, 17 completed baseline data collection, six participants had left the study by 3 months, however all participants remaining at 3 months were retained to 12 months.

3.4. Data Collection

Data will be collected using a purpose-developed, interviewer-administered telephone surveys at five-time points; baseline, and then at 3, 6, 9, and 12 months after commencing the study. Surveys will be conducted by Accredited Practicing Dietitians (APDs). The feasibility study found each survey takes approximately 30 min to complete. A measuring tape will be posted to all participants within two working days of recruitment to provide enough time to measure their waist circumference before data collection begins. Strategies including contact and scheduling methods have been shown to improve cohort retention in longitudinal studies [26]. Participants will be contacted 2 weeks prior to their next anticipated data collection round to schedule a time. All participants will be sent a reminder via their preferred contact method (email or text message) one day prior to the date of their next survey. The recruitment and contact process is outlined in Figure 1.

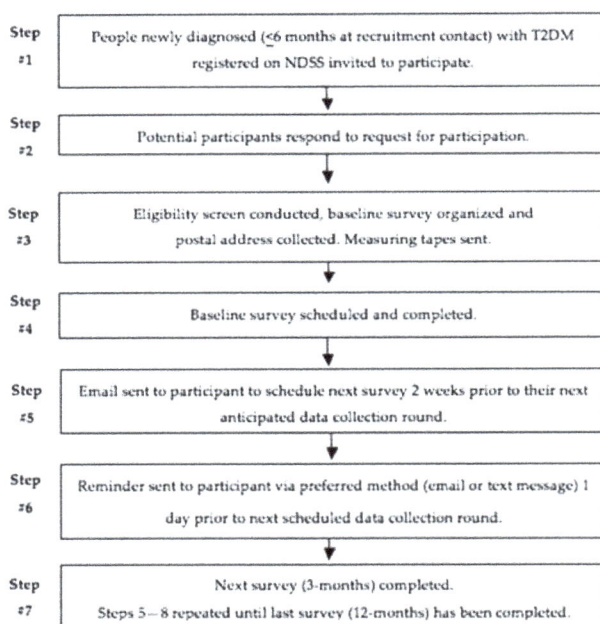

Step #1	People newly diagnosed (≤6 months at recruitment contact) with T2DM registered on NDSS invited to participate.
Step #2	Potential participants respond to request for participation.
Step #3	Eligibility screen conducted, baseline survey organized and postal address collected. Measuring tapes sent.
Step #4	Baseline survey scheduled and completed.
Step #5	Email sent to participant to schedule next survey 2 weeks prior to their next anticipated data collection round.
Step #6	Reminder sent to participant via preferred method (email or text message) 1 day prior to next scheduled data collection round.
Step #7	Next survey (3-months) completed. Steps 5–8 repeated until last survey (12-months) has been completed.

Figure 1. Recruitment and contact process for the 3D Longitudinal Study.

3.5. Survey Design

Data from all secondary outcome measures will be recorded in an online survey management system: www.limesurvey.org [27]. Item wording and response options were composed to align with the Australian Bureau of Statistics (ABS) 2016 Census and the Australian Longitudinal Study on Women's Health (ALSWH) to allow for comparison of outcomes [28,29]. Survey questions were generated using a developmental model [30] that employs five stages of questionnaire design and testing: conceptualization, design, testing, revision, and data collection. The feasibility study allowed testing of questions to ensure they were comprehendible, relevant and appropriate to participants and to confirm the survey length was suitable. Revisions were then made based on the feedback provided. For example, some participants in the feasibility study felt they were being asked the same question twice in the Healthy Eating Belief Scale. Therefore, the interviewer's scripted introduction and description of the Healthy Eating Belief Scale was modified to notify participants that there would be some repetition. The second draft was then pilot tested on three adults outside of the research team to ensure comprehensibility, suitability and flow.

3.6. Outcome Measures

Table 2 provides an overview of the primary (diet quality) and secondary outcomes and when they will be collected.

Table 2. Overview of data collection points in the 3D Longitudinal Study.

Data Collection Methods	Time Collected				
	0 Months	3 months	6 Months	9 Months	12 Months
Diet quality	✔	✔	✔	✔	✔
Glycemic control	✔	✔	✔	✔	✔
Medication use	✔	✔	✔	✔	✔
Baseline demographic factors	✔				
Physical factors	✔	✔	✔	✔	✔
Psychosocial factors	✔	✔	✔	✔	✔
Exposure to allied healthcare support	✔	✔	✔	✔	✔

3.6.1. Primary Outcome Measure: Change in Diet Quality (measured by DASH score)

Diet quality can be measured by a variety of purpose developed tools [31]. These are constructed by assigning higher scores within sub-scales based on more frequent or higher intakes of foods, nutrients or both [31]. Dietary Approaches to Stop Hypertension (DASH) is a dietary pattern high in whole-grains, fruits, and vegetables; moderate in low-fat dairy; and low in red and processed meats, added sugars, and sodium [32]. While originally developed to assist people in the prevention and management of hypertension, DASH is now recommended for the dietary management of T2D [18,33]. Adherence to DASH positively impacts on glycemic control, weight, and hypertension, which are key indicators of risk for diabetes-related complications [5,18,32]. A randomized controlled trial (RCT) conducted in adults with T2D showed that adherence to DASH improved glycated hemoglobin (HbA1c) (−1.2%), fasting blood glucose (−0.92 mmol/L), weight (−3 kg) and waist circumference (−4.8 cm) over 8 weeks when compared with a control diet [34,35]. Those following the DASH dietary pattern, also had a greater reduction in LDL cholesterol (difference from the control diet, −7.7 ± 3.3%).

A systematic review and meta-analysis of 20 RCTs found DASH significantly reduced systolic (−5·2 mmHg) and diastolic blood pressure (−2·6 mmHg) in adults with and without diabetes [36]. Another systematic review and meta-analysis of 13 RCTs revealed that adults without T2D who adhered to DASH achieved greater weight loss (−1.42 kg), reduced Body Mass Index (BMI) (−0.42 kg/m^2) and decreased waist circumference (−1.05 cm) compared with controls [37]. Considering the recognized impact on glycemic control, weight and hypertension, DASH was chosen as the dietary pattern used to assess diet quality in the present study. Participant DASH scores will be calculated using the DASH diet-quality tool which has been shown to have the highest correlation with health outcomes related to T2D compared to other tools that measure diet quality [38,39].

Change in DASH score from baseline to 3 months will be used to categorize participants as diet quality improvers or diet quality maintainers. Participants will be split into 2 groups; those who improved their DASH score by at least 3 DASH points (Diet quality improvers) and those who maintained their DASH score within 2.99 points or decreased their DASH score by at least 3 points (Diet quality maintainers). A change in DASH score of 3 points was selected based on findings from previous literature [40]. In a 20-year longitudinal study of over 40,000 adults, an average DASH score of 23.8 out of 40 was observed, and a change in score of approximately 3 points or more was sufficient to significantly influence long-term glycemic control [40].

Dietary intake data will be obtained through the Australian version of the Automated Self-Administered 24-h Dietary Assessment Tool (ASA-24). The ASA-24 is based on the validated Automated Multiple-Pass Method (AMPM) which is considered the optimal method for obtaining 24-h recall data due to its numerous probes, standardization of interviewer administration and validation against recovery biomarkers [41,42]. This method is also consistent with the methodology of the most recent population nutrition survey in Australia (the National Nutrition Survey) and has been shown to be a valid measure of dietary behavior at a given time point [43,44]. The ASA-24 is an online automated questionnaire that guides the individual through a system designed to maximize respondents' opportunities for remembering and reporting foods eaten in the previous 24 h [45]. The questionnaire is divided into five phases in line with published methodological guidelines; 'quick list', 'forgotten foods', 'time and occasion', 'detail cycle', and 'final probe' [45]. These phases encourage respondents to think about their intake in different ways and from several perspectives which has been shown to reduce bias in the estimation of dietary intake [45]. Once a specific food or beverage is reported, systematic questions are asked to capture more precise information about the food, cooking methods and quantity consumed. The ASA-24, usually a self-completed tool, will be adapted for use in a telephone survey; a researcher will ask the questions and enter the data. This will reduce participant burden and help decrease any bias associated with participant information technology literacy levels. This process was carried out successfully in a feasibility study with patients newly diagnosed with T2D. The data from the feasibility study was able to be used to assess changes in diet quality over a 12-month period.

Following data collection, participant 24-h dietary recall data will be sent from the ASA-24 program to the research team. This data will then be manually entered into FoodWorks by an experienced dietitian to allow determination of participant DASH scores. FoodWorks is a dietary analysis software program using standardized serve sizes that allows for quantification of specific food groups (e.g., vegetables) and nutrients (e.g., sodium) obtained from reported dietary intakes, recipes and meals [46]. FoodWorks draws on the national AUSNUT database [47]. AUSNUT was developed by Food Standards Australia and New Zealand and includes complete nutrient data sets of Australian foods designed specifically for nutrition surveys and is therefore suitable for use in this project [47].

DASH scores will be calculated using the standard scoring tool created by Fung et al [39]. Every tenth DASH score will be cross-checked by a second member of the research team to ensure accuracy. The standard scoring tool determines a score between 8 and 40 points, with 40 points representing optimal accordance with the DASH dietary pattern [39]. The DASH score is calculated by summing the number of daily servings of seven dietary components; fruits, vegetables, nuts and legumes, whole-grains, low-fat dairy, red and processed meats, added sugar, and sodium intake. For each of the components, participants are classified according to their intake ranking. Higher intakes of fruits, vegetables, low-fat dairy, whole-grains, and nuts and legumes receive higher scores. For example, quintile 1 is assigned 1 point and quintile 5 is assigned 5 points. Intake of sodium, red and processed meats and added sugars are scored in reverse as these are less desirable foods [39]. The lowest quintile is given a score of 5 points and the highest quintile is given a score of 1 point. The components scores are then summed to give an overall DASH score [39]. The scoring criteria for the DASH-style diet is outlined in Table 3.

Table 3. Dietary Approaches to Stop Hypertension (DASH) dietary pattern scoring criteria.

Component	Foods	Scoring Quintiles (Q) *
Fruits	All fruits and fruit juices	Q1 = 1 point
Vegetables	All vegetables except potatoes and legumes	Q2 = 2 points
Nuts and legumes	Nuts and peanut butter, dried beans, peas, tofu	Q3 = 3 points
Whole-grains	Brown rice, dark breads, cooked cereal, whole-grain cereal, other grains, popcorn, wheat germ, bran	Q4 = 4 points
Low-fat dairy	Skim milk, yogurt, cottage cheese	Q5 = 5 points
Sodium	Sum of sodium content of all foods	Q1 = 5 points
Red and processed meats	Beef, pork, lamb, deli meats, organ meats, hot dogs, bacon	Q2 = 4 points
		Q3 = 3 points
Added sugar	Foods and beverages with added sugars (i.e., sugar sweetened beverages)	Q4 = 2 points
		Q5 = 1 point

* Q1 represents low consumption and Q5 represents high consumption.

3.6.2. Secondary Outcome Measures

Secondary outcome measures will include: glycemic control, medication use, demographic factors, physical factors, psychosocial factors, and exposure to health provider support.

Glycemic Control

HbA1c reflects average plasma glucose over the previous six to eight-week period [48,49]. In Australia, it is best practice for GPs to conduct HbA1c testing on people with T2D every 3 months [8]. The test is subsidized by Medicare, the Australian Government's universal health scheme, up to four times in a 12-month period [50]. The GP on the research team will retrospectively obtain participants' HbA1c results over the 12-month study period from the relevant pathology laboratory. Other blood results collected will include; fasting blood glucose, high-density lipoprotein cholesterol, low-density lipoprotein cholesterol, and C-reactive protein.

Medication Use

Information on all medication use (name of medication and dosage) will be collected, including over-the-counter, and complementary medicines.

Demographic Factors

Demographic factors collected at baseline including; age, gender, highest education level, living arrangement, self-selected social class, household income, ability to manage on income, and smoking status. Response options will be dichotomous (e.g., gender), continuous (e.g., age) or categorical (e.g., highest educational level), consistent with categories used in the national consensus by the ABS.

Age and Gender

Participants' age at last birthday and gender will be collected. Sex response options will include three categories in line with the ABS 2016 Census; male, female and other [51].

Highest Education Level

Collecting data on highest educational level helps generate a single measure of an individual's overall educational attainment, whether it be a school or non-school qualification [51]. Participants will be asked to report their highest education level from eight categories in line with the ABS 2016 Census; postgraduate degree, graduate diploma and graduate certificate, bachelor degree, advanced diploma, diploma, certificate, year 12, or year 11 and below [51].

Living Arrangement

Data on participants' current living arrangement will be collected. In line with the ALSWH, response options will include; no one, partner/spouse, own children, someone else's children, parents, or other adults [29].

Self-Selected Social Class

Requesting information on self-selected social class allows class designation to be meaningful to participants and is more likely to reflect their actual class identity [52]. Participants will be asked to self-select their social class from one of four response options in line with the ALWHS; 'upper class', 'middle class', 'working class', or 'don't know' [52].

Household Income and Ability to Manage on Income

Gross income refers to the sum of income received from all sources before any deductions (income tax, the Medicare Levy or salary sacrificed amounts) are taken out [51]. Participants will be asked to report their average yearly gross household income from six response options in line with the ALSWH; less than $20,000, $20,001–$30,000, $30,001–$50,000, $50,001–$100,000, more than $100,000 or 'don't know/would rather not say'. Details on participants' ability to manage on their current income will also be collected. Seven response options in line with the ALSWH will include; 'impossible', 'difficult', 'always difficult', 'sometimes difficult', 'not too bad', 'easy', or 'not sure' [53].

Smoking Status

Participants will be asked to report their smoking status. Wording of the question has been developed to correspond with the ABS 2016 Census and response categories will include 'yes' or 'no' [51].

Physical Factors

Self-reported anthropometric data is valid and recommended for monitoring prevalence of obesity, particularly for large-scale studies because of its simplicity and low cost [54–56]. Physical factors will include; self-reported waist circumference, weight, and height. All response options will be continuous.

Waist Circumference

Waist circumference is a better indicator of central obesity than BMI or waist-to-hip ratio and is more strongly correlated with intra-abdominal fat content and cardiovascular risk factors [57]. Participants will be asked to self-report their waist circumference to the nearest centimeter. Participants will be asked to report results of two measures at each round of data collection, which will be averaged during data analysis. Measuring instructions adapted from the ALSWH will be provided to participants in the postal envelope [58]. Instructions will request participants to measure mid-central adiposity using the tape to measure at the level of the mid-point between the lower costal border and the iliac crest [58].

Weight

Weight will be self-reported at each data collection point to the nearest decimal point. If the participant can only report the amount in stones and pounds, a conversion factor of 2.203 will be used to convert pounds into kilograms in line with the ALSWH [52]. Participants will be asked to describe where and how their weight was measured to assess the accuracy of the information.

Height

Height will be self-reported to the nearest centimeter at baseline only. If the participant can only report the information in feet or inches, a factor of 2.54 will be used to convert inches to centimeters in line with the ALSWH [52].

BMI

BMI provides the most useful population-level measure of obesity [58,59]. Participants' BMI will be calculated after each round of data collection using the standard equation (weight (kg)/height (m)^2) [58]. Participants will be grouped into BMI categories for analysis according to the World Health Organization guidelines; underweight (<18.50 kg/m^2), normal weight (18.50–24.99 kg/m^2), overweight ($\geq$25.00 kg/m^2) and obese ($\geq$30.00 kg/m^2) [59].

Physical Activity

Regular physical activity is a key feature of international T2D management guidelines [9,60]. This is because it has been shown to improve glycemic control (regardless of whether weight loss has occurred), lipid levels, and blood pressure in people with T2D [61–63]. Participants' physical activity levels will be measured through the IPAQ-SF which is one of the most widely used physical activity assessment questionnaires and has been shown to be a valid measure of obtaining internationally comparable physical activity data [64,65]. It measures self-reported physical activity in the previous seven days and includes seven items that collect information on walking time, moderate and vigorous physical activity time and sitting time [66]. Data obtained in the IPAQ-SF will be used to estimate total metabolic equivalent (MET)-minutes per week for each participant [67].

Psychosocial Factors

Healthful Eating Beliefs

Healthy eating beliefs will be investigated at each of the five data collection points to better understand their beliefs, attitudes and intentions towards making positive dietary behaviors and how these impact on diet quality change over time. Participants' healthy eating beliefs will be assessed through the Healthful Eating Beliefs Scale. This scale is based on the TPB [68]. Standardized questions have been selected from previous Healthful Eating Beliefs Scales to suit the current study. Table 4 provides an outline of the rationale for investigation behind the questions and modes of responses. Participant scores will be generated for each of the seven subscales of the Healthful Eating Beliefs Scale by calculating the mean of the 5-point Likert scale items, with higher scores representing more positive beliefs, attitudes, and intentions towards improving dietary behaviors.

Mental Health

Mental health data will be collected at baseline, 6 and 12 months using the internationally validated K10 questionnaire [69]. This 10-item questionnaire yields a global measure of distress based on questions about anxiety and depressive symptoms experienced in the most recent four-week period [70]. It is scored using a five-level response scale based on the frequency of symptoms reported for each question. One is the minimum score for each item (none of the time) and five is the maximum score (all of the time). The maximum score is 50 indicating severe distress, the minimum score is 10 indicating no distress [70].

Table 4. Healthful Eating Beliefs Scale rationale for investigation and modes of responses.

Category	Rationale for Investigation	Area of Enquiry	Standardized Questions and Response Options	Source
Healthful Eating Beliefs Scale	To better understand healthy eating beliefs among participants and determine if they change over time.	Behavioral intention	"I intend to eat a healthful diet each day in the next 2 months," 5-pt Likert "I will try to eat a healthful diet each day in the next 2 months," 5-pt Likert "I plan to eat a healthful diet each day in the next 2 months," 5-pt Likert	[68]
		Perceived behavioral control	"I have the self-discipline to eat a healthful diet" 5-pt Likert "I have the ability to eat a healthful diet" 5-pt Likert "Me eating a healthful diet would be easy/difficult" 5-pt Likert "Whether I do or do not follow the recommendations for my diet is entirely up to me" 5-pt Likert	[71]
		Subjective norm	"People important to me think I should not/I should eat a healthful diet" 5-pt Likert "Other people expect me to follow the daily recommendations for diet" 5-pt Likert "People important to me want me to eat a healthful diet" 5-pt Likert "Other people with diabetes follow the daily recommendations for diet" 5-pt Likert	[71,72]
		Attitudes towards self-care	"Following the recommendations for my diet would be harmful/beneficial" 5-pt Likert "It would be worthless/valuable for me to follow the daily recommendations for my diet" 5-pt Likert "Following daily recommendations for diet is unnecessary/necessary" 5-pt Likert Following daily recommendations for diet is unpleasant/pleasant" 5-pt Likert	[72]

Exposure to GP and Allied Healthcare Support

Interactions with health professionals may help facilitate positive changes in dietary behaviors [73]. At each data collection point, participants will be asked about their concurrent and previous exposure to healthcare provider support (e.g., dietitian, diabetes educator). Participants will also be asked to report how useful they found the advice on a 5-point Likert scale (1 being 'not at all useful', 2 being 'slightly useful', 3 being 'neutral', 4 being 'somewhat useful' and 5 being 'extremely useful'). Question wording has been modified from previously conducted qualitative research that explored the experiences of dietary change in people with T2D [13].

3.7. Participant Confidentiality

All study related information will be de-identified and stored securely online with password-protected access systems. Daily back-ups of all electronic data will occur to minimize any risk of lost data. Only members of the research team who need to contact study patients, enter data or perform data quality control will have access to participant information.

3.8. Statistical Modeling and Sample Size

The longitudinal aspect of diet quality change will be analyzed using regression models [74]. Diet quality at 12 months (measured by the DASH score) will be the primary outcome, with glycemic control, interim diet changes (primarily at 3 months), medication use, demographic measures, physical measures, psychosocial measures, and exposure to healthcare provider support as the explanatory variables. This model will determine the relative importance of diet quality change both immediately after diagnosis and in the medium term with regards to a 12-month outcome towards sustained healthy eating.

Sample size calculations, such as those provided in Diggle et al. [74] are not readily computed for complex regression models and assessment using simulation studies would be more appropriate [75]. However, due to the relatively small participation rate in the feasibility study (22 participants/1000 invited) credible model parameters are currently unable to be formulated, and the effect differences over time cannot be reliably inferred. Additionally, current research of diet quality change post diabetes is lacking [15], therefore effects cannot be competently elicited. As a result, rather than determining an initial sample size for the study, a Bayesian updating procedure will be used to collect data. In this manner, sample size will be calculated during the early stages of data collection to yield an idea of how many samples should be collected. Additionally, using a Bayesian framework, the parameter estimates of the mixed model will be sequentially updated as batches of data are obtained, a process known as Bayesian learning [76,77].

4. Discussion

The study described in this paper, the 3D Longitudinal Study, will be the first to observe changes in diet quality in people with T2D after diagnosis and the factors (demographic, physical, and psychosocial) that influence those changes. Longitudinal studies help highlight differences or changes in the values of one or more variables between different time periods, describe participants' intra-individual and inter-individual changes over time and monitor the magnitude and patterns of those changes [78]. This is important for the proposed research because it is necessary to understand the extent to which people change their diet after a T2D diagnosis and why some people are able to sustain these changes over time and others are not. Understanding this will help to develop targeted strategies and facilitate enhanced dietary behavior support important to assist all people with T2D to have long-term success in improving their diet quality and help reduce the risk of complications. The results of this study will significantly add to the body of literature on the diet quality changes of people diagnosed with T2D, which is an under-researched area.

Limitations of the 3D Longitudinal Study are acknowledged. Recruitment through the NDSS is the most suitable way to access a large number of potential participants with T2D, however selection bias cannot be excluded as registration is voluntary, so participants may have greater diabetes self-management motivation. Self-reported dietary intake data and physical measurements may introduce misreporting bias and social desirability responses. Measurement errors associated with dietary assessment methods are also acknowledged. However, use of the ASA-24 h dietary recall (Australian version) which is a validated tool specifically designed for the Australian population, reduces risk of bias [43]. A feasibility study for this project has already determined that its recruitment capability, data collection and analysis procedures are achievable and appropriate.

Author Contributions: E.B., L.B., H.M. and L.T.W. identified the research question. All authors developed the research protocol. All authors have been involved in drafting the manuscript and revising it critically for intellectual content. All authors read and approved the final manuscript.

Funding: This research received no external funding.

Conflicts of Interest: The authors declare no conflict of interest.

References

1. Coppell, K.J.; Kataoka, M.; Williams, S.M.; Chisholm, A.W.; Vorgers, S.M.; Mann, J.I. Nutritional intervention in patients with type 2 diabetes who are hyperglycaemic despite optimised drug treatment—Lifestyle Over and Above Drugs in Diabetes (LOADD) study: Randomised controlled trial. *BMJ* **2010**, *341*, c3337. [CrossRef] [PubMed]

2. Leech, R.M.; Worsley, A.; Timperio, A.; McNaughton, S.A. Understanding meal patterns: Definitions, methodology and impact on nutrient intake and diet quality. *Nutr. Res. Rev.* **2015**, *28*, 1–21. [CrossRef] [PubMed]

3. Lockheart, M.S.K.; Steffen, L.M.; Rebnord, H.M.; Fimreite, R.L.; Ringstad, J.; Thelle, D.S.; Pedersen, J.I.; Jacobs, D.R., Jr. Dietary patterns, food groups and myocardial infarction: A case–control study. *Br. J. Nutr.* **2007**, *98*, 380–387. [CrossRef] [PubMed]

4. Drehmer, M.; Odegaard, A.O.; Schmidt, M.I.; Duncan, B.B.; Cardoso, L.D.; Matos, S.M.A.; Molina, M.D.C.B.; Barreto, S.M.; Pereira, M.A. Brazilian dietary patterns and the dietary approaches to stop hypertension (DASH) diet-relationship with metabolic syndrome and newly diagnosed diabetes in the ELSA-Brasil study. *Diabetol. Metab. Syndr.* **2017**, *9*. [CrossRef]

5. Sievenpiper, J.L.; Dworatzek, P.D.N. Food and dietary pattern-based recommendations: An emerging approach to clinical practice guidelines for nutrition therapy in diabetes. *Can. J. Diabetes* **2013**, *37*, 51–57. [CrossRef] [PubMed]

6. Mozaffarian, D.; Ludwig, D.S. Dietary guidelines in the 21st century–A time for food. *JAMA* **2010**, *304*, 681–682. [CrossRef]

7. Ley, S.H.; Hamdy, O.; Mohan, V.; Hu, F.B. Prevention and management of type 2 diabetes: Dietary components and nutritional strategies. *Lancet* **2014**, *383*, 1999–2007. [CrossRef]

8. The Royal Australian College of General Practitioners (RACGP). *General Practice Management of Type 2 Diabetes: 2016–2018*; RACGP: East Melbourne, VIC, Australia, 2016.

9. National Institute for Health and Care Excellence (NICE). *Type 2 Diabetes in Adults: Management United Kingdom*; NICE: London, UK, 2017.

10. Vitolins, M.Z. Action for Health in Diabetes (Look AHEAD) trial: Baseline evaluation of selected nutrients and food group intake. *J. Am. Diet Assoc.* **2009**, *109*, 1367–1375. [CrossRef]

11. Nelson, K.M.; Reiber, G.; Boyko, E.J. Diet and exercise among adults with type 2 diabetes: Findings from the third national health and nutrition examination survey (NHANES III). *Diabetes Care* **2002**, *25*, 1722–1728. [CrossRef]

12. Jarvandi, S.; Gougeon, R.; Bader, A.; Dasgupta, K. Differences in food intake among obese and nonobese women and men with type 2 diabetes. *J. Am. Coll. Nutr.* **2011**, *30*, 225–232. [CrossRef]

13. Ball, L.; Davmor, R.; Leveritt, M.; Desbrow, B.; Ehrlich, C.; Chaboyer, W. Understanding the nutrition care needs of patients newly diagnosed with type 2 diabetes: A need for open communication and patient-focussed consultations. *Aust J Prim Health* **2016**, *22*, 416–422. [CrossRef] [PubMed]

14. Castro-Sanchez, A.E.; Avila-Ortiz, M.N. Changing dietary habits in persons living with type 2 diabetes. *J. Nutr. Educ. Behav.* **2013**, *45*, 761–766. [CrossRef] [PubMed]

15. Burch, E.; Ball, L.; Somerville, M.; Williams, L.T. Dietary intake by food group of individuals with type 2 diabetes mellitus: A systematic review. *Diab. Res. Clin. Prac.* **2018**, *10*, 160–172. [CrossRef] [PubMed]

16. Mann, C.J. Observational research methods. Research design II: Cohort, cross sectional, and case-control studies. *Emerg. Med. J.* **2003**, *20*, 54–60. [CrossRef] [PubMed]

17. Mariani, A.W.; Pego-Fernandes, P.M. Observational studies: Why are they so important? *Sao Paulo Med. J.* **2014**, *132*, 1–2. [CrossRef] [PubMed]

18. Evert, A.B.; Boucher, J.L.; Cypress, M.; Dunbar, S.A.; Franz, M.J.; Mayer-Davis, E.J.; Neumiller, J.J.; Nwankwo, R.; Verdi, C.L.; Urbanski, P.; et al. Nutrition therapy recommendations for the management of adults with diabetes. *Diabetes Care* **2013**, *36*, 3821–3842. [CrossRef] [PubMed]

19. McEachan, R.R.C.; Conner, M.T.; Taylor, N.J.; Lawton, R. Prospective prediction of health-related behaviors with Theory of Planned Behavior: A meta-analysis. *Health Psych. Rev.* **2011**, *5*, 97–144. [CrossRef]

20. Ajzen, I. The theory of planned behavior. *Organ. Behav. Hum. Decis. Process* **1991**, *50*, 179–211. [CrossRef]

21. Kothe, E.J.; Mullan, B.A. Interaction effects in the theory of planned behavior: Predicting fruit and vegetable consumption in three prospective cohorts. *Br. J. Health Psych.* **2015**, *20*, 549–562. [CrossRef]

22. Hardeman, W.; Johnston, M.; Johnston, D.W.; Bonetti, D.; Wareham, N.; Kinmonth, A.L. Application of the theory of planned behavior in behavior change interventions: A systematic review. *Psych. Health* **2002**, *17*, 123–158. [CrossRef]

23. von Elm, E.; Altman, D.G.; Egger, M.; Pocock, S.J.; Gotzsche, P.C.; Vandenbroucke, J.P.; STROBE Initiative. The Strengthening the Reporting of Observational Studies in Epidemiology (STROBE) Statement: Guidelines for reporting observational studies. *Int. J. Surg.* **2014**, *12*, 1495–1499. [CrossRef]

24. National Diabetes Service Scheme (NDSS): Registration. Available online: https://www.ndss.com.au/registration (accessed on 20 May 2018).

25. National Diabetes Services Scheme (NDSS): Type 2 Diabetes. Available online: https://www.ndss.com.au/data-snapshots (accessed on 1 July 2018).

26. Abshire, M.; Victor, D.D.; Cajita, M.I.A.; Eakin, M.N.; Needham, D.M.; Himmelfarb, C.D. Participant retention practices in longitudinal clinical research studies with high retention rates. *BMC Med. Res. Method* **2017**, *17*, 1–10. [CrossRef]

27. LimeSurvey Organisation. Available online: https://www.limesurvey.org/ (accessed on 1 September 2018).

28. Australian Bureau of Statistics (ABS). Available online: http://www.abs.gov.au/ausstats/abs@.nsf/Lookup/bySubject/2008.0~{}2016~{}MainFeatures~{}Age~{}99 (accessed on 1 September 2018).

29. Elstgeest, L.E.M.; Mishra, G.D.; Dobson, A.J. Transitions in living arrangements are associated with changes in dietary patterns in young women. *J. Nutri.* **2012**, *142*, 1561–1567. [CrossRef] [PubMed]

30. Brancato, G.; Macchia, S.; Murgia, M.; Signore, M.; Simeoni, G.; Blanke, K.; Körner, T.; Nimmergut, A.; Lima, P.; Paulino, R.; et al. *Handbook of Recommended Practices for Questionnaire Development and Testing in the European Statistical System*; Eurostat: Luxembourg city, Luxembourg, 2004.

31. Collins, C.E.; Burrows, T.L.; Rollo, M.E.; Boggess, M.M.; Watson, J.F.; Guest, M.; Duncanson, K.; Pezdirc, K.; Hutchesson, M.J. The comparative validity and reproducibility of a diet quality index for adults: The Australian recommended food score. *Nutrients* **2015**, *7*, 785–798. [CrossRef] [PubMed]

32. Campbell, A.P. DASH eating plan: An eating pattern for diabetes management. *Diabetes Spectrum* **2017**, *30*, 76. [CrossRef] [PubMed]

33. Clark, A.L. Use of the Dietary Approaches to Stop Hypertension (DASH) eating plan for diabetes management. *Diabetes Spectrum* **2012**, *25*, 244–252. [CrossRef]

34. Salehi-Abargouei, A.; Maghsoudi, Z.; Shirani, F.; Azadbakht, L. Effects of Dietary Approaches to Stop Hypertension (DASH)-style diet on fatal or nonfatal cardiovascular diseases-incidence: A systematic review and meta-analysis on observational prospective studies. *Nutrition* **2013**, *29*, 611–618. [CrossRef]

35. Azadbakht, L.; Surkan, P.J.; Esmaillzadeh, A.; Willett, W.C. The dietary approaches to stop hypertension eating plan affects C-reactive protein, coagulation abnormalities, and hepatic function tests among type 2 diabetic patients. *J. Nutr.* **2011**, *141*, 1083–1088. [CrossRef]

36. Siervo, M.; Lara, J.; Chowdhury, S.; Ashor, A.; Oggioni, C.; Mathers, J.C. Effects of the Dietary Approach to Stop Hypertension (DASH) diet on cardiovascular risk factors: A systematic review and meta-analysis. *Brit. J. Nutri.* **2015**, *113*, 1–15. [CrossRef]

37. Soltani, S.; Shirani, F.; Chitsazi, M.J.; Salehi-Abargouei, A. The effect of dietary approaches to stop hypertension (DASH) diet on weight and body composition in adults: A systematic review and meta-analysis of randomized controlled clinical trials. *Obesi. Rev.* **2016**, *17*, 442–454. [CrossRef]

38. Alkerwi, A.; Vernier, C.; Crichton, G.E.; Sauvageot, N.; Shivappa, N.; Hebert, J.R. Cross-comparison of diet quality indices for predicting chronic disease risk: Findings from the Observation of Cardiovascular Risk Factors in Luxembourg (ORISCAV-LUX) study. *Briti. J. Nutri.* **2015**, *113*, 259–269. [CrossRef] [PubMed]

39. Fung, T.T.; Chiuve, S.E.; McCullough, M.L.; Rexrode, K.M.; Logroscino, G.; Hu, F.B. Adherence to a DASH-Style diet and risk of coronary heart disease and stroke in women. *Arch. Intern. Med.* **2008**, *168*, 713–720. [CrossRef] [PubMed]

40. de Koning, L.; Chiuve, S.E.; Fung, T.T.; Willett, W.C.; Rimm, E.B.; Hu, F.B. Diet-quality scores and the risk of type 2 diabetes in men. *Diabetes Care* **2011**, *34*. [CrossRef]

41. National Institute of Health (NIH). Available online: https://epi.grants.cancer.gov/asa24/respondent/validation.html (accessed on 1 June 2018).

42. Moshfegh, A.J.; Rhodes, D.G.; Baer, D.J.; Murayi, T.; Clemens, J.C.; Rumpler, W.V.; Paul, D.R.; Sebastian, R.S.; Kuczynski, K.J.; Ingwersen, L.A.; et al. The US department of agriculture automated multiple-pass method reduces bias in the collection of energy intakes. *Amer. J. Clin. Nutri.* **2008**, *88*, 324–332. [CrossRef] [PubMed]

43. Kirkpatrick, S.I.; Subar, A.F.; Douglass, D.; Zimmerman, T.P.; Thompson, F.E.; Kahle, L.L.; George, S.M.; Dodd, K.W.; Potischman, N.; et al. Performance of the automated self-administered 24-hour recall relative to a measure of true intakes and to an interviewer-administered 24-h recall. *Amer. J. Clin. Nutri.* **2014**, *100*, 233–240. [CrossRef] [PubMed]

44. Thompson, F.E.; Dixit-Joshi, S.; Potischman, N.; Dodd, K.W.; Kirkpatrick, S.I.; Kushi, L.H.; Alexander, G.L.; Coleman, L.A.; Zimmerman, T.P.; Sundaram, M.E.; et al. Comparison of interviewer-administered and automated self-administered 24-hour dietary recalls in 3 diverse integrated health systems. *Amer. J. Epidem.* **2015**, *181*, 970–978. [CrossRef]

45. Australian Bureau of Statistics (ABS). Available online: http://www.abs.gov.au/ausstats/abs@.nsf/mf/4363.0.55.001 (accessed on 31 May 2018).

46. Xyris Software: FoodWorks 9 Professional. Available online: https://xyris.com.au/products/foodworks-9-professional/ (accessed on 1 June 2018).

47. Food Standard Australia New Zealand (FSANZ): Food Nutrient Database FSANZ. Available online: http://www.foodstandards.gov.au/science/monitoringnutrients/ausnut/foodnutrient/Pages/default.aspx (accessed on 1 May 2018).

48. Nathan, D.M.; Turgeon, H.; Regan, S. Relationship between glycated haemoglobin levels and mean glucose levels over time. *Diabetologia* **2007**, *50*, 2239–2244. [CrossRef]

49. Schifreen, R.; Hickingbotham, J.M.; Bowers, G.N. Accuracy, precision and stability in measurement of hemoglobin A1c by "high-performance" cation-exchange chromatography. *Clin. Chem.* **1980**, *26*, 466.

50. Australian Government: Medicare Benefits Schedule online. Available online: http://www.mbsonline.gov.au (accessed on 15 June 2018).

51. Australian Bureau of Statistics (ABS). Available online: http://www.abs.gov.au/ausstats/abs@.nsf/mf/2901.0 (accessed on 28 May 2018).

52. Williams, L.; Germov, J.; Young, A. The effect of social class on mid-age women's weight control practices and weight gain. *Appetite* **2011**, *56*, 719–725. [CrossRef]

53. Australian Longitudinal Study on Women's Health (ALSWH). *Australian Longitudinal Study on Women's Health, 1946–1951 Cohort Summary 1996–2013*; ALSWH: New South Wales, Australia, 2015.

54. Spencer, E.A.; Appleby, P.N.; Davey, G.K.; Key, T.J. Validity of self-reported height and weight in 4808 EPIC–Oxford participants. *Public Health Nutri.* **2002**, *5*, 561–565. [CrossRef]

55. Booth, M.L.; Hunter, C.; Gore, C.J.; Bauman, A.; Owen, N. The relationship between body mass index and waist circumference: Implications for estimates of the population prevalence of overweight. *Intern. J. Obesity* **2000**, *24*, 1058–1061. [CrossRef]

56. Chan, N.P.T.; Choi, K.C.; Nelson, E.A.S.; Sung, R.Y.T.; Chan, J.C.N.; Kong, A.P.S. Self-reported waist circumference: A screening tool for classifying children with overweight/obesity and cardiometabolic risk factor clustering: Self-reported waist circumference. *Pediatr. Obesity* **2012**, *7*, 110–120. [CrossRef] [PubMed]

57. Ma, W.Y.; Yang, C.Y.; Shih, S.R.; Hsieh, H.J.; Hung, C.S.; Chiu, F.C.; Lin, M.S.; Liu, P.H.; Hua, C.H.; Hsein, Y.C.; et al. Measurement of Waist Circumference: Midabdominal or iliac crest? *Diabetes Care* **2013**, *36*, 1660–1666. [CrossRef] [PubMed]

58. Williams, L.; Hollis, J.; Collins, C.; Morgan, P. The 40-Something randomized controlled trial to prevent weight gain in mid-age women. *BMC Public Health* **2013**, *13*, 1007. [CrossRef]

59. World Health Organization (WHO). *Obesity: Preventing and Managing the Global Epidemic*; WHO: Geneva, Switzerland, 2000.

60. International Diabetes Federation (IDF). *IDF Clinical Practice Recommendations for Managing Type 2 Diabetes in Primary Care*; IDF: Brussels, Belgium, 2017.

61. Colberg, S.R.; Sigal, R.J.; Fernhall, B.; Regensteiner, J.G.; Blissmer, B.J.; Rubin, R.R.; Chasan-Taber, L.; Albright, A.L.; Braun, B.; American College of Sports Medicine; et al. Exercise and type 2 diabetes: The American College of Sports Medicine and the American Diabetes Association: Joint position statement. *Diabetes Care* **2010**, *33*, e147–e167. [CrossRef] [PubMed]

62. Balducci, S.; Zanuso, S.; Nicolucci, A.; De Feo, P.; Cavallo, S.; Cardelli, P.; Fallucca, S.; Alessi, E.; Fallucca, F.; Pugliese, G.; et al. Effect of an intensive exercise intervention strategy on modifiable cardiovascular risk factors in subjects with type 2 diabetes mellitus. *Arch. Internal. Med.* **2010**, *20*, 1794–1803. [PubMed]

63. Umpierre, D.; Ribeiro, P.A.; Kramer, C.K.; Leitão, C.B.; Zucatti, A.T.; Azevedo, M.J.; Gross, J.L.; Ribeiro, J.P.; Schaan, B.D. Physical activity advice only or structure exercise training and association with HbA1c levels in type 2 diabetes: A systematic review and meta-analysis. *JAMA* **2011**, *17*, 1790–1799. [CrossRef] [PubMed]

64. van Poppel, M.N.; Chinapaw, M.J.; Mokkink, L.B.; van Mechelen, W.; Terwee, C.B. Physical activity questionnaires for adults: A systematic review of measurement properties. *Sports Med.* **2010**, 565–600. [CrossRef]

65. Craig, C.L.; Marshall, A.L.; Sjostrom, M.; Bauman, A.E.; Booth, M.L.; Ainsworth, B.E. International Physical Activity Questionnaire: 12-country reliability and validity. *Med. Sci. Sports Exercise* **2003**, *35*, 1381–1395. [CrossRef]

66. International Physical Activity Group. Available online: https://sites.google.com/site/theipaq/questionnaire_links (accessed on 1 June 2018).

67. International Physical Activity Group. Available online: https://sites.google.com/site/theipaq/scoring-protocol (accessed on 1 June 2018).

68. Blue, C.L. Does the theory of planned behavior identify diabetes-related cognitions for intention to be physically active and eat a healthy diet? *Pub. Health Nurs.* **2007**, *24*, 141–150. [CrossRef]

69. Beyond Blue. Available online: https://www.beyondblue.org.au/the-facts/anxiety-and-depression-checklist-k10 (accessed on 1 June 2018).

70. Tan, L.S.; Khoo, E.Y.; Tan, C.S.; Griva, K.; Mohamed, A.; New, M.; Lee, Y.S.; Lee, J.; Tai, E.S.; Wee, H.L. Sensitivity of three widely used questionnaires. *Qual. Life Res.* **2015**, *24*, 153–162. [CrossRef] [PubMed]

71. Watanabe, T.; Berry, T.R.; Willows, N.D.; Bell, R.C. Assessing intentions to eat low-glycemic index foods by adults with diabetes using a new questionnaire based on the theory of planned behaviour. *Can. J. Diabetes* **2015**, *39*, 94–100. [CrossRef] [PubMed]

72. Gatt, S.; Sammut, R. An exploratory study of predictors of self-care behaviour in persons with type 2 diabetes. *Intern. J. Nursing Studies* **2008**, *45*, 1525–1533. [CrossRef] [PubMed]

73. Agborsangaya, C.B.; Gee, M.E.; Johnson, S.T.; Dunbar, P.; Langlois, M.F.; Leiter, L.A.; Pelletier, C.; Johnson, J.A. Determinants of lifestyle behavior in type 2 diabetes: Results of the 2011 cross-sectional survey on living with chronic diseases in Canada. *BMC Pub. Health* **2013**, *13*, 451. [CrossRef] [PubMed]

74. Diggle, P. *Analysis of Longitudinal Data*, 2nd ed.; Oxford University Press: New York, NY, USA, 2002.

75. Green, P.; MacLeod, C.J.; Nakagawa, S. SIMR: An R package for power analysis of generalized linear mixed models by simulation. *Methods Ecol. Evol.* **2016**, *7*, 493–498. [CrossRef]

76. Gill, J. *Bayesian Methods: A Social and Behavioral Sciences Approach*, 3rd ed.; CRC Press: Boca Raton, FL, USA, 2015.

77. Spiegelhalter, D.J.; Abrams, K.R.; Myles, J.P. *Bayesian Approaches to Clinical Trials and Health-Care Evaluation*, 1st ed.; John Wiley & Sons: Chichester, UK, 2004.

78. Ruspini, E. *Introduction to Longitudinal Research*, 1st ed.; Routledge: London, UK, 2002.

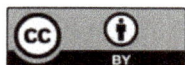

nutrients

MDPI

Review

Polyunsaturated Fatty Acids and Glycemic Control in Type 2 Diabetes

Vibeke H. Telle-Hansen, Line Gaundal and Mari C.W. Myhrstad *

Faculty of Health Sciences, Oslo Metropolitan University, Postbox 4, St. Olavsplass, 0130 Oslo, Norway;
vtelle@oslomet.no (V.H.T.-H.); linega@oslomet.no (L.G.)
* Correspondence: mmyhrsta@oslomet.no; Tel.: +47-9139-2176

Received: 1 April 2019; Accepted: 10 May 2019; Published: 14 May 2019

Abstract: The impact of dietary fat on the risk of cardiovascular disease (CVD) has been extensively studied in recent decades. Solid evidence indicates that replacing saturated fatty acids (SFAs) with polyunsaturated fatty acids (PUFAs) decreases blood cholesterol levels and prevents CVD and CVD mortality. Studies indicate that fat quality also may affect insulin sensitivity and hence, the risk of type 2 diabetes (T2D). A high intake of SFAs has shown to increase the risk of T2D in prospective studies, while a high intake of PUFAs reduces the risk. Whether PUFAs from marine or vegetable sources affect glycemic regulation differently in T2D remains to be elucidated. The aim of the present review was therefore to summarize research on human randomized, controlled intervention studies investigating the effect of dietary PUFAs on glycemic regulation in T2D. About half of the studies investigating the effect of fish, fish oils, vegetable oils, or nuts found changes related to glycemic control in people with T2D, while the other half found no effects. Even though some of the studies used SFA as controls, the majority of the included studies compared PUFAs of different quality. Considering that both marine and vegetable oils are high in PUFAs and hence both oils may affect glycemic regulation, the lack of effect in several of the included studies may be explained by the use of an inappropriate control group. It is therefore not possible to draw a firm conclusion, and more studies are needed.

Keywords: PUFA; polyunsaturated fatty acids; glycemic control; nuts; fish; fish oil; vegetable oil; type 2 diabetes

1. Introduction

The most important public health challenge in the world today is premature morbidity and mortality from non-communicable diseases (NCDs) like cancer, type 2 diabetes (T2D), and cardiovascular disease (CVD) [1]. Globally, the prevalence of T2D has increased from 108 million in 1980 to 422 million individuals in 2014 [2]. The WHO has estimated that diabetes will be the seventh most important cause of death in the world by 2030 [3]. Relative risk of CVD is increased two to four times in people with T2D compared with non-diabetic subjects, and is the primary cause of death in people with T2D [4].

The health impact of diet is well recognized, and even small dietary changes may contribute to significant health effects [5–7]. Lifestyle and diet can be highly effective in preventing and treating T2D [8–11]. A high intake of saturated fatty acids (SFAs) increases the risk of CVD due to increased low-density lipoprotein (LDL) cholesterol in the blood, while polyunsaturated fatty acids (PUFAs) have the opposite effect [5,12–15]. Studies indicate that dietary fat quality also may affect insulin sensitivity and hence, the risk of T2D. As early as 1959, Kinsell et al. reported on fat quality and insulin regulation [16]. Several studies on fat quality and glycemic regulation have been published since then [17–20]. According to observational studies, both intake of PUFAs and replacement of SFAs with

PUFAs reduce the risk of T2D [21,22]. Imamura and colleagues recently performed a comprehensive meta-analysis and systematic review of dietary fat and glycemic regulation in randomized controlled trials (RCTs). They found that replacing the intake of SFAs with PUFAs improved glycemia and insulin resistance [19]. These results are in accordance with a systematic review from 2014 [13]. However, none of these reviews distinguished between PUFAs derived from marine or vegetable sources, and both people with and without T2D were included.

In addition to the opposing health effects of saturated versus unsaturated fat, specific PUFAs may differ in their health effects. Some studies have indicated that n-6 PUFAs, but not n-3 PUFAs, may improve insulin sensitivity [13]. In a meta-analysis from 2008, n-3 PUFA supplementation in people with T2D had no significant effect on glycemic control [23], whereas vegetable PUFAs were found to reduce fasting insulin and Homeostasis Assessment Model-Insulin Resistance (HOMA-IR) in a more recent meta-analysis in healthy subjects [24]. To what degree PUFAs from different sources affect glycemic regulation in people with T2D remains unknown.

The aim of the present review was therefore to summarize the literature on human intervention studies investigating the effect of marine- and vegetable-derived PUFAs on glycemic regulation in T2D.

2. Materials and Methods

To summarize the effects of PUFAs on glycemic control in people with T2D we performed a literature search in PubMed in August 2018. Only original articles on RCTs in humans were included. Furthermore, only studies with information about glycemic control and/or T2D and/or dietary unsaturated fat were included. The search words were: "glycemic control" AND "type 2 diabetes" AND "PUFA" AND/OR "unsaturated fats" AND/OR "nuts" AND/OR "oils" AND/OR "fatty fish" AND/OR "omega 3" AND/OR "omega 6". We included studies which clearly or possibly fulfilled the following criteria: glycemic control, T2D and dietary interventions, and intake of unsaturated fat. In addition, studies with subjects referred to as non-insulin dependent diabetes mellitus (NIDDM) were also included, and hence these subjects are referred to as NIDDM in the present review. Moreover, we excluded studies that clearly fulfilled at least one of the following criteria: Non original study (for example editorial, review or conference paper), studies that did not compare the criteria measurements to a control group, animal study, articles written in languages other than English, or lack of inclusion criteria measurements (as defined previously). Interventions with ethyl esters and not available articles were excluded, and duplicate articles were removed. In addition to the literature search, two articles were included based on other reviews. In total, 31 articles were identified as eligible and included in the present article. Figure 1 shows the flow chart of the study selection.

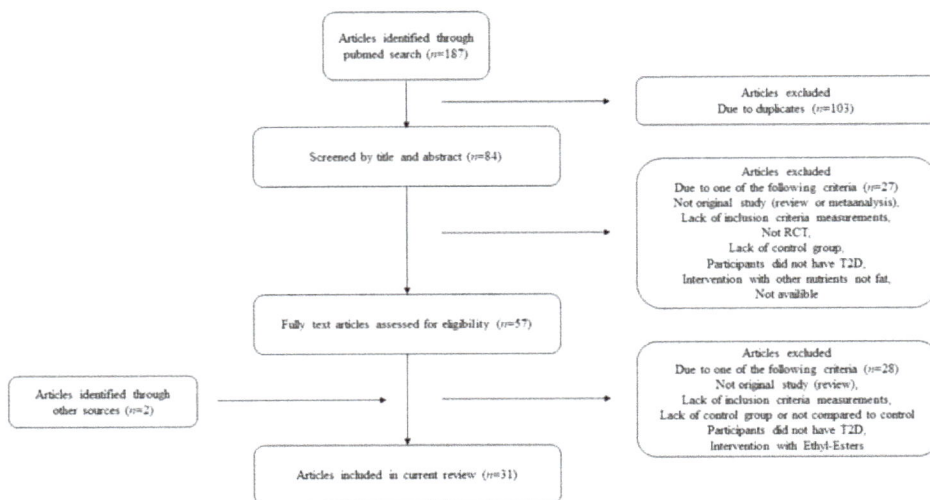

Figure 1. Flow chart of the study selection. RCT: randomized controlled trial; T2D: type 2 diabetes.

3. Results and Discussion

In the present review, we identified 31 RCTs (postprandial and short- and long-term intervention trials (lasting from 30 days to 30 weeks), parallel and crossover design) investigating the effects of PUFAs as dietary components in glycemic regulation in people with T2D or NIDDM (Tables 1–3). Of the 31 included studies, 14 studies investigated the effect of fish, fish oil, eicosapentaenoic acid (EPA) and/or docosahexaenoic acid (DHA) on glycemic regulation [25–38]; 12 studies investigated vegetable oils [39–50]; and five studies investigated the effect of nuts [51–55]. All participants were adults, male and females in the age range between 34 and 84 years (min–max), with T2D or NIDDM.

3.1. Fish and Fish Oil

A relationship between fish and/or marine n-3 fatty acids consumption and reduced risk of CVD was originally suggested by epidemiological studies among Greenland Inuits and Danes [56]. The effects of both the amount and quality of dietary fat and fish oil have since been studied intensively. Suggested mechanisms of the cardiovascular benefits from marine n-3 PUFAs include decreased plasma triglyceride levels and blood pressure, as well as anti-thrombotic, antiarrhythmic, and anti-inflammatory effects [57–59]. The effect of fish oil on glycemic regulation in T2D is less studied. In the present review, 14 intervention studies with fish or fish oil in people with T2D or NIDDM were included (Table 1).

Balfegó and coworkers investigated the effect of a standard diet with sardines on metabolic control [27]. Thirty-five subjects were randomized to follow either a T2D standard diet (control group), or a T2D standard diet enriched with 100 g of sardines per day, 5 days a week (sardine group) for 6 months. The changes in fasting glucose, glycated hemoglobin A1c (HbA1c), fasting insulin and HOMA-IR values were similar between the two groups [27]. The effects of moderate aerobic exercise and the incorporation of fish into a low-fat diet (30 energy (E) % fat) on glycemic control were examined in 49 subjects [34]. The subjects were randomly assigned to a low fat diet (30 E% fat) with or without one fish meal per day (3.6 g n-3 fatty acids) and further randomized to a moderate (55–65% VO$_2$ max) or light (heart rate <100 bpm) exercise program for eight weeks. While fasting insulin levels decreased in the fish and light exercise group compared with light exercise alone (control), there were no differences in fasting blood glucose concentration after any of the interventions compared with the control group. In the fish and light exercise group, they also demonstrated a significant rise in HbA1c compared with the control group [34].

Table 1. Effects of fish and fish oil on glycemic regulation in type 2 diabetes in randomized controlled trials. Significant results are indicated by an up/down arrow.

Study	Subject Characteristics	Study Design	Intervention	Glucose	Insulin	HbA1c	Other Markers
Wang et al. 2017, European Journal of Nutrition, China	n = 99, T2D, 65 years, M/F	6 months Parallel	(1) Corn oil (4 g/day) (2) Fish oil (4 g/day (1.34 g EPA and 1.07 g DHA))	↔	↔	↔	↔ HOMA-IR
Zheng et al. 2016, Mol. Nutr. Food Res, China	n = 166, T2D, 59 years, M/F	180 days Parallel	(1) Corn oil (1 g/day) (2) Fish oil (1 g/day (500 mg EPA + DHA, EPA:DHA = 3:2)) (3) Flaxseed oil (1 g/day (630 mg ALA))	↔	↔	(2) ↓ (3) ↔	↔ HOMA-IR
Balfegó et al. 2016, Lipids Health Dis, Spain	n = 35, T2D, 60 years, M/F	6 months Parallel	(1) Standard diet (2) Standard diet enriched with sardines 5 days a week (100 g/day)	↔	↔ *Within groups:* (1), (2) ↓	↔ *Within groups:* (1) ↓	↔ HOMA-IR *Within groups:* (1), (2) ↓ HOMA-IR
Sarbolouki et al. 2013, Singapore Med J, Iran	n = 67, T2D, 45 years, M/F	3 months Parallel	(1) Corn oil (2 g/day) (2) EPA (2 g/day)	↓	↓	↓	↓ HOMA-IR
Ogawa et al. 2013, Tohoku J Exp Med, Japan	n = 30, T2D, 80 years, M/F	3 months Parallel	(1) Liquid diet without EPA/DHA (2) Liquid diet containing EPA (25 mg/100 kcal) and DHA (17 mg/100 kcal)	↓		↓	
Crochemore et al. 2012, Nutr Clin Pract, Brazil	n = 41, T2D, 61 years, F	30 days Parallel	(1) Gelatin (500 mg/capsule) (2) Fish oil (2.5 g/day (547.5 mg EPA + 352.5 mg DHA)) (3) Fish oil (1.5 g/day (328.5 mg EPA + 211.5 mg DHA))	↔	↔	↔	↔ HOMA-IR ↔ QUICKI
Pooya et al. 2010, Nutrition, Metabolism & Cardiovascular Disease, Iran	n = 81, T2D, Control: 53 years Treatment: 56 years M/F	2 months Parallel	(1) Sunflower oil (2100 mg/day (12% SFA, 71% linoleic acid (LA), 16% MUFA)) (2) n-3 (3 g/day (1584 mg/day EPA, 828 mg/day DHA, 338 mg other n-3))	↔		↓	
Pedersen et al. 2003, EJCN, Denmark	n = 44, T2D, 63 years, M/F	8 weeks Parallel	(1) Corn oil (4 g/day) (2) Fish oil (4 g/day (2.6 g EPA + DHA))	↔ *Within groups:* (2) ↑		↔	
Luo et al. 1998, Diabetes Care, France	n = 10, T2D, 54 years, M	2 × 2 months Crossover	(1) Sunflower oil (6 g/day(65% n-6, 0.2% n-3, 24% MUFA, 11% SFA)) (2) Fish oil (6 g/day (1.8 g n-3: 18% EPA, 12% DHA, 4% n-6, 36% MUFA, 30% SFA))	↔	↔	↔	↔ euglycemic-hyperinsulinemic clamp

Table 1. Cont.

Study	Subject Characteristics	Study Design	Intervention	Glucose	Insulin	HbA1c	Other Markers
Dunstan et al. 1997, Diabetes Care, Australia	n = 49, NIDDM, 52–54 years, M/F	8 weeks parallel	(1) Light exercise (2) Fish (3.6 g n-3/day) and light exercise (3) Fish (3.6 g n-3/day) and moderate exercise (4) Moderate exercise	↔	(2) ↓ (3) (4) ↔	(2) ↑ (3) (4) ↔	
McManus et al. 1996, Diabetes Care, Canada	n = 11, T2D, 62 years, M/F	3 × 3 months Crossover	(1) Linseed oil (35 mg FA/kg body weight/day) (2) Fish oil (35 mg FA/kg body weight/day)	↔	↔	↔	↔ Insulin sensitivity ↔ Glucose effectiveness ↔ Acute insulin response to glucose
Morgan et al. 1995, Diabetes Care, USA	n = 40, NIDDM, 54 years, M/F	12 weeks Parallel	(1) Corn oil (9 g/day) (2) Corn oil (18 g/day) (3) Fish oil (9 g/day) (4) Fish oil (18 g/day)	↔		↔	
Annuzzi et al. 1991, Atherosclerosis, Italy	n = 8, NIDDM, 51 years, M	2 × 2 weeks Crossover	(1) Olive oil (10 g) (2) Fish oil (10 g (1.8 g EPA + 1.2 g DHA))	↔ daily average	↔ insulin sensitivity		↔ hyperglycemic clamp
Borkman et al. 1989 Diabetes, Australia	n = 10, NIDDM, 57 years, M/F	3 × 3 weeks Crossover	(1) Standard diabetic diet (2) Standard diabetic diet + Safflower oil (10 g) (3) Standard diabetic diet + Fish oil (10 g)	(2) (3) ↑	↔		↔ hyperinsulinemic-euglycemic clamp

Significant differences ($p \leq 0.05$) between intervention group(s) and control group are shown with ↑ or ↓, while ↔ indicates no significant difference. When several intervention groups are present, the results for each group are indicated with number. Fasting values are shown, if not otherwise stated. Control group is referred to as (1). DHA: docosahexaenoic acid; EPA: eicosapentaenoic acid; F: female; g: gram; HbA1c: glycated hemoglobin A1c; HOMA-IR: Homeostasis Assessment Model-Insulin Resistance; M: male; mg: milligram; MUFA: monounsaturated fatty acid; n: number; n-3: omega-3; NIDDM: non-insulin dependent diabetes mellitus; PUFA: polyunsaturated fatty acid; SFA: saturated fatty acid; T2D: type 2 diabetes; wt: weight.

Table 2. Effects of vegetable oils on glycemic regulation in type 2 diabetes in randomized controlled trials. Significant results are indicated by an up/down arrow.

Study	Subject Characteristics	Study Design	Intervention	Glucose	Insulin	HbA1c	Other Markers
Zibaeenezhad et al. 2016, Int J Endocrin Metab, Iran	n = 90, T2D, 55 years, M/F	3 months Parallel	(1) No oil (2) Walnut oil (15 g/day)	↓		↓	
Foster et al. 2013, Journal of Diabetes Research and Clinical Metabolism, Australia	n = 43, T2D, 65 years, F	12 weeks Parallel	(1) Olive oil (2000 mg/day + 40 mg/day zinc) (2) Zink (40 mg/d) (3) Flaxseed oil (2000 mg/day (1200 mg ALA)) (4) Zinc and flaxseed oil (40 mg/day zinc + 2000 mg/day flaxseed oil)	↔	↔ *Within groups:* (1) ↓	↔	↔ HOMA-IR *Within groups:* (1) ↓ HOMA-IR
Jenkins et al. 2014, Diabetes Care, Canada	n = 141, T2D, 59 years, M/F	3 months Parallel	(1) whole-wheat bread without canola oil (500 kcal/day) (2) low-GL diet with a canola oil-enriched bread (500 kcal/day)	↔		↓	
Taylor et al. 2010, AJCN, Canada	n = 34, T2D, 52 years, M/F	12 weeks Parallel	(1) Bakery products with no flaxseed (2) Bakery products with milled flaxseed (32 g/day) (3) Bakery products with flaxseed oil (13 g/day)	↔	↔	↔	↔ HOMA-IR ↔ QUICKI
Norris et al. 2009, AJCN, United States	n = 35, T2D, 60 years, F	2 × 16 weeks crossover	(1) Safflower oil (8 g/day) (2) CLA (c9t11 and t10c12) (8 g/day)	↑ *Within groups:* (1) ↓	↔		↑ HOMA-IR *Within groups:* (1) ↓ HOMA-IR
Barre et al. 2008, J Ole Sci, Canada	n = 32, T2D, 60 years, M/F	3 months Parallel	(1) Safflower oil 10 g/day (control) (2) Flaxseed oil 10 g/day (60 mg ALA/kg body weight/day)	↔	↔	↔	
Gerhard 2004, AJCN, United States	n = 11, T2D, 50 years, M/F	6 weeks Parallel	(1) Low-fat diet (total fat 20 E%, carbohydrates 65 E%, higher in fiber) (2) High MUFA diet (total fat 40 E%, MUFA 26 E%, carbohydrates 45 E%)	↔		↔	↔ Fructosamin

Table 2. Cont.

Study	Subject Characteristics	Study Design	Intervention	Glucose	Insulin	HbA1c	Other Markers
Brynes et al. 2000, AJCN, United Kingdom	n = 9, T2D, 56 years, M/F	2 × 3 weeks Crossover	(1) high-MUFA isoenergetic diet (olive oil) (2) high-PUFA isoenergetic diet (corn oil)	↔ ↔ iAUC	↔ ↔ iAUC	↔	↔ short insulin tolerance test (SITT)
Tsihlias et al. 2000, AJCN, Canada	n = 72, T2D, 42–79 years, M/F	6 months Parallel	(1) High-GI diet (cereals) (10% of energy) (2) Low-GI diet (cereals) (10% of energy) (3) High MUFA diet (margarine and olive oil) (10% of energy)	↔	(3) ↓ mean 8-h insulin (2) ↔ mean 8h insulin	↔	
Christiansen et al. 1997, Diabetes Care, Denmark	n = 16, NIDDM, 55 years, M/F	3 × 6 weeks Crossover	(1) SAT diet (20 E% SFA, 5 E% PUFA, 5 E% MUFA) (2) Cis-MUFA diet (20 E% cis-MUFA, 5 E% PUFA, 5 E% SFA) (3) Trans-MUFA diet (20 E% trans-MUFA, 5 E% PUFA, 5 E% SFA)	↔ ↔ AUC	↔ (2) ↓ iAUC	↔	(2) ↓ C-peptide iAUC
Lerman-Garber et al., 1994, Diabetes Care, Mexico	n = 12, NIDDM, 56 years, F	2 × 4 weeks Crossover	(1) Diet high in MUFA (HMUFA) (olive oil) (2) Diet high in complex carbohydrates (high-CHO)	↔ Within groups: (1), (2) ↓	↔ Within groups: (1), (2) ↓		↔ Fructosamine
Heine et al. 1989, AJCN, USA	n = 14, NIDDM, 52 years, M/F	2 × 30 weeks Crossover	(1) Low P:S diet (P:S ratio 0.3) (2) High P:S diet (P:S ratio 1.0)	↔ ↔ iAUC	↔	↔	↑ Metabolic clearance rate of glucose ↔ C-peptide

Significant differences ($p \leq 0.05$) between intervention group(s) and control group are shown with ↑ or ↓, while ↔ indicates no significant difference. When several intervention groups are present, the results are for each group and are indicated with number. Fasting values are shown, if not otherwise stated. Control group is referred to as (1). ALA: alpha-linolenic Acid; CHO: carbohydrates; E%: energy %; F: female; g: gram; GI: glycemic index; GL: glycemic load; HbA1c: glycated hemoglobin A1c; HOMA-%β: HOMA-percentage beta cell function; HOMA-IR: Homeostasis Assessment Model-Insulin Resistance; iAUC: incremental area under the curve; M: male; MUFA: monounsaturated fatty acid; n: number; NIDDM: non-insulin dependent diabetes mellitus; P:S: PUFA/SFA ratio; PUFA: polyunsaturated fatty acid; SAT: high saturated fatty acid diet; SFA: saturated fatty acid; T2D: type 2 diabetes; QUICKI: quantitative insulin check.

Table 3. Effects of nuts on glycemic regulation in type 2 diabetes in randomized controlled trials. Significant results are indicated by an up/down arrow.

Study	Subject Characteristics	Study Design	Intervention	Glucose	Insulin	HbA1c	Other Markers
Mohan et al. 2018, J Nutr, India	n = 269, T2D, 51 years, M/F	12 weeks Parallel	(1) Standard diabetic diet (2) Standard diabetic diet plus cashew nuts (30 g/day)	↔	↔	↔	↔ HOMA-IR
Sauder et al. 2015, Metabolism, USA	n = 30, T2D, 40–74 years, M/F	2 × 4 weeks Crossover	(1) Control diet; based on the American Heart Association's Therapeutic Lifestyle Changes diet (26.9% total fat, 6.7% saturated fat, 186 mg/day cholesterol) (2) Pistachios added to the control diet (20 % of daily energy)	↔	↔	↔	↔ HOMA-IR ↔ Matsuda ↓ Fructosamine
Parham et al. 2014, Rev Diabet Study, Iran	n = 48, T2D, 50–53 years, M/F	2 × 12 weeks Crossover	(1) Diet without nuts (2) Pistachio nuts (50 g/day)	↓		↓	
Wien et al. 2014, Nutr Journal, USA	n = 60, T2D, 34–84 years, M/F	24 weeks Parallel	(1) ADA meal plan without nuts (2) ADA meal plan with peanuts (20% of total energy (mean 46 g/day))	↔		↔	
Kendall et al. 2011, Nutrition, Metabolism & Cardiovascular Diseases, Canada	n = 24 T2D: 68 years Healthy: 36 years M/F	2-h Postprandial Crossover	(1) White bread (50 g available carbohydrate) (2) Mixed nuts (30 g) (3) Mixed nuts (60 g) (4) Mixed nuts (90 g) (5) White bread + mixed nuts (30 g) (6) White bread + mixed nuts (60 g) (7) White bread + mixed nuts (90 g)	(2), (3), (4) ↓ iAUC (healthy and T2D) (6), (7) ↓ iAUC (healthy) (7) ↓ iAUC (T2D)			

Significant differences (p ≤0.05) between intervention group(s) and control group are shown with ↑ or ↓, while ↔ indicates no significant difference. When several intervention groups are present, the results are for each group are indicated with number. Control group is referred to as (1). ADA: American Diabetes Association; d: day; F: female; g: gram; h: hour; HbA1c: glycated hemoglobin A1c; HOMA-IR: Homeostasis Assessment Model-Insulin Resistance; iAUC: incremental area under the curve; M: male; n: number; T2D: type 2 diabetes.

The effects of the marine n-3 fatty acids EPA/DHA in a liquid diet on glycemic control was investigated in a multicenter randomized trial with 30 elderly [29]. The subjects were divided into two groups receiving either an EPA/DHA-rich diet (EPA 25 mg/100 kcal and DHA 17 mg/100 kcal) or a diet without EPA/DHA (control group). A significant reduction in fasting blood glucose and HbA1c was observed after intake of EPA/DHA compared with the control diet [29]. Sarbolouki et al. included 67 men and women in a double blind, placebo-controlled randomized study to investigate the effects of EPA on glycemic regulation [28]. The participants received either EPA (2 g/day, 95% pure EPA) or placebo (2 g corn oil/day) for three months. EPA treatment reduced fasting plasma glucose, HbA1c, and HOMA-IR compared with the control group [28]. In a randomized, double blind, placebo-controlled trial, Wang and colleagues investigated the effect of 4 g fish oil per day (1.34 g EPA and 1.07 g DHA) or corn oil (control) on glucose metabolism in 99 subjects [25]. There were no significant effects on fasting serum glucose, insulin, HbA1c, or HOMA-IR after fish oil treatment for six months compared with corn oil [25]. Zhen et al. investigated the effects of n-3 PUFA from marine or vegetable sources on glycemic control in 166 subjects [26]. The study was a double blind RCT and the participants received either fish oil (2 g/day EPA + DHA), flaxseed oil (2.5 g/day alpha linolenic acid (ALA)), or corn oil (control group) for 180 days. Intake of fish oil, but not flaxseed oil, reduced HbA1c compared with corn oil. There were no effect on fasting insulin or glucose [26]. In order to determine the effects of n-3 fatty acids, a randomized, double blind, placebo-controlled trial was conducted in 81 subjects [31]. The subjects received capsules with either n-3 fatty acids (1.6 g/day EPA and 0.8 g/day DHA) or sunflower oil (control group) for two months. Treatment with n-3 fatty acids significantly decreased HbA1c, while fasting blood glucose was not significantly altered [31]. In line with these results, 6 g/day of either fish oil (1.8 g n-3 PUFAs) or sunflower oil (control) given to 10 men for two months did not show any significant changes in fasting blood glucose, insulin, or HbA1c between the groups [33]. The study had a randomized, double blind crossover design. In the same study, supplementation with fish oil did not alter basal hepatic glucose production and there were no difference in insulin suppression of hepatic glucose production nor in insulin stimulation of whole-body glucose disposal measured by the euglycemic-hyperinsulinemic clamp between the groups [33]. In a double blind RCT, Pedersen and colleagues investigated the impact of vitamin E-enriched fish oil in 44 subjects [32]. The participants received a daily dose of 4 g of either fish oil (2.6 g/day EPA + DHA) or corn oil (control) for eight weeks, in addition to an equal amount of vitamin E (53.6 g/day). There were no significant changes in fasting blood glucose or HbA1c between the groups. However, within the fish oil group, fasting blood glucose was increased [32]. In a double blind, randomized crossover study, 10 g of fish oil (1.8 g EPA + 1.2 g DHA) or olive oil (control) were given daily to eight male subjects for two weeks [37]. There were no significant changes in fasting blood glucose, average daily blood glucose, hyperglycemic clamp, nor insulin sensitivity [37]. In a double blind, randomized, crossover study, 11 subjects received supplements with fish oil, linseed oil, or olive oil (control) for three months in a dose corresponding to 35 mg fatty acids per kilogram body weight [35]. Neither fish oil nor linseed oil modulated glycemic control (fasting glucose and insulin, HbA1c, insulin sensitivity, glucose effectiveness, acute insulin response to glucose) compared with the control group [35]. Morgan and colleagues gave 40 subjects (18 men and 22 women) 9 g of fish oil, 18 g of fish oil, 9 g of corn oil, or 18 g of corn oil daily as a supplement for 12 weeks [36]. They did not detect any effect within (9 g versus 18 g) nor between (fish oil groups combined versus corn oil groups combined) the intervention groups on fasting glucose or HbA1c [36]. In a study by Borkman et al., 10 subjects were included in a three week blinded crossover study [38]. Subjects were given a standard diabetic diet supplemented with a daily dose of 10 g fish oil concentrate (30% n-3 fatty acids), 10 g safflower oil, or no supplementation (control). Fasting blood glucose increased with 14% during fish oil and 11% during safflower oil supplementation compared with control, whereas fasting insulin level remained unchanged [38].

Taken together, about half of the included studies (eight out of 14) found no significant changes related to markers of glycemic regulation such as fasting glucose, insulin, HbA1c or markers related to insulin resistance or sensitivity [25,27,30,32,33,35–37] after intervention with fish or fish oil when compared with a control group. In five of the studies a reduction in glucose [28,29], insulin [28,34] and/or HbA1c [26,28,29,31] was observed. Impaired glycemic regulation was observed in two studies, where intake of fish or fish oil increased fasting glucose [38] and an increase in HbA1c [34] was observed after intake of fish in combination with light exercise. In addition to the between groups effects, two of the studies found an additional effect on glycemic regulation within groups, in which Dunstan et al. observed increased HbA1c [34], while Balfego et al. found decreased effect on fasting insulin, HbA1c, and HOMA-IR [27]. In a recent meta-analysis of 11 RCTs including people with T2D, overweight individuals, or healthy individuals, Akinkuolie et al. showed that consumption of n-3 PUFAs did not affect insulin [60]. In line with this, a lack of association between n-3 PUFAs in blood and risk of T2D was the conclusion in the Uppsala Longitudinal Study of Adult Men (ULSAM) [61].

Since about half of the studies in the present review reported improved glycemic regulation while the other half reported no or impaired effects, it is difficult to draw a firm conclusion about fish and fish oil and glycemic regulation.

3.2. Vegetable Oils

Vegetable oils are rich in PUFAs, the main constituent being n-6 fatty acids, and in particular linoleic acid (LA). There is convincing evidence that partial replacement of SFAs with monounsaturated fatty acids (MUFAs) or PUFAs lowers fasting blood total- and LDL-cholesterol [5,13–15] and thereby reduces the risk of developing CVDs [5,6,13,14,62–64]. In addition to the cholesterol-lowering effects of PUFAs, some studies indicate that PUFAs may improve glycemic regulation [13,19]. Twelve studies investigating the effect of vegetable oils on glycemic control in people with T2D or NIDDM were included in this review (Table 2).

Foster and colleagues examined markers of glycemic control in 43 postmenopausal women after intake of flaxseed oil (high in alpha-linolenic acid (ALA)) for 12 weeks [40]. The study was a randomized, double blind, placebo-controlled trial, and the participants received either 40 mg/day zinc, 2 g/day flaxseed oil, both zinc and flaxseed oil, or olive oil (control). There were no significant changes in blood glucose, insulin, HbA1c or HOMA-IR between the intervention groups after 12 weeks. However, insulin and HOMA-IR decreased within the control group [40]. In a study by Jenkins et al., the combined effect of ALA, MUFAs, and low glycemic load on glycemic control and CVD risk factors were investigated in 141 subjects [41]. The study was a RCT with a parallel design and the subjects were provided daily with canola oil-enriched whole-wheat bread (500 kcal/day or 31 g canola oil per 2000 kcal) or whole-wheat bread without canola oil (500 kcal) (control diet). The test diet significantly reduced HbA1c compared with the control diet and the result remained statistically significant after adjustment for body weight change [41]. Barre and coworkers investigated the effect of flaxseed oil on glycemic control in 32 subjects [44]. The subjects were randomly assigned to receive 10 g/day of flaxseed oil or safflower oil for three months. The amount of ALA was approximately 60 mg/kg body weight/day in the flaxseed oil group. Flaxseed oil had no impact on fasting blood glucose, insulin, or HbA1c compared with the control group [44]. Conjugated linoleic acid (CLA), the *trans* fatty acid of LA, was compared with safflower oil high in *cis*-LA in 35 obese, postmenopausal women [43]. The participants consumed 8 g oil per day for 16 weeks in a crossover study, with four weeks washout in between the intervention periods, giving a total of 36 weeks. The aim of the study was to investigate weight reduction, and they found a significant reduction in BMI after CLA oil intake but not after safflower oil intake. Nevertheless, even though a weight reduction is associated with improved glycemic regulation, there was a significant reduction in fasting blood glucose only within the safflower oil group [43]. To investigate the long-term effects of a diet enriched in LA on insulin sensitivity, Heine and colleagues conducted a randomized, crossover study in 14 subjects [50]. The PUFA to SFA ratio (P:S ratio) of the diets were altered by substituting LA-rich fats and oils for products rich in saturated fats. The participants received a diet (total fat content of 38–39 E%) with a P:S ratio of 0.3 (low P:S diet) or 1.0 (high P:S diet) in a randomized order for 30 weeks each. Fasting blood glucose, insulin, HbA1c, glucose incremental area under the curve (iAUC), C-peptide, and insulin responses did not differ between the groups after intervention. However, the metabolic clearance rate of glucose was higher in the high P:S diet compared with the control group. This difference was only observed at the lowest infusion rate (6 mg/kg/min) [50]. A 12-week intervention with bakery products containing flaxseed oil (13 g/day), milled flaxseed (32 g/day), or no flaxseed (control group) investigated the effects on fasting blood glucose, insulin, and HbA1c in 34 adult males and females [42]. The flaxseed and flaxseed oil groups received equivalent amounts of 7.4 g ALA per day. There were no differences in fasting HbA1c, glucose and insulin after the intervention period [42]. Isocaloric diets with different fatty acid composition was investigated in a randomized crossover trial with 16 obese subjects for six weeks [48]. The energy content of carbohydrate, protein and fats were kept constant, but the diets differed in fat composition. There were no significant changes between the diets in HbA1c, fasting blood glucose, insulin, or postprandial glycemic response. However, serum insulin and C-peptide responses increased following the *trans*-MUFA and SAT diets compared with the *cis*-MUFA diet [48]. In a study by Gerhard et al., the effect of two ad libitum diets on glycemic control was investigated [45]. Eleven subjects were randomly assigned to receive an ad libitum low-fat, high-carbohydrate diet (20 E% total fat, 65 E% carbohydrates, higher in fiber), or a high-MUFA diet (40 E% total fat, 26 E% MUFAs, 45 E% carbohydrates), each for six weeks. There were no effect on fasting glucose or HbA1c after the high-MUFA diet compared with low-fat diet [45]. Brynes and coworkers investigated the effect of an isoenergetic high-MUFA diet (olive oil) compared with high-PUFA diet (corn oil), on glycemic regulation in nine overweight subjects [46]. Glycemic control remained stable throughout the study and there were no change in fasting or postprandial iAUC for glucose or insulin in response to an identical standard meal after 24 days of intervention [46]. Instead of comparing fat quality, intake of MUFAs from oil or margarine was compared with intake of carbohydrates from breakfast cereals with either a high or low glycemic index [47]. After a six-month intervention with 72 subjects there were no differences in fasting blood glucose or HbA1c between the groups. After a standard breakfast and lunch, a reduction in mean 8-h plasma insulin in the group given MUFAs compared with the cereal group was however observed [47]. During a four-week period, 12 women received an isocaloric diet high in either MUFAs (HMUFA) or complex carbohydrates (high-CHO). This crossover study had a four-week washout period during which the subjects followed the American Diabetes Association (ADA) isocaloric diet. Glycemic control, including fasting blood glucose, insulin and fructosamine did not significantly change with the different intervention diets. However, fasting blood glucose and insulin were reduced within both groups after intervention [49]. The effect of walnut oil on blood glucose in 90 subjects was investigated in a RCT, lasting for three months [39]. In the experimental group, walnut oil (15 g/day) was added to the diet, while the control group did not undergo any intervention. HbA1c level and fasting blood glucose decreased significantly in the experiment group compared with the control group [39].

In summary, six of the 12 studies investigating vegetable oils on glycemic regulation such as fasting glucose, insulin, HbA1c or markers related to insulin resistance or insulin sensitivity did not find any effects in people with T2D [40,42,44–46,49], although two of the studies found within group changes [40,49]. In the other six studies however, there were changes in glycemic regulation either between or within groups [39,41,43,47,49,50]. In contrast to the studies showing a decreasing effect on glycemic regulation after intervention, the study by Norris et al. found increased fasting glucose levels and HOMA-IR after intervention with CLA compared with safflower oil (control group). However, safflower oil reduced both fasting glucose levels and HOMA-IR within the control group [43]. Even though CLA, a *trans* fatty acid, is debated for its possible health effects [65], *trans* fatty acids in general are well known for their cholesterol increasing effects [66] and may explain the impaired effects related to glycemic regulation. Vegetable oils mainly consist of n-6 PUFAs and in particular LA, and other studies have shown a beneficial effect of n-6 PUFAs on glycemic regulation. A recent pooled analysis from prospective cohort studies demonstrated that higher levels of LA in blood were associated with a 43% reduced relative risk for T2D [67]. This is in line with the results from the ULSAM study. Men who developed T2D had a lower proportion of LA and a higher proportion of SFAs (C:14 and C:16) in serum cholesterol esters compared with those who did not develop T2D [61]. Summers et al. showed that switching from a diet rich in SFAs to a diet rich in PUFAs for 5 weeks improved insulin sensitivity in people with T2D, non-obese and obese subjects [68]. Even though others have found improved glycemic regulation after intervention with PUFAs, we are not able to draw firm conclusions based on the studies included in the present review.

3.3. Nuts

Nuts are high-energy, nutrient-dense foods that are rich in PUFAs and other bioactive components, including fiber, antioxidants, vitamins and minerals [69]. Epidemiological studies have found an inverse relationship between nut consumption and reduced risk of T2D [70,71]. In the present review, five RCTs intervening with different nuts (cashew, pistachio, peanuts or mixed nuts) in people with T2D were included (Table 3).

In the study by Mohan and coworkers, they investigated the effect of a standard diabetic diet with 30 g cashew nuts per day for 12 weeks on glycemic regulation in 300 subjects [51]. They did not find any significant differences in glycemic regulation (fasting blood glucose, insulin, HbA1c, and HOMA-IR) after the intervention [51]. In another study, by Parham et al., the effect of pistachio nut supplementation on glycemic control and inflammatory markers was investigated [53]. The study included 48 subjects in a double blind, randomized, placebo-controlled crossover trial. The subjects received either 25 g pistachio nuts twice a day or a control diet without nuts for 12 weeks, followed by an eight-week washout period, before switching interventions. A decrease in HbA1c and fasting blood glucose was observed after intake of pistachio nuts compared with the control group. There were no effects on HOMA-IR after intake of pistachio nuts [53]. Also, Sauder and coworkers investigated the effect of pistachio nuts on glycemic control [52]. They included 30 subjects in a randomized, controlled, crossover study. After a two-week run-in period, participants consumed diets with pistachio nuts (contributing with 20% of total energy) or without pistachio nuts (control group) for four weeks each, separated by a two-week washout period. Glycemic measures were assessed both fasted and during a 75-g oral glucose tolerance test. There were no effect on fasting glucose, insulin, HbA1c, HOMA-IR or glucose area under the curve (AUC) or insulin AUC after intake of nuts compared with control group [52]. Wien and colleagues investigated the effect of incorporating peanuts into the American Diabetes Association (ADA) meal plan on cardio-metabolic parameters [54]. They performed a 24-week parallel RCT with 60 subjects. The intervention group received an ADA meal plan containing about 20% of energy from peanuts, while the control group followed a peanut-free ADA meal plan. After 24 weeks of intervention, there were no differences in fasting blood glucose or HbA1c between the groups. [54]. In a study by Kendall and colleagues, the effect of nut consumption alone or in combination with white bread on postprandial glycaemia in 14 healthy compared with 10 people with T2D were examined [55]. The participants consumed 30, 60, and 90 g of mixed nuts alone or in combination with white bread (50 g available carbohydrate). All three doses of mixed nuts consumed alone significantly reduced the glycemic response compared with the control group. Adding nuts (60 g and 90 g) to white bread significantly reduced the glycemic response in healthy subjects however, significant reduction in glycemic response were only observed after adding 90 g nuts to white bread in people with T2D [55].

Taken together, three of the five studies investigating intake of nuts and glycemic regulation such as fasting blood glucose, insulin, HbA1c or markers related to insulin resistance or sensitivity found beneficial effects in T2D. Pistachio nuts reduced both fasting blood glucose levels and HbA1c [53] or fructosamine [52], and intervention with mixed nuts led to reduction in postprandial glycemic response [55]. In these studies, nut consumption benefits glycemic regulation regardless of the type of nuts, study design or duration. These results are in line with the The Prevención con Dieta Mediterránea (PREDIMED)-study, in which 30 g nuts per day (almonds, hazelnuts, and walnuts), given as supplements to a Mediterranean diet, significantly reduced the incidence of T2D compared with a low-fat diet without nut supplementation in high risk subjects [72].

4. Discussion

In the present summary, improvements related to glycemic control in people with T2D were observed in about half of the studies investigating the effect of fish, fish oil, or vegetable oil. Intake of nuts may however indicate a more beneficial effect, even though the number of studies are limited. The present review also demonstrates that the studies investigating the effect of PUFAs on glycemic control in subjects with T2D or NIDDM are quite different in design with respect to type of dietary intervention, study duration, and measurements of glycemic control, and hence the results are difficult to compare. Most importantly, the intervention and the control food differ largely between the studies. Of the included studies, mainly vegetable oils (corn, sunflower, linseed, and olives) functioned as control for both fish and fish oil interventions, and for different vegetable oils. Hence, the studies are comparing PUFAs of different quality. Considering that vegetable oils are high in PUFAs and therefore may affect glycemic regulation, the lack of effect in several of the included studies may be explained by the use of an inappropriate control group. It is therefore not possible to conclude whether intake of marine- or vegetable-derived PUFAs will have a positive effect on glycemic regulation in people with T2D. In the previous mentioned meta-analysis performed by Imamura et al., intake of PUFAs was compared with intake of SFAs. Changing the intake of SFAs with PUFAs improved glycaemia and insulin resistance [19]. SFAs may therefore represent a better control group when investigating the effect of PUFAs on glycemic regulation. The study by Imamura et al. was however not unique to T2D, as both healthy and people with T2D were included. This may explain the discrepant findings between previous studies and the present review. In addition, Coelho et al. conclude that supplementation of 0.42–5.2 g PUFAs per day for at least eight weeks may become an alternative treatment for T2D. However, only six studies were included in the review [20]. In contrast, a meta-analysis from 2011 did not find any effect of n-3 PUFA consumption on insulin sensitivity. The study included 11 studies investigating the effect in both healthy and people with T2D [60]. In addition, ALA-enriched diets did not affect HbA1c, fasting blood glucose, or insulin in a meta-analysis conducted in people with T2D. The study included eight interventions [73]. In conclusion, the reported discrepancies between other studies and this review regarding PUFAs and glycemic control are probably due to the heterogeneity of the studies.

Even though fat quality has been shown to affect glycemic regulation, it is possible that also fat quantity will be of importance. Vessby and coworkers reported that a total fat intake of more than 37 E% increases the risk of insulin resistance independent of fat quality [74]. Total fat intake were not consistently reported in the present reviewed studies, and hence we cannot rule out that a high total fat intake may have affected the results.

Limitations of the current review includes the search strategy. To ensure that the included studies had focus on glycemic regulation, the search words "glycemic control" were used. This may have affected the number of articles and we cannot rule out the possibility that some relevant studies have not been included. We did however include two studies from other reviews.

5. Conclusions

In the present review, we have identified studies that show beneficial effects of both marine and vegetable-derived PUFAs on glycemic control in people with T2D. The studies are however different in design and no firm conclusions can be drawn. In order to understand the role of PUFAs in the management of T2D, we suggest more well designed RCTs where the effect of PUFAs specifically is compared with the effect of SFAs.

Author Contributions: All authors contributed to the review. Literature search, V.H.T.-H., L.G., M.C.W.M.; Writing—Original Draft Preparation, V.H.T.-H.; Writing—Review and Editing, V.H.T.-H., L.G., M.C.W.M.

Funding: This research received no external funding.

Conflicts of Interest: The authors declare no conflict of interest.

Nutrients **2019**, 11, 1067

References

1. World Health Organization. The Top 10 Causes of Death. 2018. Available online: https://www.who.int/news-room/fact-sheets/detail/the-top-10-causes-of-death (accessed on 30 March 2019).
2. World Health Organization. *Global Report on Diabetes*; WHO: Geneva, Switzerland, 2016.
3. World Health Organization. Diabetes. 2018. Available online: https://www.who.int/en/news-room/fact-sheets/detail/diabetes (accessed on 30 March 2019).
4. Yoo, J.Y.; Kim, S.S. Probiotics and Prebiotics: Present Status and Future Perspectives on Metabolic Disorders. *Nutrients* **2016**, *8*, 173. [CrossRef] [PubMed]
5. Ulven, S.M.; Leder, L.; Elind, E.; Ottestad, I.; Christensen, J.J.; Telle-Hansen, V.H.; Skjetne, A.J.; Raael, E.; Sheikh, N.A.; Holck, M.; et al. Exchanging a few commercial, regularly consumed food items with improved fat quality reduces total cholesterol and LDL-cholesterol: A double-blind, randomised controlled trial. *Br. J. Nutr.* **2016**, *116*, 1383–1393. [CrossRef]
6. Estruch, R.; Ros, E.; Salas-Salvadó, J.; Covas, M.I.; Corella, D.; Arós, F.; Gómez-Gracia, E.; Ruiz-Gutiérrez, V.; Fiol, M.; Lapetra, J.; et al. Primary Prevention of Cardiovascular Disease with a Mediterranean Diet Supplemented with Extra-Virgin Olive Oil or Nuts. *N. Engl. J. Med.* **2018**, *379*, 1387–1389. [PubMed]
7. GBD 2015 Risk Factors Collaborators. Global, regional, and national comparative risk assessment of 79 behavioural, environmental and occupational, and metabolic risks or clusters of risks, 1990–2015: A systematic analysis for the Global Burden of Disease Study 2015. *Lancet* **2016**, *388*, 1659–1724. [CrossRef]
8. Knowler, W.C.; Barrett-Connor, E.; Fowler, S.E.; Hamman, R.F.; Lachin, J.M.; Walker, E.A.; Nathan, D.M. Reduction in the incidence of type 2 diabetes with lifestyle intervention or metformin. *N. Engl. J. Med.* **2002**, *346*, 393–403.
9. Lim, E.L.; Hollingsworth, K.G.; Aribisala, B.S.; Chen, M.J.; Mathers, J.C.; Taylor, R. Reversal of type 2 diabetes: Normalisation of beta cell function in association with decreased pancreas and liver triacylglycerol. *Diabetologia* **2011**, *54*, 2506–2514. [CrossRef] [PubMed]
10. Barnard, N.D.; Katcher, H.I.; Jenkins, D.J.; Cohen, J.; Turner-McGrievy, G. Vegetarian and vegan diets in type 2 diabetes management. *Nutr. Rev.* **2009**, *67*, 255–263. [CrossRef] [PubMed]
11. Barnard, R.J.; Jung, T.; Inkeles, S.B. Diet and exercise in the treatment of NIDDM. The need for early emphasis. *Diabetes Care* **1994**, *17*, 1469–1472. [CrossRef] [PubMed]
12. O'Flaherty, M.; Flores-Mateo, G.; Nnoaham, K.; Lloyd-Williams, F.; Capewell, S. Potential cardiovascular mortality reductions with stricter food policies in the United Kingdom of Great Britain and Northern Ireland. *Bull. World Health Organ.* **2012**, *90*, 522–531. [CrossRef]
13. Schwab, U.; Lauritzen, L.; Tholstrup, T.; Haldorsson, T.I.; Risérus, U.; Uusitupa, M.; Becker, W. Effect of the amount and type of dietary fat on cardiometabolic risk factors and risk of developing type 2 diabetes, cardiovascular diseases, and cancer: A systematic review. *Food Nutr. Res.* **2014**, *58*, 25145. [CrossRef] [PubMed]
14. Mozaffarian, D.; Micha, R.; Wallace, S. Effects on Coronary Heart Disease of Increasing Polyunsaturated Fat in Place of Saturated Fat: A Systematic Review and Meta-Analysis of Randomized Controlled Trials. *PLoS Med.* **2010**, *7*, e1000252. [CrossRef] [PubMed]
15. Jakobsen, M.U.; O'Reilly, E.J.; Heitmann, B.L.; Pereira, M.A.; Bälter, K.; Fraser, G.E.; Goldbourt, U.; Hallmans, G.; Knekt, P.; Liu, S.; et al. Major types of dietary fat and risk of coronary heart disease: A pooled analysis of 11 cohort studies123. *Am. J. Clin. Nutr.* **2009**, *89*, 1425–1432. [CrossRef]
16. Kinsell, L.W.; Michaels, G.D.; Olson, F.E.; Coelho, M.; McBride, Y.; Fukayama, G.; Conklin, J.; Walker, G. Dietary Fats and the Diabetic Patient. *N. Engl. J. Med.* **1959**, *261*, 431–434. [CrossRef] [PubMed]
17. Mann, J. Nutrition Recommendations for the Treatment and Prevention of Type 2 Diabetes and the Metabolic Syndrome: An Evidenced-Based Review. *Nutr. Rev.* **2006**, *64*, 422–427. [CrossRef]
18. Riserus, U.; Willett, W.C.; Hu, F.B. Dietary fats and prevention of type 2 diabetes. *Prog. Lipid Res.* **2009**, *48*, 44–51. [CrossRef] [PubMed]
19. Imamura, F.; Micha, R.; Wu, J.H.Y.; Otto, M.C.D.O.; Otite, F.O.; Abioye, A.I.; Mozaffarian, D. Effects of Saturated Fat, Polyunsaturated Fat, Monounsaturated Fat, and Carbohydrate on Glucose-Insulin Homeostasis: A Systematic Review and Meta-analysis of Randomised Controlled Feeding Trials. *PLoS Med.* **2016**, *13*, 1002087. [CrossRef]

20. Coelho, O.G.L.; da Silva, B.P.; Rocha, D.M.U.P.; Lopes, L.L.; Alfenas, R.C.G. Polyunsaturated fatty acids and type 2 diabetes: Impact on the glycemic control mechanism. *Crit. Rev. Food Sci. Nutr.* **2017**, *57*, 3614–3619. [CrossRef]

21. Meyer, K.A.; Kushi, L.H.; Jacobs, D.R.; Folsom, A.R. Dietary Fat and Incidence of Type 2 Diabetes in Older Iowa Women. *Diabetes Care* **2001**, *24*, 1528–1535. [CrossRef]

22. Salmerón, J.; Hu, F.B.; Manson, J.E.; Stampfer, M.J.; Colditz, G.A.; Rimm, E.B.; Willett, W.C. Dietary fat intake and risk of type 2 diabetes in women. *Am. J. Clin. Nutr.* **2001**, *73*, 1019–1026. [CrossRef] [PubMed]

23. Hartweg, J.; Perera, R.; Montori, V.M.; Dinneen, S.F.; Neil, A.H.; Farmer, A.J. Omega-3 polyunsaturated fatty acids (PUFA) for type 2 diabetes mellitus. *Cochrane Database Syst. Rev.* **2008**. [CrossRef] [PubMed]

24. Wanders, A.J.; Blom, W.A.M.; Zock, P.L.; Geleijnse, J.M.; Brouwer, I.A.; Alssema, M. Plant-derived polyunsaturated fatty acids and markers of glucose metabolism and insulin resistance: A meta-analysis of randomized controlled feeding trials. *BMJ Open Diabetes Res. Care* **2019**, *7*, e000585. [CrossRef]

25. Wang, F.; Wang, Y.; Zhu, Y.; Liu, X.; Xia, H.; Yang, X.; Sun, G. Treatment for 6 months with fish oil-derived n-3 polyunsaturated fatty acids has neutral effects on glycemic control but improves dyslipidemia in type 2 diabetic patients with abdominal obesity: A randomized, double-blind, placebo-controlled trial. *Eur. J. Nutr.* **2017**, *56*, 2415–2422. [CrossRef] [PubMed]

26. Zheng, J.S.; Lin, M.; Fang, L.; Yu, Y.; Yuan, L.; Jin, Y.; Feng, J.; Wang, L.; Yang, H.; Chen, W.; et al. Effects of n-3 fatty acid supplements on glycemic traits in Chinese type 2 diabetic patients: A double-blind randomized controlled trial. *Mol. Nutr. Food Res.* **2016**, *60*, 2176–2184. [CrossRef]

27. Balfegó, M.; Canivell, S.; Hanzu, F.A.; Sala-Vila, A.; Martínez-Medina, M.; Murillo, S.; Mur, T.; Ruano, E.G.; Linares, F.; Porras, N.; et al. Effects of sardine-enriched diet on metabolic control, inflammation and gut microbiota in drug-naïve patients with type 2 diabetes: A pilot randomized trial. *Lipids Heal.* **2016**, *15*, 78. [CrossRef] [PubMed]

28. Sarbolouki, S.; Javanbakht, M.; Derakhshanian, H.; Hosseinzadeh, P.; Zareei, M.; Hashemi, S.; Dorosty, A.; Eshraghian, M.; Djalali, M. Eicosapentaenoic acid improves insulin sensitivity and blood sugar in overweight type 2 diabetes mellitus patients: A double-blind randomised clinical trial. *Singap. Med. J.* **2013**, *54*, 387–390. [CrossRef]

29. Ogawa, S.; Abe, T.; Nako, K.; Okamura, M.; Senda, M.; Sakamoto, T.; Ito, S. Eicosapentaenoic Acid Improves Glycemic Control in Elderly Bedridden Patients with Type 2 Diabetes. *Tohoku J. Exp. Med.* **2013**, *231*, 63–74. [CrossRef]

30. Crochemore, I.C.C.; Souza, A.F.; de Souza, A.C.; Rosado, E.L. Omega-3 polyunsaturated fatty acid supplementation does not influence body composition, insulin resistance, and lipemia in women with type 2 diabetes and obesity. *Nutr. Clin. Pract.* **2012**, *27*, 553–560. [CrossRef]

31. Pooya, S.; Jalali, M.D.; Jazayery, A.D.; Saedisomeolia, A.; Eshraghian, M.R.; Toorang, F. The efficacy of omega-3 fatty acid supplementation on plasma homocysteine and malondialdehyde levels of type 2 diabetic patients. *Nutr. Metab. Cardiovasc. Dis.* **2010**, *20*, 326–331. [CrossRef] [PubMed]

32. Pedersen, H.; Petersen, M.; Major-Pedersen, A.; Jensen, T.; Nielsen, N.S.; Lauridsen, S.T.; Marckmann, P. Influence of fish oil supplementation on in vivo and in vitro oxidation resistance of low-density lipoprotein in type 2 diabetes. *Eur. J. Clin. Nutr.* **2003**, *57*, 713–720. [CrossRef]

33. Luo, J.; Rizkalla, S.W.; Vidal, H.; Oppert, J.-M.; Colas, C.; Boussairi, A.; Guerre-Millo, M.; Chapuis, A.-S.; Chevalier, A.; Durand, G.; et al. Moderate Intake of n-3 Fatty Acids for 2 Months Has No Detrimental Effect on Glucose Metabolism and Could Ameliorate the Lipid Profile in Type 2 Diabetic Men: Results of a controlled study. *Diabetes Care* **1998**, *21*, 717–724. [CrossRef]

34. Dunstan, D.W.; Mori, T.A.; Puddey, I.B.; Beilin, L.J.; Burke, V.; Morton, A.R.; Stanton, K.G. The Independent and Combined Effects of Aerobic Exercise and Dietary Fish Intake on Serum Lipids and Glycemic Control in NIDDM: A randomized controlled study. *Diabetes Care* **1997**, *20*, 913–921. [CrossRef]

35. McManus, R.M.; Jumpson, J.; Finegood, D.T.; Clandinin, M.T.; Ryan, E.A. A Comparison of the Effects of n-3 Fatty Acids from Linseed Oil and Fish Oil in Well-Controlled Type II Diabetes. *Diabetes Care* **1996**, *19*, 463–467. [CrossRef]

36. Morgan, W.A.; Raskin, P.; Rosenstock, J. A Comparison of Fish Oil or Corn Oil Supplements in Hyperlipidemic Subjects with NIDDM. *Diabetes Care* **1995**, *18*, 83–86. [CrossRef]

37. Annuzzi, G.; Rivellese, A.; Capaldo, B.; Di Marino, L.; Iovine, C.; Marotta, G.; Riccardi, G. A controlled study on the effects of n − 3 fatty acids on lipid and glucose metabolism in non-insulin-dependent diabetic patients. *Atherosclerosis* **1991**, *87*, 65–73. [CrossRef]

38. Borkman, M.; Chisholm, D.J.; Furler, S.M.; Storlien, L.H.; Kraegen, E.W.; Simons, L.A.; Chesterman, C.N. Effects of Fish Oil Supplementation on Glucose and Lipid Metabolism in NIDDM. *Diabetes* **1989**, *38*, 1314–1319. [CrossRef]

39. Zibaeenezhad, M.; Aghasadeghi, K.; Hakimi, H.; Yarmohammadi, H.; Nikaein, F. The Effect of Walnut Oil Consumption on Blood Sugar in Patients with Diabetes Mellitus Type 2. *Int. J. Endocrinol. Metab.* **2016**, *14*, e34889.

40. Foster, M.; Petocz, P.; Caterson, I.D.; Samman, S. Effects of zinc and α-linolenic acid supplementation on glycemia and lipidemia in women with type 2 diabetes mellitus: A randomized, double-blind, placebo-controlled trial. *J. Diabetes Res. Clin. Metab.* **2013**, *2*, 3–9. [CrossRef]

41. Jenkins, D.J.; Kendall, C.W.; Vuksan, V.; Faulkner, D.; Augustin, L.S.; Mitchell, S.; Ireland, C.; Srichaikul, K.; Mirrahimi, A.; Chiavaroli, L.; et al. Effect of Lowering the Glycemic Load With Canola Oil on Glycemic Control and Cardiovascular Risk Factors: A Randomized Controlled Trial. *Diabetes Care* **2014**, *37*, 1806–1814. [CrossRef]

42. Taylor, C.G.; Noto, A.D.; Stringer, D.M.; Froese, S.; Malcolmson, L. Dietary Milled Flaxseed and Flaxseed Oil Improve N-3 Fatty Acid Status and Do Not Affect Glycemic Control in Individuals with Well-Controlled Type 2 Diabetes. *J. Am. Nutr.* **2010**, *29*, 72–80. [CrossRef]

43. Norris, L.E.; Collene, A.L.; Asp, M.L.; Hsu, J.C.; Liu, L.-F.; Richardson, J.R.; Li, D.; Bell, D.; Osei, K.; Jackson, R.D.; et al. Comparison of dietary conjugated linoleic acid with safflower oil on body composition in obese postmenopausal women with type 2 diabetes mellitus1234. *Am. J. Clin. Nutr.* **2009**, *90*, 468–476. [CrossRef]

44. Barre, D.E.; Mizier-Barre, K.A.; Griscti, O.; Hafez, K. High Dose Flaxseed Oil Supplementation May Affect Fasting Blood Serum Glucose Management in Human Type 2 Diabetics. *J. Oleo Sci.* **2008**, *57*, 269–273. [CrossRef]

45. Gerhard, G.T.; Ahmann, A.; Meeuws, K.; McMurry, M.P.; Duell, P.B.; Connor, W.E. Effects of a low-fat diet compared with those of a high-monounsaturated fat diet on body weight, plasma lipids and lipoproteins, and glycemic control in type 2 diabetes. *Am. J. Clin. Nutr.* **2004**, *80*, 668–673. [CrossRef] [PubMed]

46. Brynes, A.E.; Edwards, C.M.; Jadhav, A.; Ghatei, M.A.; Bloom, S.R.; Frost, G.S. Diet-induced change in fatty acid composition of plasma triacylglycerols is not associated with change in glucagon-like peptide 1 or insulin sensitivity in people with type 2 diabetes. *Am. J. Clin. Nutr.* **2000**, *72*, 1111–1118. [CrossRef]

47. Tsihlias, E.B.; Gibbs, A.L.; McBurney, M.I.; Wolever, T.M. Comparison of high- and low-glycemic-index breakfast cereals with monounsaturated fat in the long-term dietary management of type 2 diabetes. *Am. J. Clin. Nutr.* **2000**, *72*, 439–449. [CrossRef] [PubMed]

48. Christiansen, E.; Schnider, S.; Palmvig, B.; Tauber-Lassen, E.; Pedersen, O. Intake of a Diet High in Trans Monounsaturated Fatty Acids or Saturated Fatty Acids: Effects on postprandial insulinemia and glycemia in obese patients with NIDDM. *Diabetes Care* **1997**, *20*, 881–887. [CrossRef]

49. Lerman-Garber, I.; Ichazo-Cerro, S.; Cardoso-Saldaña, G.; Posadas-Romero, C.; Zamora-Gonzalez, J. Effect of a High-Monounsaturated Fat Diet Enriched With Avocado in NIDDM Patients. *Diabetes Care* **1994**, *17*, 311–315. [CrossRef]

50. Heine, R.J.; Mulder, C.; Popp-Snijders, C.; Van Der Meer, J.; Van Der Veen, E.A. Linoleic-acid-enriched diet: Long-term effects on serum lipoprotein and apolipoprotein concentrations and insulin sensitivity in noninsulin-dependent diabetic patients. *Am. J. Clin. Nutr.* **1989**, *49*, 448–456. [CrossRef]

51. Mohan, V.; Gayathri, R.; Lakshmipriya, N.; Anjana, R.M.; Spiegelman, D.; Jeevan, R.G.; Balasubramaniam, K.K.; Jayanthan, M.; Gopinath, V.; Divya, S.; et al. Cashew Nut Consumption Increases HDL Cholesterol and Reduces Systolic Blood Pressure in Asian Indians with Type 2 Diabetes: A 12-Week Randomized Controlled Trial. *J. Nutr.* **2018**, *148*, 63–69. [CrossRef]

52. Sauder, K.A.; McCrea, C.E.; Ulbrecht, J.S.; Kris-Etherton, P.M.; West, S.G.; Kris-Ethertonb, S.G.W.P.M. Effects of pistachios on the lipid/lipoprotein profile, glycemic control, inflammation, and endothelial function in type 2 diabetes: A randomized trial. *Metab. Clin. Exp.* **2015**, *64*, 1521–1529. [CrossRef]

53. Parham, M.; Heidari, S.; Khorramirad, A.; Hozoori, M.; Hosseinzadeh, F.; Bakhtyari, L.; Vafaeimanesh, J. Effects of Pistachio Nut Supplementation on Blood Glucose in Patients with Type 2 Diabetes: A Randomized Crossover Trial. *Diabetes Stud.* **2014**, *11*, 190–196. [CrossRef]
54. Wien, M.; Oda, K.; Sabaté, J. A randomized controlled trial to evaluate the effect of incorporating peanuts into an American Diabetes Association meal plan on the nutrient profile of the total diet and cardiometabolic parameters of adults with type 2 diabetes. *Nutr. J.* **2014**, *13*, 10. [CrossRef] [PubMed]
55. Kendall, C.; Esfahani, A.; Josse, A.; Augustin, L.; Vidgen, E.; Jenkins, D. The glycemic effect of nut-enriched meals in healthy and diabetic subjects. *Nutr. Metab. Cardiovasc. Dis.* **2011**, *21*, S34–S39. [CrossRef]
56. Bang, H.O.; Dyerberg, J. Plasma lipids and lipoproteins in Greenlandic west coast Eskimos. *Acta Med. Scand.* **1972**, *192*, 85–94. [CrossRef] [PubMed]
57. Mozaffarian, D.; Wu, J.H. Omega-3 fatty acids and cardiovascular disease: Effects on risk factors, molecular pathways, and clinical events. *J. Am. Coll. Cardiol.* **2011**, *58*, 2047–2067. [CrossRef]
58. Delany, J.P.; Vivian, V.M.; Snook, J.T.; Anderson, P.A. Effects of fish oil on serum lipids in men during a controlled feeding trial. *Am. J. Clin. Nutr.* **1990**, *52*, 477–485. [CrossRef]
59. Saynor, R.; Verel, D.; Gillott, T. The long-term effect of dietary supplementation with fish lipid concentrate on serum lipids, bleeding time, platelets and angina. *Atherosclerosis* **1984**, *50*, 3–10. [CrossRef]
60. Akinkuolie, A.O.; Ngwa, J.S.; Meigs, J.B.; Djoussé, L. Omega-3 polyunsaturated fatty acid and insulin sensitivity: A meta-analysis of randomized controlled trials. *Clin. Nutr.* **2011**, *30*, 702–707. [CrossRef]
61. Vessby, B.; Aro, A.; Skarfors, E.; Berglund, L.; Salminen, I.; Lithell, H. The Risk to Develop NIDDM Is Related to the Fatty Acid Composition of the Serum Cholesterol Esters. *Diabetes* **1994**, *43*, 1353–1357. [CrossRef]
62. Sacks, F.M.; Campos, H. Polyunsaturated Fatty Acids, Inflammation, and Cardiovascular Disease: Time to Widen Our View of the Mechanisms. *J. Clin. Endocrinol. Metab.* **2006**, *91*, 398–400. [CrossRef]
63. Farvid, M.S.; Ding, M.; Pan, A.; Sun, Q.; Chiuve, S.E.; Steffen, L.M.; Willett, W.C.; Hu, F.B. Dietary Linoleic Acid and Risk of Coronary Heart Disease: A Systematic Review and Meta-Analysis of Prospective Cohort Studies. *Circulation* **2014**, *130*, 1568–1578. [CrossRef]
64. Warensjö, E.; Sundström, J.; Vessby, B.; Cederholm, T.; Risérus, U. Markers of dietary fat quality and fatty acid desaturation as predictors of total and cardiovascular mortality: A population-based prospective study. *Am. J. Clin. Nutr.* **2008**, *88*, 203–209. [CrossRef]
65. Kim, J.H.; Kim, Y.; Kim, Y.J.; Park, Y. Conjugated Linoleic Acid: Potential Health Benefits as a Functional Food Ingredient. *Annu. Rev. Food Sci. Technol.* **2016**, *7*, 221–244. [CrossRef]
66. Brouwer, I.A.; Wanders, A.J.; Katan, M.B. Trans fatty acids and cardiovascular health: Research completed? *Eur. J. Clin. Nutr.* **2013**, *67*, 541–547. [CrossRef]
67. Wu, J.H.Y.; Marklund, M.; Imamura, F.; Tintle, N.; Korat, A.V.A.; De Goede, J.; Zhou, X.; Yang, W.-S.; Otto, M.C.D.O.; Kröger, J.; et al. Omega-6 fatty acid biomarkers and incident type 2 diabetes: Pooled analysis of individual-level data for 39 740 adults from 20 prospective cohort studies. *Lancet Diabetes Endocrinol.* **2017**, *5*, 965–974. [CrossRef]
68. Summers, L.K.M.; Fielding, B.A.; Bradshaw, H.A.; Ilic, V.; Beysen, C.; Clark, M.L.; Moore, N.R.; Frayn, K.N. Substituting dietary saturated fat with polyunsaturated fat changes abdominal fat distribution and improves insulin sensitivity. *Diabetologia* **2002**, *45*, 369–377. [CrossRef]
69. Ros, E. Nuts and CVD. *Br. J. Nutr.* **2015**, *113* (Suppl. 2), S111–S120. [CrossRef]
70. Luo, C.; Zhang, Y.; Ding, Y.; Shan, Z.; Chen, S.; Yu, M.; Hu, F.B.; Liu, L. Nut consumption and risk of type 2 diabetes, cardiovascular disease, and all-cause mortality: A systematic review and meta-analysis. *Am. J. Clin. Nutr.* **2014**, *100*, 256–269. [CrossRef]
71. Jiang, R.; Manson, J.E.; Stampfer, M.J.; Liu, S.; Willett, W.C.; Hu, F.B. Nut and Peanut Butter Consumption and Risk of Type 2 Diabetes in Women. *JAMA* **2002**, *288*, 2554–2560. [CrossRef]
72. Salas-Salvadó, J.; Bulló, M.; Babio, N.; Martínez-González, M.Á.; Ibarrola-Jurado, N.; Basora, J.; Estruch, R.; Covas, M.I.; Corella, D.; Arós, F.; et al. Reduction in the incidence of type 2 diabetes with the Mediterranean diet: Results of the PREDIMED-Reus nutrition intervention randomized trial. *Diabetes Care* **2011**, *34*, 14–19. [CrossRef]

73. Jovanovski, E.; Li, D.; Ho, H.V.T.; Djedovic, V.; Marques, A.D.C.R.; Shishtar, E.; Mejia, S.B.; Sievenpiper, J.L.; De Souza, R.J.; Duvnjak, L.; et al. The effect of alpha-linolenic acid on glycemic control in individuals with type 2 diabetes: A systematic review and meta-analysis of randomized controlled clinical trials. *Medicine* **2017**, *96*, e6531. [CrossRef]

74. Vessby, B.; Uusitupa, M.; Hermansen, K.; Riccardi, G.; Rivellese, A.A.; Tapsell, L.C.; Nälsén, C.; Berglund, L.; Louheranta, A.; Rasmussen, B.M.; et al. Substituting dietary saturated for monounsaturated fat impairs insulin sensitivity in healthy men and women: The KANWU study. *Diabetologia* **2001**, *44*, 312–319. [CrossRef] [PubMed]

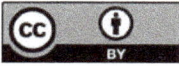

Review

nutrients

MDPI

The Effects of a Low GI Diet on Cardiometabolic and Inflammatory Parameters in Patients with Type 2 and Gestational Diabetes: A Systematic Review and Meta-Analysis of Randomised Controlled Trials

Omorogieva Ojo [1,*], Osarhumwese Osaretin Ojo [2], Xiao-Hua Wang [3] and Amanda Rodrigues Amorim Adegboye [4]

[1] Faculty of Education and Health, Department of Adult Nursing and Paramedic Science, University of Greenwich, London SE9 2UG, UK
[2] South London and Maudsley NHS Foundation Trust, University Hospital, Lewisham High Street, London SE13 6LH, UK
[3] The School of Nursing, Soochow University, Suzhou 215006, China
[4] Faculty of Education and Health, Department of Psychology, Social Work & Counselling, University of Greenwich, London SE9 2UG, UK
* Correspondence: o.ojo@greenwich.ac.uk; Tel.: +44-020-8331-8626; Fax: +44-020-8331-8060

Received: 31 May 2019; Accepted: 5 July 2019; Published: 12 July 2019

Abstract: The prevalence of diabetes is increasing globally, and its effect on patients and the healthcare system can be significant. Gestational diabetes mellitus (GDM) and type 2 diabetes are well established risk factors for cardiovascular disease, and strategies for managing these conditions include dietary interventions, such as the use of a low glycemic index (GI) diet. Aims: This review aimed to evaluate the effects of a low GI diet on the cardio-metabolic and inflammatory parameters in patients with type 2 diabetes and women with GDM and assess whether the effects are different in these conditions. Methods: This review was based on the preferred reporting items for systematic reviews and meta-analyses (PRISMA) guidelines. Three databases (EMBASE, Pubmed, and PsycINFO) were searched from inception to 20 February 2019 using search terms that included synonyms and Medical Subject Headings (MeSH) in line with the population, intervention, comparator, outcomes, and studies (PICOS) framework. Studies were evaluated for the quality and risk of bias. Results: 10 randomised controlled studies were included in the systematic review, while 9 were selected for the meta-analysis. Two distinct areas were identified: the effect of a low GI diet on lipid profile and the effect of a low GI diet on inflammatory parameters. The results of the meta-analysis showed that there were no significant differences ($p > 0.05$) between the low GI and higher GI diets with respect to total cholesterol, HDL, and LDL cholesterol in patients with type 2 diabetes. However, there was a significant difference ($p = 0.027$) with respect to triglyceride which increased by a mean of 0.06 mmol/L (0.01, 0.11) in patients with type 2 diabetes on higher GI diet. With respect to the women with GDM, the findings from the systematic review were not consistent in terms of the effect of a low GI diet on the lipid profile. The results of the meta-analysis did not show significant differences ($p > 0.05$) between low GI and higher GI diets with respect to adiponectin and C-reactive proteins in patients with type 2 diabetes, but a significant difference ($p < 0.001$) was observed between the two groups in relation to interleukin–6. Conclusion: This systematic review and meta-analysis have demonstrated that there were no significant differences ($p > 0.05$) between the low GI and higher GI diets in relation to total cholesterol—HDL and LDL cholesterol—in patients with type 2 diabetes. However, a significant difference ($p < 0.05$) was observed between the two groups with respect to triglyceride in patients with type 2 diabetes. The results of the effect of a low GI diet on the lipid profile in patients with GDM were not consistent. With respect to the inflammatory parameters, the low GI diet significantly decreased interleukin–6 in patients with type 2 diabetes compared to the higher GI diet. More studies are needed in this area of research.

Nutrients **2019**, 11, 1584

Keywords: type 2 diabetes; gestational diabetes; glycemic index; randomised controlled trial; lipid profile; inflammatory parameters

1. Introduction

Globally, there is an increasing prevalence of diabetes, with over 420 million people living with the condition. This number has significant implications for health care provisions due to the impact of diabetes and its complications on those who have the condition [1,2]. Type 2 diabetes is usually characterised by insulin deficiency due to beta cell dysfunction and often involves insulin resistance [3]. On the other hand, hyperglycaemia first detected at any time during pregnancy is classified either as diabetes in pregnancy or Gestational Diabetes Mellitus (GDM), and are usually diagnosed based on the fasting and/or 2 h plasma glucose following a 75 g oral glucose load [4].

Both type 2 diabetes and GDM have implications for carbohydrate, protein and fat metabolism and may predispose individuals to acute and long-term complications [5]. About half of the women diagnosed with GDM proceed to develop type 2 diabetes within 5 to 10 years after giving birth [6]. Due to changing lifestyles, type 2 diabetes is increasingly diagnosed in children [7]. In 2013, over 3.2 million adults were diagnosed with diabetes in England and Wales, with prevalence rates of 6% and 6.7% in England and Wales, respectively [7]. In addition, about 90% of adults who are currently diagnosed with diabetes have type 2 diabetes, with the burden of the disease disproportionally affecting ethnic minorities, particularly Africans, African-Caribbeans, and South Asians [7].

GDM presents adverse risks to the mother and child during the pre- and post–natal period [4]. It was estimated that 21.3 million live births had some form of raised blood glucose or hyperglycaemia in 2017, and about 85.1% of these were due to GDM [6]. This represented about one in every seven births affected by GDM [6]. In England and Wales, of the estimated 700,000 women who give birth every year, about 5% have either pre-existing diabetes or GDM [8]. About 87.5% of these women who have diabetes during pregnancy have GDM [8]. Therefore, management strategies, including dietary interventions such as the use of a low glycemic index (GI) diet, have been recommended instead of a higher GI diet, in order to manage hyperglycaemia and mitigate related complications [8]. In our previous review on the effect of a low GI diet in patients with type 2 diabetes, Ojo et al. [9] found that a low GI diet was more effective in controlling glycated haemoglobin and fasting blood glucose compared with a higher GI diet in these patients. Therefore, this current review builds on the earlier systematic review and meta-analysis [9] by assessing the impact of a low GI diet on lipid profile and inflammatory markers.

Why is it important to do this review? GDM is closely associated with type 2 diabetes, as they share many key pathophysiological characteristics including progressive insulin resistance [3,10]. In addition, people who develop either type 2 diabetes or GDM have similar risk factors, such as ethnicity (South Asian or Afro–Caribbean), a high body mass index (BMI), family history, and advanced age [5,10].

Although low grade inflammation and insulin resistance are part of normal physiological adaptation of pregnancy, these processes are exacerbated in patients with GDM and obesity [11]. Elevated levels of inflammatory components, such as tumour necrosis factor alpha (TNF-α), have been shown to correlate with progressive insulin resistance in pregnancy and are associated with hyperinsulinaemia in obesity and in patients with type 2 diabetes [10]. The risks associated with GDM, including postpartum type 2 diabetes, increase with progressive hyperglycaemia [8,12]. Furthermore, both GDM and type 2 diabetes are well established risk factors for cardiovascular diseases [3,5,13].

This calls for scrutiny and a greater understanding of the role of low GI diets on inflammatory parameters and lipid profiles (cardiometabolic parameters) in these patients, as the biomarkers have implications for insulin resistance and cardiovascular mortality. We know this based on the knowledge that dietary interventions are useful approaches to managing type 2 diabetes and GDM.

Therefore, a study should involve an evaluation of the effect, and quality and quantity of the macro and micronutrients in the foods consumed. Of particular interest is the quality of carbohydrate in the diets of people with type 2 diabetes or GDM, often linked to its glycemic index (GI). Foods with low GI may improve glycemic control including the reduction in glycated haemoglobin (HbA1c) through improvement in peripheral insulin sensitivity [14–19]. However, the evidence regarding the effect of a low GI diet on lipid profiles is still conflicting.

Bouchie et al. [20] revealed that 5 weeks of a low GI diet was useful in improving plasma lipids in non-diabetic men who were moderately overweight. However, in normolipidemic well controlled patients with type 2 diabetes, Brand et al. [21] observed that low GI diets did not provide improvement in plasma lipids. Clar et al. [22], in their meta–analysis, noted that there is, presently, no compelling evidence that shows that low GI diets have significant beneficial effects on blood lipids. On the other hand, Schwingshacki and Hoffman [23] demonstrated that a low GI diet has beneficial effects with respect to pro–inflammatory markers, such as C–reactive protein (CRP) which may be useful in preventing obesity associated diseases. This study involved both patients who had type 2 diabetes and participants who were non–diabetic. The systematic reviews by Goff et al. [13], Clar et al. [22], and Fleming and Godwin [24] were based on assessing the effect of low GI diets on lipid profiles on either general participants or those with cardiovascular diseases. No previous review has assessed the effect of a low GI diet on both lipids and the inflammatory profile of patients with type 2 diabetes and/or GDM. Therefore, the current review evaluates the impact of a low GI diet on the cardio-metabolic and inflammatory parameters in patients with type 2 diabetes and GDM. This is based on the understanding that the control of cardio-metabolic parameters is a useful approach in managing patients with type 2 diabetes and women with GDM [4,25].

Objectives:

This is a systematic review and meta-analysis which:

- Evaluates the effect of a low GI diet on cardio-metabolic and inflammatory parameters in patients with type 2 diabetes and women with GDM.

2. Methods

This systematic review and meta-analysis was written according to the preferred reporting items for systematic reviews and meta-analyses (PRISMA) guidelines [26]. The eligibility criteria for paper inclusion according to type of study, participants, intervention, and outcomes are described below.

Types of Studies:

Randomised controlled studies were the only studies included in this review (Tables 1 and 2).

Type of Participants:

Patients with type 2 diabetes or pregnant women with gestational diabetes were the participants of interest in all the studies selected (Table 2).

Type of Interventions:

Diets with low GI were compared with diets with higher GI in patients with type 2 diabetes and in women with GDM. The classification of diets as having either low GI or higher GI was based on the lower GI values of the intervention diets (low GI diet).

2.1. Outcomes of Interest

The primary measures of interest were:

- Cardio-metabolic parameters: total cholesterol (TC) mmol/L, low density lipoprotein (LDL) cholesterol mmol/L, high density lipoprotein (HDL) cholesterol mmol/L, and triglycerides (TG) mmol/L.

The secondary outcome measures were:

- Inflammatory parameters: C–reactive protein (CRP) mg/L, Adiponectin mg/L, and Interleukin–6 (IL-6) mg/L.

2.2. Search Terms and Search Strategy

The process of searching for articles for this review relied on the Population, Intervention, Comparator, Outcome, and Study design (PICOS) approach [27] and involved electronic databases (EMBASE, Pubmed, and PsycINFO) from inception to 20 February 2019. A number of articles were identified through this process by using search terms, including Medical Subject Headings (MeSH) and synonyms. Boolean operators (AND/OR) were used to combine words and search terms (Table 1). The reference lists of included articles were manually searched for relevant papers.

2.3. Inclusion and Exclusion Criteria

The criteria for selecting studies are outlined in Table 2. No time or language restriction was applied. Only primary research studies that were randomised controlled trials were selected for this review. In addition, studies involving patients with type 2 diabetes or GDM and the use of low GI diets across the world were included. Those studies not meeting the criteria set out in Table 2 and the text were excluded from this review. In this regard, studies that had animals, patients with type 1 diabetes, children with diabetes, or healthy adults without diabetes were excluded from the current review (Table 2). In addition, observational studies and those involving dietary supplements were excluded. Therefore, a total of 9 studies were included in the meta-analysis (Figure 1).

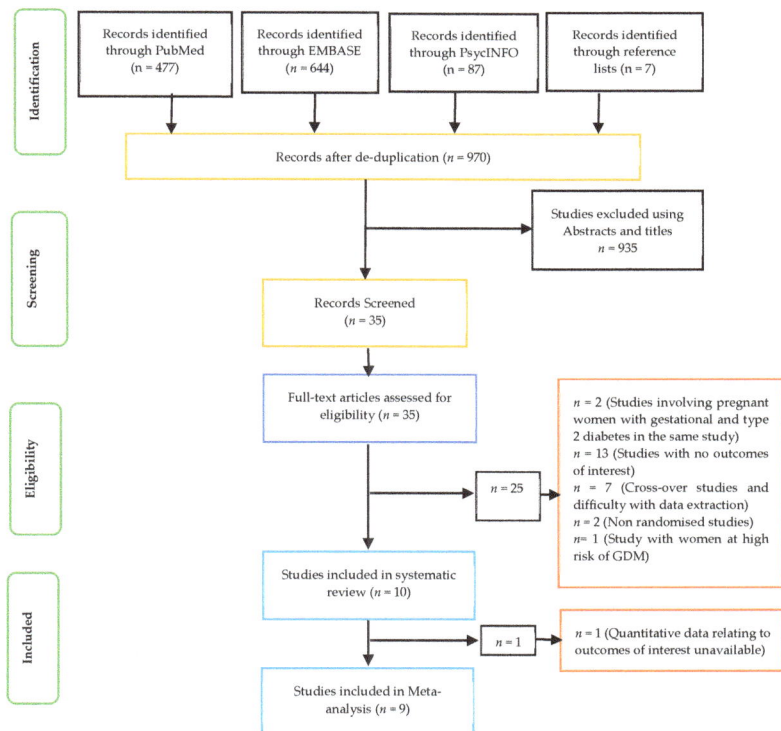

Figure 1. Prisma flow chart showing the studies included.

Table 1. Search Strategy and Search Terms.

Population	Intervention	Comparator	Study Designs	Combining Search Terms
Patients with Diabetes	**Low Glycemic Index (GI) Diet**	**Higher GI Diet**	**Randomised Controlled Trial**	
Type 2 diabetes OR diabetes OR Patients with diabetes OR diabetes mellitus OR Gestational diabetes OR gestational diabetes mellitus (GDM) OR gestational diabetes mellitus OR diabetes mellitus, gestational OR diabetes in pregnancy	GI diet OR glycemic index OR Glycemic Index Numbers OR glycemic load OR Glycemic Indices OR Glycemic Index Number		#1 Controlled clinical trial OR Randomised controlled trial OR placebo OR randomized OR groups OR drug therapy OR randomly OR trial	Column 1 AND Column 2 AND Column 3
			#2 "Animals" NOT "Humans"	
			#3 #1 NOT #2	

Table 2. Inclusion and Exclusion Criteria Based on PICOS Framework.

	Inclusion Criteria	Exclusion Criteria
Population	Patients with gestational diabetes or patients with type 2 diabetes	Studies involving participants with type 1 diabetes and animal studies. Studies that include children that have diabetes or adults that are healthy. Pre-existing diabetes in patients who are pregnant
Intervention	Low GI diet	Studies involving dietary supplements
Comparator	higher GI diet	Studies involving additional supplements
Outcomes	Primary outcome measures of interest: Cardio-metabolic: total cholesterol, low density lipoprotein (LDL) cholesterol, high density lipoprotein (HDL) cholesterol, triglycerides. Secondary outcome measures of interest: Inflammatory parameters: C–reactive protein, Adiponectin and Interleukin–6	Qualitative outcomes
Types of Study: Quantitative	Randomised controlled trials	Observational studies Letters Comments Reviews Editorials

2.4. Quality Assessment and Risk of Bias of Included Studies

The Critical Appraisal Skills Programme (CASP) checklist for randomised controlled trials [28] was used to evaluate the studies. In addition, the Cochrane risk of bias tool [29,30] was used to assess the methodological quality of the included studies. A grade (or score) was allocated to each trial on the basis of selection bias, performance bias, detection bias, attrition bias, and reporting bias. This process involved reviewing details about the similarity at baseline of the groups being compared, the blindness of the outcome measurement and participants, the randomisation method, dropout rates, selective reporting, and compliance with the intervention. On the basis of this information, studies were categorised into three groups: (a) low risk of bias, (b) unclear risk of bias, and (c) high risk of bias.

2.5. Data Extraction and Management

Statistical Analysis

Treatment effects were summarized as the weighted mean difference (WMD) with standard deviation by using the absolute change values from baseline to post-intervention for control and intervention groups. The meta-analysis was performed in stata (version 15.0, Stata Corp, College Station, TX, USA). Fixed-effects models were applied to estimate the overall weighted mean difference.

All results were presented with a 95% confidence interval (CI) and displayed on a forest plot and table, and the null hypothesis of no effect was rejected at $p \leq 0.05$. In addition to the forest plots, I^2 statistics were assessed to quantify the degree of heterogeneity. Values <25% were considered to be low, 25%–50% moderate, and >50% high. Q statistics was also used to assess heterogeneity. The null hypothesis of homogeneity was rejected if $p < 0.1$, given the low power of the test [29].

2.6. Data Inclusion Decisions

Gomes et al. [31] expressed their results as the median and interquartile ranges, which were converted to means and standard deviations [29]. In addition, for the meta-analysis, the units of measurements for the lipid parameters were converted to mmol/L, while for the inflammatory markers, they were converted to mg/L. The Grant et al. [32] study was not included in the meta-analysis, as the information provided showed that there were no significant differences ($p > 0.05$) between the low GI and the higher GI groups in terms of lipids and inflammatory markers. However, these results were not expressed in quantitative terms.

3. Results

Ten studies were selected for the systematic review (Table 3), and nine studies were included in the meta-analysis (Table 4). In addition, while four of the studies were conducted in Canada, two were carried out in China and one study each was carried out in Brazil, Greece, Malaysia, and the USA. The total number of subjects in the eight studies included in the meta-analysis in patients with type 2 diabetes involved 394 participants in the low GI group and 388 participants in the higher GI group. There were 41 subjects in the low GI group compared with 42 participants in the higher GI group in the only study on women with GDM.

Based on the systematic review (Tables 3 and 4) and meta-analysis, two distinct areas have been identified: the effect of a low GI diet on lipid profiles and the effect of a low GI diet on inflammatory parameters.

Table 3. The summary of studies selected for the review.

Citation	Country	Type of Diabetes	Length of Study	Study Type	Age (Years)	Sample Size	Interventions/Glycemic Index (GI) Values	Results/Conclusion
Gomes et al. [31]	Brazil	Type 2 diabetes	1 month	Parallel Design	42.4 ± 5.1	$n = 20$	Low GI diet v. higher GI diet (Mean ± SD) Baseline Higher GI: 66 ± 4 Low GI: 63 ± 6 Post-intervention Higher GI: 72 ± 3 Low GI: 54 ± 4	Serum non esterified fatty acid level increased in the higher GI group compared to the low GI group after intervention ($p = 0.032$). Low GI diet prevented the inflammatory responses induced by higher GI diet.
Grant et al. [32]	Canada	GDM	From 28 weeks gestation until delivery	Parallel Design	Higher GI: 34 ± 1.1 Low GI: 34 ± 0.1	Low GI: $n = 23$ Higher GI: $n = 24$	Higher GI v. Low GI (Mean ± SD) Higher GI: 58 ± 0.5 Low GI: 49 ± 0.8	The difference between the low GI and higher GI groups in respect of lipids and CRP were not statistically significant ($p > 0.05$).
Ma et al. [33]	China	GDM	12–14 Weeks	Parallel Design	Higher GI: 30.0 ± 3.5 Low GI: 30.1 ± 3.8 $p = 0.901$	Higher GI: $n = 42$ Low GI: $n = 41$	Higher GI v. Low GI (Mean ± SD) Baseline Higher GI: 56.1 ± 2.4 Low GI: 56.0 ± 2.1 Post-intervention Higher GI: 53.8 ± 2.5 Low GI: 50.1 ± 2.2	The increases in TC, TG and the decrease in HDL cholesterol were significantly lower ($p < 0.05$) in the low GI group compared with the higher GI group.
Jenkins et al. [34]	Canada	Type 2 diabetes	6 months	Parallel Design	(Mean ± SD) High-cereal fibre diet = 61 ± 9 Low-GI diet = 60 ± 10	210	Low GI diet v. high-cereal fibre diet Mean (95% CI) Baseline Higher GI: 81.5 (80.4-82.7) Low GI: 80.8 (79.6-82.0) Post-intervention Higher GI: 83.5 (82.4-84.7) Low GI: 69.6 (67.7-71.4)	HDL cholesterol increased by 1.7 mg/dL in the low GI group and decreased by -0.2 mg/dL in the higher GI group ($p = 0.005$). Reductions of the CRP were similar in the low GI and higher GI groups.
Jenkins et al. [35]	Canada	Type 2 diabetes	3 months	Parallel Design	(Mean ± SEM) High-wheat fibre diet: 61 ± 1.0 Low-GI legume diet: 58 ± 1.3	121	Low GI legume diet v. high-wheat fibre diet Mean (95% CI) Baseline Higher GI: 78 (77–80) Low GI: 80 (79–82) Post-intervention Higher GI: 82 (81–83) Low GI: 66 (64–67)	Low GI legume produced significant decreases in TC ($p < 0.001$) and TG ($p < 0.001$) with no significant change in HDL cholesterol ($p = 0.19$). The relative reduction in TC and HDL cholesterol were greater in the low GI legume diet group compared with the higher GI diet group. No other lipid treatment differences were significant.

Table 3. *Cont.*

Citation	Country	Type of Diabetes	Length of Study	Study Type	Age (Years)	Sample Size	Interventions/Glycemic Index (GI) Values	Results/Conclusion
Ma et al. [36]	USA	Type 2 diabetes	12 months	Parallel Design	(Mean ± SD) 53.53 ± 8.40	40	Low GI diet v. American Diabetes Association diet (ADA) (Mean ± SEM) Baseline ADA: 82.03 ± 1.31 Low GI: 79.35 ± 1.36 Post-intervention ADA: 80.36 ± 1.40 Low GI: 76.64 ± 1.46	There were no significant differences between low GI and higher GI groups with respect to TC, HDL, and TG.
Wolever et al. [37]	Canada	Type 2 diabetes	12 months	Parallel Design	(Mean ± SEM) Higher GI diet: 60.4 ± 1.1 Low GI diet: 60.6 ± 1.0	162	Low GI diet v. higher GI diet (Mean ± SEM) Baseline Higher GI: 61.5 ± 0.4 Low GI: 60.3 ± 0.4 Post-intervention Higher GI: 63.2 ± 0.4 Low GI: 55.1 ± 0.4	There were no significant effects for TC. With the low GI diet, mean triacylglycerol was 12% higher, HDL was 4% lower, the higher GI values were intermediate. The CRP with the low GI diet was 29% less than the higher GI diet ($p < 0.05$).
Yusof et al. [38]	Malaysia	Type 2 diabetes	12 weeks	Parallel Design	Not data	104	Low GI diet v. conventional carbohydrate exchange (CCE) (Mean ± SD) Baseline Higher GI: 64 ± 6 Low GI: 63 ± 5 Post-intervention Higher GI: 64 ± 5 Low GI: 57 ± 6	TG increased at week 4, then decreased at week 12 in the Low GI group and this was reversed in the CCE group. Serum HDL cholesterol increased significantly in both groups over time, although no significant differences were found between the two groups.
Argiana et al. [39]	Greece	Type 2 diabetes	12 weeks	Parallel Design	Control: 63.0 ± 1.3 Low GI: 61.3 ± 1.4	n = 61	Low GI diet v. Higher GI diet	The differences between the low GI diet and control diet with respect to HDL cholesterol at the end of the study was statistically significant ($p = 0.007$). A significant decrease ($p = 0.02$) in CRP was found in participants in the low GI diet group and the differences between the low GI and the higher GI groups were significant ($p = 0.007$) after the study. Serum IL–6 and adiponectin did not differ significantly in both groups at week 0 and week 12.
Cai et al. [40]	China	Type 2 diabetes	12 months	Parallel Design	56.7 ± 3.5	n = 130	Low GI diet v. Higher GI diet	After intervention, the levels of CRP-reactive protein and IL–6 in the low GI diet were significantly lower than the control group ($p < 0.05$).

Abbreviations: CCE (conventional carbohydrate exchange); Higher GI (Higher glycemic index); Low GI (Low glycemic index); *n* (Number); TC: total cholesterol; TG: triglyceride; CRP: C-reactive protein; IL–6: interleukin 6; v. (Versus).

Table 4. Cardio–metabolic and inflammatory parameters of studies included.

Citation	Baseline Versus Post-Intervention	HDL Cholesterol	LDL Cholesterol	Total Cholesterol	Triglyceride	C-Reactive Protein	Adiponectin	Interleukin-6
Gomes et al. [31]	Baseline mg/dL Median (Minimum/Maximum) Post-intervention	Higher GI: 43 (30/59) Low GI: 38 (27.6/45.2) Higher GI: 40 (30/54) Low GI: 41 (24.5/47)	No Data	Higher GI: 210.1 (180/273.5) Low GI: 200.4 (123/248.1) Higher GI: 211 (172/284) Low GI: 214.1 (145/288.5)	Higher GI: 180.2 (88.7/287) Low GI: 195 (68/372) Higher GI: 175.3 (132/311.2) Low GI: 205.1 (63/384.1)	(mg/L) Higher GI: 2.6 (0.8/7.3) Low GI: 2.7 (0.5/5.5) Higher GI: 2.8 (0.6/6.13) Low GI: 2.5 (0.1/6.9) $p = 0.44$	ng/mL Higher GI: 30.9 (29.8/31.4 Low GI: 30.1 (29.4/31.3) Higher GI: 30.8 (30.2/31.6) Low GI: 30.5 (26.7/93) $p = 0.74$	No Data
Ma et al. [33]	Baseline mmol/L (Mean ± SD) Post-intervention	Higher GI: 1.96 ± 0.39 Low GI: 1.89 ± 0.33 Higher GI: 1.85 ± 0.36 Low GI: 1.87 ± 0.34	Higher GI: 2.13 ± 0.60 Low GI: 2.19 ± 0.58 Higher GI: 2.16 ± 0.81 Low GI: 2.20 ± 0.54	Higher GI: 5.74 ± 0.74 Low GI: 5.79 ± 1.01 Higher GI: 5.97 ± 0.89 Low GI: 5.96 ± 1.02	Higher GI: 2.20 ± 0.60 Low GI:2.67 ± 1.27 Higher GI: 3.14 ± 1.05 Low GI: 3.09 ± 1.14	No Data	No Data	No Data
Jenkins et al. [34]	Baseline mg/dL (Mean) Post-intervention	Higher GI: 43.1 Low GI: 41.9 Higher GI: 42.8 Low GI: 43.6	Higher GI: 101.1 Low GI: 96.9 Higher GI: 101.3 Low GI: 95.3	Higher GI: 168.4 Low GI: 164.3 Higher GI: 168.4 Low GI: 162.6	Higher GI: 122.0 Low GI: 128.1 Higher GI: 122.2 Low GI: 124.6	Higher GI: 4.59 Low GI: 4.62 Higher GI: 2.82 Low GI: 3.02	No Data	No Data
Jenkins et al. [35]	Baseline mg/dL (95%CI) Post-intervention	Higher GI: 47 (44, 50) Low GI: 43 (40, 46) Higher GI: 48 (45, 52) Low GI: 43 (40, 45)	Higher GI: 91 (81, 101) Low GI: 84 (77, 92) Higher GI: 90 (81, 99) Low GI: 81 (74, 89)	Higher GI: 163 (151, 174) Low GI: 158 (147, 168) Higher GI: 161 (150, 172) Low GI: 149 (139, 160)	Higher GI: 124 (104, 145) Low GI: 149 (125, 173) Higher GI: 115 (96, 133) Low GI: 128 (107, 148)	No Data	No Data	No Data
Ma et al. [36]	Baseline mg/dL (Mean ± SEM) Post-intervention	Higher GI: 42.95 ± 2.26 Low GI: 45.42 ± 2.38 Higher GI: 44.29 ± 2.30 Low GI: 47.53 ± 2.43	Higher GI: 88.95 ± 7.52 Low GI: 93.16 ± 8.07 Higher GI: 71.49 ± 7.81 Low GI: 94.50 ± 8.32	Higher GI: 168.10 ± 9.06 Low GI: 175.58 ± 9.53 Higher GI: 149.71 ± 9.35 Low GI: 173.63 ± 0.06 $p = 0.09$	* Higher GI: 5.05 (0.14) Low GI: 4.99 (0.15) Higher GI: 4.93 (0.15) Low GI: 4.90 (0.16)	No Data	No Data	No Data
Wolever et al. [37]	Baseline mmol/L (Mean ± SEM) Post-intervention	Higher GI: 1.14 ± 0.05 Low GI: 1.21 ± 0.03 Higher GI: 1.19 ± 0.03 Low GI: 1.16 ± 0.03	Higher GI: 2.82 ± 0.13 Low GI: 3.02 ± 0.13 Higher GI: 3.0 ± 0.08 Low GI: 2.92 ± 0.05	Higher GI: 4.86 ± 0.16 Low GI: 5.09 ± 0.13 Higher GI: 5.04 ± 0.08 Low GI: 5.04 ± 0.08	Higher GI: 2.07 ± 0.15 Low GI: 1.87 ± 0.10 Higher GI: 2.0 ± 0.07 Low GI: 2.17 ± 0.07	** Higher GI: 3.34 (2.56, 4.26) Low GI: 2.64 (1.89, 3.70) Higher GI: 2.75 (2.33, 3.24) Low GI: 1.95 (1.68, 2.27)	No Data	No Data
Yusof et al. [38]	Baseline mmol/L (Mean ± SEM) Post-intervention	Higher GI: 1.18 ± 0.34 Low GI: 1.08 ± 0.30 Higher GI: 1.21 ± 0.05 Low GI: 1.14 ± 0.04	Higher GI: 2.78 ± 0.67 Low GI: 2.78 ± 0.67 Higher GI: 2.93 ± 0.14 Low GI: 2.67 ± 0.11	Higher GI: 4.56 ± 0.80 Low GI: 4.54 ± 0.75 Higher GI: 4.80 ± 0.16 Low GI: 4.54 ± 0.12	Higher GI: 1.35 ± 0.53 Low GI: 1.5 ± 0.47 Higher GI: 1.46 ± 0.08 Low GI: 1.59 ± 0.10	No Data	No Data	No Data
Argiana et al. [39]	Baseline mg/dL (Mean ± SEM) Post-intervention	Higher GI: 46.4 ± 1.8 Low GI: 43.1 ± 1.3 Higher GI: 46.1 ± 1.7 Low GI: 43.3 ± 1.2	Higher GI: 104.9 ± 5.1 Low GI: 107.0 ± 5.5 Higher GI: 104.2 ± 5.2 Low GI: 97.2 ± 6.2	Higher GI: 176.6 ± 5.2 Low GI: 173.9 ± 6.4 Higher GI: 175.8 ± 5.2 Low GI: 167.0 ± 4.1	Higher GI: 126.5 ± 10.8 Low GI: 119.2 ± 11.6 Higher GI: 127.5 ± 10.3 Low GI: 122 ± 9.3	*** Higher GI: 2.1 ± 0.5 Low GI: 4.4 ± 1.2 Higher GI: 2.8 ± 0.6 Low GI: 3.0 ± 0.8	*** Higher GI: 7.4 ± 1.6 Low GI: 12.2 ± 3.4 Higher GI: 8.3 ± 2.1 Low GI: 12.5 ± 1.5	**** Higher GI: 1.3 ± 0.2 Low GI: 1.4 ± 0.3 Higher GI: 2.0 ± 0.5 Low GI: 1.3 ± 0.2
Cai et al. [40]	Baseline mg/L (Not stated whether Mean or SD) Post-intervention	No Data	No Data	No Data	No Data	Higher GI: 8.03 ± 0.72 Low GI: 8.04 ± 0.75 Higher GI: 5.01 ± 0.32 Low GI: 3.68 ± 0.29	No Data	**** Higher GI: 12.26 ± 1.57 Low GI: 12.29 ± 1.44 Higher GI: 9.01 ± 0.83 Low GI: 7.97 ± 0.86

Abbreviations: CCE (conventional carbohydrate exchange); Higher GI (Higher glycemic index); Low GI (Low glycemic indexn (Number); TC: total cholesterol; TG: triglyceride; CRP: C-reactive protein; IL−6: interleukin 6. * mmol/L (Natural Logarithm); ** mg/L (Mean, 95% CIs); *** μg/mL (Mean ± SEM); *** pg/mL (Mean ± SEM); v. (Versus).

3.1. Evaluation of the Risk of Bias of the Studies Selected

Most of the studies demonstrated either a low risk of bias or an unclear risk of bias in all the domains evaluated (selection bias, performance bias, detection bias, attrition bias, and reporting bias) (Figure 2). However, Jenkins et al. [34] showed high risk of bias in the area of selection bias (Figure 3).

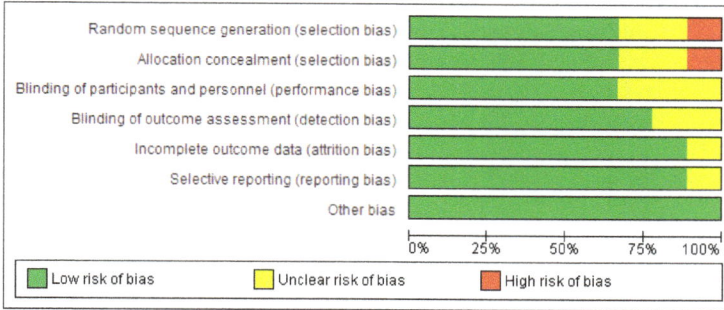

Figure 2. A summary risk of bias graph of included studies.

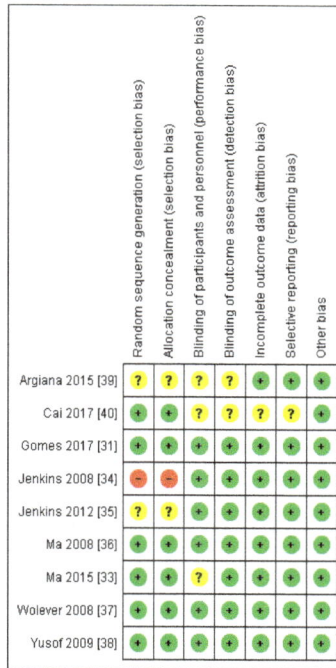

Figure 3. A risk of bias graph for each included study.

3.2. The Effect of a Low GI Diet on Lipid Profile

Grant et al. [32] found no significant differences ($p > 0.05$) between the low GI group compared to the higher GI group, with respect to the lipid profile in women with GDM (Table 3). In their study, Ma et al. [33] observed that the increases in total cholesterol (0.12 versus 0.23 mmol/L) and triglyceride

(0.41 versus 0.56 mmol/L), and the decrease in HDL cholesterol (−0.01 versus −0.11), were significantly lower ($p < 0.05$) than the higher GI group in women with GDM (Table 4).

In patients with type 2 diabetes, the results of the meta-analysis showed no significant differences ($p > 0.05$) between the low GI and higher GI groups with respect to HDL with a mean difference of 0.00 mmol/L (−0.02, 0.02) and LDL cholesterol with a mean difference of −0.14 mmol/L (−0.37, 0.09) (Figures 4 and 5, respectively).

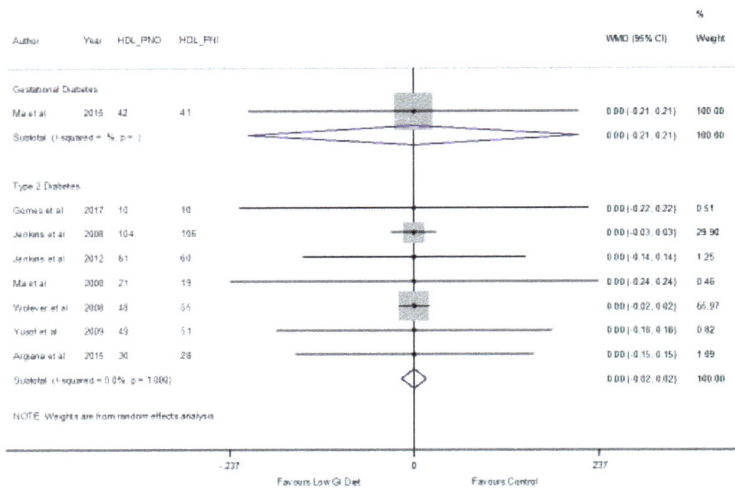

Figure 4. A forest plot showing the effects of a low GI diet on HDL cholesterol (mmol/L).

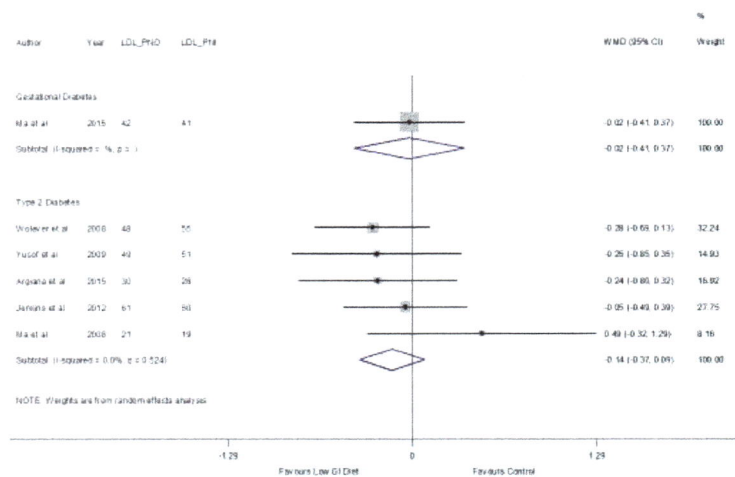

Figure 5. A forest plot showing the effect of a low GI diet on LDL cholesterol (mmol/L).

In addition, the findings from the meta-analysis found no significant difference ($p > 0.05$) between the two groups in relation to the total cholesterol which decreased by a mean of −0.08 mmol/L (−0.31, 0.16) (Figure 6) in the low GI group. The results showed that there was a significant difference ($p = 0.027$) with respect to triglycerides, which increased by a mean of 0.06 mmol/L (0.01, 0.11) in patients with type 2 diabetes in the higher GI group (Figure 7).

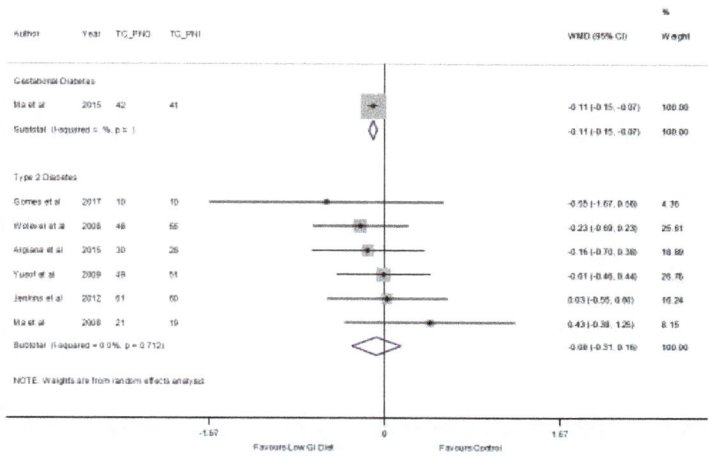

Figure 6. A forest plot depicting the effect of a low GI diet on Total Cholesterol (mmol/L).

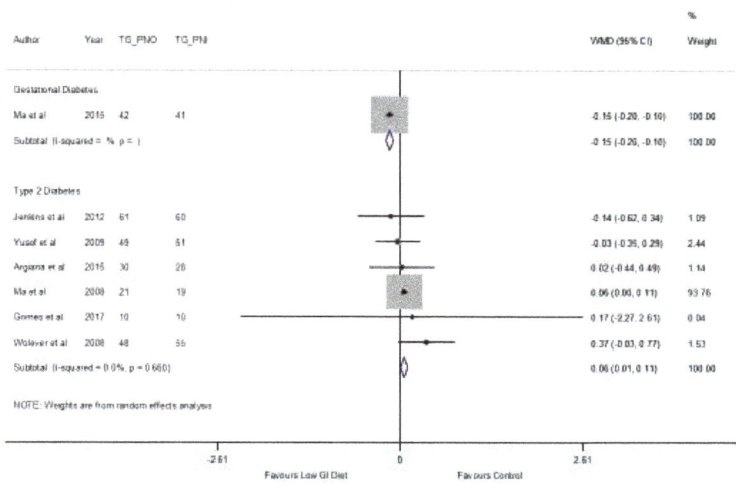

Figure 7. A forest plot depicting the effect of a low GI diet on Triglyceride (mmol/L).

3.3. The Effect of a Low GI Diet on Inflammatory Parameters

According to Grant et al. [32], there was no significant difference ($p > 0.05$) between the low GI and higher GI groups in relation to the C–reactive protein in women with GDM. In patients with type 2 diabetes, Gomes et al. [31] and Cai et al. [40] found that a low GI diet can reduce or prevent the inflammatory responses induced by a high GI diet. In addition, a low GI diet has been shown to reduce C–reactive protein levels significantly compared to a high GI diet [37,39].

With respect to serum interleukin–6 and adiponectin, Argiana et al. [39] did not find significant differences in both groups between week 0 and week 12 in patients with type 2 diabetes. The results of the meta-analysis did not show significant differences ($p > 0.05$) between low GI and higher GI diets with respect to adiponectin and C-reactive protein in patients with type 2 diabetes (Table 5). However, a significant difference ($p < 0.001$) was observed between the two groups in relation to interleukin–6 (Table 5), with the low GI diet decreasing interleukin–6 by a mean of -1.01 mg/L (-1.55, -0.48). A meta-analysis was not conducted for the patients with GDM with respect to inflammatory parameters due to the limited number of studies.

Table 5. Results of a meta-analysis of the effect of a low GI diet on inflammatory parameters.

Outcomes	Patients with Type 2 Diabetes			
	N Studies	Weighted Mean Difference (95% CI) mg/L	*p*-Value	I^2 %
Interleukin–6	2	-1.01 (-1.55, -0.48)	0.001	0.0
C–eactive Protein	5	-0.32 (-1.17, 0.53)	0.467	0.0
Adiponectin	2	0.01 (-0.00, 0.03)	0.072	0.0

4. Discussion

The results of the two studies [32,33] that evaluated the effects of low GI diets on lipid profiles in women with GDM were not consistent. While Grant et al. [32] did not find significant differences ($p > 0.05$) between the low GI and higher GI groups in relation to lipids, Ma et al. [33] found significant differences ($p < 0.05$) between the two groups with respect to total cholesterol, triglycerides, and HDL cholesterol. On the other hand, the results of the meta-analysis showed that there were no significant differences ($p > 0.05$) between the low GI diet and higher GI group with respect to total cholesterol, HDL, and LDL cholesterol in patients with type 2 diabetes (although the difference was statistically significant ($p < 0.05$) in relation to triglycerides, with higher GI diet increasing triglyceride levels). The differences observed between the effects of a low GI in patients with GDM compared to patients with type 2 diabetes in some of the metabolites may due to the limited number of studies in the current review and the differences in the pathophysiology of both conditions. In a previous meta-analysis, Fleming and Godwin [24] revealed that a low GI diet may help lower total cholesterol and LDL cholesterol. In addition, Goff et al. [13] found that low GI diets reduced total and LDL cholesterol and had no effect on HDL cholesterol and triglycerides. It is possible that the differences between the current review and the previous reviews in relation to some of the metabolites may be due to the participants included in the studies. While this review was based only on patients with GDM and type 2 diabetes, the earlier reviews were based on the general population [24] or included participants without diabetes [13].

The results of the effect of a low GI diet on inflammatory markers were variable in the studies selected in patients with GDM. However, the results of the meta-analysis showed that differences between low GI and higher GI groups were only significant ($p < 0.05$) in relation to interleukin–6, which decreased in the low GI group in patients with type 2 diabetes. These results are discussed below.

4.1. The Effect of a Low GI Diet on Lipid Profile

There appears to be controversy regarding the role of low GI diets in the prevention of cardiovascular diseases. The effect of GI on total cholesterol, LDL, and HDL cholesterol is not quite clear [39,41]. For example, in women with GDM, Grant et al. [32] reported no significant differences ($p > 0.05$) between the low GI and higher GI groups with respect to the lipids in women with GDM. However, Ma et al. [33] found that low GI diets improved blood lipids.

In patients with type 2 diabetes, Gomes et al. [31] found that a low GI diet reduced body fat. In the study by Jenkins et al. [34], it was observed that HDL cholesterol increased by 1.7 mg/dL in the low GI group and decreased by −0.2 mg/dL in the higher GI group ($p = 0.005$). In contrast, Wolever et al. [37] noted that HDL cholesterol was 4% lower in the low GI group, while the higher GI values were intermediate. Other studies [35,36,38] demonstrated no significant difference between the low GI and higher GI groups in relation to HDL cholesterol.

According to Jenkins et al. [35], low GI legumes produced significant decreases in total cholesterol level ($p < 0.001$) in patients with type 2 diabetes. The relative reduction in total cholesterol level was greater in the low GI legume diet group compared with the higher GI group [35]. However, Ma et al. [36] and Wolever et al. [37] did not find a significant difference between low GI and higher GI diets with respect to the total cholesterol in patients with type 2 diabetes.

Jenkins et al. [35] demonstrated that a low GI legume produced significant decreases in triglycerides ($p < 0.001$) in patients with type 2 diabetes. Decreases in triglycerides in the low GI group were also reported by Yusof et al. [38], although Wolever et al. [37] showed increased levels of triglycerides in the low GI group. On the other hand, Ma et al. [36] found no significant difference between low GI and higher GI with respect to triglycerides.

The mechanism by which dietary GI influences blood lipids has not been entirely elucidated [42]. This may explain the differences in the findings of the various studies. However, it has been suggested that high GI diets increase non esterified fatty acid concentrations after intervention compared to baseline, and increased levels of non-esterified fatty acids can cause beta cell dysfunction, insulin resistance, and reduced glucose uptake [31]. In other words, elevated levels of blood glucose, insulin, and free fatty acids following a high GI diet can induce insulin resistance, which could lead to increased triglyceride, a greater inflammatory response, and a decrease in HDL cholesterol [43,44].

Hyperinsulinaemia and insulin resistance are significantly correlated to dyslipidaemia and contribute to the changes in the plasma lipid profile [45]. Therefore, the potential effects of a low GI diet on cardiometabolic parameters may be caused by a reduction of hyperglycaemia, hyperinsulinaemia and levels of free fatty acids, which could lead to a reduced risk of insulin resistance, beta cell dysfunction, dyslipidaemia, and inflammatory response [45,46].

4.2. The Effect of a Low GI Diet on Inflammatory Parameters

Based on the findings of the meta-analysis in relation to the inflammatory parameters, low GI diets significantly decreased ($p < 0.05$) levels of interleukin-6 compared with the higher GI diets in patients with type 2 diabetes. Differences between the two groups were not statistically significant ($p > 0.05$) with respect to C-reactive proteins. The mechanism for this finding, with respect to interleukin-6, may due to hyperglycaemia in the higher GI group, which induces the release of inflammatory cytokines from monocytes [47]. Furthermore, the exposure of endothelial cells to varying levels of glucose concentration can increase the risk of oxidative stress and apoptosis and thus lead to the production of pro-inflammatory cytokines [39,48,49]. The results of this review confirm the findings of a previous study by Juanola-Falgaroma et al. [50], which found that subjects allocated a low GI diet showed significantly higher decreases in interleukin–6 after intervention.

This review has both clinical and public health implications in terms of our understanding of the role low GI diets in the management of cardiometabolic and inflammatory parameters in patients with diabetes.

5. Limitations

Although a total of nine studies were included in the meta-analysis, this number was limited by the two sub-groups of GDM and type 2 diabetes. More studies in each of the sub-groups would have further enhanced the wider application of the findings of this review. In addition, the lack of a consensus on what constitutes a low GI diet, and the variation in the GI levels of dietary interventions in the studies included, may have impacted the analysis of the findings of this review.

6. Conclusions

This systematic review and meta-analysis have demonstrated that there were no significant differences ($p > 0.05$) between low GI and higher GI diets in relation to total cholesterol, HDL, and LDL cholesterol in patients with type 2 diabetes. However, a significant difference ($p < 0.05$) was observed between the two groups with respect to triglycerides in patients with type 2 diabetes. The results of the effect of a low GI diet on the lipid profile in patients with GDM were not consistent. With respect to the inflammatory parameters, the low GI diet significantly decreased interleukin–6 in patients with type 2 diabetes than the higher GI diet. More studies are needed in this area of research.

Author Contributions: Conceptualization, O.O., O.O.O., X.-H.W., A.R.A.A.; methodology, O.O., O.O.O., X.-H.W., A.R.A.A.; validation, O.O., O.O.O., X.-H.W., A.R.A.A.; formal analysis, A.R.A.A. and O.O. and reviewed by O.O.O. and X.-H.W.; writing—original draft preparation, O.O.; writing—review and editing, O.O., O.O.O., X.-H.W., A.R.A.A.

Funding: This research received no external funding.

Conflicts of Interest: The authors declare no conflict of interest.

References

1. International Diabetes Federation. Promoting Diabetes Care, Prevention and a Cure Worldwide. 2019. Available online: https://www.idf.org/ (accessed on 16 March 2019).
2. National Collaborating Centre for Chronic Conditions (NCCCC). *Type 2 Diabetes: National Clinical Guideline for Management in Primary and Secondary Care (Update)*; Royal College of Physicians: London, UK, 2008.
3. Poulakos, P.; Mintziori, G.; Tsirou, E.; Taousani, E.; Savvaki, D.; Harizopoulou, V.; Goulis, D.G. Comments on gestational diabetes mellitus: From pathophysiology to clinical practice. *Hormones (Athens, Greece)* **2015**, *14*, 335–344. [CrossRef] [PubMed]
4. World Health Organisation. Diagnostic Criteria and Classification of Hyperglycaemia First Detected in Pregnancy. 2013. Available online: http://apps.who.int/iris/bitstream/handle/10665/85975/WHO_NMH_MND_13.2_eng.pdf;jsessionid=09A82B923EF7A55CC6AB690976A1A1F3?sequence=1 (accessed on 16 March 2019).
5. Abell, S.K.; De Courten, B.; Boyle, J.A.; Teede, H.J. Inflammatory and Other Biomarkers: Role in Pathophysiology and Prediction of Gestational Diabetes Mellitus. *Int. J. Mol. Sci.* **2015**, *16*, 13442–13473. [CrossRef] [PubMed]
6. International Diabetes Federation. Care and Prevention Improving the Quality of Life of People with Diabetes and Those at Risk. 2019. Available online: https://www.idf.org/our-activities/care-prevention/gdm (accessed on 16 March 2019).
7. National Institute for Health and Care Excellence (NICE). Type 2 Diabetes in Adults: Management. 2015. Available online: nice.org.uk/guidance/ng28 (accessed on 1 March 2019).
8. National Institute for Health and Care Excellence (NICE). Diabetes in Pregnancy: Management from Preconception to the Postnatal Period. 2015. Available online: http://nice.org.uk/guidance/ng3 (accessed on 16 March 2018).
9. Ojo, O.; Ojo, O.O.; Adebowale, F.; Wang, X.-H. The Effect of Dietary Glycaemic Index on Glycaemia in Patients with Type 2 Diabetes: A Systematic Review and Meta-Analysis of Randomized Controlled Trials. *Nutrients* **2018**, *10*, 373. [CrossRef] [PubMed]
10. Hodson, K.; Robson, S.; Taylor, R. Gestational diabetes: Emerging concepts in pathophysiology. *Obstet. Med.* **2010**, *3*, 128–132. [CrossRef] [PubMed]
11. Daher, S. Gestational diabetes, inflammation and obesity: New insights into genetic markers and phenotype. *J. Reprod. Immunol.* **2012**, *94*, 6. [CrossRef]
12. American Diabetes Association. Life style management: Standards of Medical Care in Diabetes–2018. *Diabetes Care* **2018**, *41* (Suppl. 1), S38–S50. [CrossRef] [PubMed]

13. Goff, L.M.; Cowland, D.E.; Hooper, L.; Frost, G.S. Low glycaemic index diets and blood lipids: A systematic review and meta-analysis of randomised controlled trials. *Nutr. Metab. Cardiovasc. Dis.* **2013**, *23*, 1–10. [CrossRef]
14. Similä, M.E.; Valsta, L.M.; Kontto, J.P.; Albanes, D.; Virtamo, J. Low-, medium-and high-glycaemic index carbohydrates and risk of type 2 diabetes in men. *Br. J. Nutr.* **2011**, *105*, 1258–1264. [CrossRef]
15. Esfahani, A.; Wong, J.W.; Mirrahimi, A.; Villa, C.R.; Kendall, C.C. The application of the glycemic index and glycemic load in weight loss: A review of the clinical evidence. *IUBMB Life* **2011**, *63*, 7–13. [CrossRef]
16. Food and Agricultural Organisation (FAO). *Carbohydrates in Human Nutrition. Report of a Joint FAO/WHO Expert Consultation*; FAO (Food and Nutrition paper–66); FAO: Rome, Italy, 1998. Available online: http://www.fao.org/docrep/w8079e/w8079e00.htm (accessed on 16 January 2019).
17. Chiu, C.; Taylor, A. Dietary hyperglycemia, glycemic index and metabolic retinal diseases. *Prog. Retin. Eye Res.* **2011**, *30*, 18–53. [CrossRef]
18. Chang, K.T.; Lampe, J.W.; Schwarz, Y.; Breymeyer, K.L.; Noar, K.A.; Song, X.; Neuhouser, M.L. Low Glycemic Load Experimental Diet More Satiating Than High Glycemic Load Diet. *Nutr. Cancer* **2012**, *64*, 666–673. [CrossRef] [PubMed]
19. Russell, W.R.; Baka, A.; Björck, I.; Delzenne, N.; Gao, D.; Griffiths, H.R.; Weickert, M.O. Impact of Diet Composition on Blood Glucose Regulation. *Crit. Rev. Food Sci. Nutr.* **2016**, *56*, 541–590. [CrossRef] [PubMed]
20. Bouché, C.; Rizkalla, S.W.; Luo, J.; Vidal, H.; Veronese, A.; Pacher, N.; Fouquet, C.; Lang, V.; Slama, G. Five-week, low-glycemic index diet decreases total fat mass and improves plasma lipid profile in moderately overweight nondiabetic men. *Diabetes Care* **2002**, *25*, 822–828. [CrossRef] [PubMed]
21. Brand, J.C.; Colagiuri, S.; Crossman, S.; Allen, A.; Roberts, D.C.; Truswell, A.S. Low-glycemic index foods improve long-term glycemic control in NIDDM. *Diabetes Care* **1991**, *14*, 95–101. [CrossRef] [PubMed]
22. Clar, C.; Al-Khudairy, L.; Loveman, E.; Kelly, S.A.; Hartley, L.; Flowers, N.; Germanò, R.; Frost, G.; Rees, K. Low glycaemic index diets for the prevention of cardiovascular disease. *Cochrane Database Syst. Rev.* **2017**, *7*, CD004467. [CrossRef]
23. Schwingshackl, L.; Hoffmann, G. Long-term effects of low glycemic index/load vs. high glycemic index/load diets on parameters of obesity and obesity-associated risks: A systematic review and meta-analysis. *Nutr. Metab. Cardiovasc. Dis. NMCD* **2013**, *23*, 699–706. [CrossRef]
24. Fleming, P.; Godwin, M. Low-glycaemic index diets in the management of blood lipids: A systematic review and meta-analysis. *Fam. Pract.* **2013**, *30*, 485–491. [CrossRef]
25. Mendes, N.; Tavares Ribeiro, R.; Serrano, F. Beyond self-monitored plasma glucose and HbA1c: The role of non-traditional glycaemic markers in gestational diabetes mellitus. *J. Obstet. Gynaecol.* **2018**, *38*, 762–769. [CrossRef]
26. Moher, D.; Liberati, A.; Tetzlaff, J.; Altman, D.G. The PRISMA Group Preferred Reporting Items for Systematic Reviews and Meta-Analyses: The PRISMA Statement. *PLoS Med.* **2009**, *6*, e1000097. [CrossRef]
27. Methley, A.M.; Campbell, S.; Chew-Graham, C.; McNally, R.; Cheraghi-Sohi, S. PICO, PICOS and SPIDER: A comparison study of specificity and sensitivity in three search tools for qualitative systematic reviews. *BMC Health Serv. Res.* **2014**, *14*, 579. [CrossRef]
28. Critical Appraisal Skills Programme (CASP). Randomised Controlled Trial Checklist. 2017. Available online: https://casp-uk.net/wp-content/uploads/2018/01/CASP-Randomised-Controlled-Trial-Checklist-2018.pdf (accessed on 18 January 2019).
29. Higgins, J.P.T.; Green, S. *Cochrane Handbook for Systematic Reviews of Interventions*; Wiley-Blackwell: Hoboken, NJ, USA, 2009.
30. The Nordic Cochrane Centre. *Review Manager (RevMan) [Computer Program]*, Version 5.3.; The Nordic Cochrane Centre, The Cochrane Collaboration: Copenhagen, Denmark, 2014.
31. Gomes, J.G.; Fabrini, S.P.; Alfenas, R.G. Low glycemic index diet reduces body fat and attenuates inflammatory and metabolic responses in patients with Type 2 diabetes. *Arch. Endocrinol. Metab.* **2017**, *61*, 137–144. [CrossRef] [PubMed]
32. Grant, S.M.; Wolever, T.M.; O'Connor, D.L.; Nisenbaum, R.; Josse, R.G. Effect of a low glycaemic index diet on blood glucose in women with gestational hyperglycaemia. *Diabetes Res. Clin. Pract.* **2011**, *91*, 15–22. [CrossRef] [PubMed]
33. Ma, W.J.; Huang, Z.H.; Huang, B.X.; Qi, B.H.; Zhang, Y.J.; Xiao, B.X.; Li, Y.H.; Chen, L.; Zhu, H.L. Intensive low-glycaemic-load dietary intervention for the management of glycaemia and serum lipids among women with gestational diabetes: A randomized control trial. *Public Health Nutr.* **2015**, *18*, 1506–1513. [CrossRef] [PubMed]

34. Jenkins, D.A.; Kendall, C.C.; McKeown-Eyssen, G.; Josse, R.G.; Silverberg, J.; Booth, G.L.; Leiter, L.A. Effect of a low-glycemic index or a high-cereal fiber diet on Type 2 diabetes: A randomized trial. *JAMA* **2008**, *300*, 2742–2753. [CrossRef] [PubMed]

35. Jenkins, D.A.; Kendall, C.C.; Augustin, L.A.; Mitchell, S.; Sahye-Pudaruth, S.; Blanco Mejia, S.; Josse, R.G. Effect of legumes as part of a low glycemic index diet on glycemic control and cardiovascular risk factors in type 2 diabetes mellitus: A randomized controlled trial. *Arch. Intern. Med.* **2012**, *172*, 1653–1660. [CrossRef] [PubMed]

36. Ma, Y.; Olendzki, B.C.; Merriam, P.A.; Chiriboga, D.E.; Culver, A.L.; Li, W.; Pagoto, S.L. A randomized clinical trial comparing low-glycemic index versus ADA dietary education among individuals with type 2 diabetes. *Nutrition* **2008**, *24*, 45–56. [CrossRef]

37. Wolever, T.; Gibbs, A.; Mehling, C.; Chiasson, J.; Connelly, P.; Josse, R.; Ryan, E. The Canadian Trial of Carbohydrates in Diabetes (CCD), a 1-y controlled trial of low-glycemic-index dietary carbohydrate in type 2 diabetes: No effect on glycated hemoglobin but reduction in C-reactive protein. *Am. J. Clin. Nutr.* **2008**, *87*, 114–125. [CrossRef] [PubMed]

38. Yusof, B.M.; Talib, R.A.; Kamaruddin, N.A.; Karim, N.A.; Chinna, K.; Gilbertson, H. A low-GI diet is associated with a short-term improvement of glycaemic control in Asian patients with Type 2 diabetes. *Diabetes Obes. Metab.* **2009**, *11*, 387–396. [CrossRef]

39. Argiana, V.; Kanellos, P.T.; Makrilakis, K.; Eleftheriadou, I.; Tsitsinakis, G.; Kokkinos, A.; Perrea, D.; Tentolouris, N. The effect of consumption of low-glycemic-index and low-glycemic-load desserts on anthropometric parameters and inflammatory markers in patients with Type 2 diabetes mellitus. *Eur. J. Nutr.* **2015**, *54*, 1173–1180. [CrossRef]

40. Cai, X.; Wang, L.; Wang, X.; Liu, S. Effect of high dietary fiber low glycemic index diet on intestinal flora, blood glucose and inflammatory response in T2DM patients. *Biomed. Res.* **2017**, *28*, 9371–9375.

41. Pelkman, C.L. Effects of the glycemic index of foods on serum concentrations of high-density lipoprotein cholesterol and triglycerides. *Curr. Atheroscler. Rep.* **2001**, *3*, 456–461. [CrossRef] [PubMed]

42. Huffman, F.G.; Zarini, G.G.; Cooper, V. Dietary glycemic index and load in relation to cardiovascular disease risk factors in Cuban American population. *Int. J. Food Sci. Nutr.* **2010**, *61*, 690–701. [CrossRef] [PubMed]

43. Reaven, G.M. Pathophysiology of insulin resistance in human disease. *Physiol. Rev.* **1995**, *75*, 473–486. [CrossRef] [PubMed]

44. Ludwig, D.S. The glycemic index: Physiological mechanisms relating to obesity, diabetes, and cardiovascular disease. *JAMA* **2002**, *287*, 2414–2423. [CrossRef] [PubMed]

45. Radulian, G.; Rusu, E.; Dragomir, A.; Posea, M. Metabolic effects of low glycaemic index diets. *Nutr. J.* **2009**, *8*, 1–8. [CrossRef] [PubMed]

46. Aston, L.M. Glycaemic index and metabolic disease risk. *Proc. Nutr. Soc.* **2006**, *65*, 125–134. [CrossRef] [PubMed]

47. Devaraj, S.; Venugopal, S.K.; Singh, U.; Jialal, I. Hyperglycemia induces monocytic release of interleukin-6 via induction of protein kinase c-{alpha} and -{beta}. *Diabetes* **2005**, *54*, 85–91. [CrossRef]

48. Leiter, L.A.; Ceriello, A.; Davidson, J.A.; Hanefeld, M.; Monnier, L.; Owens, D.R.; Tajima, N.; Tuomilehto, J. Postprandial glucose regulation: New data and new implications. *Clin. Ther.* **2005**, *27* (Suppl. B), S42–S56. [CrossRef]

49. Risso, A.; Mercuri, F.; Quagliaro, L.; Damante, G.; Ceriello, A. Intermittent high glucose enhances apoptosis in human umbilical vein endothelial cells in culture. *Am. J. Physiol. Endocrinol. Metab.* **2001**, *281*, E924–E930. [CrossRef]

50. Juanola-Falgarona, M.; Salas-Salvadó, J.; Ibarrola-Jurado, N.; Rabassa-Soler, A.; Díaz-Lopez, A.; Guasch-Ferré, M.; Hernández-Alonso, P.; Balanza, R.; Bullo, M. Effect of the glycemic index of the diet on weight loss, modulation of satiety, inflammation, and other metabolic risk factors: A randomized controlled trial. *Am. J. Clin. Nutr.* **2014**, *100*, 27–35. [CrossRef]

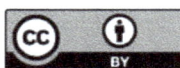

nutrients

MDPI

Review

Insulin in Type 1 and Type 2 Diabetes—Should the Dose of Insulin Before a Meal be Based on Glycemia or Meal Content?

Janusz Krzymien and Piotr Ladyzynski *

Nalecz Institute of Biocybernetics and Biomedical Engineering of the Polish Academy of Sciences, 4 Trojdena Street, 02-109 Warsaw, Poland; janusz.krzymien@hotmail.com
* Correspondence: pladyzynski@ibib.waw.pl; Tel.: +48-22-592-59-42

Received: 30 January 2019; Accepted: 8 March 2019; Published: 13 March 2019

Abstract: The aim of this review was to investigate existing guidelines and scientific evidence on determining insulin dosage in people with type 1 and type 2 diabetes, and in particular to check whether the prandial insulin dose should be calculated based on glycemia or the meal composition, including the carbohydrates, protein and fat content in a meal. By exploring the effect of the meal composition on postprandial glycemia we demonstrated that several factors may influence the increase in glycemia after the meal, which creates significant practical difficulties in determining the appropriate prandial insulin dose. Then we reviewed effects of the existing insulin therapy regimens on glycemic control. We demonstrated that in most existing algorithms aimed at calculating prandial insulin doses in type 1 diabetes only carbohydrates are counted, whereas in type 2 diabetes the meal content is often not taken into consideration. We conclude that prandial insulin doses in treatment of people with diabetes should take into account the pre-meal glycemia as well as the size and composition of meals. However, there are still open questions regarding the optimal way to adjust a prandial insulin dose to a meal and the possible benefits for people with type 1 and type 2 diabetes if particular parameters of the meal are taken into account while calculating the prandial insulin dose. The answers to these questions may vary depending on the type of diabetes.

Keywords: carbohydrate counting; protein and fat counting; insulin dosage; glucose monitoring; diabetes mellitus; type 1 diabetes; type 2 diabetes

---

1. Introduction

In healthy people, fasting plasma glucose rarely reaches 5.5 mmol/L (100 mg/dL) and the highest values after meals do not exceed 7.8 mmol/L (140 mg/dL), and quickly return to the starting level [1]. Hyperglycemia defines diabetes, and glycemic control plays an important role in the treatment of diabetes. Type 1 and type 2 diabetes are the two main types of the disease, which affects more than 425 million people worldwide [2]. Consistent hyperglycemia can lead to serious micro- and macrovascular complications, which cause diseases affecting the heart and blood vessels, kidneys, eyes, nerves and teeth. In addition, people with diabetes also have a higher risk of developing infections. In almost all high-income countries, diabetes is a leading cause of cardiovascular disease, blindness, kidney failure, and lower limb amputation. The premature morbidity, mortality, reduced life expectancy, and financial and social costs of diabetes make it one of the most important public health conditions [3]. The goals of treatment for diabetes are to prevent or delay complications, decrease mortality and maintain quality of life. An adequate glycemic control is a way of achieving these goals. In the American Diabetes Association (ADA) recommendations [4] for the majority of adults with diabetes (excluding pregnant women), the glycated hemoglobin A1c (HbA1c) below 7.0% (53 mmol/mol), preprandial blood glucose concentration in the range from 4.4 to 7.2 mmol/L (from

80 to 130 mg/dL) and after meals—below 10.0 mmol/L (180 mg/dL) were accepted as target values. At the same time, the recommendations underline that more or less stringent targets may be taken into account. They should be individualized depending on the duration of diabetes, age, life expectancy, co-morbid medical conditions, cardiovascular complications or advanced microvascular complications, occurrence of the hypoglycemic unawareness, as well as the individual expectations of the person with diabetes. It should be noted that in recent years, organizations such as The National Institute for Health and Care Excellence (NICE) [5], Institute for Clinical Systems Improvement (ICSI) [6], American Association of Clinical Endocrinologists and American College of Endocrinology (AACE/ACE) [7,8], Scottish Intercollegiate Guidelines Network (SIGN) [9], and the U.S Veterans Affairs/Department of Defense (SIGN) [10] have indicated that the target values of HbA1c are differentiated depending on the individual characteristics of people with diabetes. In its recently published recommendations, the American College of Physicians proposed target values of HbA1c for most people with type 2 diabetes in the range of 7.0% to 8.0% (53 to 64 mmol/mol) [11]. In a commentary from Diabetes Care, Matthew C. Riddle and colleagues [12] indicate the necessity to evaluate established and newer therapeutic options based on many years of observation, which will optimize the individualization of both goals and methods of therapy. The therapeutic goals set by ADA seem balanced and reasonable, they are broadly in line with the guidelines of other scientific societies. The HbA1c concentration below 7.0% (53 mmol/mol) is the accepted target value for the majority of patients with diabetes, excluding pregnant women. The possibility of achieving a more stringent goal of treatment, i.e., HbA1c below 6.5% (48 mmol/mol) for a group of patients who can achieve this goal without an increased risk of hypoglycemia or other adverse effects of the treatment as well as taking into account less stringent values of HbA1c, e.g., below 8.0% (64 mmol/mol) for older people are good examples of individualized therapeutic goals. Recommendations of the Polish Diabetes Association include similar individualized therapeutic goals [13]. Therapy adjustments should be made to maximize the proportion of time that glycemia is within the optimal range, i.e., between 3.9 and 10.0 mmol/L (70 and 180 mg/dL) for most patients [14]. A study of Bode et al. in people with type 1 and type 2 diabetes with HbA1c of 7.5% (58 mmol/mol) showed that 29% of blood glucose values exceeded 10.0 mmol/L (180 mg/dL) [15]. The postprandial blood glucose testing and evaluation is particularly important if the HbA1c target is not achieved despite satisfactory pre-meal glycemia. The postprandial glucose measurements should be made 1–2 h after the beginning of the meal and using treatments aimed at reducing postprandial plasma glucose values to <10.0 mmol/L (180 mg/dL) may help to lower HbA1c [4].

What is the real effect of the diet on the postprandial glycemia? Can we assess the effect of carbohydrates, fat and protein, and meals with a high or low glycemic index (GI) on postprandial glycemia? Are there differences that are related to the type of diabetes? In this review, we have attempted to answer these questions, based on the existing guidelines and available scientific evidence, to see if the prandial insulin dose should be calculated based on glycemia or the size and composition of a meal including carbohydrates, protein and fat content in the meal. We investigated the effect of macronutrient content in a meal on postprandial glycemia and we identified factors that may make it difficult to determine the appropriate dose of insulin to compensate for food intake in people with diabetes. Then we reviewed effects of the existing insulin therapy regimens on glycemic control and we assessed existing algorithms aimed at calculating prandial insulin doses in people with type 1 and type 2 diabetes. Finally, we concluded the work and asked questions which are still waiting for answers.

2. Effect of Fat, Protein and Carbohydrates in a Meal on Postprandial Glycemia

In type 1 diabetes, fat reduces the early glucose response (the first 2–3 h after the meal) and delays the peak blood glucose due to the delayed gastric emptying. In type 1 diabetes, fat leads to late post meal (>3 h) hyperglycemia [16]. In children with type 1 diabetes, adding 35 g of fat to the meal can increase the blood glucose level by 2.3 mmol/L (41 mg/dL) [17]. Fat consumption increases the need for insulin and requires an individual increase of the insulin dose with caution, and the calculation of the necessary insulin dose should take into account the duration of insulin action [18]. While paying attention to prevent late after-meal hyperglycemia, one should remember the risk of early hypoglycemia immediately after the meal. Campbell et al. demonstrated in type 1 diabetic patients that increasing the mealtime insulin is not an efficient strategy alone because it may increase the risk of early postprandial hypoglycemia [19].

Total and saturated fat intake were associated with a higher risk of type 2 diabetes, but these associations were not independent of obesity [20]. Dietary fat and free fatty acids (FFA) are known to impair insulin sensitivity and enhance hepatic glucose production [21]. Limited results are available on the fat effects on gastric emptying and postprandial glycemia in people with type 2 diabetes. Gentilcore et al. demonstrated that ingestion of fat before a carbohydrate meal resulted in slower gastric emptying and attenuated postprandial rises in glucose, insulin, and glucose-dependent insulinotropic polypeptide but it stimulated glucagon-like peptide-1 (GLP-1) in type 2 diabetes [22].

Protein consumption affects the blood glucose concentration in the late postprandial period. In people with type 1 diabetes using intensive insulin therapy 75 g or more of protein alone significantly increases postprandial glycemia from 3 to 5 h in people with type 1 diabetes [23]. Moreover, protein has different effects when consumed with and without carbohydrates, e.g., 30 g of protein with carbohydrates will affect blood glucose [16,17].

In type 2 diabetes, protein when consumed without carbohydrates has a very small effect on the level of glucose in the blood. In people with type 2 diabetes, after ingesting 50 g of protein the glucose response to protein remains stable for 2 h and then begins to decline [24]. Protein does not result in an increase of the blood glucose concentration, and it results in only a modest increase in the rate of glucose disappearance [25].

Meals with a high GI cause a rapid increase in glycemia. An inadequate insulin dose that does not take into account the rapid absorption of carbohydrates after consuming foods with a high GI may lead to a rapid increase in the blood glucose concentration.

Foods with a low GI cause a smaller increase in the glucose level, reducing the peak of glycemia, but at the same time it was demonstrated that such foods increase the risk of hypoglycemia after the meal in people with type 1 diabetes if taken with inadequate doses of insulin [16]. Three studies in people with type 1 diabetes suggested that the risk of mild hypoglycemia is greater with low GI than with high GI foods when the usual carbohydrate-to-insulin ratio is used [26–28]. However, low GI diets can significantly improve metabolic control in less than optimally controlled people with type 1 and type 2 diabetes, as indicated by the results of a meta-analysis reported by Thomas and Elliott [29]. The twelve included studies in this meta-analysis involved a total of 612 participants. Three studies had participants with type 1 diabetes, 8 studies had participants with type 2 diabetes, and one study had participants with either type 1 or type 2 diabetes. Low GI diets lower HbA1c levels by 0.4% compared with comparison diets, i.e., high GI diet in 10 studies, measured carbohydrate exchange diet in one study, and a high-cereal fiber diet in another study. Nevertheless, it should be remembered that eating a large amount of high carbohydrate foods with a low GI can lead to a significant increase in glycemia. A similar effect is observed after eating foods with a low GI but with a high content of fructose or sucrose, e.g., fruit juices.

The following questions should be asked: what do we know about the effects of individual components of the diet on postprandial glycemia in people with diabetes and is this knowledge necessary for us to effectively control it?

In a study reported in 2004, the effect of two diets on a 24-h glycemia and insulinemia profiles was compared in people with untreated type 2 diabetes [30]. The control diet was developed in accordance with the recommendations of the American Heart Association and the US Department of Agriculture, and it consisted of 55% carbohydrates with emphasis on products containing starch, 15% protein and 30% fat, including 10% monounsaturated, 10% polyunsaturated and 10% saturated fatty acids. The test diet was designed to consist of 20% carbohydrates, 30% protein and 50% fat. The content of saturated fatty acids in this diet was ~10% of the total food energy. Mean blood glucose values determined after 5 weeks of the dietary treatment were significantly lower in patients using the test diet compared to those using the control diet, 7.0 mmol/L (126 mg/dL) vs. 10.5 mmol/L (190 mg/dL). The control diet caused a higher increase of the insulin concentration in the blood. Thus, the diet with the carbohydrate restriction consumed for 5 weeks dramatically reduced blood glucose levels in people with type 2 diabetes. However, it should be emphasized that the study was conducted in people with untreated diabetes. Studies on the effect of various diets on glycemic control in people with type 2 diabetes treated with insulin have not been conducted so far, and thus—are required. Low-carbohydrate diets (LCD) are recognized as "no side effects" diets in the newest consensus report of ADA and the European Association for the Study of Diabetes (EASD) [31]. However, in the same consensus report the systematic literature review and meta-analysis of Sainsbury et al. is cited, which indicates that LCDs (26% of total energy) in people with type 1 and type 2 diabetes produce substantial reductions in HbA1c at 3 months and 6 months, with diminishing effects at 12 and 24 months and that no benefit of moderate carbohydrate restriction (26%–45%) was observed in 25 randomized controlled trials involving 2415 participants that were included in the meta-analysis [32]. Moreover, Mizidi et al. demonstrated the unfavorable effect of LCDs on total and cause-specific mortality, based on both individual data and pooling previous cohort studies. These authors concluded that given the fact that LCDs may be unsafe, it would be currently preferable not to recommend such diets [33]. On the other hand, several cohort studies showed that high carbohydrate diets (HCD) might be associated with higher risk of total mortality and cardiovascular disease [34,35].

The composition of the diet isn't the only factor that affects the blood glucose after a meal. In people with poorly controlled type 2 diabetes, reducing consumption of carbohydrates during breakfast and increasing it during lunch helps to improve glycemic control. By choosing one of meals with the highest carbohydrate content, while keeping the same daily intake of carbohydrates, a different therapeutic effect can be obtained [36].

The order in which foods containing various amounts of carbohydrates, protein and fat are consumed also affects the postprandial glucose level. Shukla et al. studied people with type 2 diabetes, who have been receiving the same meal consisting of carbohydrates, protein and vegetables for three days and consumed it in a random order: first carbohydrates, then after 10 min protein and vegetables or first protein and vegetables, then after 10 min carbohydrates or all components of the meal at the same time. It was shown that peaks of the glucose rise after the meal were more than 50% lower, with a simultaneously lower increase of insulinemia and higher secretion of GLP-1 when carbohydrates had been consumed as the last part of the meal in comparison with consumption of carbohydrates at the beginning of the meal [37]. The order of consuming food products affects also concentration of ghrelin—the "hunger hormone" which has orexigenic and adipogenic properties and is thought to play an important role in regulating food intake and body weight. Shukla et al. showed that the intake of carbohydrates at the beginning of the meal led to the restoration of postprandial ghrelin concentration in the postprandial period [38]. This effect was not found when the meal was started by serving protein and vegetables. Ghrelin secretion is suppressed immediately after a meal, the depth and duration of the suppression being proportional to the energy intake. Insulin may suppress circulating ghrelin independently of glucose [39]. Taking carbohydrates at the beginning of a meal shortens the period of suppression of ghrelin, which may result in shortening the period of feeling satiety, speeding up the next meal, and consequently leading to weight gain.

All these data indicate that a few factors may influence the increase in glycemia after the meal, which creates significant practical difficulties in determining the appropriate dose of insulin to compensate for food intake in people with diabetes.

3. Automatic Bolus Calculators in People with Type 1 Diabetes

People with type 1 diabetes treated with insulin pumps may use an automatic bolus calculator that allows them to determine the insulin dose based on the amount of carbohydrates consumed in the meal and an individual insulin sensitivity. The use of the bolus calculator in patients treated with multiple insulin injections resulted in a significant improvement of the metabolic control while the number of hypoglycemic episodes was slightly reduced [40]. There are some promising new applications of the emerging technologies in this field like the expert system using the automatic speech-to-text conversion, which is able to determine the caloricity, the content of carbohydrates, fat and protein in the meal in a fairly accurate way based on its voice description provided by the user. Such a system is an easy-to-use support tool in the type 1 diabetes treatment that makes it possible to improve the postprandial glycemic control [41,42]. This system can also be useful in people with type 2 diabetes to control the amount of food consumed or adjust insulin dosage. Other systems that attempt to calculate the meal content based on its digital image [43,44] or the monitoring of activities related to consumption of the meal, e.g., swallowing or chewing [45] are also under development and testing. Regardless of how the meal content is determined and entered, each automatic bolus calculator must implement an algorithm determining the insulin dose, which should be able to control postprandial glucose concentration. The review of such algorithms for people with type 1 diabetes can be found for example in a report of Krzymien et al. [46].

In people with type 1 diabetes, prandial insulin doses are individualized using parameters such as the insulin-to-carbohydrates ratio, and much less frequently, the circadian fluctuations of this parameter. However, in most algorithms the meal is characterized just by carbohydrate content despite the fact that new insights concerning the effect of dietary macronutrients on postprandial glycemia confirm that fat and protein content should be taken into consideration while calculating prandial insulin doses [16,47,48]. Pankowska and Blazik showed that the insulin bolus calculator with an algorithm accounting for carbohydrates and protein and/or fat in the meal could effectively suggest a normal or a square-wave bolus and indicate the timing of the square-wave bolus in the insulin pump users [49]. The same authors demonstrated in a 3-month open label randomized control study that the use of this system by educated children and adolescents with type 1 diabetes was safe and reduced 2-h postprandial blood glucose level and glucose variability [50].

Summing up, the improvement in the postprandial plasma glucose control in people with type 1 diabetes depends primarily on properly adjusting the insulin dose to the meal being consumed.

4. Inter-Subject Variability of a Response to Meals

The algorithms that have been implemented in automatic bolus calculators so far have not accounted for variability in the response to meals with identical carbohydrate content. In 2015, Zeevi et al. demonstrated on an 800-person cohort of individuals aged 18–70 not previously diagnosed with diabetes that people eating identical meals presented high variability in post-meal blood glucose responses. These authors showed that personalized diets created with the help of an accurate predictor of the blood glucose response integrating parameters such as dietary habits, physical activity, and gut microbiota might successfully lower postprandial blood glucose concentration and its long-term metabolic consequences [51]. In the same report authors developed a machine-learning algorithm accurately predicting personalized postprandial glycemic responses to real-life meals based on blood parameters, dietary habits, anthropometrics, physical activity, and the gut microbiota. These results indicate that it may be beneficial to incorporate such a personalized meal-dependent predictor of the postprandial glycemia into automatic insulin bolus calculators. However, we must emphasize that in the work of Zeevi et al., the study group consisted of a healthy population and it should be confirmed that the findings are equally valid in people with diabetes before they can be used to optimize the diabetes treatment. Recently, Rozendaal et al. demonstrated that the large variability in postprandial glycemic response dynamics to different types of food is inadequately predicted by existing glycemic measures such as the Glycemic Index, the Glycemic Load and the Glycemic Glucose Equivalents [52]. They quantitatively described the postprandial glycemic response dynamics using a physiology-based dynamic model. Although both these reports were based on data of people without diabetes, their conclusions admittedly should be applicable also to people with type 1 diabetes. The conclusions from the recent studies on variability of postprandial glucose response, if confirmed in people with diabetes, should result in more personalized algorithms for prandial insulin dose calculation in the future.

5. Insulin Therapy in People with Type 2 Diabetes

Insulin therapy in people with type 2 diabetes is significantly different from that used to treat people with type 1 diabetes. Typically, the treatment starts with the basal insulin and is directed to the fasting blood glucose control [53]. The fasting glucose is closely controlled by regulating hepatic glucose production with variable release of insulin into the portal vein, and with modulation of insulin action in the liver by glucagon and FFA [54,55]. In type 2 diabetes, the basal insulin secretion is impaired, and FFA and the fasting glucagon levels are high. An injection of long-acting insulin inhibits glucose production in the liver by acting directly on the liver and indirectly by reducing the release of FFA from adipose tissue [56,57]. In untreated type 2 diabetes, the HbA1c level depends primarily on fasting glycemia. The postprandial glucose concentration is less influential, especially in cases where the HbA1c level is greater than 8.0% (64 mmol/mol) [58]. In type 2 diabetes, most of the hypoglycemic agents used allow effective control of the fasting blood glucose. Metformin, sulfonylureas, thiazolidinediones and basal insulins (human NPH and insulin glargine, detemir, degludec) have little effect on postprandial hyperglycemia. Starting the basal insulin therapy is very simple. Normally, oral medications that have been used before initiation of the insulin therapy are given with insulin at a dose of 10 U or 0.1–0.2 U/kg of the body weight. The daily dose is then adjusted based on the fasting glycemia to obtain an individually determined fasting glucose target by increasing it in steps of 10% to 15% or 2 to 4 U once or twice a week. In the case of hypoglycemia, the dose is usually reduced by 4 U or 10% to 15% [59]. Yki-Järvinen et al. performed a study in patients with type 2 diabetes treated with one or two oral preparations with an average baseline HbA1c value of 9.5% (80 mmol/mol). After 36 weeks of active administration of insulin glargine and metformin, a significant improvement in metabolic control and a reduction in the fasting glucose was achieved. During the last 12 weeks the fasting plasma glucose averaged 5.8 mmol/L (104 mg/dL), and the mean HbA1c value was 7.14% (54 mmol/mol) at the end of the study period implying that half of the study group remained inadequately controlled (HbA1c > 7%), mainly due to hyperglycemia during the day [60]. The insulin treatment of people with type 2 diabetes requires normalization of both fasting and postprandial glycemia [61]. Failure to achieve HbA1c targets requires intensification of the therapy by choosing one of two therapeutic options, administering insulin mixtures twice a day, or administering fast-acting insulin before the largest meal.

For the treatment with insulin mixtures, the following principles established by ADA should be followed in the majority of people with type 2 diabetes [59]:

- Initially, the usual dose of the basal insulin should be divided, and 2/3 of the dose should be administered before the morning and 1/3 of the dose before the evening meal.
- The insulin dose should be adjusted by adding 1 to 2 U or 10% to 15% once or twice a week until the target values in the glucose self-monitoring are obtained. In case of 4 blood glucose measurements per day, the insulin dose before the breakfast should be adjusted to control the blood glucose concentration after lunch and before supper, and the dose administered before the dinner should be changed to control the blood glucose measured before bedtime and before breakfast.
- If hypoglycemia occurs, the appropriate insulin dose should be reduced by 2 to 4 U or 10% to 20%.

Recommendations for choosing dosage of insulin mixtures are similar to those of basal insulin, and dose adjustments depend on the results of blood glucose measurements. It is assumed that patients treated with insulin mixtures should eat meals at a similar rate of calories. It should also be noted what part of the mixture is short-acting or fast-acting insulin. A randomized study performed by Chen et al. showed that insulin mixtures containing 50% of the fast-acting analogue are much more effective in treating patients using higher carbohydrate diets [62]. This is reflected in the summary of clinical recommendations on the use of insulin mixtures in the treatment of type 2 diabetes, indicating that in some patients Mix50 mixtures may be more appropriate than Mix25/30 mixtures, and clinicians should consider not only efficacy and safety, but also traits and patient preferences during insulin treatment of people with type 2 diabetes [63].

In healthy people after eating a meal, insulin releases quickly and significantly increases, which is accompanied by an increase in the secretion of amylin (another hormone besides insulin, which is produced by β cells), which inhibits the secretion of glucagon, slows gastric emptying and causes a feeling of satiety. An important role is also played by various gastro-intestinal peptides, including GLP-1, which also inhibit the release of glucagon, such as amylin, and slow the emptying of the stomach and lead to a feeling of fullness. In people with type 2 diabetes, the release of insulin after a meal is slower, no increase is observed as in healthy people, the peak of insulin secretion occurs 90 to 120 min after starting the meal whereas in healthy people it is observed within the first 30 min. The increase in amylin secretion is also delayed and reduced, which, as a consequence, does not lead to suppression of glucagon, slowing gastric emptying and limiting food intake (no feeling of fullness). The secretion or action of GLP-1 may also be impaired [64]. Many individuals with type 2 diabetes may require mealtime bolus insulin dosing in addition to basal insulin. The dose and duration of action of prandial insulin should correspond to the need for adequate glycemic control. In many cases, meals vary greatly in terms of composition, size and time of consumption. Inappropriate therapeutic decisions regarding insulin dosing may lead to significant hyperglycemia or hypoglycemia. It should also be remembered that the exogenous insulin injection leads to inhibition of endogenous insulin and amylin secretion, reducing the feeling of satiety, leading to increased food intake and the body weight gain. In the case of a significant reduction in endogenous insulin and amylin secretion, treatment with insulin administered before meals is very difficult.

A lack of ability to achieve adequate glycemic control (HbA1c) during the treatment with basal insulin is a signal, besides the possibility of treatment with insulin mixtures, for administration of a fast-acting analogue before the largest meal, i.e., the use of the basal-plus insulin regimen. Usually an analogue is administered at a dose of 4 U, 0.1 U/kg or 10% of the basal insulin dose. If HbA1c is lower than 8.0% (64 mmol/mol) during this period, a reduction in the basal insulin dose should be considered. Then the dose should be adjusted by 1 to 2 U or 10% to 15% once or twice a week until the target values in self-control are achieved. In the presence of hypoglycemia and the diagnosis of the cause, the dose is reduced by 2 to 4 U or by 10% to 20%. It is a simple treatment that is easily accepted by patients [59]. On average, after adding a single dose before one meal, a reduction of HbA1c by 0.3 to 0.5% (3.3 to 5.5 mmol/mol) is observed. At the beginning of the treatment, the addition of a single injection of insulin is usually just as effective as using two injections, but with a lower risk of hypoglycemia and similar glycemic control is achievable as in the case of insulin delivery in multiple injections [65,66]. A good therapeutic effect can be obtained regardless of the rate of change in adjusting insulin doses [67]. Hence, just like in the case of insulin mixtures, the dose setting depends on the results of glycemic measurements and it is not based on adjusting the doses to the meal. Along with the time from the diagnosis of type 2 diabetes, the postprandial hyperglycemia control becomes more and more difficult. Many patients require early significant intensification of therapy to ensure further decades of active life. In particular, earlier intensification of the treatment due to a rapid deterioration of metabolic control is required in relatively young people with type 2 diabetes [68]. However, intensification of insulin therapy increases the risk of weight gain and hypoglycemia. Many patients reach a state where further insulin dose increase does not improve glycemic control. In addition, as demonstrated in studies evaluating the results of intensification of insulin therapy in people with type 2 diabetes, the basal-bolus regimen provides a small further improvement in HbA1c levels compared to simpler insulin delivery regimens [69,70].

The ADA states in its recommendations that the postprandial glucose increase may be better controlled by adjusting the time of insulin administration before a meal, indicating that the type of insulin used (short acting insulin or a fast-acting analog) should be taken into account while adjusting the time of insulin administration. Insulin doses set before meals should depend on the measured blood glucose levels and meal times. In this case, ADA also draws attention to the adjustment of the dose according to the carbohydrates consumed. However, this is only a note, because in the published recommendations the results of glycemia have a major impact on the setting of insulin doses [59].

For over a dozen years, research has been undertaken to assess the effectiveness of insulin therapy in people with type 2 diabetes based on adjusting insulin doses to meals. In 2008, Bergenstal et al. published the results of a multicenter, controlled, open label, randomized study that compared the use of two algorithms, i.e., Simple Algorithm vs. Carbohydrates Count, for adjusting mealtime insulin along with a simple algorithm for adjusting glargine insulin in a group of people with type 2 diabetes. The study involved 273 participants aged 18–70 years, with type 2 diabetes for at least 6 months, with HbA1c in the range of 7.0 to 10.0% (53 to 86 mmol/mol), taking at least 2 insulin injections per day for at least 3 months before the study. All patients recorded results of the self-monitored blood glucose before meals and at bedtime, insulin doses, menus, information on hypoglycemia, physical activity levels as well as the results of a 7-point blood glucose profile performed on week 0, 12, 18, and 24. The study established fairly stringent blood glucose targets that were as follows: fasting < 5.3 mmol/L (95 mg/dL), preprandial (before lunch and dinner) < 5.6 mmol/L (100 mg/dL) and before sleep < 7.2 mmol/L (130 mg/dL). In the Carbohydrates Count group, depending on the sensitivity to insulin, from 1 U per 20 g of carbohydrates to 3 U per 15 g of carbohydrates were given. In this group, a slightly greater but not statistically significant reduction in HbA1c, i.e., -1.59 vs. -1.46% (-17.5 vs. -16.1 mmol/mol) was obtained, lower daily doses of insulin were used, and a tendency towards less weight gain was observed [71]. In AACE/ACE Consensus Statement it has been declared that "carbohydrate counting was not more effective than a simplified bolus insulin dosage algorithm based on pre-meal and bedtime glucose patterns" based on results of this trial [8]. However, Hirose et al. conducted tests in a hospital setting in a small group of patients comparing the results of dose setting based on glycemia and based on carbohydrate content counting. After 14 days of treatment, better glycemic control was obtained in the carbohydrate counting group ($p < 0.001$) [72]. These results were not confirmed by the authors of another randomized study, which compared the fixed meal insulin dosing with flexible meal dosing based on carbohydrate counting in hospitalized people with type 2 diabetes requiring at least 20 U of insulin per day. In the flexible meal dosing group, the algorithm used to treat type 1 diabetes with insulin pumps was adopted. The constant dose group required much larger amounts of basal insulin, but both groups achieved similar glycemic control [73]. During the last EASD meeting in Berlin (2018), a group of Danish researchers announced the results of the evaluation of efficacy of advanced carbohydrate counting and the use of an automated bolus calculator compared with mental insulin bolus calculation in people with type 2 diabetes on the basal-bolus insulin therapy. In conclusion they stated that the advanced carbohydrate counting and insulin bolus calculation is an efficient, low cost tool to reduce HbA1c in people with type 2 diabetes on the basal-bolus insulin regimen. Similar effects were observed regardless of whether the automated bolus calculator or the mental bolus calculations were used. The blinded continuous glucose monitoring revealed decreased glycemic variability with both options, whereas only the group using the automated bolus calculator increased the time in the euglycemic range [74].

Practically, the system based on the results of both glycemic and glycemic-after-prone tests is a combined treatment with GLP-1 agonist and the basal insulin. However, this treatment is effective only in those people with type 2 diabetes who have preserved endogenous insulin secretion.

6. Conclusions

It seems reasonable to conclude that in the insulin treatment of people with diabetes prandial doses of insulin should take into account the result of pre-meal glycemia as well as the composition and size of meals. There are still open questions regarding the optimal way to adjust a prandial insulin dose to a meal and the possible benefits for people with type 1 and type 2 diabetes if particular parameters of the meal are taken into account while calculating the prandial insulin dose (e.g., content of all macronutrients in a meal, the proportion and order of consumption of various foods during a meal, inter-subject variability of response to the meal in respect to the postprandial blood glucose etc.). It should be emphasized that the answers to these questions may vary depending on the type of diabetes. In type 1 diabetes, it is generally accepted and considered to be beneficial to take into account the carbohydrate content of the meals when adjusting the prandial insulin doses. There is also evidence that protein and fat counting is advantageous in children and adolescents with type 1 diabetes treated with insulin pumps. However, there is no data available on this topic for adults with type 1 diabetes or people with type 2 diabetes. Hence, we should emphasize that the following questions are still waiting for answers:

- Is the calculation of carbohydrate exchangers sufficient to achieve improved postprandial glycemic control in adults with type 1 diabetes and people with type 2 diabetes or should the intake of protein and fat be also taken into account?
- What other factors should be taken into consideration when determining doses of insulin administered before meals in people with diabetes?
- Is it possible to develop a simple algorithm for prandial insulin dose adjustment based on the blood glucose measurements and counting all macronutrients in the meal?

Author Contributions: Conceptualization, writing—original draft preparation, J.K.; data curation, investigation, methodology, validation, J.K. and P.L.; project administration, supervision, writing—review and editing, P.L. Both authors approved the final version of the paper.

Funding: This study, including the costs to publish in open access, was partially funded by the National Center for Research and Development (grant No. PBS1/B9/13/2012).

Conflicts of Interest: The authors declare no conflict of interest.

References

1. Mazze, R.S.; Strock, E.; Wesley, D.; Borgman, S.; Morgan, B.; Bergenstal, R.; Cuddihy, R. Characterizing glucose exposure for individuals with normal glucose tolerance using continuous glucose monitoring and ambulatory glucose profile analysis. *Diabetes Technol.* **2008**, *10*, 149–159. [CrossRef] [PubMed]
2. International Diabetes Federation. Diabetes Atlas Eighth Edition 2018. Available online: http://diabetesatlas.org/resources/2017-atlas.html (accessed on 15 February 2019).
3. Forouhi, N.G.; Wareham, N.J. Epidemiology of diabetes. *Medicine (Abingdon)* **2014**, *42*, 698–702. [CrossRef]
4. American Diabetes Association. Glycemic targets: Standards of medical care in diabetes—2019. *Diabetes Care* **2019**, *42*, S61–S70. [CrossRef] [PubMed]
5. National Institute for Health and Care Excellence. Type 2 Diabetes in Adults: Management. Available online: http://www.nice.org.uk/guidance/ng28/resources/type-2-diabetes-in-adults-management-pdf-1837338615493 (accessed on 28 January 2019).
6. Redmon, B.; Caccamo, D.; Flavin, P.; Michels, R.; Myers, C.; O'Connor, P.; Roberts, J.; Setterlund, L.; Smith, S.; Sperl-Hillen, J.; Institute for Clinical Systems Improvement. Diagnosis and Management of Type 2 Diabetes Mellitus in Adults. Updated July 2014. Available online: https://www.icsi.org/_asset/3rrm36/Diabetes.pdf (accessed on 28 January 2019).
7. Handelsman, Y.; Bloomgarden, Z.T.; Grunberger, G.; Umpierrez, G.; Zimmerman, R.S.; Bailey, T.S.; Blonde, L.; Bray, G.A.; Cohen, A.J.; Dagogo-Jack, S.; et al. American Association of Clinical Endocrinologists and American College of Endocrinology—Clinical practice guidelines for developing a diabetes mellitus comprehensive care plan—2015. *Endocr. Pract.* **2015**, *21*, 1–87. [CrossRef] [PubMed]
8. Consensus Statement by the American Association of Clinical Endocrinologists and American College of Endocrinology on the comprehensive type 2 diabetes management algorithm—2018 Executive summary. *Endocr. Pract.* **2018**, *24*, 91–120. [CrossRef] [PubMed]
9. Scottish Intercollegiate Guidelines Network Management of Diabetes. *A National Clinical Guidelinei*; SIGN Publication No. 116; Scottish Intercollegiate Guidelines Network: Edinburgh, UK, 2013; pp. 1–161.
10. The Management of Type 2 Diabetes Mellitus in Primary Care Work Group. VA/DoD Clinical Practice Guideline for the Management of Type 2 Diabetes Mellitus in Primary Care. April 2017. Available online: http://www.healthquality.va.gov/guidelines/CD/diabetes/VADoDDMCPGFinal508.pdf (accessed on 28 January 2019).

11. Qaseem, A.; Wilt, T.J.; Kansagara, D.; Horwitch, C.; Barry, M.J.; Forciea, M.A.; Clinical Guidelines Committee of the American College of Physicians. Hemoglobin A1c Targets for glycemic control with pharmacologic therapy for nonpregnant adults with type 2 diabetes mellitus: A Guidance Statement Update from the American College of Physicians. *Ann. Intern. Med.* **2018**, *168*, 569–576. [CrossRef] [PubMed]

12. Riddle, M.C.; Gerstein, H.C.; Holman, R.R.; Inzucchi, S.E.; Zinman, B.; Zoungas, S.; Cefalu, W.T. A1c targets should be personalized to maximize benefits while limiting risks. *Diabetes Care* **2018**, *41*, 1121–1124. [CrossRef] [PubMed]

13. Polish Diabetes Association. Guidelines on the management of diabetic patients. Diabetes and pregnancy. *Clin. Diabetes* **2017**, *3*, A53–A56.

14. Fonseca, V.A.; Grunberger, G.; Anhalt, H.; Bailey, T.S.; Blevins, T.; Garg, S.K.; Handelsman, Y.; Hirsch, I.B.; Orzeck, E.A.; Consensus Conference Writing Committee; et al. Continuous glucose monitoring: A consensus conference of the American Association of Clinical Endocrinologists and American College of Endocrinology. *Endocr. Pract.* **2016**, *22*, 1008–1021. [CrossRef]

15. Bode, B.W.; Schwartz, S.; Stubbs, H.A.; Block, J.E. Glycemic characteristics in continuously monitored patients with type 1 and type 2 diabetes. *Diabetes Care* **2005**, *28*, 2361–2366. [CrossRef]

16. Bell, K.J.; Carmel, E.; Smart, C.E.; Steil, G.M.; Brand-Miller, J.C.; King, B.; Wolper, H.A. Impact of fat, protein, and glycemic index on postprandial glucose control in type 1 diabetes: Implications for intensive diabetes management in the continuous glucose monitoring era. *Diabetes Care* **2015**, *38*, 1008–1015. [CrossRef]

17. Smart, C.E.; Evans, M.; O'Connell, S.M.; McElduff, P.; Lopez, P.E.; Jones, T.W.; Davis, E.A.; King, B.R. Both dietary protein and fat increase postprandial glucose excursions in children with type 1 diabetes, and the effect is additive. *Diabetes Care* **2013**, *36*, 3897–3902. [CrossRef]

18. Wolpert, H.A.; Atakov-Castillo, A.; Smith, S.A.; Steil, G.M. Dietary fat acutely increases glucose concentrations and insulin requirements in patients with type 1 diabetes: Implications for carbohydrate-based bolus dose calculation and intensive diabetes management. *Diabetes Care* **2013**, *36*, 810–816. [CrossRef]

19. Campbell, M.D.; Walker, M.; King, D.; Gonzalez, J.T.; Allerton, D.; Stevenson, E.J.; Shaw, J.A.; West, D.J. Carbohydrate counting at meal time followed by a small secondary postprandial bolus injection at 3 hours prevents late hyperglycemia, without hypoglycemia, after a high-carbohydrate, high-fat meal in type 1 diabetes. *Diabetes Care* **2016**, *39*, e141–e142. [CrossRef]

20. Van Dam, R.M.; Willett, W.C.; Rimm, E.B.; Stampfer, M.J.; Hu, F.B. Dietary fat and meat intake in relation to risk of type 2 diabetes in men. *Diabetes Care* **2002**, *25*, 417–424. [CrossRef]

21. Savage, D.B.; Petersen, K.F.; Shulman, G.I. Disordered lipid metabolism and the pathogenesis of insulin resistance. *Physiol. Rev.* **2007**, *87*, 507–520. [CrossRef]

22. Gentilcore, D.; Chaikomin, R.; Jones, K.L.; Russo, A.; Feinle-Bisset, C.; Wishart, J.M.; Rayner, C.K.; Horowitz, M. Effects of fat on gastric emptying of and the glycemic, insulin, and incretin responses to a carbohydrate meal in type 2 diabetes. *J. Clin. Endocrinol. Metab.* **2006**, *91*, 2062–2067. [CrossRef]

23. Paterson, M.A.; Smart, C.E.; Lopez, P.E.; McElduff, P.; Attia, J.; Morbey, C.; King, B.R. Influence of pure protein on postprandial blood glucose levels in individuals with type 1 diabetes mellitus. *Diabet Med.* **2016**, *33*, 592–598. [CrossRef]

24. Nuttall, F.Q.; Mooradian, A.D.; Gannon, M.C.; Billington, C.J.; Krezowski, P.A. Effect of protein ingestion on the glucose and insulin response to a standardized oral glucose load. *Diabetes Care* **1984**, *7*, 465–470. [CrossRef]

25. Gannon, M.C.; Nuttall, J.A.; Damberg, G.; Gupta, V.; Nuttall, F.Q. Effect of protein ingestion on the glucose appearance rate in people with type 2 diabetes. *J. Clin. Endocrinol. Metab.* **2001**, *86*, 1040–1047. [CrossRef]

26. Lafrance, L.; Rabasa-Lhoret, R.; Poisson, D.; Ducros, F.; Chiasson, J.L. Effects of different glycaemic index foods and dietary fibre intake on glycaemic control in type 1 diabetic patients on intensive insulin therapy. *Diabet Med.* **1998**, *15*, 972–978. [CrossRef]

27. Mohammed, N.H.; Wolever, T.M.S. Effect of carbohydrate source on post-prandial blood glucose in subjects with type 1 diabetes treated with insulin lispro. *Diabetes Res. Clin. Pract.* **2004**, *65*, 29–35. [CrossRef]

28. Nansel, T.R.; Gellar, L.; McGill, A. Effect of varying glycemic index meals on blood glucose control assessed with continuous glucose monitoring in youth with type 1 diabetes on basal-bolus insulin regimens. *Diabetes Care* **2008**, *31*, 695–697. [CrossRef]

29. Thomas, D.E.; Elliott, E.J. The use of low-glycaemic index diets in diabetes control. *Br. J. Nutr.* **2010**, *104*, 797–802. [CrossRef]

30. Gannon, M.C.; Nuttall, F.Q. Effect of a high-protein, low-carbohydrate diet on blood glucose control in people with type 2 diabetes. *Diabetes* **2004**, *53*, 2375–2382. [CrossRef]

31. Davs, M.J.; D'Alessio, D.A.; Fradkin, J.; Kernan, W.N.; Mathieu, C.; Mingrone, G.; Rossing, P.; Tsapas, A.; Wexler, D.J.; Buse, J.B. Management of hyperglycemia in type 2 diabetes, 2018. A Consensus Report by the American Diabetes Association (ADA) and the European Association for the Study of Diabetes (EASD). *Diabetes Care* **2018**, *41*, 2669–2701. [CrossRef]

32. Sainsbury, E.; Kizirian, N.V.; Partridge, S.R.; Gill, T.; Colagiuri, S.; Gibson, A.A. Effect of dietary carbohydrate restriction on glycemic control in adults with diabetes: A systematic review and metaanalysis. *Diabetes Res. Clin. Pract.* **2018**, *139*, 239–252. [CrossRef]

33. Mazidi, M.; Katsiki, N.; Mikhailidis, D.P.; Banach, M.; International Lipid Expert Panel (ILEP). Low-carbohydrate diets and all-cause and cause-specific mortality: A population-based cohort study and pooling prospective studies. *Eur. Heart J.* **2018**, *39*, 289–298. [CrossRef]

34. Yu, D.; Shu, X.-O.; Li, H.; Xiang, Y.B.; Yang, G.; Gao, Y.T.; Zheng, W.; Zhang, X. Dietary carbohydrates, refined grains, glycemic load, and risk of coronary heart disease in Chinese adults. *Am. J. Epidemiol.* **2013**, *178*, 1542–1549. [CrossRef]

35. Dehghan, M.; Mente, A.; Zhang, X.; Swaminathan, S.; Li, W.; Mohan, V.; Iqbal, R.; Kumar, R.; Wentzel-Viljoen, E.; Rosengren, A.; et al. Associations of fats and carbohydrate intake with cardiovascular disease and mortality in 18 countries from five continents (PURE): A prospective cohort study. *Lancet* **2017**, *390*, 2050–2062. [CrossRef]

36. Pearce, K.L.; Noakes, M.; Keogh, J.; Clifton, P.M. Effect of carbohydrate distribution on postprandial glucose peaks with the use of continuous glucose monitoring in type 2 diabetes. *Am. J. Clin. Nutr.* **2008**, *87*, 638–644. [CrossRef] [PubMed]

37. Shukla, A.P.; Andono, J.; Touhamy, S.H.; Casper, A.; Iliescu, R.G.; Mauer, E.; Zhu, Y.S.; Ludwig, D.S.; Aronne, L.J. Carbohydrate-last meal pattern lowers postprandial glucose and insulin excursions in type 2 diabetes. *BMJ Open Diab. Res. Care* **2017**, *5*, e000440. [CrossRef] [PubMed]

38. Shukla, A.P.; Mauer, E.; Igel, L.I.; Truong, W.; Casper, A.; Kumar, R.B.; Saunders, K.H.; Aronne, L.J. Effect of food order on ghrelin suppression. *Diabetes Care* **2018**, *41*, e76–e77. [CrossRef] [PubMed]

39. Flanagan, D.E.; Evans, M.L.; Monsod, T.P.; Rife, F.; Heptulla, R.A.; Tamborlane, W.V.; Sherwin, R.S. The influence of insulin on circulating ghrelin. *Am. J. Physiol. Endocrinol. Metab.* **2003**, *284*, E313–E316. [CrossRef] [PubMed]

40. Vallejo-Mora, M.D.; Carreira-Soler, M.; Linares-Parrado, F.; Olveira, G.; Rojo-Martínez, G.; Domínguez-López, M.; Ruiz-de-Adana-Navas, M.S.; González-Romero, M.S. The Calculating Boluses on Multiple Daily Injections (CBMDI) study: A randomized controlled trial on the effect on metabolic control of adding a bolus calculator to multiple daily injections in people with type 1 diabetes. *J. Diabetes* **2017**, *9*, 24–33. [CrossRef] [PubMed]

41. Ladyzynski, P.; Krzymien, J.; Foltynski, P.; Rachuta, M.; Bonalska, B. Accuracy of automatic carbohydrate, protein, fat and calorie counting based on voice descriptions of meals in people with type 1 diabetes. *Nutrients* **2018**, *10*, 518. [CrossRef] [PubMed]

42. Foltynski, P.; Ladyzynski, P.; Pankowska, E.; Mazurczak, K. Efficacy of automatic bolus calculator with automatic speech recognition in patients with type 1 diabetes: A randomized cross-over trial. *J. Diabetes* **2018**, *10*, 600–608. [CrossRef] [PubMed]

43. Bally, L.; Dehais, J.; Nakas, C.T.; Anthimopoulos, M.; Laimer, M.; Rhyner, D.; Rosenberg, G.; Zueger, T.; Diem, P.; Mougiakakou, S.; et al. Carbohydrate estimation supported by the GoCARB system in individuals with type 1 diabetes: A randomized prospective pilot study. *Diabetes Care* **2017**, *40*, e6–e7. [CrossRef] [PubMed]

44. Wang, Y.; He, Y.; Boushey, C.J.; Zhu, F.; Delp, E.J. Context based image analysis with application in dietary assessment and evaluation. *Multimed. Tools Appl.* **2018**, *77*, 19769–19794. [CrossRef] [PubMed]

45. Schiboni, G.; Amft, O. Automatic dietary monitoring using wearable accessories. In *Seamless Healthcare Monitoring. Advances in Wearable, Attachable and Invisible Devices*; Tamura, T., Chen, W., Eds.; Springer Int. Publ.: Cham, Switzerland, 2018; pp. 369–412. [CrossRef]

46. Krzymien, J.; Rachuta, M.; Kozlowska, I.; Ladyzynski, P.; Foltynski, P. Treatment of patients with type 1 diabetes—Insulin pumps or multiple injections? *Biocybern. Biomed. Eng.* **2016**, *29*, 1–8. [CrossRef]
47. Tascini, G.; Berioli, M.G.; Cerquiglini, L.; Santi, E.; Mancini, G.; Rogari, F.; Toni, G.; Esposito, S. Carbohydrate counting in children and adolescents with type 1 diabetes. *Nutrients* **2018**, *10*, 109. [CrossRef] [PubMed]
48. Kordonouri, O.; Hartmann, R.; Remus, K.; Bläsig, S.; Sadeghian, E.; Danne, T. Benefit of supplementary fat plus protein counting as compared with conventional carbohydrate counting for insulin bolus calculation in children with pump therapy. *Pediatr. Diabetes* **2012**, *13*, 540–544. [CrossRef] [PubMed]
49. Pankowska, E.; Blazik, M. Bolus calculator with nutrition database software, a new concept of prandial insulin programming for pump users. *J. Diabetes Sci. Technol.* **2010**, *4*, 571–576. [CrossRef] [PubMed]
50. Blazik, M.; Pankowska, E. The effect of bolus and food calculator Diabetics on glucose variability in children with type 1 diabetes treated with insulin pump: The results of RCT. *Pediatr. Diabetes* **2012**, *13*, 534–539. [CrossRef] [PubMed]
51. Zeevi, D.; Korem, T.; Zmora, N.; Israeli, D.; Rothschild, D.; Weinberger, A.; Ben-Yacov, O.; Lador, D.; Avnit-Sagi, T.; Lotan-Pompan, M.; et al. Personalized nutrition by prediction of glycemic responses. *Cell* **2015**, *163*, 1079–1094. [CrossRef] [PubMed]
52. Rozendaal, Y.J.; Maas, A.H.; van Pul, C.; Cottaar, E.J.; Haak, H.R.; Hilbers, P.A.; van Riel, N.A. Model-based analysis of postprandial glycemic response dynamics for different types of food. *Clin. Nutr. Exp.* **2018**, *19*, 32–45. [CrossRef]
53. Blonde, L.; Merilainen, M.; Karwe, V.; Raskin, P.; TITRATE Study Group. Patient-directed titration for achieving glycaemic goals using a once-daily basal insulin analogue: An assessment of two different fasting plasma glucose targets—the TITRATE study. *Diabetes Obes. Metab.* **2009**, *11*, 623–631. [CrossRef] [PubMed]
54. Faerch, K.; Borch-Johnsen, K.; Holst, J.J.; Vaag, A. Pathophysiology and aetiology of impaired fasting glycaemia and impaired glucose tolerance: Does it matter for prevention and treatment of type 2 diabetes? *Diabetologia* **2009**, *52*, 1714–1723. [CrossRef] [PubMed]
55. Varghese, R.T.; Dalla Man, C.; Sharma, A.; Viegas, I.; Barosa, C.; Marques, C.; Shah, M.; Miles, J.M.; Rizza, R.A.; Jones, J.G.; et al. Mechanisms underlying the pathogenesis of isolated impaired glucose tolerance in humans. *J. Clin. Endocrinol. Metab.* **2016**, *101*, 4816–4824. [CrossRef] [PubMed]
56. Porcellati, F.; Lucidi, P.; Cioli, P.; Candeloro, P.; Andreoli, A.M.; Marzotti, S.; Ambrogi, M.; Bolli, G.B.; Carmine, G.; Fanelli, C.G. Pharmacokinetics and pharmacodynamics of insulin glargine given in the evening as compared with in the morning in type 2 diabetes. *Diabetes Care* **2015**, *38*, 503–512. [CrossRef] [PubMed]
57. Wang, Z.; Hedrington, M.S.; Gogitidze Joy, N.; Briscoe, V.J.; Richardson, M.A.; Younk, L.; Nicholson, W.; Tate, D.B.; Davis, S.N. Dose-response effects of insulin glargine in type 2 diabetes. *Diabetes Care* **2010**, *33*, 1555–1560. [CrossRef] [PubMed]
58. Monnier, L.; Lapinski, H.; Colette, C. Contributions of fasting and postprandial plasma glucose increments to the overall diurnal hyperglycemia of type 2 diabetic patients. *Diabetes Care* **2003**, *26*, 881–885. [CrossRef] [PubMed]
59. The American Diabetes Association (ADA). Pharmacologic approaches to glycemic treatment: Standards of medical care in diabetes—2018. *Diabetes Care* **2018**, *41*, S73–S85. [CrossRef] [PubMed]
60. Yki-Järvinen, H.; Kauppinen-Mäkelin, R.; Tiikkainen, M.; Vähätalo, M.; Virtamo, H.; Nikkilä, K.; Tulokas, T.; Hulme, S.; Hardy, K.; McNulty, S.; et al. Insulin glargine or NPH combined with metformin in type 2 diabetes: The LANMET study. *Diabetologia* **2006**, *49*, 442–451. [CrossRef] [PubMed]
61. Matthew Riddle, M.; Umpierrez, G.; DiGenio, A.; Zhou, R.; Rosenstock, J. Contributions of basal and postprandial hyperglycemia over a wide range of A1c levels before and after treatment intensification in type 2 diabetes. *Diabetes Care* **2011**, *34*, 2508–2514. [CrossRef] [PubMed]
62. Chen, W.; Qian, L.; Watada, H.; Li, P.F.; Iwamoto, N.; Imori, M.; Yang, W.Y. Impact of diet on the efficacy of insulin lispro mix 25 and insulin lispro mix 50 as starter insulin in East Asian patients with type 2 diabetes: Subgroup analysis of the comparison between low mixed insulin and mid mixed insulin as starter insulin for patients with type 2 diabetes mellitus (CLASSIFY Study) randomized trial. *J. Diabetes Investig.* **2017**, *8*, 75–83. [PubMed]
63. Deed, G.; Kilov, G.; Dunning, T.; Cutfield, R.; Overland, J.; Wu, T. Use of 50/50 Premixed insulin analogs in type 2 diabetes: Systematic review and clinical recommendations. *Diabetes* **2017**, *8*, 1265–1296. [CrossRef] [PubMed]

64. Aronoff, S.L.; Berkowitz, K.; Shreiner, B.; Want, L. Glucose metabolism and regulation: Beyond insulin and glucagon. *Diabetes Spectr.* **2004**, *17*, 183–190. [CrossRef]

65. Meece, J. Basal insulin intensification in patients with type 2 diabetes: A review. *Diabetes Ther.* **2018**, *9*, 877–890. [CrossRef] [PubMed]

66. Rodbard, H.W.; Visco, V.E.; Andersen, H.; Hiort, L.C.; Shu, D.H.W. Treatment intensification with stepwise addition of prandial insulin aspart boluses compared with full basal-bolus therapy (FullSTEP Study): A randomised.; treat-to-target clinical trial. *Lancet Diabetes Endrocinol.* **2014**, *2*, 30–37. [CrossRef]

67. Edelman, S.V.; Liu, R.; Johnson, J.; Glass, L.C. AUTONOMY: The first randomized trial comparing two patient-driven approaches to initiate and titrate prandial insulin lispro in type 2 diabetes. *Diabetes Care* **2014**, *37*, 2132–2140. [CrossRef] [PubMed]

68. Donnelly, L.A.; Zhou, K.; Doney, A.S.F.; Jennison, C.; Franks, P.W.; Pearson, E.R. Rates of glycaemic deterioration in a real-world population with type 2 diabetes. *Diabetologia* **2018**, *61*, 607–615. [CrossRef] [PubMed]

69. Holman, R.R.; Farmer, A.J.; Davies, M.J.; Levy, J.C.; Darbyshire, J.L.; Keenan, J.F.; Paul, S.K.; 4-T Study Group. Three-year efficacy of complex insulin regimens in type 2 diabetes. *N. Engl. J. Med.* **2009**, *361*, 1736–1747. [CrossRef] [PubMed]

70. Riddle, M.C.; Rosenstock, J.; Vlajnic, A.; Gao, L. Randomized, 1-year comparison of three ways to initiate and advance insulin for type 2 diabetes: Twice-daily premixed insulin versus basal insulin with either basal-plus one prandial insulin or basal-bolus up to three prandial injections. *Diabetes Obes. Metab.* **2014**, *16*, 396–402. [CrossRef] [PubMed]

71. Bergenstal, R.M.; Johnson, M.; Powers, M.A.; Wynne, A.; Vlajnic, A.; Hollander, P.; Rendell, M. Adjust to target in type 2 diabetes: Comparison of a simple algorithm with carbohydrate counting for adjustment of mealtime insulin glulisine. *Diabetes Care* **2008**, *31*, 1305–1310. [CrossRef]

72. Hirose, M.; Yamanaka, H.; Ishikawa, E.; Sai, A.; Kawamura, T. Easy and flexible carbohydrate counting sliding scale reduces blood glucose of hospitalized diabetic patient in safety. *Diabetes Res. Clin. Pract.* **2011**, *93*, 404–409. [CrossRef] [PubMed]

73. Dungan, K.M.; Sagrilla, C.; Abdel-Rasoul, M.; Osei, K. Prandial insulin dosing using the carbohydrate counting technique in hospitalized patients with type 2 diabetes. *Diabetes Care* **2013**, *36*, 3476–3482. [CrossRef]

74. Christensen, M.B.; Serifovski, N.; Herz, A.M.; Schmidt, S.; Gaede, P.; Hommel, E.; Raimond, L.; Gotfredsen, A.; Nørgaard, K. Efficacy of advanced carbohydrate counting and automated insulin bolus calculators in type 2 diabetes: The BolusCal2 study. An open-label randomised controlled trial. *Diabetologia* **2018**, *61*, 819.

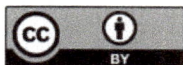

nutrients

MDPI

Article

Glycemia Lowering Effect of an Aqueous Extract of *Hedychium coronarium* Leaves in Diabetic Rodent Models

Ling-Shan Tse [1], Po-Lin Liao [2], Chi-Hao Tsai [1,3], Ching-Hao Li [4], Jiunn-Wang Liao [5],
Jaw-Jou Kang [2] and Yu-Wen Cheng [1,*]

[1] School of Pharmacy, College of Pharmacy, Taipei Medical University, Taipei 110, Taiwan;
    zoetsels@gmail.com (L.-S.T.); d01447001@ntu.edu.tw (C.-H.T.)
[2] Institute of Food Safety and Health Risk Assessment, School of Pharmaceutical Sciences,
    National Yang-Ming University, Taipei 112, Taiwan; plliao0825@gmail.com (P.-L.L.);
    jjkang@ym.edu.tw (J.-J.K.)
[3] Institute of Toxicology, College of Medicine, National Taiwan University, Taipei 100, Taiwan
[4] Department of Physiology, School of Medicine, Graduate Institute of Medical Sciences, College of Medicine,
    Taipei Medical University, Taipei 110, Taiwan; bros22@tmu.edu.tw
[5] Graduate Institute of Veterinary Pathobiology, National Chung Hsing University, Taichung 402, Taiwan;
    jwliao@dragon.nchu.edu.tw
* Correspondence: ywcheng@tmu.edu.tw; Tel.: +886-2-2736-1661 (ext. 6123); Fax: +886-2-2737-4622

Received: 7 February 2019; Accepted: 11 March 2019; Published: 14 March 2019

Abstract: *Hedychium coronarium* has a long history of use worldwide as a food and in folk medicine. In this study, we aimed to investigate the effect of an aqueous extract of *H. coronarium* leaves (HC) on type 2 diabetes mellitus (T2DM). Two types of animal models were used in this study: Streptozotocin (STZ)-induced T2DM (Wistar rats; $N = 8$) and C57BKSdb/db mice ($N = 5$). After treatment with HC for 28 days, glucose tolerance improved in both of the diabetic animal models. As significant effects were shown after 14 days of treatment in the STZ-induced T2DM model, we carried out the experiments with it. After 28 days of treatment with HC, the levels of cholesterol, triglyceride, high-density lipoprotein, and low-density lipoprotein were significantly improved in the STZ-induced T2DM model. The lesions degree of islet β-cells was decreased after the HC treatment. Although the insulin level increased moderately, the aldosterone level was significantly decreased in the HC-treated groups, suggesting that aldosterone might play an important role in this effect. In summary, HC is a natural product and it is worth exploring its effect on T2DM.

Keywords: *Hedychium coronarium*; type 2 diabetes; aldosterone; streptozotocin; metabolic syndrome; folk medicine

1. Introduction

Diabetes is a chronic progressive disease and one of the ten leading causes of death worldwide [1]. In the past three decades, the prevalence of type 2 diabetes mellitus (T2DM) has increased dramatically in countries of all income levels. Over time, diabetes causes various complications: It starts by damaging blood vessels, reducing the blood flow, with sequelae that may be macrovascular (heart attack, stroke, and heart failure) [2–4], or microvascular (blindness [5–7] and kidney failure [8]), or causing neuropathies (lower limb amputation). When diabetes is not controlled, not only is the patient quality of life affected and present a burden on medical resources, but the condition may also lead to death. In 2015, the World Health Organization (WHO) declared diabetes as one of the four priority noncommunicable diseases (NCDs) and established a diabetes program to reduce the impact of diabetes by 2020. The management of diabetes consists of two main steps: Preventing (decreasing the possible risk factors) and stabilizing the disease progress (early diagnosis, medication, and intake management) [9]. To stabilize the disease, it is crucial to adopt effective measures for surveillance and treatment strategies (pharmacologic and non-pharmacologic interventions) [10,11]. In addition to the development of novel drugs, the use of traditional medicine and food supplements for the treatment of T2DM should be investigated.

Traditional medicine (also known as folk medicine) has been used globally for centuries. Although the medicinal properties of resources such as mollusks and plants rely on the inheritance of experience, they have been gradually accepted in modern medicine. A food supplement is a dosed formulation of food and herbs, and provides medical benefits through its biologically active components [12]. Therefore, both traditional medicine and food supplements can be part of the treatment strategies for diabetes.

Extensive research has focused on the rhizome of *Hedychium coronarium*. However, the pharmacological benefits of *H. coronarium* leaf appear overlooked. *H. coronarium* is highly accessible and its leaf is a common vegetable in Taiwan. Therefore, in this study, two types of animal models were used to evaluate the lowering blood glucose level benefits of an aqueous extract of *H. coronarium* leaves (HC). A new supplement was developed, called SugarOut (SO), which contained 15% red yeast rice (RYR) and 7.2% *H. coronarium*. Red yeast rice (RYR) is a fermentation product that is traditionally used in East Asia to dye and preserve food. Its main pharmacologically active compound is monacolin-K (also called lovastatin).

H. coronarium (also called ginger lily), a plant approximately 1–3 m in height and has a long history of use in food and traditional folk medicine. For example, it is used in beauty products in Hawaii and Japan, as an essential oil in Vietnam, and as a vegetable in Malaysia. It can help ease indigestion, inflammation, insomnia, and pain in the muscles, joints, and abdomen [13,14]. In Brazil, *H. coronarium* leaf is considered a diuretic [15] and is used for the treatment of hypertension [16]. In India, the rhizome is used for the treatment of diabetes [17]. Many different bioactive compounds have been isolated from *H. coronarium* and their pharmacological effects have been established. For example, diterpenoids and a diarylheptanoid showed anti-angiogenic activity and suppressed the growth of different cancer cell types [18]. Coronarin D shows active resistance to Gram-positive bacteria and fungi [19], induces G2/M arrest, apoptosis, and autophagy [20]. Hedychilactones A, B, and C inhibit increases in nitric oxide (NO) production and the induction of inducible NO synthase [21]. Quercetin-3-*O*-glucuronide (Q3GA) has been reported to show beneficial effects in the reduction and prevention of various diseases, including neurodegenerative diseases, and to exert anti-inflammatory and antioxidant activities [22].

2. Material and Methods

2.1. Preparation of Aqueous Extract of Hedychium coronarium and SugarOut

The HC (containing 1.4% Q3GA) was a deep brown powder. Fresh overground parts (leaves and stems) of *H. coronarium* were collected in Pingtung, Taiwan. The dried leaves and stems of *H. coronarium* (100 kg) were extracted in 100% water at room temperature (25–35 °C). The 100% water extracts were concentrated in vacuo and then lyophilized to obtain a dark brown powder (8.4% yield).

SO was a prototype supplement (dark red powder) developed from *H. coronarium* that assisted with blood glucose regulation. It contained two main extracts: The RYR extract (15%) and the HC (7.2%). The two main bioactive compounds were monacolin K 1.8 mg ($\pm$20%) and Q3GA 0.6 mg ($\pm$20%).

Both test substances were provided by Vinovo Inc. The HC was stored at 4 °C and the SO was stored at room temperature. Both test substances were freshly dissolved in distilled water and administered by oral gavage daily to all rodents in the morning.

2.2. Animal Study

The Streptozotocin (STZ)-induced T2DM model was established in Wistar rats obtained from BioLASCO Ltd. (Taipei, Taiwan) and C57BKS$^{db/db}$ mice (termed db/db here) were obtained from the National Laboratory Animal Center (Taipei, Taiwan). All procedures involving the use of animals were in compliance with the Guide for the Care and Use of Laboratory Animals (Press, 1996) and approved by the Institutional Animal Care and Use Committee at our institution (Approval no. LAC-2016-0168). The preliminary data suggested that the effective dose of SO was 246 mg/kg in the db/db model. As bioavailability differs between rodent species, based on FDA Guidance, the conversion factors for the rat Wistar STZ model and the mouse db/db model were 6.2 and 12.3, respectively [23]. Therefore, 124 mg/kg SO was administered to the STZ-T2DM rats and 246 mg/kg was administered to the C57BKS$^{db/db}$ mice by oral gavage.

2.2.1. C57BKS$^{db/db}$ Mice (db/db Model)

The C57BKS$^{db/db}$ mouse is a model of diabetes with a spontaneous mutation (Lepr^{db}) resulting in morbid obesity, chronic hyperglycemia, pancreatic beta cell atrophy, and low insulin [24]. The diabetes model is determined to be well-established when the blood glucose level is >230 mg/dL after 18 h fasting. Fifteen male mice (25–30 g) were divided into the following three groups (N = 5): Control (treated with distilled water); HC (17.71 mg/kg); and SO (246 mg/kg) [23] (Figure 1).

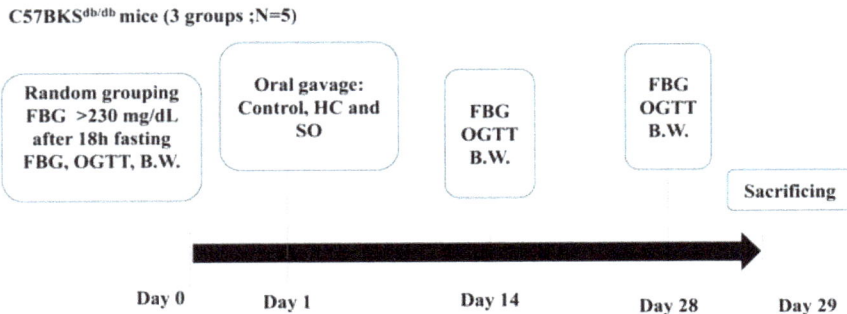

Figure 1. Study procedure for the C57BKS$^{db/db}$ mice (termed db/db here). Fifteen male db/db mice were randomly divided into three groups (N = 5): Control, treatment with *Hedychium coronarium* leaves (HC), or SugarOut (SO) supplement. FBG, fasting blood glucose; OGTT, oral glucose tolerance test; B.W., Body Weight.

2.2.2. STZ-Induced Type 2 Diabetes Model

T2DM was induced in 24 6-week-old male Wistar rats by the administration of 65 mg/kg STZ in 0.1 M citrate solution 15 min after nicotinamide injection (230 mg/kg in saline; intraperitoneally) [25–28]. The rats were caged (two animals per cage) in a controlled environment (12 h light/dark cycle, 23 ± 1 °C, and 39–43% relative humidity). The fasting glucose level was measured 1 week after the injections. The T2DM model was determined to be well-established when the blood glucose level was >230 mg/dL after 18 h of fasting. After T2DM was established, the rats were randomly divided into three groups of eight rats: Control; HC (8.928 mg/kg); and SO (124 mg/kg). An additional eight Wistar rats were used as the sham control (Figure 2).

6-week old male wistar (3 groups; N=8)

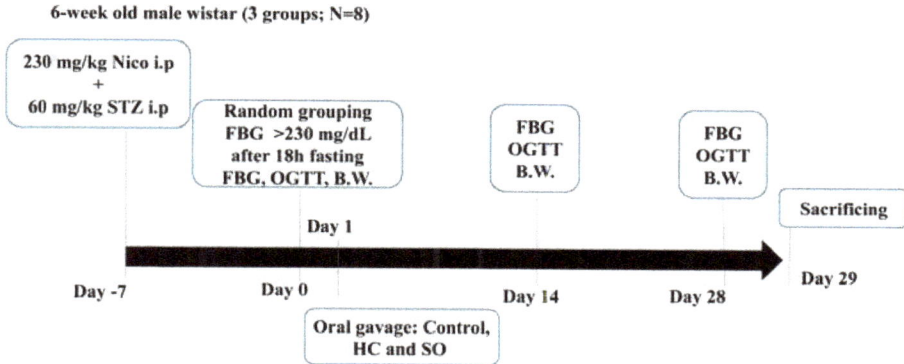

Figure 2. Study procedure for Streptozotocin (STZ)-induced type 2 diabetes rats. Diabetes was induced in 24 male Wistar rats, which were then randomly divided into three groups (Control, HC, and SO; *N* = 8).

2.3. Fasting Blood Glucose and Oral Glucose Tolerance Test

All rodents were administered the test substances daily. The body weight and fasting blood glucose (FBG) was measured on day 0, 14, and 28. The oral glucose tolerance test (OGTT) was performed on day 14 and 28. Each rodent fasted for 16 h before the FBG measurement. The test substances were administered 30 min before glucose challenge (1 g/kg), and then the blood glucose was tested 0, 30, 60, 90, and 120 min after the challenge by using IME-DC glucose test strips (IME-DC, Berlin, Germany).

2.4. Aldosterone and Insulin Levels

Serum samples were collected on day 29 after the T2DM rats were sacrificed. Insulin was quantified through the measurement of the optical density at 450 nm by using a Mercodia Ultrasensitive rat insulin ELISA kit (Mercodia AB, Uppsala, Sweden) and aldosterone was quantified through the measurement of the optical density at 405 nm corrected by the measurement at 590 nm by using an aldosterone ELISA kit (ab136933; Abcam, Cambridge, UK).

2.5. Histopathological Analysis

The pancreas was excised from T2DM rats after they were sacrificed on day 29. The samples were fixed in 10% neutral buffered formalin, and then prepared and examined by a professional pathologist from the Graduate Institute of Veterinary Pathobiology, National Chung Hsing University, Taichung, Taiwan. The severity of lesions in the islet β-cells of the pancreas was graded according to the methods described by Shackelford et al. [29]. The degree of lesions was graded from one to five, depending on severity: 1 = minimal (<1%); 2 = slight (1–25%); 3 = moderate (26–50%); 4 = moderately severe (51–75%); 5 = severe/high (76–100%).

2.6. Serum Biochemical Analysis

Blood samples from the T2DM rats were collected at the end of the 28-day oral administration period and then analyzed by using an Express Plus automatic clinical chemistry analyzer (Siemens Healthineers, Erlangen, Germany).

2.7. Statistical Analysis

All values are expressed as the mean ± standard deviation (SD) in tables and the mean ± standard error (SE) in figures. The comparisons between groups were performed by one-way analysis of variance (ANOVA) followed by Scheffe multiple comparison tests using SPSS Statistical Software (IBM, New York, NY, USA). Values of $p < 0.05$ were considered significant.

3. Results

3.1. HC Improved Fasting Blood Glucose and Glucose Tolerance in Both Diabetic Animal Models After 28 Days of Treatment

In the db/db model, after oral gavage of SO and HC, mice gained weight slower than the control group (Figure 3A). The HC decreased the FBG (Figure 3B) and increased the glucose tolerance after treatment for 14 days (Figure 3C); a significant difference was observed after treatment for 28 days (Figure 3D). SO also affected the FBG and glucose tolerance, however, the effects of SO were not as remarkable as those of the HC.

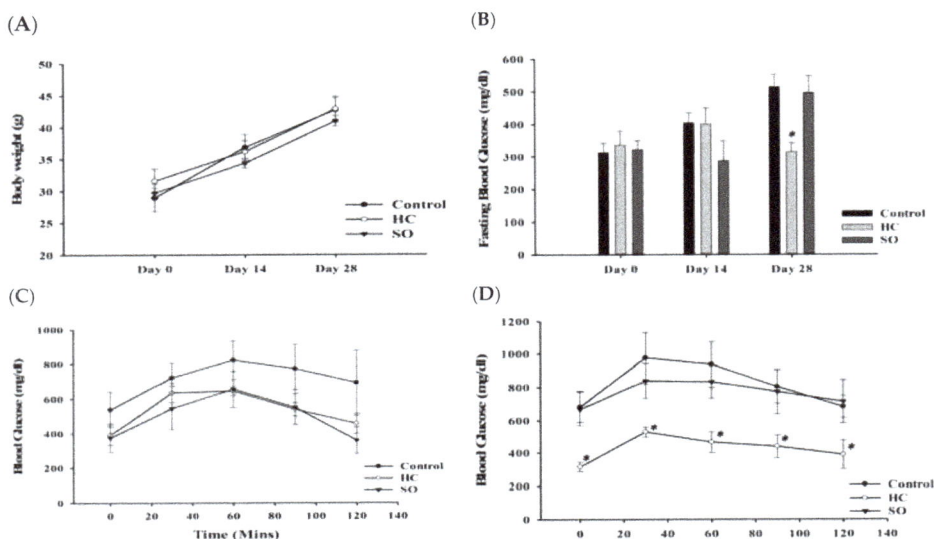

Figure 3. Effects of HC and SO in C57BKS$^{db/db}$ mice ($N = 5$). (**A**) Changes in body weight. (**B**) Changes in fasting blood glucose (FBG) after treatment with HC and SO for 14 days and 28 days. (**C**) Oral glucose tolerance test (OGTT) after administration of HC and SO for 14 days. (**D**) OGTT after administration of HC and SO for 28 days. Significant difference between the control-treated group at * $p < 0.05$, by one-way ANOVA.

In general, the STZ-induced T2DM model shows a significant weight reduction [30]. In this study, after oral gavage of SO and HC for 28 days, the body weights of mice receiving HC and SO was increased compared to that in the control group (Figure 4A) and the FBG was slightly lower in the SO group on day 28 (Figure 4B). After 14 days of oral administration of HC and SO, the blood glucose level in the HC and SO groups was significantly decreased compared with that in the control group at 60, 90, and 120 min after intake of 1 g/kg glucose (Figure 4C; p-value in Supplementary Table S1). After administration of HC and SO for 28 days (Figure 4D), the glucose level in the SO group was significantly lower than that in control group from 30 to 120 min after the intake of 1 g/kg glucose (p-value in Supplementary Table S1), however, the HC only resulted in a significant difference at 30 min after glucose intake. The area under the curve (AUC) of both the SO and HC groups was significantly lower than that of the control group (Table 1). These results suggested that HC could improve the FBG and glucose tolerance after 28 days in the db/db mice. A notable increase in glucose tolerance was observed in both the HC and SO groups after 14 days of administration, and a significant increase in glucose tolerance was observed after 28 days of administration in the T2DM model. Therefore, the following experiments focused on the STZ-induced T2DM model.

(A)

(B)

(C)

(D)

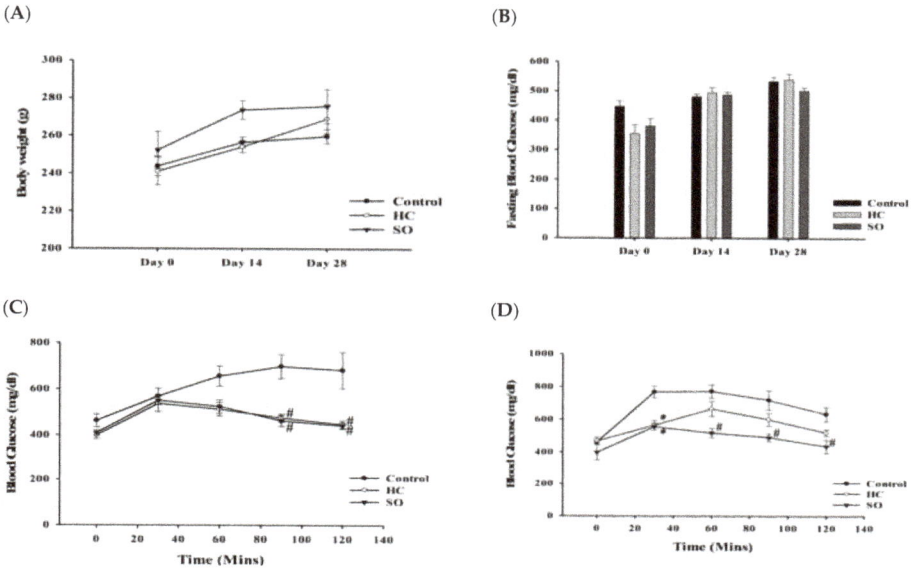

Figure 4. STZ-induced type 2 diabetes model (T2DM; $N = 8$) after the administration of HC and SO for 14 and 28 days. (**A**) Changes in body weight. (**B**) Changes in fasting blood glucose. (**C**) OGTT after administration of HC and SO for 14 days. (**D**) OGTT after administration of HC and SO for 28 days. Significant difference between control-treated group at * $p < 0.05$, # $p < 0.01$ by one-way ANOVA.

Table 1. Area under the curve (AUC) of blood glucose in the oral glucose tolerance test (OGTT).

AUC	14 Days	28 Days
Sham	8898.75 ± 1816.12	1666.88 ± 3399.66
Control	23,578.13 ± 9636.76	32,130.00 ± 8133.19
H. coronarium leaves (HC)	11,730.00 ± 5959.70	14,979.38 ± 5656.03 *
SugarOut (SO)	10,301.25 ± 5884.57	11,945.63 ± 13,782.89 **

Sham = wild-type Wistar rats treated with distilled water. $N = 8$ in each group. The data are expressed as the mean ± standard deviation (SD). Significant difference between the control-treated group at * $p < 0.05$, ** $p < 0.01$ by one-way ANOVA.

3.2. H. coronarium Attenuated STZ-Induced Pancreatic Damage and Ameliorated the Markers of Metabolic Syndrome

The levels of cholesterol, triglyceride, high-density lipoprotein (HDL), and low-density lipoprotein (LDL) were significantly decreased in the STZ-induced T2DM model compared with the control group. In the HC group, creatinine and blood urea nitrogen (BUN) were lower than the control group and similar to the sham group. The SO group did not show any significant differences compared with the control group, but the laboratory results tended to be similar to those in the sham group (Tables 2 and S2). STZ caused a severe decrease in islet β-cells (Figure 5B) and severe atrophy of acinar cells in the pancreas (Figure 5B; Figure 6B). Biopsy sections of the HC (Figure 5C; Figure 6C) and SO (Figure 5D; Figure 6D) groups showed that the morphology of the islet β-cells and acinar cells of the pancreas tended to be similar to the sham group (Figure 5A; Figure 6A). According to the degree of lesions (Table 3) after 28 days treatment, HC (0.79-fold) and SO (0.68-fold) prevented the decrease of islet cells and the atrophy of acinar cells (HC, 0.85-fold; SO 0.70-fold). HC and SO had moderate protective effects against the damage caused by STZ and regulated lipid markers (Table 2). However, the mechanism underlying the beneficial effects of HC on T2DM remains to be elucidated.

Table 2. Biochemical analysis of T2DM rat model after treatment with HC and SO for 28 days.

Group		Sham	Control	HC	SO
Number of Animals		8	8	8	8
Cholesterol	mg/dL	69.28 ± 25.71	161.50 ± 63.79	76.63 ± 15.30 **	111.63 ± 51.48
Triglycerides	mg/dL	58.13 ± 23.93	753.38 ± 434.92	105.13 ± 33.31 **	480.75 ± 410.14
HDL	mmol/L	27.13 ± 12.16	33.38 ± 13.23	42.75 ± 13.10	38.50 ± 12.31
LDL	mmol/L	7.63 ± 1.77	37.63 ± 19.83	10.50 ± 2.56 **	22.25 ± 21.02

HDL: low-density lipoproteins cholesterol; LDL: low-density lipoproteins cholesterol. Data are expressed as the mean ± SD. Significant difference between the control-treated group at ** $p < 0.01$ by one-way ANOVA.

(A)   (B)   (C)   (D)

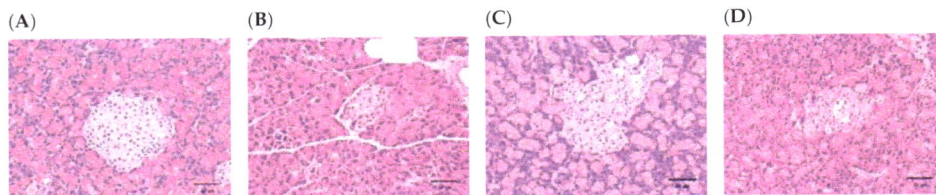

Figure 5. Histopathological changes by hemotoxylin and eosin (H & E) staining (400×) of the islets of the pancreas in rats with STZ-induced β-cell toxicity. (**A**) Sham control. Normal architecture of the β-cells in the islets of the pancreas. STZ induced a slight to moderate/severe decrease of β-cells in the islets of the pancreas in (**B**) T2DM control model. (**C**) T2DM model treated with HC for 28 days. (**D**) T2DM model treated with SO for 28 days. Scale bar = 50 μm.

(A)   (B)   (C)   (D)

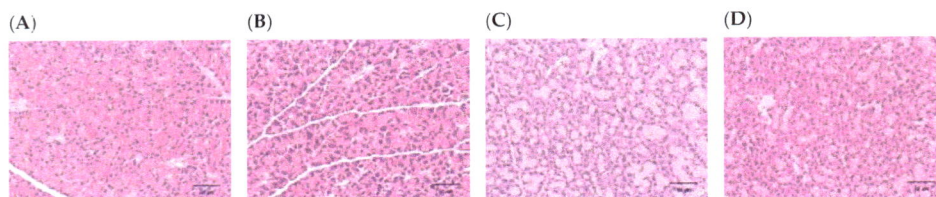

Figure 6. Histopathological changes (H & E staining, 400×) of the acinar cells in the pancreas in rats with STZ-induced β-cell toxicity. (**A**) Sham control. Normal architecture of the β-cells in the islets of the pancreas. STZ induced a slight to moderate/severe decrease of β-cells in the islets of the pancreas in (**B**) T2DM control model. (**C**) T2DM model treated with HC for 28 days. (**D**) T2DM model treated with SO for 28 days. Scale bar = 50 μm.

Table 3. Degree of lesions in the pancreas of the T2DM model animals after treatment with HC and SO for 28 days.

Pancreas	Control	HC	SO
Decrease, β-cell, islet, focal	3.80 ± 0.45	3.00 ± 0.71	2.60 ± 0.55
Atrophy, acinar cell, diffuse	4.00 ± 0.00	3.40 ± 0.89	2.80 ± 1.10

The degree of lesions was graded from one to five depending on severity: 1 = minimal (<1%); 2 = slight (1–25%); 3 = moderate (26–50%); 4 = moderate/severe (51–75%); 5 = severe/high (76–100%).

3.3. HC Altered Insulin and Aldosterone Content in Blood

Insulin levels in the HC (1.32-fold) and SO (1.29-fold) groups increased moderately compared with the control group (Figure 7). Much research has shown that the renin-angiotensin-aldosterone system (RAAS) plays a critical role in diabetes [31–33]. In our previous study, the oral administration of *H. coronarium* aqueous extract (3 g/kg) to Sprague Dawley rats for 90 days, resulted in a decrease of aldosterone levels in the serum. Therefore, we measured the aldosterone level in the present study. Aldosterone was significantly decreased in both HC (0.59-fold) and SO (0.61-fold) groups compared with that in the control group (Figure 8).

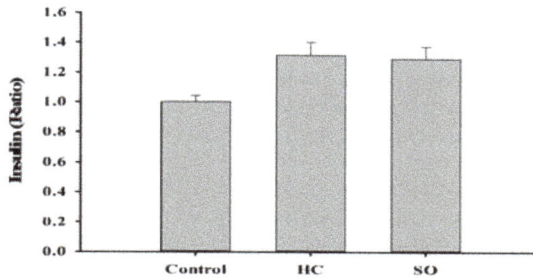

Figure 7. Insulin level in T2DM model rats after 28 days of treatment. No significant difference was found between the control-treated group by one-way ANOVA.

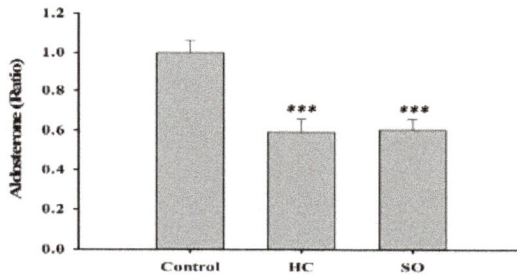

Figure 8. Aldosterone level in T2DM model rats after 28 days of treatment. Significant difference between the control-treated group at *** $p < 0.001$ by one-way ANOVA.

4. Discussion and Conclusions

In this study, we aimed to explore a natural product, *H. coronarium*, and determine if it would benefit people with diabetes. Two types of diabetic rodent models were used to determine the glycemia lowering effect of an aqueous extract of *H. coronarium* leaves. We found that HC significantly increased glucose tolerance in both diabetic models, improved the lipid profile, moderately increased insulin, benefited β-cell structure, and decreased the aldosterone level in an STZ-induced T2DM model. Although HC has been used as a folk medicine worldwide—as a diuretic and for the treatment of inflammation, hypertension, and diabetes—its mechanism of action is yet to be elucidated.

Previous studies have reported that the RAAS has played a major role in diabetes; aldosterone is significantly increased in primary hyperaldosteronism, diabetes, and other metabolic syndromes. An increase in aldosterone causes impaired glucose tolerance, decreased pancreatic β-cell function, and tissue insulin sensitivity [31,34,35]. Aldosterone is a mineralocorticoid hormone that is produced from cholesterol in the cortex of the adrenal gland. It interacts with the mineralocorticoid receptor (MR) to regulate blood pressure, water sodium, and potassium homeostasis [36]. In addition, it has genomic and non-genomic actions. The genomic actions occur through the binding of aldosterone to cytoplasmic MR, and the aldosterone-MR complex translocates to the nucleus and modulates nuclear transcription [37]. As for the rapid non-genomic action, aldosterone increases intracellular Ca^{2+} and protein kinase C (PKC) activation. In addition, aldosterone activates and stimulates Na^+/K^+-ATPase, $Na^+/K^+/2Cl^+$, NHE1, and NBCe1 [38–40], and other pathways, such as the Mitogen-activated protein (MAP) kinases pathway, adenylate cyclase, tyrosine kinase, and cAMP-dependent protein kinase. Therefore, understanding the complete regulation of aldosterone biosynthesis will allow medicinal interventions for the management of hypertension, congestive heart failure, renal disease, and diabetes mellitus [41]. In this study, both HC and SO significantly decreased aldosterone levels and increased glucose tolerance in the STZ-induced T2DM model. These findings suggest that T2DM may be improved by alteration of the aldosterone levels, but more studies are recommended to understand the regulation of this pathway.

Flavonoids may play a role in many metabolic processes involved in T2DM, and Q3GA (also known as miquelianin) is a flavonol glucuronide. Q3GA has been proven to inhibit the production of reactive oxygen species (ROS), low-density lipoprotein (LDL) oxidation [42,43], act as an anti-inflammatory, and improve insulin resistance in skeletal cells [44]. Q3GA also inhibited angiotensin II (Ang II)-induced increases in the DNA binding activity of activator protein (AP)-1, a downstream transcription factor of c-Jun N-terminal kinases (JNK), composed of the c-Jun homo/heterodimer [45]. Angiotensin II interacts with the angiotensin receptor (AT1) membrane receptor that is coupled to cellular second messengers, it is important in the regulation of aldosterone secretion [46]. As Q3GA can reduce the effect of Ang II, it may also contribute to the regulation of aldosterone.

As we would like to develop a new supplement containing HC, we also examined the effect of SO in this study. RYR has been reported to exert anti-inflammatory, hypotensive, cholesterol-lowering, cardioprotective, anticancer, and osteogenic activities [47]. In a previous study, RYR extract (300 mg/kg/day) was reported to decrease the FBG, increase insulin secretion, and protect islet cells in db/db mice [48]. Therefore, we selected RYR for the development of a food supplement containing HC. When the two compounds were combined, we expected an additional effect. In the present study, we also tested the efficacy of SO. SO slightly lowered fasting blood glucose after 28 days of treatment in the STZ-induced T2DM model (Figure 4B). The glucose tolerance (Figure 4C,D) in the SO treatment group was moderately increased compared with that in the HC group after 28 days. However, no differences in insulin, aldosterone, and histopathological findings were observed when the SO group was compared with the HC group. We found that HC exerts beneficial effects in diabetes through modulation of the aldosterone level in the blood to improve glucose tolerance. SO may slightly assist in the improvement of glucose tolerance, although the supplement formula requires improvement. SO also showed effects in two animal models, however, the efficacy of SO in the db/db model was not as strong as HC. The db/db model is known to have as defects in the leptin receptor, leading to increases in insulin and blood glucose, insulin resistance, and obesity [49]. In contrast, STZ is a DNA alkylating agent that targets β-cells [25–28]. As shown by the lipid profile in the STZ model, SO has the ability to ameliorate lipid markers, although not to the same extent as HC (Table 2). This explained how SO lowered the FBG and increased the glucose tolerance after 14 days of treatment, but was not as effective as HC during day 28 in db/db model (Figure 3).

In summary, we treated two types of diabetic rodent models with HC and SO, and found that both HC and SO exerted beneficial effects on T2DM. However, SO treatment did not show a significant difference compared with the HC treatment. The underlying mechanisms of HC, and the interactions of HC and RYR combined, are not wholly investigated yet. Therefore, we suggest that HC could be a suitable candidate for the development of drugs and food supplements for the treatment of T2DM, but more studies should be performed in order to understand the profound mechanism.

Supplementary Materials: The following are available online at http://www.mdpi.com/2072-6643/11/3/629/s1, Table S1: *p*-Value of oral glucose tolerance test (OGTT) after administrating *Hedychium coronarium* (HC) and SugarOut (SO) in STZ-induced type 2 diabetes model (T2DM; *N* = 8); Table S2: Biochemistry analysis of STZ-T2DM after treating HC and SO for 28 days.

Author Contributions: Y.-W.C., C.-H.L. and J.-J.K. planned the experiments; P.-L.L., C.-H.T., and L.-S.T. performed the experiments; L.-S.T. performed data analysis and wrote the manuscript; J.-W.L. is the main pathologist. All authors reviewed the manuscript.

Funding: This study was sponsored by Vitnovo Inc. and the Ministry of Science and Technology of Taiwan (MOST106-2320-B-038-015-MY3, MOST107-2320-B-038-064).

Conflicts of Interest: The authors declare no conflict of interest. The study design, operation, data analyses, and conclusions were not influenced by the sponsor.

Abbreviations

T2DM   type 2 diabetes;
HDL   high-density lipoproteins cholesterol;
LDL   low-density lipoproteins cholesterol;
OGTT   oral glucose tolerance test'
FBG   fasting blood glucose

References

1.   World Health Organization. The Top 10 Causes of Death. Available online: https://www.who.int/news-room/fact-sheets/detail/the-top-10-causes-of-death (accessed on 24 May 2018).

2.   Bajaj, H.S.; Zinman, B. Glucose lowering strategies for cardiac benefits: Pathophysiological mechanisms. *Physiology (Bethesda)* **2018**, *33*, 197–210. [CrossRef]

3.   Kannel, W.B.; Hjortland, M.; Castelli, W.P. Role of diabetes in congestive heart failure: The Framingham study. *Am. J. Cardiol.* **1974**, *34*, 29–34. [CrossRef]

4.   Kannel, W.B.; McGee, D.L. Diabetes and cardiovascular disease. The Framingham study. *JAMA* **1979**, *241*, 2035–2038. [CrossRef] [PubMed]

5.   Petropoulos, I.N.; Green, P.; Chan, A.W.; Alam, U.; Fadavi, H.; Marshall, A.; Asghar, O.; Efron, N.; Tavakoli, M.; Malik, R.A. Corneal confocal microscopy detects neuropathy in patients with type 1 diabetes without retinopathy or microalbuminuria. *PLoS ONE* **2015**, *10*, e0123517. [CrossRef] [PubMed]

6.   Yorek, M.A. Vascular impairment of epineurial arterioles of the sciatic nerve: Implications for diabetic peripheral neuropathy. *Rev. Diabet. Stud.* **2015**, *12*, 13–28. [CrossRef] [PubMed]

7.   Javed, S.; Alam, U.; Malik, R.A. Treating diabetic neuropathy: Present strategies and emerging solutions. *Rev. Diabet. Stud.* **2015**, *12*, 63–83. [CrossRef]

8.   Manski-Nankervis, J.A.; Thuraisingam, S.; Sluggett, J.K.; Kilov, G.; Furler, J.; O'Neal, D.; Jenkins, A. Prescribing of diabetes medications to people with type 2 diabetes and chronic kidney disease: A national cross-sectional study. *BMC Fam. Pract.* **2019**, *20*, 29. [CrossRef] [PubMed]

9.   Schrijvers, G. Disease management: A proposal for a new definition. *Int. J. Integr. Care* **2009**, *9*, e06. [CrossRef] [PubMed]

10. Raveendran, A.V.; Chacko, E.C.; Pappachan, J.M. Non-pharmacological treatment options in the management of diabetes mellitus. *Eur. Endocrinol.* **2018**, *14*, 31–39. [CrossRef] [PubMed]

11. World Health Organization. *Global Report on Diabetes*; WHO: Geneva, Switzerland, 2016.

12. Perera, P.K.; Li, Y. Functional herbal food ingredients used in type 2 diabetes mellitus. *Pharmacogn. Rev.* **2012**, *6*, 37–45. [PubMed]

13. Van Thanh, B.; Dai, D.N.; Thang, T.D.; Binh, N.Q.; Anh, L.D.; Ogunwande, I.A. Composition of essential oils of four Hedychium species from Vietnam. *Chem. Cent. J.* **2014**, *8*, 54. [CrossRef] [PubMed]

14. Ibrahim, H. *Hedychium*; Backhuys Publisher: Leiden, The Netherlands, 2001; Volume 2, pp. 290–295.

15. Ribeiro Rde, A.; de Barros, F.; de Melo, M.M.; Muniz, C.; Chieia, S.; Wanderley M das, G.; Gomes, C.; Trolin, G. Acute diuretic effects in conscious rats produced by some medicinal plants used in the state of São Paulo, Brasil. *J. Ethnopharmacol.* **1988**, *24*, 19–29. [CrossRef]

16. Ribeiro Rde, A.; Fiuza de Melo, M.M.; De Barros, F.; Gomes, C.; Trolin, G. Acute antihypertensive effect in conscious rats produced by some medicinal plants used in the state of São Paulo. *J. Ethnopharmacol.* **1986**, *15*, 261–269. [CrossRef]

17. Bhandary, M.J.; Chandrashekar, K.R.; Kaveriappa, K.M. Medical ethnobotany of the siddis of Uttara-Kannada District, Karnataka, India. *J. Ethnopharmacol.* **1995**, *47*, 149–158. [CrossRef]

18. Zhan, Z.J.; Wen, Y.T.; Ren, F.Y.; Rao, G.W.; Shan, W.G.; Li, C.P. Diterpenoids and a diarylheptanoid from Hedychium coronarium with significant anti-angiogenic and cytotoxic activities. *Chem. Biodivers.* **2012**, *9*, 2754–2760. [CrossRef] [PubMed]

19. Reuk-ngam, N.; Chimnoi, N.; Khunnawutmanotham, N.; Techasakul, S. Antimicrobial activity of coronarin D and its synergistic potential with antibiotics. *Biomed. Res. Int.* **2014**, *2014*, 581985. [CrossRef] [PubMed]

20. Chen, J.C.; Hsieh, M.C.; Lin, S.H.; Lin, C.C.; Hsi, Y.T.; Lo, Y.S.; Chuang, Y.C.; Hsieh, M.J.; Chen, M.K. Coronarin D induces reactive oxygen species-mediated cell death in human nasopharyngeal cancer cells through inhibition of p38 MAPK and activation of JNK. *Oncotarget* **2017**, *8*, 108006–108019. [CrossRef] [PubMed]

21. Matsuda, H.; Morikawa, T.; Sakamoto, Y.; Toguchida, I.; Yoshikawa, M. Labdane-type diterpenes with inhibitory effects on increase in vascular permeability and nitric oxide production from Hedychium coronarium. *Bioorg. Med. Chem.* **2002**, *10*, 2527–2534. [CrossRef]

22. Li, F.; Sun, X.Y.; Li, X.W.; Yang, T.; Qi, L.W. Enrichment and separation of quercetin-3-*O*-beta-d-glucuronide from lotus leaves (nelumbo nucifera gaertn.) and evaluation of its anti-inflammatory effect. *J. Chromatogr. B Anal. Technol. Biomed. Life Sci.* **2017**, *1040*, 186–191. [CrossRef]

23. Food and Drug Administration. *Guidance for Industry-Estimating the Maximum Safe Starting Dose in Initial Clinical Trials for Therapeutic in Adult Healthy Volunteers*; Center for Drug Evaluation and Research, Ed.; Food and Drug Administration: Rockville, MD, USA, 2005.

24. *BKS.Cg-Dock7m +/+ Leprdb/J*; The Jackson Laboratory: Bar Harbor, ME, USA, 2019.

25. Szkudelski, T. The mechanism of alloxan and streptozotocin action in B cells of the rat pancreas. *Physiol. Res.* **2001**, *50*, 537–546.

26. Szkudelski, T. Streptozotocin-nicotinamide-induced diabetes in the rat. Characteristics of the experimental model. *Exp. Biol. Med. (Maywood)* **2012**, *237*, 481–490. [CrossRef]

27. Islam, M.S.; Wilson, R.D. Experimentally induced rodent models of type 2 diabetes. *Methods Mol. Biol.* **2012**, *933*, 161–174. [PubMed]

28. Ghasemi, A.; Khalifi, S.; Jedi, S. Streptozotocin-nicotinamide-induced rat model of type 2 diabetes. *Acta Physiol. Hung.* **2014**, *101*, 408–420. [CrossRef] [PubMed]

29. Shackelford, C.; Long, G.; Wolf, J.; Okerberg, C.; Herbert, R. Qualitative and quantitative analysis of nonneoplastic lesions in toxicology studies. *Toxicol. Pathol.* **2002**, *30*, 93–96. [CrossRef] [PubMed]

30. Akbarzadeh, A.; Norouzian, D.; Mehrabi, M.R.; Jamshidi, S.; Farhangi, A.; Verdi, A.A.; Mofidian, S.M.; Rad, B.L. Induction of diabetes by Streptozotocin in rats. *Indian J. Clin. Biochem.* **2007**, *22*, 60–64. [CrossRef] [PubMed]

31. Joseph, J.J.; Echouffo-Tcheugui, J.B.; Kalyani, R.R.; Yeh, H.C.; Bertoni, A.G.; Effoe, V.S.; Casanova, R.; Sims, M.; Correa, A.; Wu, W.C.; et al. Aldosterone, renin, and diabetes mellitus in African Americans: The jackson heart study. *J. Clin. Endocrinol. Metab.* **2016**, *101*, 1770–1778. [CrossRef]

32. Lovshin, J.A.; Lytvyn, Y.; Lovblom, L.E.; Katz, A.; Boulet, G.; Bjornstad, P.; Lai, V.; Cham, L.; Tse, J.; Orszag, A.; et al. Retinopathy and RAAS activation: Results from the Canadian study of longevity in type 1 diabetes. *Diabetes Care* **2019**, *42*, 273–280. [CrossRef] [PubMed]

33. Griffin, T.P.; Islam, M.N.; Blake, L.; Bell, M.; Griffin, M.D.; O'Shea, P.M. Effect of sodium glucose co-transporter-2 inhibition on the aldosterone/renin ratio in type 2 diabetes mellitus. *Horm. Metab. Res.* **2018**, *51*, 91–99. [CrossRef] [PubMed]

34. Mosso, L.M.; Carvajal, C.A.; Maiz, A.; Ortiz, E.H.; Castillo, C.R.; Artigas, R.A.; Fardella, C.E. A possible association between primary aldosteronism and a lower beta-cell function. *J. Hypertens.* **2007**, *25*, 2125–2130. [CrossRef] [PubMed]

35. Widimsky, J., Jr.; Sindelka, G.; Haas, T.; Prazny, M.; Hilgertova, J.; Skrha, J. Impaired insulin action in primary hyperaldosteronism. *Physiol. Res.* **2000**, *49*, 241–244. [PubMed]

36. Schmidt, B.M. Rapid non-genomic effects of aldosterone on the renal vasculature. *Steroids* **2008**, *73*, 961–965. [CrossRef] [PubMed]

37. Hermidorff, M.M.; de Assis, L.V.; Isoldi, M.C. Genomic and rapid effects of aldosterone: What we know and do not know thus far. *Heart Fail. Rev.* **2017**, *22*, 65–89. [CrossRef]

38. Alzamora, R.; Brown, L.R.; Harvey, B.J. Direct binding and activation of protein kinase C isoforms by aldosterone and 17beta-estradiol. *Mol. Endocrinol.* **2007**, *21*, 2637–2650. [CrossRef]

39. Mihailidou, A.S.; Mardini, M.; Funder, J.W. Rapid, nongenomic effects of aldosterone in the heart mediated by epsilon protein kinase C. *Endocrinology* **2004**, *145*, 773–780. [CrossRef] [PubMed]

40. Yoshida, T.; Shin-ya, H.; Nakai, S.; Yorimoto, A.; Morimoto, T.; Suyama, T.; Sakurai, M. Genomic and non-genomic effects of aldosterone on the individual variation of the sweat Na^+ concentration during exercise in trained athletes. *Eur. J. Appl. Physiol.* **2006**, *98*, 466–471. [CrossRef]

41. Bollag, W.B. Regulation of aldosterone synthesis and secretion. *Compr. Physiol.* **2014**, *4*, 1017–1055. [PubMed]

42. Terao, J.; Yamaguchi, S.; Shirai, M.; Miyoshi, M.; Moon, J.H.; Oshima, S.; Inakuma, T.; Tsushida, T.; Kato, Y. Protection by quercetin and quercetin 3-*O*-beta-D-glucuronide of peroxynitrite-induced antioxidant consumption in human plasma low-density lipoprotein. *Free Rad. Res.* **2001**, *35*, 925–931. [CrossRef]
43. Moon, J.H.; Tsushida, T.; Nakahara, K.; Terao, J. Identification of quercetin 3-*O*-beta-D-glucuronide as an antioxidative metabolite in rat plasma after oral administration of quercetin. *Free Rad. Biol. Med.* **2001**, *30*, 1274–1285. [CrossRef]
44. Liu, K.; Mei, F.; Wang, Y.; Xiao, N.; Yang, L.; Wang, Y.; Li, J.; Huang, F.; Kou, J.; Liu, B.; et al. Quercetin oppositely regulates insulin-mediated glucose disposal in skeletal muscle under normal and inflammatory conditions: The dual roles of AMPK activation. *Mol. Nutr. Food Res.* **2016**, *60*, 551–565. [CrossRef] [PubMed]
45. Ishizawa, K.; Yoshizumi, M.; Kawai, Y.; Terao, J.; Kihira, Y.; Ikeda, Y.; Tomita, S.; Minakuchi, K.; Tsuchiya, K.; Tamaki, T. Pharmacology in health food: Metabolism of quercetin in vivo and its protective effect against arteriosclerosis. *J. Pharmacol. Sci.* **2011**, *115*, 466–470. [CrossRef]
46. Mulrow, P.J. Angiotensin II and aldosterone regulation. *Regul. Pept.* **1999**, *80*, 27–32. [CrossRef]
47. Patel, S. Functional food red yeast rice (RYR) for metabolic syndrome amelioration: A review on pros and cons. *World J. Microbiol. Biotechnol.* **2016**, *32*, 87. [CrossRef] [PubMed]
48. Wang, J.; Jiang, W.; Zhong, Y.; Lu, B.; Shao, J.; Jiang, S.; Gu, P. Xuezhikang attenuated the functional and morphological impairment of pancreatic islets in diabetic mice via the inhibition of oxidative stress. *J. Cardiovasc. Pharmacol.* **2014**, *63*, 282–289. [CrossRef] [PubMed]
49. Tao, Y.-X. *Glucose Homeostatis and the Pathogenesis of Diabetes Mellitus*, 1st ed.; Academic Press: Cambridge, MA, USA, 2014.

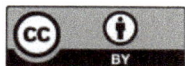

nutrients

MDPI

Article

Attenuation of Free Fatty Acid-Induced Muscle Insulin Resistance by Rosemary Extract

Filip Vlavcheski [1] and Evangelia Tsiani [1,2,*]

[1] Department of Health Sciences, Brock University, St. Catharines, ON L2S 3A1, Canada;
    fvlavcheski@brocku.ca
[2] Centre for Bone and Muscle Health, Brock University, St Catharines, ON L2S 3A1, Canada
*   Correspondence: ltsiani@brocku.ca; Tel.: +1(905)-688-5550 (ext. 3881)

Received: 18 September 2018; Accepted: 29 October 2018; Published: 2 November 2018

Abstract: Elevated blood free fatty acids (FFAs), as seen in obesity, impair muscle insulin action leading to insulin resistance and Type 2 diabetes mellitus. Serine phosphorylation of the insulin receptor substrate (IRS) is linked to insulin resistance and a number of serine/threonine kinases including JNK, mTOR and p70 S6K have been implicated in this process. Activation of the energy sensor AMP-activated protein kinase (AMPK) increases muscle glucose uptake, and in recent years AMPK has been viewed as an important target to counteract insulin resistance. We reported recently that rosemary extract (RE) increased muscle cell glucose uptake and activated AMPK. However, the effect of RE on FFA-induced muscle insulin resistance has never been examined. In the current study, we investigated the effect of RE in palmitate-induced insulin resistant L6 myotubes. Exposure of myotubes to palmitate reduced the insulin-stimulated glucose uptake, increased serine phosphorylation of IRS-1, and decreased the insulin-stimulated phosphorylation of Akt. Importantly, exposure to RE abolished these effects and the insulin-stimulated glucose uptake was restored. Treatment with palmitate increased the phosphorylation/activation of JNK, mTOR and p70 S6K whereas RE completely abolished these effects. RE increased the phosphorylation of AMPK even in the presence of palmitate. Our data indicate that rosemary extract has the potential to counteract the palmitate-induced muscle cell insulin resistance and further studies are required to explore its antidiabetic properties.

Keywords: muscle; insulin resistance; free fatty acids (FFA); diabetes; rosemary extract; AMPK

1. Introduction

Insulin plays a critical role in maintaining blood glucose homeostasis. The increase in postprandial glucose levels causes the release of insulin by the β cells of the pancreas which is delivered to its target tissues via the bloodstream. In skeletal muscle and adipose tissue, insulin promotes the transport, utilization and storage of glucose [1,2], while in the liver, insulin inhibits endogenous glucose production. The end result of these actions of insulin is to return the plasma glucose levels to a physiological range of 4–7 millimolar (mM).

The action of insulin in muscle cells is initiated by binding to its receptor, leading to tyrosine phosphorylation of the receptor and insulin receptor substrate (IRS-1), activation of the lipid kinase phosphatidylinositol-3 kinase (PI3K) and the serine threonine kinase Akt resulting in GLUT4 glucose transporter translocation from an intracellular pool to the plasma membrane and increase in glucose uptake [3,4]. Impairments in the PI3K-Akt cascade leads to insulin resistance and type 2 diabetes mellitus (T2DM) [1,2,5].

Skeletal muscle accounts for around 80% of postprandial glucose uptake and is quantitatively the most important insulin target tissue, and therefore muscle insulin resistance is a major contributor to decreased glucose tolerance and T2DM. Insulin resistance is strongly associated with obesity and increased plasma lipid levels. In vitro studies have shown that exposure of muscle cells to the free fatty acids (FFA) palmitate induces insulin resistance [6]. In addition, evidence from in vivo animals studies have shown that lipid infusion [7,8] or increased plasma lipid levels by high fat diet results in muscle insulin resistance [7,9]. Studies have shown that serine phosphorylation of IRS-1 leads to impairment in the insulin-signaling pathway and contributes to insulin resistance [6,10,11]. Signaling molecules such as mammalian target of rapamycin (mTOR) [12,13], ribosomal protein S6 kinase (p70 S6K) [14,15], glycogen synthase kinase 3 (GSK3) [16], c-Jun N-terminal kinase (JNK) [17] and protein kinase C (PKCs) [18] have been implicated in the serine phosphorylation of IRS-1 [19].

Adenosine monophosphate (AMP)-activated protein kinase (AMPK) is a serine/threonine kinase acting as a cellular energy sensor and activated by increased AMP/ATP ratio and/or via phosphorylation by its upstream kinases, liver kinase B1 (LKB1), calmodulin-dependent protein kinase (CaMKKs) and transforming growth factor-β (TGF-β)-activated kinase 1 (TAK1) [20,21]. Muscle AMPK is activated by muscle contraction/exercise [21] and several compounds including metformin [22], thiazolidineones [23] and polyphenols such as resveratrol [24] and naringenin [25] leading to increased glucose uptake. In recent years, AMPK activators have been recognized as promising pharmacological intervention for the prevention and treatment of T2DM [21,26–28].

Rosemary (*Rosmarinus officinalis* L.) is an aromatic evergreen plant reported to have antioxidant [29,30], anticancer [19,20] and antidiabetic properties [31–36]. Rosemary extract (RE) contains different classes of polyphenols including phenolic acids, flavonoids and phenolic terpenes [37]. The polyphenols found in the highest quantity in RE are carnosic acid (CA), carnosol (COH) and rosmarinic acid (RA) and their production is influenced by growth conditions such as soil quality, water availability and sunlight exposure. Furthermore, the choice of solvent and extraction method affects the chemical composition of the extract with the possibility of losing lipid soluble chemicals by an aqueous-based extraction method and water-soluble chemicals by non-polar solvent (ethanol, methanol)-based extraction.

Previous studies by our group found a significant increase in muscle glucose uptake and AMPK activation by RE treatment [38]. In addition, administration of RE decreased plasma glucose levels in streptozotocin-induced diabetic mice [31], rats [33,35,36], alloxan-induced diabetic rabbits [32], genetic [34], and dietary [36,39–41] animal models of obesity and insulin resistance.

According to the World Health Organization and the International Diabetes Federation (IDF) estimates, T2DM is a disease on the rise [42] and with huge economic burden to health care systems around the globe. Although many different strategies currently exist for the prevention and treatment of insulin resistance and T2DM, they are lacking in efficacy and, therefore, there is a need for new preventative measures and targeted therapies. In recent years, chemicals found in plants/herbs have attracted attention for their use as functional foods or nutraceuticals for preventing and treating insulin resistance and T2DM.

In the present study, we focused on RE and examined its potential to counteract the palmitate-induced insulin resistance in muscle cells.

2. Materials and Methods

2.1. Materials

Fetal bovine serum (FBS), dimethyl sulfoxide (DMSO), palmitate, bovine serum albumin (BSA) and cytochalasin B, were purchased from Sigma Life Sciences (St. Louis, MO, USA). Materials for cell culture and trypan blue solution 0.4% were purchased from GIBCO Life Technologies (Burlington, ON, USA). Phospho—and total AMPK (CAT 2531 and 2532, respectively), Akt (CAT 9271 and 9272 respectively), JNK (CAT 9251 and 9252, respectively), mTOR (CAT 2971 and 2972, respectively), p70 S6K (CAT 9205 and 2708, respectively) and HRP-conjugated anti-rabbit antibodies (CAT 7074) were purchased from New England BioLabs (NEB) (Missisauga, ON, Canada). Insulin (Humulin R) was from Eli Lilly (Indianapolis, IN, USA). Luminol Enhancer reagents, polyvinylidene difluoride (PVDF) membrane, reagents for electrophoresis and Bradford protein assay reagent were purchased from BioRad (Hercules, CA, USA). [3H]-2-deoxy-D-glucose was purchased from PerkinElmer (Boston, MA, USA).

2.2. Preparation of Rosemary Extract (RE)

Following previously established protocols by our group [38] whole dried rosemary leaves (*Rosmarinus officinalis* L.) (Compliments, Sobey's Missisauga, ON, Canada) were grounded and passed through a mesh sieve. 5 grams of ground leaves were steeped for 16 h in dichloromethane-methanol (1:1) (30 mL). Under a slight vacuum the filtrate was collected followed by methanol (30 mL) extraction for 30 min. The solvent was removed using rotary evaporator. Aliquots of the extract dissolved in dimethyl sulfoxide (DMSO) were prepared (100 µg/mL) and were stored at $-20\,^{\circ}$C. All experiments were performed using the same batch of RE.

2.3. Preparation of Palmitate Stock Solution

Stock palmitate solution was prepared by conjugating palmitate with fatty acid-free BSA as previously reported [6]. In brief palmitic acid was dissolved in 0.1N NaOH and diluted in 9.7% *(w/v)* BSA solution that was previously warmed (45–50 $^{\circ}$C) to give a stock solution of 8 mM palmitate. The final molar ratio of free palmitate/BSA was 6:1.

2.4. Cell Culture, Treatment and Glucose Uptake

L6 rat muscle cells were used in all experiments. Myoblasts were grown and differentiated into myotubes, as previously established [5,24]. Briefly, cells were grown in α-Minimum Essential Medium (MEM) media containing 2% *v/v* FBS until fully differentiated. Myotube stage was reached at approximately 6 to 7 days after seeding. All treatments were performed using serum-free media. The fully differentiated myotubes were treated with 0.2 mM palmitate in the absence or presence of 5 µg/mL RE for 16 h followed by treatment without or with 100 nM insulin for 0.5 h. A vehicle-treated control DMSO group was used in parallel with the treated groups. Following the treatment, the cells were rinsed using HEPES-buffered saline (HBS) and exposed to HBS containing 10 µM [3H]-2-deoxy-D-glucose for 10 min to measure glucose uptake, as previously described [24,43]. Cytochalasin B (10 µM) was used to determine the non-specific glucose uptake. Cells were seeded in 12-well plates and 3 wells were used for each treatment group. The first two wells were used to measure the total glucose uptake and the third used to measure the non-specific (treated with cytochalasin B). The two total glucose uptake values were averaged, and the non-specific value was subtracted to obtain the specific. At the end of the assay, the cells were rinsed with 0.9% NaCl solution and lysed using 0.05 N NaOH. The radioactivity was measured by liquid scintillation counter and the Bradford assay was used to examine the cellular protein content.

2.5. Immunoblotting

After treatment, the cells were quickly washed with ice cold HBS solution and lysed using cold lysis buffer. Whole cell lysates were prepared using lysis buffer containing 20 mM Tris (PH 7.5), 150 mM NaCI, 1 mM ethylenediaminetetraacetic acid (EDTA), 1 mM ethylene glycol-bis β-aminoethyl ether/egtazic acid (EGTA), 1% Triton X-100, 2.5 mM sodium pyrophosphate, 1 mM p-glycerolphosphate, 1mM sodium orthovanadate (Na_3VO_4), 1 µg/mL leupeptin. Phenylmethylsulfonyl fluoride (PMSF) was added, to a final concentration of 1 mM, prior to use. The lysates were stored at $-20\,^{\circ}$C. The protein samples (20 µg) were separated using sodium dodecyl sulfate polyacrylamide gel electrophoresis (SDS-PAGE) followed by a transfer to a PVDF membrane. The membranes were blocked using blocking buffer (5% *(w/v)* dry milk powder in Tris-buffered saline) followed by overnight incubation at 4 $^{\circ}$C with the primary antibody. The primary antibody was detected using HRP-conjugated anti-rabbit secondary antibody followed by exposure to

LumiGLOW reagent. The corresponding bands were visualized with FluroChem software (Thermo Fisher, Waltham, MA, USA).

2.6. Statistical Analysis

Statistical analysis was completed using GraphPad Prism software 5.3 manufactured from Graphpad Software Inc. (La Jolla, CA, USA). The data from several experiments were pooled and presented as mean ± standard error (SE). The means of all the groups were obtained and compared to the control group using one-way analysis of variance (ANOVA) which was followed by Tukey's post hoc test for multiple comparisons.

3. Results

3.1. Rosemary Extract Restores the Insulin-Stimulated Glucose Uptake in Palmitate-Treated Muscle Cells

All the experiments were performed using L6 cells in their differentiated myotube stage (Figure 1). In our lab we have used L6 myotubes for different studies extensively for more than 20 years and differentiation of the cells is assessed microscopically. We are certain that all experiments were performed using differentiated cells/myotubes. Upon differentiation of L6 cells, the expression of the insulin receptor and GLUT4 transporters dramatically increases which results in a 2-fold increase in insulin responsiveness. We examined routinely the response of the cells to insulin (100 nM for 30 min) and we got a 2-fold increase in glucose uptake an indirect measurement of differentiation. Altogether with (1) the microscopic evaluation and (2) the biological evaluation/ insulin responsiveness/glucose uptake assay we are absolutely sure that the cells used in the present study were at the myotube stage.

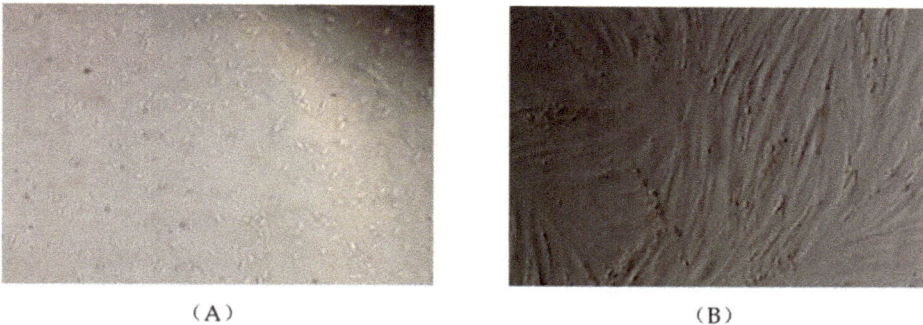

(A) (B)

Figure 1. L6 muscle cells in the myoblast (**A**) and fully differentiated myotube (**B**) stage. L6 cells were seeded and cultured in 2% fetal bovine serum (FBS)-containing α-MEM culture media (day 1, **A**) and upon reaching confluency were spontaneously differentiated into myotubes (day 7, **B**). Photographs were taken using EVOS XL Core imaging system at magnification ×10 and ×20.

The effects of the free-fatty acid palmitate in the absence or the presence of RE on the insulin-stimulated glucose uptake was examined. Acute stimulation of L6 myotubes with insulin (100 nM, 30 min) significantly increased glucose uptake (201 ± 1.21% of control, $p < 0.0001$, Figure 2). Exposure of the cells to palmitate (0.2 mM, 16 h) although did not have any effect on the basal glucose uptake (103 ± 2.7% of control) (Figure 2), it resulted in significant reduction of the insulin-stimulated glucose uptake (117 ± 15.6% of control) indicating insulin resistance. Most importantly in palmitate-treated cells, exposure to RE resulted in significant restoration of insulin-stimulated glucose uptake (179 ± 10.5% of control, $p = 0.0001$, Figure 2). Exposure of the cells to RE (5 μg/mL) alone resulted in significant increase in glucose uptake (208 ± 15.6% of control, $p < 0.0001$). Treatment with RE and palmitate did not have a significant effect on glucose uptake (122 ± 7.6% of control). Moreover, combined treatment with RE and insulin (202 ± 8.0% of control, $p < 0.0001$)

did not result in greater response than each treatment alone. These data indicate that the negative effect imposed by palmitate treatment on insulin responsiveness is abolished by the presence of RE.

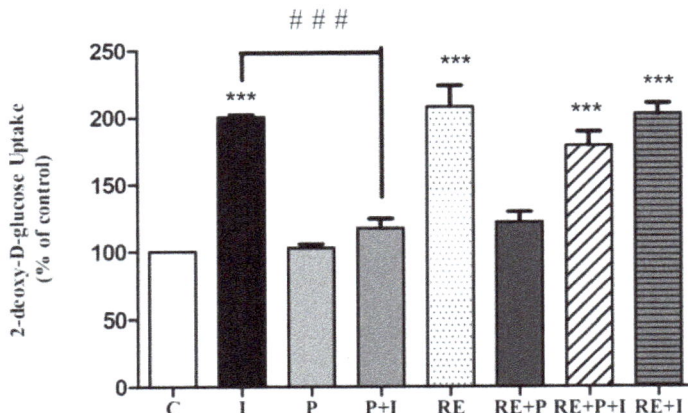

Figure 2. Rosemary extract (RE) restores the insulin-stimulated glucose uptake in palmitate treated muscle cells. Fully differentiated L6 myotubes were treated without (control, C) or with 0.2 mM palmitate (P) for 16 h in the absence or the presence of 5 μg/mL RE followed by stimulation without or with 100 nM insulin (I) for 30 min and [$3H$]-2-deoxy-D-glucose uptake measurements. The results are the mean ± standard error (SE) of 4–7 independent experiments, expressed as percent of control (*** $p < 0.001$ vs. control, ### $p < 0.001$ vs. insulin alone).

To investigate any potential cell-damaging effects of palmitate and RE treatment, we examined cell morphology and cell viability. No changes in cell morphology was seen with any of the treatments. Additionally, we utilized the trypan blue exclusion assay to examine cell viability. No effect on cell viability (RE: 98%, P: 97%, P + RE: 99% of control) was seen.

3.2. Rosemary Extract Prevents the Palmitate-Induced Ser307 and Ser636/639 Phosphorylation of IRS-1

Previous studies conducted in L6 muscle cells in vitro and rat muscle in vivo have indicated that increased phosphorylation levels of Ser307 and Ser636/639 of IRS-1 leads to impairment in the insulin signaling leading to insulin resistance [44,45]. Therefore, next we investigated the effects of palmitate and RE downstream of the insulin receptor and examined IRS-1 phosphorylation and expression. Exposure of L6 myotubes to 0.2 mM palmitate resulted in significant increase in Ser307 and Ser636/639 phosphorylation of IRS-1 (199.4 ± 24.98%, 162 ± 6.74% of control, $p = 0.0005$, $p < 0.0091$ respectively) (Figure 3A,B). Treatment with 5 μg/mL RE did not have any effect on the basal Ser307 or Ser636/639 phosphorylation (118 ± 11.24%, 105 ± 3.51% of control respectively) but completely abolished the palmitate-induced increase in Ser307 and Ser636/639 phosphorylation of IRS-1 (108 ± 16.91% of control and 107 ± 7.32% of control, respectively), (Figure 3A,B). The total levels of IRS-1 were not impacted by any treatment (P: 103.3 ± 8.63, RE: 98.82 ± 13.21, RE + P: 108 ± 9.33) (Figure 3C). The ratio of phosphorylated levels of IRS-1 (Ser307 and Ser636/639) over the total levels of IRS-1 is shown on Figure 3D. Treatment with palmitate significantly increased the ratio of phosphorylated Ser307 and Ser636/639 /total IRS-1(202.2 ± 43.7, 157.7 ± 7.7% of control, $p < 0.0009$ respectively). RE did not have an effect on the ratio of basal Ser307 and Ser636/639 phosphorylation of IRS-1/ total IRS-1 (123.8 ± 20 and 111.4 ± 19.4% of control respectively) but completely abolished the palmitate-induced response (101.1 ± 12.6 and 99.3 ± 5.1% of control, $p = 0.0008$ and $p = 0.0086$ respectively).

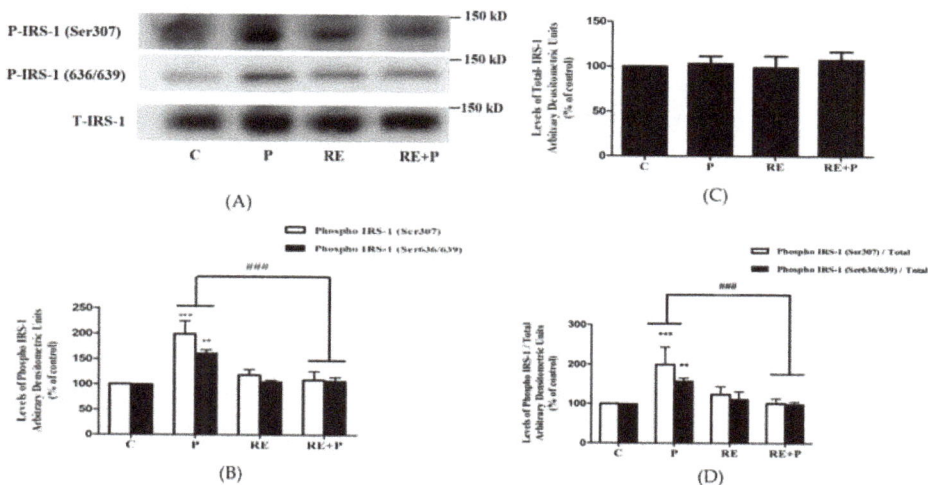

Figure 3. Effects of palmitate and RE on IRS-1 expression and Ser307, Ser636/639 phosphorylation. Fully differentiated myotubes were treated without (control, C) or with 0.2 mM palmitate (P) in the absence or the presence of 5 µg/mL RE for 16 h. After treatment, the cells were lysed, and sodium dodecyl sulfate polyacrylamide gel electrophoresis (SDS-PAGE) was performed, followed by immunoblotting with specific antibodies that recognize phosphorylated (Ser307, Ser636/639) or total IRS-1 (T-IRS-1). Representative immunoblots are shown (**A**). The densitometry of the bands was measured and expressed in arbitrary units (**B–D**). The data are the mean $\pm$ SE of three separate experiments (*** $p < 0.001$, ** $p < 0.01$ vs. control, ### $p < 0.001$ vs. palmitate alone).

3.3. Rosemary Extract Restores the Insulin-Stimulated Akt Phosphorylation in Palmitate Treated Myotubes

Next, we investigated the effect of palmitate and RE treatment on insulin-stimulated Akt phosphorylation and expression. Treatment of L6 myotubes with insulin resulted in a significant increase in Akt Ser473 and Thr308 phosphorylation (I: 312 ± 19.21 and $289 \pm 23.12\%$ of control, $p = 0.0006$, $p = 0.0009$, respectively) (Figure 4A,B). Treatment of the cells with palmitate abolished the insulin-stimulated Akt phosphorylation on Ser473 and Thr308 residues (P + I: 121.9 ± 31.30 and $131 \pm 35.90\%$ of control respectively, $p = 0.0008$) (Figure 4A,B). Palmitate and RE each alone or in combination did not have any effect on the basal Ser473 or Thr308 Akt phosphorylation (P: 98.2 ± 3.02, 95 ± 6.20, RE: 103 ± 4.10, $105 \pm 6.2\%$, RE + P: 109.1 ± 9.06, $111 \pm 5.92\%$ of control, respectively). However, in the presence of RE, the decline in the insulin-stimulated Akt phosphorylation on Ser473 and Thr308 seen with palmitate was completely prevented (RE + P + I: 346.7 ± 66 and $312 \pm 30.31\%$ of control respectively, $p < 0.001$ (Figure 4A,B). The total levels of Akt were not significantly affected by any of the treatments (I: 108 ± 8.4, P: 99 ± 5.9, P + I: 101 ± 11.6, RE: 94 ± 5.72, RE + P: 93.6 ± 7.2, RE + P + I: $93 \pm 15.23\%$ of control) (Figure 4C).

3.4. Rosemary Extract Prevents the Palmitate-Induced Phosphorylation of C-Jun N-Terminal Kinase (JNK) in L6 Myotubes

Following the establishment that chronic exposure to palmitate increases the phosphorylation of Ser307 and Ser636/639 of IRS-1, we examined the signaling molecules that may be involved. JNK is a serine/threonine kinase shown to increase serine phosphorylation of IRS-1 and involved in insulin resistance [46,47]. We hypothesized that the levels of JNK phosphorylation and/or expression would be increased by palmitate. Indeed, exposure of the cells to palmitate (0.2 mM) significantly increased JNK phosphorylation ($250 \pm 9.77\%$ of control, $p = 0.0007$) and treatment with RE completely abolished the palmitate-induced phosphorylation of JNK ($114 \pm 12.90\%$ of control, $p = 0.0006$) (Figure 5A,B).

RE alone did not affect the phosphorylation of JNK (98 ± 7.44% of control). Moreover, the total levels of JNK were not significantly changed by any treatment: P: 107 ± 7.21, RE: 104 ± 7.53 and RE + P: 105 ± 8.76% of control (Figure 5C).

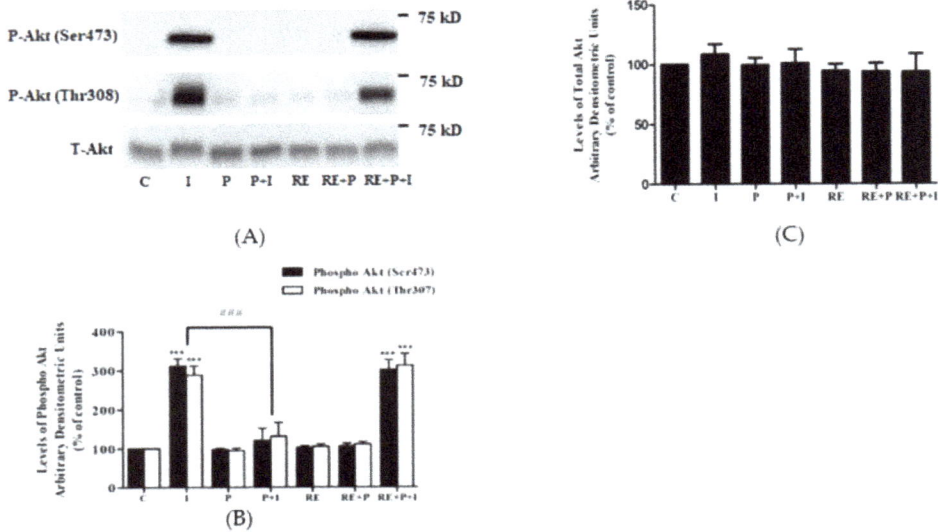

(A)

(C)

(B)

Figure 4. Effects of palmitate and RE on Akt expression and Ser473 and Thr308 phosphorylation. Fully differentiated L6 myotubes were treated without (control, C) or with 0.2 mM palmitate (P) for 16 h in the absence or the presence of 5 µg/mL RE followed by stimulation without or with 100 nM insulin (I) for 15 min. After treatment, the cells were lysed, and SDS-PAGE was performed, followed by immunoblotting with specific antibodies that recognize phosphorylated Ser473, Thr308 or total Akt. Representative immunoblots are shown (**A**). The densitometry of the bands was measured and expressed in arbitrary units (**B,C**). The data are the mean ± SE of three separate experiments (*** $p < 0.001$ vs. control, ### $p < 0.001$ vs. insulin alone).

3.5. Rosemary Extract Prevents the Palmitate-Induced Phosphorylation of mTOR and p70 S6K in L6 Myotubes

Another kinase implicated in serine phosphorylation of IRS-1 is mTOR and, therefore, we examined the effects of palmitate on mTOR phosphorylation/activation and expression. Exposure of the cells to 0.2 mM palmitate significantly increased mTOR and p70 S6K phosphorylation (403 ± 85.60 and 200 ± 42.55% of control, $p < 0.0001$, respectively) (Figure 6A–C). Treatment with RE alone did not affect the basal mTOR or p70 S6K phosphorylation (104 ± 13.71 and 82.12 ± 6.04% of control, respectively) while completely abolished the palmitate-induced phosphorylation of mTOR and p70 S6K (60 ± 20.53% and 90 ± 7.11% of control, $p = 0.0002$ and $p = 0.0005$, respectively), (Figure 6A–C). The total levels of mTOR and p70 S6K were not significantly changed by any treatment: P: 104 ± 3.01, 105 ± 5.83, RE: 93 ± 2.44, 97 ± 2.21 and RE + P: 88 ± 3.85, 92.22 ± 4.23% of control, respectively (Figure 6A–C).

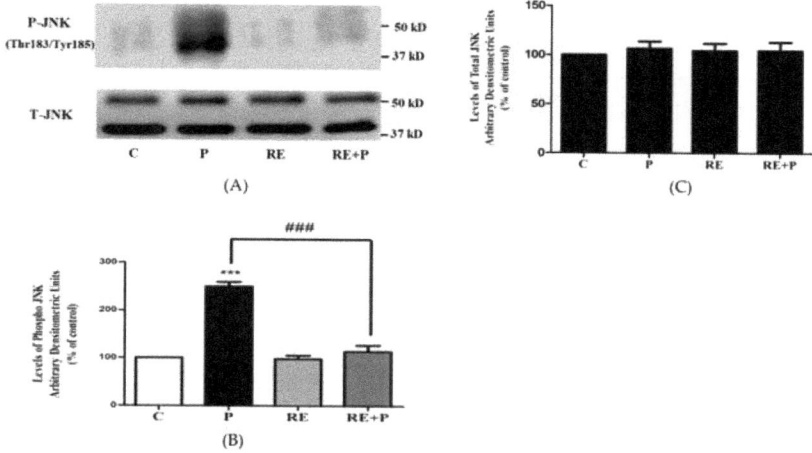

Figure 5. Effects of palmitate and RE on JNK expression and phosphorylation. Fully differentiated myotubes were treated without (control, C) or with 0.2 mM palmitate (P) for 16 h in the absence or the presence of 5 μg/mL RE. After treatment, the cells were lysed, and SDS-PAGE was performed, followed by immunoblotting with specific antibodies that recognize phosphorylated Thr183/Tyr185 or total JNK. Representative immunoblots are shown (**A**). The densitometry of the bands was measured and expressed in arbitrary units (**B,C**). The data are the mean ± SE of three separate experiments (*** $p < 0.001$ vs. control, ### $p < 0.001$ vs. palmitate alone).

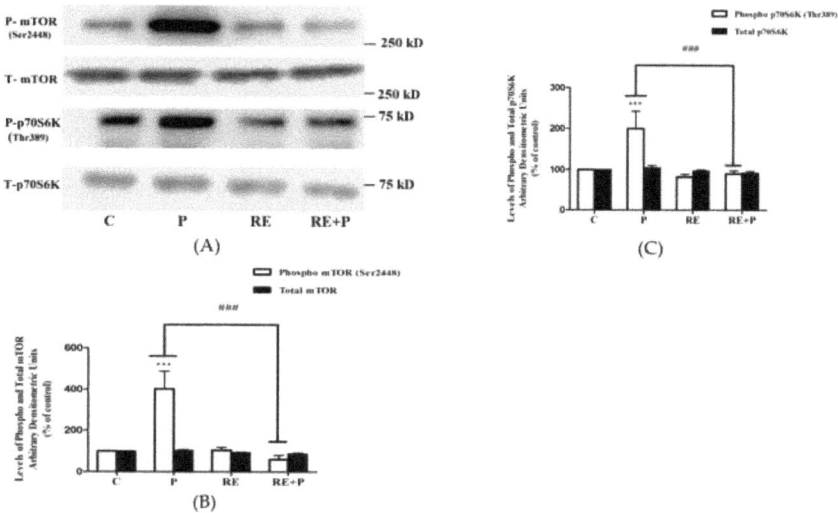

Figure 6. Effects of palmitate and RE on mTOR and p70 S6K expression and phosphorylation. Fully differentiated myotubes were treated without (control, C) or with 0.2 mM palmitate (P) for 16 h in the absence or the presence of 5 μg/mL RE. After treatment, the cells were lysed, and SDS-PAGE was performed, followed by immunoblotting with specific antibodies that recognize phosphorylated Ser2448 or total mTOR or phosphorylated Thr389 or total p70 S6K. Representative immunoblots are shown (**A**). The densitometry of the bands was measured and expressed in arbitrary units (**B,C**). The data are the mean ± SE of three separate experiments (*** $p < 0.001$ vs. control, ### $p < 0.001$ vs. palmitate alone).

3.6. Rosemary Extract increases the Phosphorylation of AMPK in the Presence of Palmitate

Previous studies by our group showed that rosemary extract and rosemary extract polyphenols increased glucose uptake and phosphorylated/activated AMPK in L6 muscle cells [38,48–50]. Here we investigated the chronic effect of RE on AMPK as well as the effect of RE on AMPK in an environment of elevated FFA. Treatment with 5 µg/mL RE significantly increased the phosphorylation of AMPK ($295 \pm 26.94\%$ of control, $p < 0.0001$) (Figure 7A,B). Most importantly, RE increased phosphorylation of AMPK even in the presence of 0.2 mM of palmitate ($270 \pm 22.54\%$ of control, $p < 0.0001$), (Figure 7A,B). Treatment with palmitate alone did not have any significant effect on the phosphorylation of AMPK ($150 \pm 14.32\%$ of control). Furthermore, the total levels of AMPK were not affected by any treatment (P: 103 ± 8.63, RE: 99 ± 13.21, RE + P: $108 \pm 9.33\%$ of control) (Figure 7C).

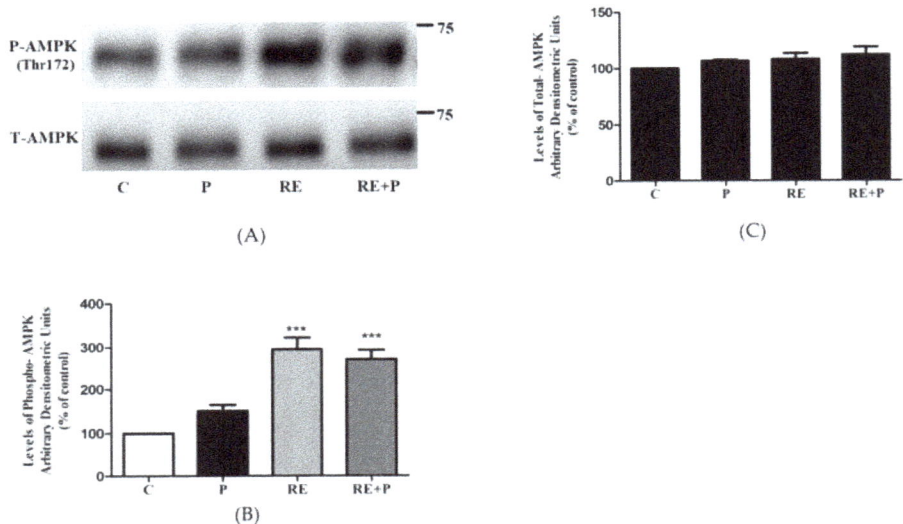

(A)

(C)

(B)

Figure 7. Effects of palmitate and RE on AMPK expression and phosphorylation. Fully differentiated myotubes were treated without (control, C) or with 0.2 mM palmitate (P) for 16 h in the absence or the presence of 5 µg/mL RE. After treatment, the cells were lysed, and SDS-PAGE was performed, followed by immunoblotting with specific antibodies that recognize phosphorylated Thr172 or total AMPK. Representative immunoblots are shown (**A**). The densitometry of the bands was measured and expressed in arbitrary units (**B,C**). The data are the mean $\pm$ SE of three separate experiments (*** $p < 0.001$ vs. control).

4. Discussion

Obesity and elevated FFAs are highly correlated with insulin resistance and are major risk factors for the development of type 2 diabetes mellitus [19], a disease affecting millions of people globally. The search of compounds with the potential to counteract insulin resistance is the focus of many research groups worldwide and such compounds will provide huge benefits.

In the present study, we found that exposure of L6 myotubes to palmitate, to mimic the elevated plasma FFA levels seen in obesity in vivo, significantly decreased the insulin-stimulated glucose uptake indicating the induction of insulin resistance. These data are in agreement with previous studies showing that exposure of skeletal muscle cells to similar concentrations of palmitate induced insulin resistance [6,51–53]. Most importantly, in the presence of rosemary extract the palmitate-induced insulin resistance was prevented and the insulin-stimulated glucose uptake was restored to levels comparable to the response seen with insulin alone. These findings are the first to show that RE can counteract the palmitate-induced insulin resistance. It should be noted that although all the experiments in the present study were performed using the same batch of RE, in our lab we prepared a total of 3 different batches of RE using the same source of whole dried rosemary leaves (compliments of Sobey's Mississauga, ON, Canada) and we tested them; all 3 batches gave us the same response, significantly increased L6 muscle cell glucose uptake and activated AMPK. We found that exposure of L6 cells to palmitate for 16 h increased Ser307 and Ser636/639 phosphorylation of IRS-1 in agreement with other studies showing increased Ser307 and Ser636/639 phosphorylation of IRS-1 by palmitate exposure in L6 [52,54] and C2C12 [55]. Our data are in agreement with in vivo animal studies showing increased serine phosphorylation of muscle tissue IRS-1 by high fat diet [15,17,56]. Increased phosphorylation of these serine residues of IRS-1 lead to a decreased PI3K-Akt downstream signaling and reduced glucose uptake [57]. Importantly our data show that treatment with RE prevented the palmitate-induced serine phosphorylation of IRS-1. This effect of RE is similar to metformin, the first line of treatment for T2DM, found to decrease the palmitate-induced Ser307 phosphorylation of IRS-1 in L6 muscle cells [58].

Furthermore, our data showed that exposure of the cells to palmitate significantly attenuated the insulin-stimulated phosphorylation of Akt. These data are in agreement with other in vitro studies using L6 [59], or C2C12 [60] cells and in vivo studies showing attenuation of the insulin-induced phosphorylation of Akt in isolated soleus muscle from animals fed a high-fat diet [61]. Interestingly, in the presence of RE the insulin-induced phosphorylation of Akt was restored indicating that RE has a potential to counteract the deleterious effects of palmitate and act similarly to metformin shown to counteract the effects of palmitate and restore insulin-induced Akt phosphorylation in L6 muscle cells [62].

Exposure of L6 muscle cells to palmitate significantly increased the phosphorylation of JNK in agreement with other studies in L6 [63] and C2C12 [64] muscle cells as well as findings from in vivo studies showing increased phosphorylation of JNK in muscle tissue from animals fed a high-fat diet [46,65]. Our data show that treatment with RE prevented the palmitate-induced phosphorylation of JNK in L6 muscle cells and are in agreement with a study showing quercetin, a polyphenol from the flavonoid group, to significantly attenuate the palmitate-induced phosphorylation of JNK in L6 muscle cells and in muscles obtained from ob/ob mice [63].

Furthermore, exposure of L6 cells to palmitate significantly increased the phosphorylation of mTOR and its downstream effector p70 S6K and treatment with RE abolished the palmitate effects. Although increased mTOR and p70 S6K phosphorylation by palmitate has been reported previously in L6 [66] and C2C12 cells [67] and in muscle tissue from animals fed a high-fat diet [66,68], our study is the first to show that RE has the potential to block these effects. Our data indicate the potential of RE, similar to metformin, to block the palmitate-induced mTOR and p70 S6K phosphorylation in C2C12 muscle cells [69].

Furthermore, we investigated the total and phosphorylated levels of AMPK. Previously, we found that treatment of L6 myotubes with RE [38] and the RE polyphenols carnosic acid (CA) [48], rosmarinic acid [49] and carnosol [50] significantly increased the phosphorylation of AMPK. In the present study, we found that 0.2 mM palmitate for 16 h did not affect AMPK phosphorylation or expression. Treatment with RE increased the phosphorylation/activation of AMPK even in the presence of palmitate, an effect similar to metformin which has been shown to phosphorylate/activate AMPK in the presence of palmitate in C2C12 and L6 muscle cells [62,69]. Studies have indicated that activation of AMPK significantly lowers the activity of mTOR and its downstream effector p70 S6K [70,71] and, therefore, the inhibition of mTOR and p70 S6K phosphorylation by RE treatment, seen in our study, may be mediated by AMPK. Studies using strategies to inhibit AMPK such as using an inhibitor of AMPK (Compound C) or siRNA techniques should be performed in the future to explore this further. To our surprise, exposure of the cells to RE and palmitate did not have a significant effect on the glucose uptake, indicating that in the presence of palmitate not only the acute insulin response was abolished but also the effect of RE is attenuated (Figure 2). It should be noted that RE in the presence of palmitate, resulted in a significant increase in AMPK phosphorylation and our data indicate that this increase was enough to abolish the palmitate-induced phosphorylation of mTOR and p70 S6K leading to a decrease in serine phosphorylation of IRS-1 but not sufficient to increase the glucose uptake in the cells (Figure 7, RE + P increased AMPK phosphorylation; Figure 2: RE + P no significant increase in glucose uptake). We have investigated previously the effects of RE, CA and RA on glucose transporters in GLUT4 and GLUT1 overexpressing cells and found no effect on glucose transporter translocation [38,48,49], and we had proposed that RE may increase glucose uptake by affecting GLUT3 translocation or by affecting glucose transporter activity. The lack of a significant increase in glucose uptake by RE in the presence of palmitate (Figure 2: RE + P) indicates that palmitate may affect a signaling step downstream of AMPK such as TBC1D1 that prevents the increase in glucose transporter activity/glucose uptake.

A limited number of studies have also examined the antidiabetic effects of RE and its polyphenols in vivo. In high-fat diet-induced diabetic mice, the administration of RE significantly decreased the fasting plasma glucose levels (72%), decreased total cholesterol (68%), total fat fecal excretion (1–2 fold) and body weight, thereby improving the lipid profile of the mice [39]. Another study found that RE enriched with CA significantly ameliorated high-fat diet-induced obesity and metabolic syndrome in mice [72]. The administration of RE enriched with CA in obese rats resulted in significant attenuation of TNFα and interleukin 1α indicating the anti-inflammatory effects of RE [73]. Additional studies showed that dietary supplementation of RE enriched with CA resulted in body weight and epidydimal fat reduction [74], as well as suppression of hepatic steatosis [75]. In high-fat diet-induced diabetic rats, the administration of RA dose-dependently ameliorated hyperglycemia and insulin resistance in addition to increasing GLUT4 translocation to the plasma membrane in muscle [36]. Moreover, a recent study conducted in humans administered dried rosemary leaf powder have shown significant improvement in the blood lipid profile, antioxidant levels, and decrease in fasting plasma glucose levels [76]. These studies demonstrate that RE and its polyphenols exhibit antihyperglycemic and antidiabetic properties in vivo and are in agreement with our findings. However, there are currently no studies that elucidate the mechanism involved in the effects of RE and its polyphenols. The present study found increased serine phosphorylation of IRS-1, and increased phosphorylation of mTOR, p70 S6K and JNK by palmitate and an effect of RE treatment to inhibit them and restore the insulin-stimulated Akt phosphorylation and the insulin-stimulated glucose uptake.

5. Conclusions

The prevalence of T2DM is constantly increasing and according to the International Diabetes Federation it is expected to affect 420 million people worldwide by the year 2040 [42]. Additionally, insulin resistance and T2DM are highly correlated with the development of other pathological states including cardiovascular disease and cancer [19]. As a result, new strategies to aid in the prevention and management of T2DM will provide huge benefits to our society. As previously indicated, increased levels of FFA and obesity mediate insulin resistance in muscle cells. The present study has shown that the exposure of muscle cells to the FFA palmitate, to mimic the elevated FFA levels seen in obesity, induced insulin resistance. Palmitate increased the serine phosphorylation of IRS-1 and phosphorylation of JNK, mTOR and p70 S6K, while the insulin-stimulated Akt phosphorylation and the insulin-stimulated glucose uptake were significantly reduced. Importantly, these effects of palmitate were attenuated by rosemary extract and the insulin-stimulated glucose uptake was restored. In addition, rosemary extract increased the phosphorylation/activation of the energy sensor AMPK, the activation of which has recently been recognized as a targeted approach to counteract insulin resistance and T2DM. Our study is the first to show that rosemary extract has the potential to counteract the palmitate-induced muscle cell insulin resistance, and further studies are required to explore its antidiabetic properties and to elucidate the exact cellular mechanisms involved.

Author Contributions: E.T. was responsible for the conception and design of the study, data presentation and manuscript preparation. F.V. performed all the experiments, data analysis, figure preparation and contributed to the manuscript preparation. Both authors read and approved the manuscript.

Funding: This work was supported by a Natural Sciences and Engineering Research Council of Canada (NSERC) grant to E.T.

Acknowledgments: Parental, L6 cells were a kind gift from A Klip (Hospital for Sick Children, Toronto, ON, Canada). This work was supported by a Natural Sciences and Engineering Research Council of Canada (NSERC) grant to E.T.

Conflicts of Interest: The authors declare no conflict of interest.

References

1. Kahn, B.B.; Flier, J.S. Obesity and insulin resistance. *J. Clin. Investig.* **2000**, *106*, 473–481. [CrossRef] [PubMed]
2. Guo, S. Mechanisms of Obesity: Molecular basis of insulin resistance: The role of IRS and Foxo1 in the control of diabetes mellitus and its complications. *Drug Discov. Today Dis. Mech.* **2013**, *10*, e27–e33. [CrossRef] [PubMed]
3. Manning, B.D.; Cantley, L.C. AKT/PKB Signaling: Navigating Downstream. *Cell* **2007**, *129*, 1261–1274. [CrossRef] [PubMed]
4. Taniguchi, C.M.; Emanuelli, B.; Kahn, C.R. Critical nodes in signalling pathways: Insights into insulin action. *Nat. Rev. Mol. Cell. Biol.* **2006**, *7*, 85–96. [CrossRef] [PubMed]
5. Tripathy, D.; Chavez, A.O. Defects in insulin secretion and action in the pathogenesis of type 2 diabetes mellitus. *Curr. Diab. Rep.* **2010**, *10*, 184–191. [CrossRef] [PubMed]
6. Sinha, S.; Perdomo, G.; Brown, N.F.; O'Doherty, R.M. Fatty acid-induced insulin resistance in L6 myotubes is prevented by inhibition of activation and nuclear localization of nuclear factor kappa B. *J. Biol. Chem.* **2004**, *279*, 41294–41301. [CrossRef] [PubMed]
7. Samuel, V.T.; Petersen, K.F.; Shulman, G.I. Lipid-induced insulin resistance: Unravelling the mechanism. *Lancet* **2010**, *375*, 2267–2277. [CrossRef]
8. Pereira, S.; Park, E.; Moore, J.; Faubert, B.; Breen, D.M.; Oprescu, A.I.; Nahle, A.; Kwan, D.; Giacca, A.; Tsiani, E. Resveratrol prevents insulin resistance caused by short-term elevation of free fatty acids in vivo. *Appl. Physiol. Nutr. Metab.* **2015**, *40*, 1129–1136. [CrossRef] [PubMed]
9. Hancock, C.R.; Han, D.-H.; Chen, M.; Terada, S.; Yasuda, T.; Wright, D.C.; Holloszy, J.O. High-fat diets cause insulin resistance despite an increase in muscle mitochondria. *Proc. Natl. Acad. Sci. USA* **2008**, *105*, 7815–7820. [CrossRef] [PubMed]
10. Kanety, H.; Feinstein, R.; Papa, M.Z.; Hemi, R.; Karasik, A. Tumor necrosis factor alpha-induced phosphorylation of insulin receptor substrate-1 (IRS-1). Possible mechanism for suppression of insulin-stimulated tyrosine phosphorylation of IRS-1. *J. Biol. Chem.* **1995**, *270*, 23780–23784. [CrossRef] [PubMed]
11. Ueno, M.; Carvalheira, J.B.C.; Tambascia, R.C.; Bezerra, R.M.N.; Amaral, M.E.; Carneiro, E.M.; Folli, F.; Franchini, K.G.; Saad, M.J.A. Regulation of insulin signalling by hyperinsulinaemia: Role of IRS-1/2 serine phosphorylation and the mTOR/p70 S6K pathway. *Diabetologia* **2005**, *48*, 506–518. [CrossRef] [PubMed]
12. Mordier, S.; Iynedjian, P.B. Activation of mammalian target of rapamycin complex 1 and insulin resistance induced by palmitate in hepatocytes. *Biochem. Biophys. Res. Commun.* **2007**, *362*, 206–211. [CrossRef] [PubMed]
13. Carlson, C.J.; White, M.F.; Rondinone, C.M. Mammalian target of rapamycin regulates IRS-1 serine 307 phosphorylation. *Biochem. Biophys. Res. Commun.* **2004**, *316*, 533–539. [CrossRef] [PubMed]
14. Manning, B.D. Balancing Akt with S6K: Implications for both metabolic diseases and tumorigenesis. *J. Cell. Biol.* **2004**, *167*, 399–403. [CrossRef] [PubMed]
15. Um, S.H.; Frigerio, F.; Watanabe, M.; Picard, F.; Joaquin, M.; Sticker, M.; Fumagalli, S.; Allegrini, P.R.; Kozma, S.C.; Auwerx, J.; et al. Absence of S6K1 protects against age- and diet-induced obesity while enhancing insulin sensitivity. *Nature* **2004**, *431*, 200–205. [CrossRef] [PubMed]
16. Lee, J.; Kim, M.-S. The role of GSK3 in glucose homeostasis and the development of insulin resistance. *Diabetes Res. Clin. Pract.* **2007**, *77* (Suppl. 1), S49–S57. [CrossRef] [PubMed]
17. Hirosumi, J.; Tuncman, G.; Chang, L.; Görgün, C.Z.; Uysal, K.T.; Maeda, K.; Karin, M.; Hotamisligil, G.S. A central role for JNK in obesity and insulin resistance. *Nature* **2002**, *420*, 333–336. [CrossRef] [PubMed]

18. Li, Y.; Soos, T.J.; Li, X.; Wu, J.; Degennaro, M.; Sun, X.; Littman, D.R.; Birnbaum, M.J.; Polakiewicz, R.D. Protein kinase C Theta inhibits insulin signaling by phosphorylating IRS1 at Ser(1101). *J. Biol. Chem.* **2004**, *279*, 45304–45307. [CrossRef] [PubMed]

19. Hulver, M.W.; Dohm, G.L. The molecular mechanism linking muscle fat accumulation to insulin resistance. *Proc. Nutr. Soc.* **2004**, *63*, 375–380. [CrossRef] [PubMed]

20. Xie, M.; Zhang, D.; Dyck, J.R.B.; Li, Y.; Zhang, H.; Morishima, M.; Mann, D.L.; Taffet, G.E.; Baldini, A.; Khoury, D.S.; et al. A pivotal role for endogenous TGF-beta-activated kinase-1 in the LKB1/AMP-activated protein kinase energy-sensor pathway. *Proc. Natl. Acad. Sci. USA* **2006**, *103*, 17378–17383. [CrossRef] [PubMed]

21. Towler, M.C.; Hardie, D.G. AMP-activated protein kinase in metabolic control and insulin signaling. *Circ. Res.* **2007**, *100*, 328–341. [CrossRef] [PubMed]

22. Zhou, G.; Myers, R.; Li, Y.; Chen, Y.; Shen, X.; Fenyk-Melody, J.; Wu, M.; Ventre, J.; Doebber, T.; Fujii, N.; et al. Role of AMP-activated protein kinase in mechanism of metformin action. *J. Clin. Investig.* **2001**, *108*, 1167–1174. [CrossRef] [PubMed]

23. Fryer, L.G.D.; Parbu-Patel, A.; Carling, D. The anti-diabetic drugs rosiglitazone and metformin stimulate AMP-activated protein kinase through distinct signaling pathways. *J. Biol. Chem.* **2002**, *277*, 25226–25232. [CrossRef] [PubMed]

24. Breen, D.M.; Sanli, T.; Giacca, A.; Tsiani, E. Stimulation of muscle cell glucose uptake by resveratrol through sirtuins and AMPK. *Biochem. Biophys. Res. Commun.* **2008**, *374*, 117–122. [CrossRef] [PubMed]

25. Zygmunt, K.; Faubert, B.; MacNeil, J.; Tsiani, E. Naringenin, a citrus flavonoid, increases muscle cell glucose uptake via AMPK. *Biochem. Biophys. Res. Commun.* **2010**, *398*, 178–183. [CrossRef] [PubMed]

26. Hardie, D.G. AMP-activated protein kinase: An energy sensor that regulates all aspects of cell function. *Genes Dev.* **2011**, *25*, 1895–1908. [CrossRef] [PubMed]

27. Hardie, D.G.; Ross, F.A.; Hawley, S.A. AMPK: A nutrient and energy sensor that maintains energy homeostasis. *Nat. Rev. Mol. Cell. Biol.* **2012**, *13*, 251–262. [CrossRef] [PubMed]

28. Gasparrini, M.; Giampieri, F.; Alvarez Suarez, J.M.; Mazzoni, L.; Forbes Hernandez, T.Y.; Quiles, J.L.; Bullon, P.; Battino, M. AMPK as a New Attractive Therapeutic Target for Disease Prevention: The Role of Dietary Compounds AMPK and Disease Prevention. *Curr. Drug Targets* **2016**, *17*, 865–889. [CrossRef] [PubMed]

29. Cheung, S.; Tai, J. Anti-proliferative and antioxidant properties of rosemary *Rosmarinus officinalis*. *Oncol. Rep.* **2007**, *17*, 1525–1531. [CrossRef] [PubMed]

30. Moore, J.; Yousef, M.; Tsiani, E. Anticancer Effects of Rosemary (*Rosmarinus officinalis* L.) Extract and Rosemary Extract Polyphenols. *Nutrients* **2016**, *8*, 731. [CrossRef] [PubMed]

31. Erenmemisoglu, A. Effect of a *Rosmarinus officinalis* leave extract on plasma glucose levels in normoglycaemic and diabetic mice. *Pharmazie* **1997**, *52*, 645–646. [PubMed]

32. Bakirel, T.; Bakirel, U.; Keles, O.U.; Ulgen, S.G.; Yardibi, H. In vivo assessment of antidiabetic and antioxidant activities of rosemary (*Rosmarinus officinalis*) in alloxan-diabetic rabbits. *J. Ethnopharmacol.* **2008**, *116*, 64–73. [CrossRef] [PubMed]

33. Emam, M. Comparative evaluation of antidiabetic activity of *Rosmarinus officinalis* L. and Chamomile recutita in streptozotocin induced diabetic rats. *Agric. Biol. J. N. Am.* **2012**, *3*, 247–252. [CrossRef]

34. Romo Vaquero, M.; Yáñez-Gascón, M.-J.; García Villalba, R.; Larrosa, M.; Fromentin, E.; Ibarra, A.; Roller, M.; Tomás-Barberán, F.; Espín de Gea, J.C.; García-Conesa, M.-T. Inhibition of Gastric Lipase as a Mechanism for Body Weight and Plasma Lipids Reduction in Zucker Rats Fed a Rosemary Extract Rich in Carnosic Acid. *PLoS ONE* **2012**, *7*. [CrossRef] [PubMed]

35. Ramadan, K.S.; Khalil, O.A.; Danial, E.N.; Alnahdi, H.S.; Ayaz, N.O. Hypoglycemic and hepatoprotective activity of *Rosmarinus officinalis* extract in diabetic rats. *J. Physiol. Biochem.* **2013**, *69*, 779–783. [CrossRef] [PubMed]

36. Runtuwene, J.; Cheng, K.-C.; Asakawa, A.; Amitani, H.; Amitani, M.; Morinaga, A.; Takimoto, Y.; Kairupan, B.H.R.; Inui, A. Rosmarinic acid ameliorates hyperglycemia and insulin sensitivity in diabetic rats, potentially by modulating the expression of PEPCK and GLUT4. *Drug Des. Dev. Ther.* **2016**, *10*, 2193–2202. [CrossRef]

37. Naimi, M.; Vlavcheski, F.; Shamshoum, H.; Tsiani, E. Rosemary Extract as a Potential Anti-Hyperglycemic Agent: Current Evidence and Future Perspectives. *Nutrients* **2017**, *9*, 968. [CrossRef] [PubMed]

38. Naimi, M.; Tsakiridis, T.; Stamatatos, T.C.; Alexandropoulos, D.I.; Tsiani, E. Increased skeletal muscle glucose uptake by rosemary extract through AMPK activation. *Appl. Physiol. Nutr. Metab.* **2015**, *40*, 407–413. [CrossRef] [PubMed]

39. Ibarra, A.; Cases, J.; Roller, M.; Chiralt-Boix, A.; Coussaert, A.; Ripoll, C. Carnosic acid-rich rosemary (*Rosmarinus officinalis* L.) leaf extract limits weight gain and improves cholesterol levels and glycaemia in mice on a high-fat diet. *Br. J. Nutr.* **2011**, *106*, 1182–1189. [CrossRef] [PubMed]

40. Afonso, M.S.; de O Silva, A.M.; Carvalho, E.B.; Rivelli, D.P.; Barros, S.B.; Rogero, M.M.; Lottenberg, A.M.; Torres, R.P.; Mancini-Filho, J. Phenolic compounds from Rosemary (*Rosmarinus officinalis* L.) attenuate oxidative stress and reduce blood cholesterol concentrations in diet-induced hypercholesterolemic rats. *Nutr. Metab.* **2013**, *10*, 19. [CrossRef] [PubMed]

41. Ma, P.; Yao, L.; Lin, X.; Gu, T.; Rong, X.; Batey, R.; Yamahara, J.; Wang, J.; Li, Y. A mixture of apple pomace and rosemary extract improves fructose consumption-induced insulin resistance in rats: modulation of sarcolemmal CD36 and glucose transporter-4. *Am. J. Transl. Res.* **2016**, *8*, 3791–3801. [PubMed]

42. International Diabetes Federation. *IDF Diabetes Atlas*, 7th ed.; Belgium International Diabetes Federation: Brussels, Belgium, 2015.

43. Johnson, J.J. Carnosol: A promising anti-cancer and anti-inflammatory agent. *Cancer Lett.* **2011**, *305*, 1–7. [CrossRef] [PubMed]

44. Yu, C.; Chen, Y.; Cline, G.W.; Zhang, D.; Zong, H.; Wang, Y.; Bergeron, R.; Kim, J.K.; Cushman, S.W.; Cooney, G.J.; et al. Mechanism by which fatty acids inhibit insulin activation of insulin receptor substrate-1 (IRS-1)-associated phosphatidylinositol 3-kinase activity in muscle. *J. Biol. Chem.* **2002**, *277*, 50230–50236. [CrossRef] [PubMed]

45. Le Marchand-Brustel, Y.; Gual, P.; Grémeaux, T.; Gonzalez, T.; Barrès, R.; Tanti, J.-F. Fatty acid-induced insulin resistance: Role of insulin receptor substrate 1 serine phosphorylation in the retroregulation of insulin signalling. *Biochem. Soc. Trans.* **2003**, *31*, 1152–1156. [CrossRef] [PubMed]

46. Prada, P.; Zecchin, H.; Gasparetti, A.; Torsoni, M.; Ueno, M.; Hirata, A.; do Amaral, M.; Hoer, N.; Boschero, A.; Saad, M. Western diet modulates insulin signaling, c-jun N-terminal kinase activity, and insulin receptor substrate-1(ser307) phosphorylation in a tissue-specific fashion. *Endocrinology* **2005**, *146*, 1576–1587. [CrossRef] [PubMed]

47. Solinas, G.; Naugler, W.; Galimi, F.; Lee, M.-S.; Karin, M. Saturated fatty acids inhibit induction of insulin gene transcription by JNK-mediated phosphorylation of insulin-receptor substrates. *Proc. Natl. Acad. Sci. USA* **2006**, *103*, 16454–16459. [CrossRef] [PubMed]

48. Naimi, M.; Vlavcheski, F.; Murphy, B.; Hudlicky, T.; Tsiani, E. Carnosic acid as a component of rosemary extract stimulates skeletal muscle cell glucose uptake via AMPK activation. *Clin. Exp. Pharmacol. Physiol.* **2016**. [CrossRef] [PubMed]

49. Vlavcheski, F.; Naimi, M.; Murphy, B.; Hudlicky, T.; Tsiani, E. Rosmarinic Acid, a Rosemary Extract Polyphenol, Increases Skeletal Muscle Cell Glucose Uptake and Activates AMPK. *Mol. Basel. Switz.* **2017**, *22*, 1669. [CrossRef] [PubMed]

50. Vlavcheski, F.; Baron, D.; Vlachogiannis, I.A.; MacPherson, R.E.K.; Tsiani, E. Carnosol Increases Skeletal Muscle Cell Glucose Uptake via AMPK-Dependent GLUT4 Glucose Transporter Translocation. *Int. J. Mol. Sci.* **2018**, *19*, 1321. [CrossRef] [PubMed]

51. Perdomo, G.; Commerford, S.R.; Richard, A.-M.T.; Adams, S.H.; Corkey, B.E.; O'Doherty, R.M.; Brown, N.F. Increased beta-oxidation in muscle cells enhances insulin-stimulated glucose metabolism and protects against fatty acid-induced insulin resistance despite intramyocellular lipid accumulation. *J. Biol. Chem.* **2004**, *279*, 27177–27186. [CrossRef] [PubMed]

52. Dimopoulos, N.; Watson, M.; Sakamoto, K.; Hundal, H.S. Differential effects of palmitate and palmitoleate on insulin action and glucose utilization in rat L6 skeletal muscle cells. *Biochem. J.* **2006**, *399*, 473–481. [CrossRef] [PubMed]

53. Lang, C.H. Elevated plasma free fatty acids decrease basal protein synthesis, but not the anabolic effect of leucine, in skeletal muscle. *Am. J. Physiol. Endocrinol. Metab.* **2006**, *291*, E666–E674. [CrossRef] [PubMed]

54. Jaiswal, N.; Gunaganti, N.; Maurya, C.K.; Narender, T.; Tamrakar, A.K. Free fatty acid induced impairment of insulin signaling is prevented by the diastereomeric mixture of calophyllic acid and isocalophyllic acid in skeletal muscle cells. *Eur. J. Pharmacol.* **2015**, *746*, 70–77. [CrossRef] [PubMed]

55. Deng, Y.-T.; Chang, T.-W.; Lee, M.-S.; Lin, J.-K. Suppression of Free Fatty Acid-Induced Insulin Resistance by Phytopolyphenols in C2C12 Mouse Skeletal Muscle Cells. *J. Agric. Food Chem.* **2012**, *60*, 1059–1066. [CrossRef] [PubMed]

56. Le Bacquer, O.; Petroulakis, E.; Paglialunga, S.; Poulin, F.; Richard, D.; Cianflone, K.; Sonenberg, N. Elevated sensitivity to diet-induced obesity and insulin resistance in mice lacking 4E-BP1 and 4E-BP2. *J. Clin. Investig.* **2007**, *117*, 387–396. [CrossRef] [PubMed]

57. Gual, P.; Le Marchand-Brustel, Y.; Tanti, J.-F. Positive and negative regulation of insulin signaling through IRS-1 phosphorylation. *Biochimie* **2005**, *87*, 99–109. [CrossRef] [PubMed]

58. Bogachus, L.D.; Turcotte, L.P. Genetic downregulation of AMPK-α isoforms uncovers the mechanism by which metformin decreases FA uptake and oxidation in skeletal muscle cells. *Am. J. Physiol. Cell Physiol.* **2010**, *299*, C1549–C1561. [CrossRef] [PubMed]

59. Powell, D.J.; Turban, S.; Gray, A.; Hajduch, E.; Hundal, H.S. Intracellular ceramide synthesis and protein kinase Czeta activation play an essential role in palmitate-induced insulin resistance in rat L6 skeletal muscle cells. *Biochem. J.* **2004**, *382*, 619–629. [CrossRef] [PubMed]

60. Capel, F.; Cheraiti, N.; Acquaviva, C.; Hénique, C.; Bertrand-Michel, J.; Vianey-Saban, C.; Prip-Buus, C.; Morio, B. Oleate dose-dependently regulates palmitate metabolism and insulin signaling in C2C12 myotubes. *Biochim. Biophys. Acta* **2016**, *1861*, 2000–2010. [CrossRef] [PubMed]

61. Jung, T.W.; Kim, H.-C.; Abd El-Aty, A.M.; Jeong, J.H. Protectin DX ameliorates palmitate- or high-fat diet-induced insulin resistance and inflammation through an AMPK-PPARα-dependent pathway in mice. *Sci. Rep.* **2017**, *7*. [CrossRef] [PubMed]

62. Wu, W.; Tang, S.; Shi, J.; Yin, W.; Cao, S.; Bu, R.; Zhu, D.; Bi, Y. Metformin attenuates palmitic acid-induced insulin resistance in L6 cells through the AMP-activated protein kinase/sterol regulatory element-binding protein-1c pathway. *Int. J. Mol. Med.* **2015**, *35*, 1734–1740. [CrossRef] [PubMed]

63. Anhê, G.F.; Okamoto, M.M.; Kinote, A.; Sollon, C.; Lellis-Santos, C.; Anhê, F.F.; Lima, G.A.; Hirabara, S.M.; Velloso, L.A.; Bordin, S.; et al. Quercetin decreases inflammatory response and increases insulin action in skeletal muscle of ob/ob mice and in L6 myotubes. *Eur. J. Pharmacol.* **2012**, *689*, 285–293. [CrossRef] [PubMed]

64. Sadeghi, A.; Seyyed Ebrahimi, S.S.; Golestani, A.; Meshkani, R. Resveratrol Ameliorates Palmitate-Induced Inflammation in Skeletal Muscle Cells by Attenuating Oxidative Stress and JNK/NF-κB Pathway in a SIRT1-Independent Mechanism. *J. Cell. Biochem.* **2017**, *118*, 2654–2663. [CrossRef] [PubMed]

65. Araújo, E.P.; De Souza, C.T.; Ueno, M.; Cintra, D.E.; Bertolo, M.B.; Carvalheira, J.B.; Saad, M.J.; Velloso, L.A. Infliximab Restores Glucose Homeostasis in an Animal Model of Diet-Induced Obesity and Diabetes. *Endocrinology* **2007**, *148*, 5991–5997. [CrossRef] [PubMed]

66. Rivas, D.A.; Yaspelkis, B.B.; Hawley, J.A.; Lessard, S.J. Lipid-induced mTOR activation in rat skeletal muscle reversed by exercise and 5′-aminoimidazole-4-carboxamide-1-beta-D-ribofuranoside. *J. Endocrinol.* **2009**, *202*, 441–451. [CrossRef] [PubMed]

67. Wang, X.; Yu, W.; Nawaz, A.; Guan, F.; Sun, S.; Wang, C. Palmitate Induced Insulin Resistance by PKCtheta-Dependent Activation of mTOR/S6K Pathway in C2C12 Myotubes. *Exp. Clin. Endocrinol. Diabetes* **2010**, *118*, 657–661. [CrossRef] [PubMed]

68. Woo, J.H.; Shin, K.O.; Lee, Y.H.; Jang, K.S.; Bae, J.Y.; Roh, H.T. Effects of treadmill exercise on skeletal muscle mTOR signaling pathway in high-fat diet-induced obese mice. *J. Phys. Ther. Sci.* **2016**, *28*, 1260–1265. [CrossRef] [PubMed]

69. Kwon, B.; Querfurth, H.W. Palmitate activates mTOR/p70S6K through AMPK inhibition and hypophosphorylation of raptor in skeletal muscle cells: Reversal by oleate is similar to metformin. *Biochimie* **2015**, *118*, 141–150. [CrossRef] [PubMed]

70. Cantó, C.; Auwerx, J. AMP-activated protein kinase and its downstream transcriptional pathways. *Cell. Mol. Life Sci.* **2010**, *67*, 3407–3423. [CrossRef] [PubMed]

71. Mihaylova, M.M.; Shaw, R.J. The AMP-activated protein kinase (AMPK) signaling pathway coordinates cell growth, autophagy, & metabolism. *Nat. Cell. Biol.* **2011**, *13*, 1016–1023. [CrossRef] [PubMed]

72. Zhao, Y.; Sedighi, R.; Wang, P.; Chen, H.; Zhu, Y.; Sang, S. Carnosic acid as a major bioactive component in rosemary extract ameliorates high-fat-diet-induced obesity and metabolic syndrome in mice. *J. Agric. Food Chem.* **2015**, *63*, 4843–4852. [CrossRef] [PubMed]

Nutrients **2018**, *10*, 1623

73. Romo-Vaquero, M.; Larrosa, M.; Yáñez-Gascón, M.J.; Issaly, N.; Flanagan, J.; Roller, M.; Tomás-Barberán, F.A.; Espín, J.C.; García-Conesa, M.-T. A rosemary extract enriched in carnosic acid improves circulating adipocytokines and modulates key metabolic sensors in lean Zucker rats: Critical and contrasting differences in the obese genotype. *Mol. Nutr. Food Res.* **2014**, *58*, 942–953. [CrossRef] [PubMed]

74. Ninomiya, K.; Matsuda, H.; Shimoda, H.; Norihisa, N.; Kasajima, N.; Yoshino, T.; Morikawa, T.; Yoshikawa, M. Carnosic acid, a new class of lipid absorption inhibitor from sage. *Bioorg. Med. Chem. Lett.* **2004**, *14*, 1943–1946. [CrossRef] [PubMed]

75. Park, M.-Y.; Mun, S.T. Dietary carnosic acid suppresses hepatic steatosis formation via regulation of hepatic fatty acid metabolism in high-fat diet-fed mice. *Nutr. Res. Pract.* **2013**, *7*, 294–301. [CrossRef] [PubMed]

76. Labban, L.; Mustafa, U.E.-S.; Ibrahim, Y.M. The Effects of Rosemary (*Rosmarinus officinalis*) Leaves Powder on Glucose Level, Lipid Profile and Lipid Perodoxation. *Int. J. Clin. Med.* **2014**, *05*, 297–304. [CrossRef]

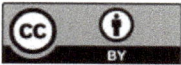

![nutrients logo] *nutrients*

MDPI

Article

Effects of Tempeh Fermentation with *Lactobacillus plantarum* and *Rhizopus oligosporus* on Streptozotocin-Induced Type II Diabetes Mellitus in Rats

Ying-Che Huang [1] [ORCID], Bo-Hua Wu [2], Yung-Lin Chu [3], Wen-Chang Chang [4,†] and Ming-Chang Wu [1,2,*,†]

1   Graduate Institute of Bioresources, National Pingtung University of Science and Technology, Pingtung 91201, Taiwan; huangleo0811@gmail.com
2   Department of Food Science, National Pingtung University of Science and Technology, Pingtung 91201, Taiwan; david9097@yahoo.com.tw
3   International Master's Degree Program in Food Science, International College, National Pingtung University of Science and Technology, Pingtung 91201, Taiwan; ylchu@mail.npust.edu.tw
4   Department of Food Science, National Chiayi University, Chiayi 60004, Taiwan; d99641001@ntu.edu.tw
*   Correspondence: mcwu@mail.npust.edu.tw; Tel.: +886-8-7740240 (ext. 7035); Fax: +886-8-7740378
†   These authors contributed equally to this work.

Received: 28 July 2018; Accepted: 17 August 2018; Published: 22 August 2018

Abstract: The increased consumption of high fat-containing foods has been linked to the prevalence of obesity and abnormal metabolic syndromes. *Rhizopus oligosporus*, a fungus in the family Mucoraceae, is widely used as a starter for homemade tempeh. Although *R. oligosporus* can prevent the growth of other microorganisms, it grows well with lactic acid bacteria (LAB). *Lactobacillus plantarum* can produce β-glucosidase, which catalyzes the hydrolysis of glucoside isoflavones into aglycones (with greater bioavailability). Therefore, the development of a soybean-based functional food by the co-inoculation of *R. oligosporus* and *L. plantarum* is a promising approach to increase the bioactivity of tempeh. In this study, the ameliorative effect of *L. plantarum* in soy tempeh on abnormal carbohydrate metabolism in high-fat diet (HFD)-induced hyperglycemic rats was evaluated. The co-incubation of *L. plantarum* with *R. oligosporus* during soy tempeh fermentation reduced the homeostatic model assessment of insulin resistance, HbA1c, serum glucose, total cholesterol, triglyceride, free fatty acid, insulin, and low-density lipoprotein contents, and significantly increased the high-density lipoprotein content in HFD rats. It also increased the LAB counts, as well as the bile acid, cholesterol, triglyceride, and short-chain fatty acid contents in the feces of HFD rats. Our results suggested that the modulation of serum glucose and lipid levels by LAB occurs via alterations in the internal microbiota, leading to the inhibition of cholesterol synthesis and promotion of lipolysis. Tempeh, which was produced with both *L. plantarum* and *R. oligosporus*, might be a beneficial dietary supplement for individuals with abnormal carbohydrate metabolism.

Keywords: tempeh; lactic acid bacteria; short chain fatty acids; metabolic syndrome; high fat diet; feces

---

1. Introduction

The consumption of fast food, fried food, and high-fat foods is increasing along with changes in lifestyle. Therefore, the incidence of metabolic syndrome is increasing and is expected to become a major issue worldwide. It is characterized by high blood pressure, high blood sugar, hypertriglyceridemia, obesity, and low high-density lipoprotein (HDL) levels in the blood. In addition, metabolic syndrome is associated with an increased risk of type II diabetes and cardiovascular diseases. Therefore, the WHO predicts that the prevalence of diabetes mellitus (DM) will increase to 5.92 billion individuals by 2035, and Asia is one of the regions with the highest patient population [1]. Preliminary estimates are predicted to increase to 42.3 million for patients with diabetes mellitus in Asia in 2080 from 20.8 million populations in 2000, and economic development, high-fat foods, fried food, etc., are likely to be the primary underlying causes [1].

Lactobacillus has wide applications in probiotics and has many advantages among humans and animals. It will be beneficial to administer active microorganisms to hosts when probiotics are supplied in sufficient quantity [2]. The study also shows that probiotics play an important role in preventing and treating chronic metabolic diseases or immune-related diseases. Many studies have shown that lactic acid bacteria (LAB) are beneficial for human health, e.g., they could decrease the total cholesterol in blood and they have favorable effects in patients with type II diabetes [2]. It remarkably increased fecal and bile acid cholesterol levels after administration of *Lactobacillus plantarum*. Furthermore, it helped decrease the total blood cholesterol levels after moderate intake of *Lactobacillus plantarum* [2,3]. Recently, numerous phytochemicals have been reported in soybeans and fermented soybean products. In particular, isoflavones genistein and daidzein are beneficial for humans and isoflavones can prevent cardiovascular diseases, cancers, metabolic syndrome, or help to treat osteoporosis because it can mimic estrogen in humans [2,4]. Furthermore, certain animal studies reported that isoflavones can either decrease body weight or increase insulin levels; moreover, it plays an important role in modulating serum glucose levels in diabetic rats [2]. Numerous complex compounds are metabolized/decomposed by microorganisms to generate compounds of higher nutritional value, such as increasing aglycone during soybean fermentation [4].

Tempeh is a fermented soybean product that originated in Indonesia. Tempeh is rich in soy protein and genistein, which have beneficial effects on the regulation of high blood sugar and prevent diabetes [5]. The processing of tempeh involves the addition of *Rhizopus* spp. to cooked, peeled soybeans for fermentation at 37 °C for five days. The weather in Indonesia is wet and hot, and accordingly, tempeh can be made at room temperature [6]. Some studies have reported that tempeh, which prevents diarrhea and anemia and is richer in vitamins and minerals than unfermented soybean, contains many vitamins B_{12} and antioxidants [4]. Furthermore, genistein, daidzein, and β-sitosterol in tempeh prevent cancers, cardiovascular diseases, type II diabetes, and blood glucose regulation [7]. Tempeh also significantly decreases phytic acid and trypsin (antinutritive factors) levels during fermentation. This is one of the reasons why tempeh is popular, especially among vegetarians, in Asia, Europe, and the Americas because of its beneficial functions [4,7,8].

Many studies have shown that fermented soybean and LAB are effective for the prevention of type II diabetes [9,10]. However, the effects of the co-fermentation of *Lactobacillus plantarum* and *Rhizopus oligosporus* on type II diabetes have not been evaluated. Therefore, we prepared tempeh while using both *L. plantarum* and *R. oligosporus* (a common fungus used as a starter for tempeh) and administered it to rat models of diabetes, with HFD-induced high serum glucose and cholesterol. The objective of this study was to develop a strategy to improve the quality of life in patients with metabolic syndrome based on alternative food therapy.

2. Materials and Methods

2.1. Sample Preparation

Kaohsiung Number 9 soybeans were used for co-fermented tempeh. Soybeans were washed and soaked for 12 h and the outer membranes were removed. After drying, water (twice the weight of soybeans) and 1% lactic acid were added, followed by cooking at 100 °C for 30 min. Next, *L. plantarum* and *R. oligosporus* were inoculated at 30 °C in a fermentative environment for 48 h after samples were cooled. Normal tempeh was prepared according to the same procedure with only *R. oligosporus*. All of the samples were stored at −20 °C in a refrigerator until the central temperature reached −18 °C, and samples were then freeze-dried for 48 h. After the water was removed, samples were milled and stored at $-20°C$. In addition, normal diet (LabDiet 5001) was purchased from Young Li Trading Co., Ltd. (New Taipei, Taiwan) The composition of the HFD was normal diet: cholesterol: coconut oil = 73:2:25 [11].

2.2. Animals and Diets

Eight-week-old male Sprague–Dawley (SD) rats were obtained from BioLASCO Taiwan Co., Ltd. (Taipei, Taiwan). The animals were housed in a room with an alternate light/dark cycle (12 h), a temperature of 25 ± 2 °C, and a relative humidity of $55-60\%$. All rats were fed experimental diets ad libitum with free access to drinking water at all times. After two weeks of adaptive feeding, the rats were randomly assigned to groups of eight animals each and fed different experimental diets as follows: rats in the control group were fed a normal chow diet with 13.5% kcal fat (Laboratory Rodent Diet 5001; Lab Diet/PMI Nutrition International, Purina Mills LLC, Gray Summit, MO, USA) and rats in the negative control group and treatment groups were fed the HFD (coconut oil 25%, cholesterol 2%, feed powder 73%) modified, as described in Gandhi et al. [11]. Diabetes was induced by treatment with 30 mg/kg STZ and 45 mg/kg nicotinamide for four weeks. Rats were induced by 20 mg/kg STZ again if their serum glucose levels did not reach 150 mg/dL after one week of induction. Rats in the treatment groups (8 rats/group) were separated into the normal diet group (control group), negative control group (HFD, SH group), and positive control group fed pioglitazone (10 mg/kg body weight/day, SHP group) in the last four weeks. The other rats were orally administered cooked soybean (40 mg/kg body weight/day, SHS group), tempeh (40 mg/kg body weight/day, SHL group), or probiotic fermented tempeh (40 mg/kg body weight/day, SHTL group) in the last four weeks. The total study period was 14 weeks for all groups. Food intake and body weight were measured weekly for the duration of the experiment. The animals were maintained in accordance with the National Pingtung University of Science and Technology and Tajen University guidelines for the care and use of laboratory animals. The animal study protocols were approved by the Ethics Committee at the Tajen University (Approval No. 105-10).

2.3. Serum Samples

All blood samples were solidified at room temperature for 30 min after collection. Centrifugation at $3000\times g$ for 20 min, the supernatant was obtained and stored at $-80°C$ before analysis.

2.4. Fasting Serum Glucose

Before the fasting serum glucose test, all rats were fasted overnight (14–16 h). Blood from the tail artery was collected (0.1 mL/rat) and analyzed while using a blood-glucose meter.

2.5. Oral Glucose Tolerance Test (OGTT)

The OGTT assay followed a similar protocol to that of the fasting serum glucose test. All of the rats were fasted overnight (14–16 h) and weighed. Blood was then collected from the tail artery (0.1 mL/rat) and analyzed using a blood-glucose meter. All animals received 1.5 g of glucose/kg body weight. Blood was sampled from the tail vessels of conscious animals before the load ($t = 0$) and 30, 60, 90, and 120 min after glucose administration. The samples were allowed to clot for 30 min, centrifuged ($3000\times g$, 20 min), and evaluated while using a blood-glucose meter.

2.6. Biochemical Measurements

Commercial kits for determining the levels of free fatty acids (FFA), HbA1c, high-density-lipoprotein-cholesterol (HDL-C), insulin, and low-density-lipoprotein-cholesterol (LDL-C) in rats were obtained from Randox Laboratories (Crumlin, Co., Antrim, UK). The biochemical assays were performed according to the protocols provided by Randox Laboratories.

2.7. Homeostasis Model Assessment-Insulin Resistance (HOMA-IR)

The homeostasis model assessment for insulin resistance (HOMA-IR) was calculated via the following equation: fasting serum insulin (mU/L) × fasting glucose (mmol/L)/22.5 [12].

2.8. Stool Assay

Total LAB in stool samples were determined while using a 1.0-g stool sample diluted 10–1000 times with double distilled endotoxin-free water. Next, 1.0 mL of the sample was added to Lactic Acid Bacteria Count Plates 6461 (3M Petrifilm, St. Paul, MN, USA). Samples were analyzed after incubation for 48 h at 37 °C. For short chain fatty acid (SCFA) detection, the protocol described by Holben [13] was used, with modifications. First, 910 µL of absolute alcohol and 90 µL of pivalic acid (5 mg/mL) were added to 0.5 g of the stool sample and vortexed for 2 min. Next, 500 µL of 0.8 M perchloric acid was added and vortexed for 5 min, followed by centrifugation for 1 min at 13,000 rpm. Then, 0.5 mL of the supernatant was mixed with 50 µL of 4 M KOH for 5 min, and 250 µL of oxalic acid solution was added at 4 °C for 60 min. Finally, the sample was centrifuged for 1 min at 13000 rpm again and the supernatant was passed through a 0.22-µm filter. All of the samples were analyzed while using Mass Selective Detector 5973Network, HP-INNOWax (Capillary column: 30 m, inner diameter: 0.25 mm, particle size: 0.25 µm, detector: Mass Selective Detector 5973Network, gas: Helium, split rate: 5:1, column flow rate: 2 mL/min, total flow rate: 15 mL/min, injector temperature = 200 °C, oven temperature = 100 °C, detector temperature = 200 °C, initial temperature = 100 °C for 1 min, heating procedure of 2 °C/min until reaching 110 °C for 2 min, then 3 °C/min until reaching 170 °C for 1 min, final heating at 10 °C/min until reaching 200 °C for 2 min). Each sample (1 µL) was used for gas chromatography injection for 32 min, and then a mass spectrometer was used to compare acetic acid, propionate, and butyrate, as described previously [13]. Cholesterol, triglycerides, and cholic acid were analyzed while using ELISA kits (BioVision Inc., Milpitas, CA, USA). All tests were performed according to the protocols provided by BioVision Inc.

2.9. Next-Generation Sequencing Analysis of Stool Samples

2.9.1. Amplicon Library Construction and Sequencing

Total bacterial DNA from 5 g of rat feces was isolated and purified using the PowerSoil® DNA Isolation Kit (Mo Bio, Qiagen, Hilden, Germany). A 16S rDNA region (V3–V5 hypervariable region) from purified total bacterial DNA was amplified via PCR to produce 400-bp DNA fragments for further purification. The specific PCR primers were as follows: forward primer overhang adaptor (5′–TCGTCGGCAGCGTCAGATGTGTATAA GAGACAG–3′) and reverse primer overhang adaptor (5′–GTCTCGTGGGCTCGGAGATGTG TATAAGAGACAG–3′). Amplicons were generated while using a high-fidelity polymerase (AccuPrime; Invitrogen, Carlsbad, CA, USA), purified using a Magnetic Bead Capture Kit (Ampure; Agencourt, Beverly, MA, USA), and quantified using a fluorometric kit (QuantIT PicoGreen; Invitrogen, Carlsbad, CA, USA). PCR conditions were 30 cycles of 30 s at 95 °C, 30 s at 55 °C, and 30 s at 72 °C, and a final extension for 5 min at 72 °C. The purified amplicons were then pooled in equimolar concentrations using a SequalPrep Plate Normalization Kit (Invitrogen, Carlsbad, CA, USA). The final concentration of the library was determined using an SYBR Green Quantitative PCR (qPCR) assay and the size distribution of the library was determined using Caliper LabChip. 16S rRNA-specific regions were then sequenced using a MiSeq sequencer (Illumina, San Diego, CA, USA).

2.9.2. Bioinformatic Analysis

Raw reads from the MiSeq sequencer for the metagenomic workflow were analyzed while using QIIME (http://qiime.org/). Reference sequences in Greengenes gg_13_8 (99_otus.fasta) were used in the analysis (Greengenes database, http://greengenes.lbl.gov/). The Ribosomal Database Project (RDP) classifier (http://rdp.cme.msu.edu/classifier/) was used to classify the 16S rDNA sequences into distinct taxonomic categories that are based on sequence alignments. The operational taxonomic units (OTUs) for Lactobacillus species were determined by BLAST searches and groups were preliminarily assigned by alignments with the NCBI genome database. All 16S rDNA sequences were mapped to the RDP database while using QIIME and divided into groups corresponding to their taxonomy at the level of order and were then assigned to OTUs. A sequence similarity exceeding 0.95 was the threshold for OTUs, according to the value for species distinction in microbiology.

2.10. Statistical Analysis

All results are reported as means ± SD and the differences between the control and tempeh-treated groups were analyzed by one-way analysis of variance (ANOVA) and Duncan's multiple range tests (IBM SPSS Statistics 19, North Castle, NY, USA) with a significance threshold of $p < 0.05$.

3. Results

3.1. Hyperglycemic Rat Model

We induced DM in rats by STZ after 10 weeks of feeding on the HFD. The fasting serum glucose level was significantly higher ($p < 0.05$) in the STZ treatment group than in normal rats provided the chow diet (Figure 1).

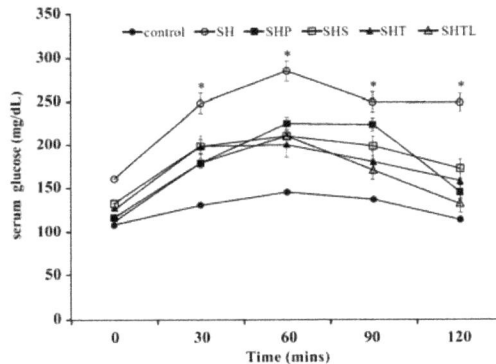

Figure 1. Oral glucose tolerance test (OGTT) for streptozotocin (STZ)-induced diabetic rats fed a high-fat diet for 14 weeks and administered *Lactobacillus plantarum* co-fermented tempeh orally during the last 4 weeks. Control: normal diet; SH: Streptozotocin (STZ 30 mg/kg, Nicotinamide 45 mg/kg) + High fat diet (Coconut oil 25%, Cholesterol 2%, Feed powder 73%); SHP: Streptozotocin (STZ 30 mg/kg, Nicotinamide 45 mg/kg) + High fat diet (Coconut oil 25%, Cholesterol 2%, Feed powder 73%) + Pioglitazone (10 mg/kg body weight); SHS: Streptozotocin (STZ 30 mg/kg, Nicotinamide 45 mg/kg) + High fat diet (Coconut oil 25%, Cholesterol 2%, Feed powder 73%) + Unfermented soybean (40 mg/kg body weight); SHT: Streptozotocin (STZ 30 mg/kg: Nicotinamide 45 mg/kg) + High fat diet (Coconut oil 25%, Cholesterol 2%, Feed powder 73%) + Tempeh (40 mg/kg body weight); SHTL: Streptozotocin (STZ 30 mg/kg, Nicotinamide 45 mg/kg) + High fat diet (Coconut oil 25%, Cholesterol 2%, Feed powder 73%) + Tempeh + *Lactobacillus plantarum* (40 mg/kg body weight). * Indicates a significant difference ($p < 0.05$) compared with the control group at the same time point. Results are expressed as mean values ± SD. ($n = 8$/group).

3.2. Oral Glucose Tolerance Test

In the treatment groups, serum glucose levels were ameliorated in DM rats after 14 weeks of HFD feeding (Figure 1). The serum glucose levels in the SH group (HFD) after the oral administration of glucose at 30, 60, 90, and 120 min were significantly higher than those of other treatment groups

($p < 0.05$). In addition, the OGTT showed that 40 mg/kg soybean (SHS group) and 40 mg/kg tempeh (SHT group) reduced the serum glucose level in STZ-induced DM rats. Moreover, the SHTL treatment group (40 mg/kg) exhibited significantly lower serum glucose levels than those in other treatment groups that are based on the OGTT ($p < 0.05$).

3.3. Effects of Various Treatments on Serum Biochemistry in DM Rats

In our serum biochemistry analysis, we observed significantly increased TG, cholesterol, LDL, FFA, serum glucose, HbA1C, and insulin levels, but reduced HDL levels in DM rats in the SH group after 14 weeks of the HFD ($p < 0.05$) (Table 1). The SH group achieved insulin resistance based on the HOMA-IR values. However, the SHS (40 mg/kg), SHT (40 mg/kg), and SHTL (40 mg/kg) treatments resulted in significant decreases in TG, cholesterol, LDL, FFA, serum glucose, HbA1C, and insulin levels, but increased HDL levels in DM rats ($p < 0.05$). In addition, the SHTL (40 mg/kg) treatment group exhibited the greatest improvements in all serum biochemical parameters, indicating that it could alleviate the symptoms of DM in rats; this group also exhibited improved insulin-resistance based on the HOMA-IR calculation.

Table 1. Selected serum biochemical parameters for STZ-induced diabetic rats fed a high-fat diet for 14 weeks and administered *Lactobacillus plantarum* co-fermented tempeh orally during the last 4 weeks.

Items/Groups	Control	SH	SHP	SHS	SHT	SHTL
Triglyceride (mg/dL)	55.11 ± 20.0 [bcd]	118.1 ± 35.8 [a]	49.30 ± 8.52 [cd]	71.50 ± 17.2 [bc]	76.40 ± 24.7 [b]	47.90 ± 9.95 [d]
Cholesterol-total (mg/dL)	53.50 ± 6.86 [c]	90.33 ± 11.1 [a]	66.50 ± 13.4 [bc]	79.67 ± 14.4 [ab]	69.67 ± 14.4 [bc]	65.50 ± 9.98 [bc]
HDL-cholesterol (mg/dL)	40.56 ± 7.78 [ab]	35.71 ± 4.59 [b]	34.20 ± 6.16 [b]	45.13 ± 10.3 [a]	40.29 ± 4.08 [ab]	40.14 ± 3.42 [ab]
Cholesterol/HDL-C	1.41 ± 0.07 [b]	2.12 ± 0.35 [a]	2.04 ± 0.36 [a]	2.02 ± 0.15 [a]	1.94 ± 0.16 [a]	2.01 ± 0.17 [a]
LDL-cholesterol (mg/dL)	7.89 ± 2.23 [c]	36.00 ± 8.68 [a]	23.63 ± 7.20 [b]	28.75 ± 9.77 [b]	24.78 ± 6.29 [b]	25.00 ± 5.24 [b]
Free-fatty acid (mmol/L)	1.43 ± 0.61 [b]	2.31 ± 0.25 [a]	1.16 ± 0.06 [b]	1.55 ± 0.23 [b]	1.36 ± 0.31 [b]	1.41 ± 0.24 [b]
Glucose AC (mg/dL)	100 ± 8.4 [c]	199 ± 42.3 [a]	125 ± 34.6 [bc]	151 ± 25.5 [b]	141 ± 24.8 [b]	109 ± 17.3 [c]
HbA1C (%)	4.02 ± 0.13 [d]	6.96 ± 1.05 [a]	5.17 ± 0.97 [bc]	5.58 ± 1.42 [b]	5.51 ± 1.25 [b]	4.42 ± 0.32 [cd]
Insulin (ng/mL)	2.48 ± 2.11 [b]	9.99 ± 5.46 [a]	1.61 ± 0.81 [b]	2.11 ± 0.67 [b]	2.61 ± 0.53 [b]	1.65 ± 0.53 [b]
HOMA-IR	0.55 ± 0.18 [c]	4.46 ± 0.95 [a]	0.54 ± 0.19 [c]	0.89 ± 0.17 [bc]	1.07 ± 0.36 [b]	0.59 ± 0.16 [c]

Control: normal diet; SH: Streptozotocin (STZ 30 mg/kg, Nicotinamide 45 mg/kg) + High fat diet (Coconut oil 25%, Cholesterol 2%, Feed powder 73%); SHP: Streptozotocin (STZ 30 mg/kg, Nicotinamide 45 mg/kg) + High fat diet (Coconut oil 25%, Cholesterol 2%, Feed powder 73%) + Pioglitazone (10 mg/kg body weight); SHS: Streptozotocin (STZ 30 mg/kg, Nicotinamide 45 mg/kg) + High fat diet (Coconut oil 25%, Cholesterol 2%, Feed powder 73%) + Unfermented soybean (40 mg/kg body weight); SHT: Streptozotocin (STZ 30 mg/kg: Nicotinamide 45 mg/kg) + High fat diet (Coconut oil 25%, Cholesterol 2%, Feed powder 73%) + Tempeh (40 mg/kg body weight); SHTL: Streptozotocin (STZ 30 mg/kg, Nicotinamide 45 mg/kg) + High fat diet (Coconut oil 25%, Cholesterol 2%, Feed powder 73%) + Tempeh + *Lactobacillus plantarum* (40 mg/kg body weight). a~d letters are significantly different from all samples tested ($p < 0.05$). Results are expressed as mean values ± SD. ($n = 8$/group).

3.4. Changes in Total Lactic Acid Bacteria in Diabetes Mellitus (DM) Rat Stools

There were no significant differences in the total LAB content in the rat stool samples before treatment among groups (Table 2). However, the total LAB content was lower in the SH group than in the Normal group. The total LAB contents were significantly higher in the SHT and SHTL groups than in the SH group in DM rats ($p < 0.05$). The total LAB content in the stool sample in the SHTL group was higher than those in other groups. However, the total LAB content in stool samples in the SHP group was significantly lower than those in all DM rats ($p < 0.05$).

Table 2. Lactic acid bacteria counts (Log CFU/g) in STZ-induced diabetic rats in different treatment groups.

Items/Groups	Control	SH	SHP	SHS	SHT	SHTL
Week 0	7.66 ± 0.04 [a]	7.65 ± 0.09 [a]	7.64 ± 0.01 [a]	7.59 ± 0.05 [a]	7.75 ± 0.08 [ab]	7.67 ± 0.05 [a]
Week 4	8.91 ± 0.07 [a]	8.09 ± 0.06 [c]	7.71 ± 0.27 [d]	8.04 ± 0.16 [c]	8.31 ± 0.04 [bc]	8.44 ± 0.05 [b]

Control: normal diet; SH: Streptozotocin (STZ 30 mg/kg, Nicotinamide 45 mg/kg) + High fat diet (Coconut oil 25%, Cholesterol 2%, Feed powder 73%); SHP: Streptozotocin (STZ 30 mg/kg, Nicotinamide 45 mg/kg) + High fat diet (Coconut oil 25%, Cholesterol 2%, Feed powder 73%) + Pioglitazone (10 mg/kg body weight); SHS: Streptozotocin (STZ 30 mg/kg, Nicotinamide 45 mg/kg) + High fat diet (Coconut oil 25%, Cholesterol 2%, Feed powder 73%) + Unfermented soybean (40 mg/kg body weight); SHT: Streptozotocin (STZ 30 mg/kg: Nicotinamide 45 mg/kg) + High fat diet (Coconut oil 25%, Cholesterol 2%, Feed powder 73%) + Tempeh (40 mg/kg body weight); SHTL: Streptozotocin (STZ 30 mg/kg, Nicotinamide 45 mg/kg) + High fat diet (Coconut oil 25%, Cholesterol 2%, Feed powder 73%) + Tempeh + *Lactobacillus plantarum* (40 mg/kg body weight). a~d letters are significantly different from all samples tested ($p < 0.05$). Results are expressed as mean values ± SD. ($n = 8$/group).

3.5. Changes in Short Chain Fatty Acids (SCFAs) in DM Rat Stools

For STZ-induced DM rat groups within two weeks, there were no significant differences in acetic acid, propionic acid, and butyric acid in comparison with those in the SH group in DM rats (data not shown). However, the DM rats had higher SCFA contents than the rats fed a normal diet (Table 3). After four weeks of oral administration, the SHTL group exhibited significantly increased acetic acid, propionic acid, butyric acid, and valeric acid in stool samples compared with those in the SH group in DM rats ($p < 0.05$). The increases in acetic acid, propionic acid, and butyric acid in the SHTL group were the greatest when compared with those of other treatment groups.

Table 3. Changes in short- and medium-chain fatty acid in the feces in STZ-induced diabetic rats fed a high-fat diet for 14 weeks and administered *Lactobacillus plantarum* co-fermented tempeh orally during the last four weeks.

Week	Items	Groups					
		Control	SH	SHP	SHS	SHT	SHTL
	Acetic acid_C2	4.16 ± 0.41 [d]	5.21 ± 0.11 [c]	5.30 ± 0.29 [c]	5.93 ± 0.31 [c]	6.86 ± 0.28 [b]	7.86 ± 0.64 [a]
	Propanoic acid_C3	0.55 ± 0.11 [c]	0.70 ± 0.17 [bc]	0.84 ± 0.19 [abc]	1.01 ± 0.16 [ab]	0.87 ± 0.07 [ab]	1.13 ± 0.07 [a]
	Butyric acid_C4	0.51 ± 0.06 [abc]	0.27 ± 0.02 [c]	0.45 ± 0.06 [bc]	0.70 ± 0.21 [ab]	0.57 ± 0.28 [abc]	0.83 ± 0.11 [a]
4	Isobutyric acid_C4t	0.00 ± 0.01 [a]	0.04 ± 0.05 [a]	0.02 ± 0.01 [a]	0.01 ± 0.02 [a]	0.04 ± 0.02 [a]	0.05 ± 0.01 [a]
	Valeric acid_C5	0.03 ± 0.01 [ab]	0.00 ± 0.00 [b]	0.01 ± 0.02 [b]	0.09 ± 0.07 [ab]	0.05 ± 0.03 [ab]	0.11 ± 0.04 [a]
	Isovaleric acid_C5t	0.02 ± 0.01 [a]	0.05 ± 0.06 [a]	0.05 ± 0.01 [a]	0.05 ± 0.01 [a]	0.06 ± 0.03 [a]	0.08 ± 0.02 [a]
	Caproic acid_C6	0.00 ± 0.00 [a]	0.00 ± 0.00 [a]	0.00 ± 0.00 [a]	0.00 ± 0.00 [a]	0.01 ± 0.01 [a]	0.01 ± 0.02 [a]

Control: normal diet; SH: Streptozotocin (STZ 30 mg/kg, Nicotinamide 45 mg/kg) + High fat diet (Coconut oil 25%, Cholesterol 2%, Feed powder 73%); SHP: Streptozotocin (STZ 30 mg/kg, Nicotinamide 45 mg/kg) + High fat diet (Coconut oil 25%, Cholesterol 2%, Feed powder 73%) + Pioglitazone (10 mg/kg body weight); SHS: Streptozotocin (STZ 30 mg/kg, Nicotinamide 45 mg/kg) + High fat diet (Coconut oil 25%, Cholesterol 2%, Feed powder 73%) + Unfermented soybean (40 mg/kg body weight); SHT: Streptozotocin (STZ 30 mg/kg: Nicotinamide 45 mg/kg) + High fat diet (Coconut oil 25%, Cholesterol 2%, Feed powder 73%) + Tempeh (40 mg/kg body weight); SHTL: Streptozotocin (STZ 30 mg/kg, Nicotinamide 45 mg/kg) + High fat diet (Coconut oil 25%, Cholesterol 2%, Feed powder 73%) + Tempeh + *Lactobacillus plantarum* (40 mg/kg body weight). a~d letters are significantly different from all samples tested ($p < 0.05$). Results are expressed as mean values ± SD. ($n = 8$/group).

3.6. Changes in Total Cholesterol, Bile Acid, and TG in DM Rat Stools

As shown in Table 4, there were no significant differences in stool weight, cholesterol (TC), bile acid, and TG before treatment among samples. However, the SH group had the lowest weights and excretion of TC and bile acid from the stool at 14 weeks among all the DM groups ($p < 0.05$). The SHT and SHTL groups exhibit greater bile acid contents than those of other groups in stool samples ($p < 0.05$), especially the SHTL group, which exhibited the highest bile acid excretion at 14 weeks in the DM rats ($p < 0.05$). The TG content in the SH group was significantly lower than those in the control, SHP, SHT, and SHTL groups. The excretion of TC, bile acid, and TG in the SHTL group was significantly higher than that in the SH group ($p < 0.05$).

Table 4. Changes in weight, cholesterol, bile acid, and triglyceride contents in feces in STZ-induced diabetic rats fed a high-fat diet for 14 weeks and administered *Lactobacillus plantarum* co-fermented tempeh orally during the last 4 weeks.

Week	Items	Groups					
		Control	SH	SHP	SHS	SHT	SHTL
Week 0							
	Feces weight (g)	81.7 ± 1.75	81.0 ± 5.00	81.7 ± 3.06	80.7 ± 3.73	80.3 ± 4.30	81.7 ± 4.16
	cholesterol content (mg/g)	1.56 ± 0.31	1.47 ± 0.57	1.67 ± 0.16	1.66 ± 0.34	1.60 ± 0.26	1.43 ± 0.18
	Bile acid content (µg/g)	6.35 ± 0.51	6.22 ± 0.49	6.54 ± 0.41	6.84 ± 0.59	6.48 ± 0.35	6.56 ± 0.36
	Triglyceride content (µg/g)	57.52 ± 2.85	57.14 ± 3.48	58.12 ± 4.98	58.28 ± 2.78	57.04 ± 4.62	57.28 ± 2.14
Week 4							
	Feces weight (g)	81.7 ± 3.80 [c]	79.7 ± 3.06 [c]	83.0 ± 9.8 [bc]	96.7 ± 4.16 [ab]	100.0 ± 6.00 [a]	104.0 ± 6.27 [a]
	cholesterol content (mg/g)	4.90 ± 1.32 [d]	27.5 ± 0.93 [c]	29.2 ± 2.62 [bc]	29.0 ± 3.13 [bc]	32.1 ± 2.44 [b]	35.6 ± 1.34 [a]
	Bile acid content (µg/g)	4.63 ± 0.55 [d]	176.4 ± 0.44 [b]	247.7 ± 3.73 [a]	115.9 ± 2.76 [c]	173.0 ± 6.78 [b]	248.2 ± 3.86 [a]
	Triglyceride content (µg/g)	68.97 ± 1.76 [a]	47.63 ± 3.45 [c]	57.48 ± 2.01 [b]	43.11 ± 0.24 [c]	67.16 ± 3.15 [a]	72.29 ± 8.87 [a]

Control: normal diet; SH: Streptozotocin (STZ 30 mg/kg, Nicotinamide 45 mg/kg) + High fat diet (Coconut oil 25%, Cholesterol 2%, Feed powder 73%); SHP: Streptozotocin (STZ 30 mg/kg, Nicotinamide 45 mg/kg) + High fat diet (Coconut oil 25%, Cholesterol 2%, Feed powder 73%) + Pioglitazone (10 mg/kg body weight); SHS: Streptozotocin (STZ 30 mg/kg, Nicotinamide 45 mg/kg) + High fat diet (Coconut oil 25%, Cholesterol 2%, Feed powder 73%) + Unfermented soybean (40 mg/kg body weight); SHT: Streptozotocin (STZ 30 mg/kg: Nicotinamide 45 mg/kg) + High fat diet (Coconut oil 25%, Cholesterol 2%, Feed powder 73%) + Tempeh (40 mg/kg body weight); SHTL: Streptozotocin (STZ 30 mg/kg, Nicotinamide 45 mg/kg) + High fat diet (Coconut oil 25%, Cholesterol 2%, Feed powder 73%) + Tempeh + *Lactobacillus plantarum* (40 mg/kg body weight). a~d letters are significantly different from all samples tested ($p < 0.05$). Results are expressed as mean values ± SD. ($n = 8$/group).

3.7. Microbiota Analysis of DM Rats

We evaluated the distribution of gut bacteria by next-generation sequencing. The SH, SHP, SHS, and SHT groups exhibited a change in the dominant bacteria to Bacteroides in STZ-induced DM rats, and the second most dominant bacteria changed to Prevotella (Figure 2). Interestingly, in the SHTL group, the dominant bacteria in the stool samples was Lactobacillus (36.29%) after the oral administration of tempeh co-fermented with *L. plantarum* (40 mg/kg) in DM rats. The second most dominant bacterium in the SHTL group was Bacteroides (29.58%). The Lactobacillus content in the SHTL group was greater than that in the SH group by 34.2%.

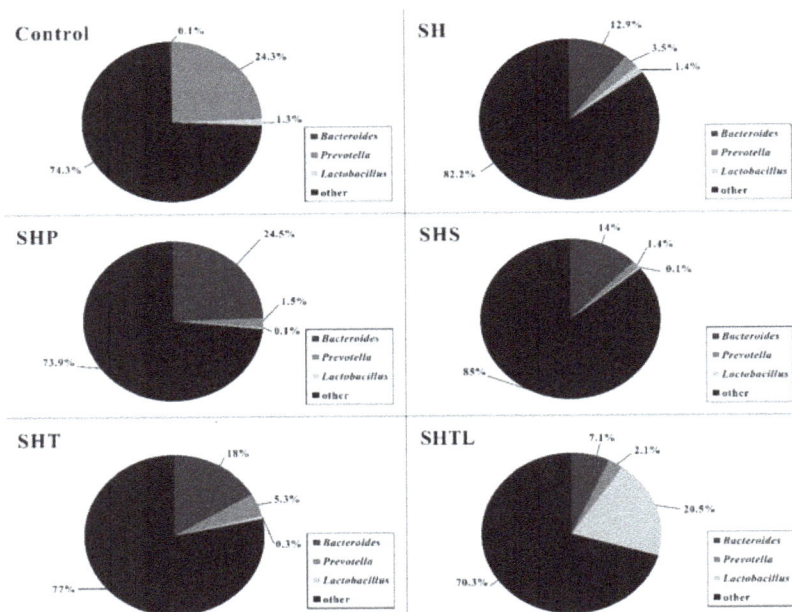

Figure 2. Changes in bacterial distribution in feces in STZ-induced diabetic rats fed a high-fat diet for 14 weeks and administered *Lactobacillus plantarum* co-fermented tempeh orally during the last 4 weeks. Control: normal diet; SH: Streptozotocin (STZ 30 mg/kg, Nicotinamide 45 mg/kg) + High fat diet (Coconut oil 25%, Cholesterol 2%, Feed powder 73%); SHP: Streptozotocin (STZ 30 mg/kg, Nicotinamide 45 mg/kg) + High fat diet (Coconut oil 25%, Cholesterol 2%, Feed powder 73%) + Pioglitazone (10 mg/kg body weight); SHS: Streptozotocin (STZ 30 mg/kg, Nicotinamide 45 mg/kg) + High fat diet (Coconut oil 25%, Cholesterol 2%, Feed powder 73%) + Unfermented soybean (40 mg/kg body weight); SHT: Streptozotocin (STZ 30 mg/kg: Nicotinamide 45 mg/kg) + High fat diet (Coconut oil 25%, Cholesterol 2%, Feed powder 73%) + Tempeh (40 mg/kg body weight); SHTL: Streptozotocin (STZ 30 mg/kg, Nicotinamide 45 mg/kg) + High fat diet (Coconut oil 25%, Cholesterol 2%, Feed powder 73%) + Tempeh + *Lactobacillus plantarum* (40 mg/kg body weight). Results are expressed as mean values ± SD. (n = 8/group).

4. Discussion

High serum glucose is a symptom of diabetes, and postprandial hyperglycemia is a metabolic phenomenon in type II diabetes [14,15]. Therefore, the objective of diabetes therapy is to control the fasting and postprandial serum glucose concentrations. Soybean isoflavones can be transformed from glycosides to aglycones by probiotics, and aglycone-isoflavones have better bioavailability in humans [16]. After treatment for four weeks, rats in each group were fasted for 12 h and then evaluated by OGTT (Figure 1). In our study, the SHTL group had better OGGT results in the late stage, and this was attributed to the high bioavailability of isoflavones from *L. plantarum* fermented with *Rhizopus oryzae* in tempeh in DM rats. Although the SHS and SHT groups had isoflavones, they exhibited decreased serum glucose in the OGTT. The higher serum glucose levels that were observed in the SHTL group than in other groups may reflect the higher aglycone-isoflavone content in the SHTL group. These results are consistent with previous findings [17].

The syndromes of insulin resistance are caused by abnormal responses of human tissues (such as the muscle, liver, adipocyte, and central nervous system tissues) to insulin, thereby inducing dysfunctions in glucose and lipid metabolism [18–22]. Insulin resistance normally co-exists with high blood pressure, hypertriglyceridemia, decreased HDL, increased LDL, and multiple metabolic disorder syndromes in animals. Hence, these syndromes could induce severe complications in patients with type II diabetes [23,24]. Animal and human studies consistently demonstrate that Lactobacillus can reduce the total cholesterol and LDL levels in the blood [25–27]. In addition, epidemiological and other studies have shown that isoflavonoids (genistein) in soybean could improve type II DM by regulating the metabolism of glucose and lipids [28,29]. Many studies have shown that isoflavonoids and daidzein of the soybean could reduce serum glucose levels in animals with DM [30–32]. As shown in Table 1, the SHLT co-fermentative group had better bioavailability, decreased TG and LDL levels, and increased HDL levels in the serum. Additionally, serum glucose and HbA1C levels were effectively regulated in the SHLT group. However, isoflavonoids (genistein) not only improved the metabolism of serum glucose, but also reduced the HOMA-IR value in DM rats. Our results were similar to those of Kwon (2010), who showed that fermented soybean can decrease TC and TG levels in the liver and can regulate the metabolism of serum glucose in SD rats [33].

Microbes that are beneficial to hosts are referred to as probiotics [34]. These probiotics, including LAB, need to survive in gastric acid and bile acid conditions in animals [35]. LAB can inhibit potential pathogen proliferation, decrease serum cholesterol levels, and regulate the immune system [36]. Furthermore, LAB in the stool can protect against gastric acid and bile acid damage. The consumption of soybean products also increases SCFAs, lactic acid bacteria, and the volume of stool [37]. Table 2 shows that total LAB increased significantly in soybean-fed groups. In particular, the SHLT group had the highest total LAB count in the stool. These findings are consistent with those of Panasevich [37].

Many studies have shown that increased dietary fiber intake can improve stool excretion, stimulate segmented colon movement, and improve blood sugar control [38–43]. Probiotics can produce active metabolites, such as SCFAs, in the gut. SCFAs are also a product of dietary fiber fermentation. They include acetate, propionate, and butyrate [44,45]. Some studies have shown that acetate is the most abundant SCFA in the serum and it can regulate inflammation and protect against the invasion of pathogens [46–48]. Propionate can decrease total cholesterol levels [49]. Butyrate can improve HFD-induced obesity and insulin sensitivity [50,51]. Table 3 demonstrates that the SHLT group exhibited increased acetate, propionate, and butyrate in the stool when compared with the levels in other groups. The results of Schneider (2006) supported our results for stool SCFAs [52].

Protein, isoflavones, or dietary fiber in soybeans would affect the metabolism of cholesterol [53–55]. LAB can improve the absorption of isoflavones by regulating β-galactosidase and glucosidase activity [56]. Glucosides of isoflavones are transformed to aglycone-isoflavones with better bioavailability via Lactobacillus [57]. In addition, increased consumption of aglycone-isoflavones improves fatty liver diseases [58]. Some results have demonstrated that the intake of soy products with dietary fiber can decrease serum total cholesterol and LDL-C levels, and the interaction of bile acid and microbes also regulates liver fat and the metabolism of cholesterol [59–61]. Recent studies have shown that the gut microbiota can affect intestinal-liver circulation and bile acid metabolism because it can produce new bile acid via decarboxylation, replacing the bile acid that is consumed by intestinal-liver circulation and decreasing the serum cholesterol level [62,63]. The consumption of dietary soy products can increase Lactobacillus spp. in the stool and promotes the activity of bile hydrolase [64]. Nagata (1982) also found that soy products could increase the bile acid content in rat feces and affects the metabolism of liver cholesterol, since bile acid synthesis requires cholesterol [65,66]. These results may be explained by the stimulation of bile acid secretion and the activity of 7α-hydroxylase cholesterol synthesis induced by LAB and isoflavones [67–69].

Prebiotics are a good source of probiotics and regulate cholesterol and blood sugar. They are typically derived from cereal fibers, such as β-dextran, arabinoxylan, inulin, galactose, and fructooligosaccharides [70,71]. Wang (2012) found that hemicellulose from cereals is composed of β-dextran, which can compete with cholesterol binding sites on LDL. Therefore, the consumption of dietary cereal fiber can decrease the serum levels of LDL and cholesterol [72,73]. Moreover, LAB can reduce blood cholesterol by various mechanisms, e.g., the inhibition of cholesterol synthesis enzymes, stimulation of cholesterol excretion in feces, and inhibition of cholesterol recycling, which can increase the synthesis of cholic acid [74]. Table 4 shows that the SHLT group exhibited dramatically increased levels of stool cholesterol and triglycerides. It is possible that LAB decreased cholesterol by each of these mechanisms, but it decreases blood cholesterol by increasing bile acid synthesis.

The gut microbiota is substantially influenced by the diet and it affects human health via microbial metabolism [75]. The gut microbiota in the human colon is also affected by the diet and induces metabolic diseases, like type II diabetes. In other words, dietary changes can improve physiological metabolism in humans by modifying microbial metabolic processes [76,77]. In a comparison of the gut microbiota, 53% of children in the African countryside, but not in Europe, had Prevotella. This may be explained by dietary differences since children in the African countryside consume cereal, soy, and vegetables and European children consume more protein and animal fat (and exhibit abundant Bacteroides in the gut) [78]. Prevotella and Bacteroides are major microbes in the human colon, and their distribution and metabolic activity are related to the diet. For example, Prevotella is abundant in those who eat a high fiber diet, but Bacteroides is abundant in those who eat high protein and high-fat diets [77]. Figure 2 also shows that the dominant bacteria in our HFD group were Bacteroides, but those in the normal control group were Prevotella.

Stool samples of children in the African countryside have four times higher levels of propionate and butyrate than those of samples from European children [78], and this difference might reflect the consumption of soy products, which increases Lactobacillus in stool samples [79]. Probiotics can increase SCFA production [79]. As shown in Figure 2, Lactobacillus was more abundant in the SHTL group than in other groups. Accordingly, the acetate, propionate, and butyrate contents were the highest in the stool samples of the SHTL group. These findings suggest that the SHTL group exhibits decreased serum glucose via increases in the proliferation of Lactobacillus and improvements in SCFA excretion.

5. Conclusions

The effects of *L. plantarum* co-incubated with *R. oligosporus* to produce soy tempeh on diabetes have not been evaluated. The present results demonstrate that *L. plantarum* co-incubation in soy tempeh ameliorates hyperglycemia, hyperlipidemia, and hyperinsulinemia by altering the intestinal bacterial distribution and increasing intestinal SCFA release in HFD-fed rats. These findings suggest that soy tempeh that is produced by co-incubation with *L. plantarum* has therapeutic effects and is a potential dietary supplement for preventing the progression of DM.

Author Contributions: Conceptualization, W.-C.C.; Data curation, Y.-C.H. and B.-H.W.; Funding acquisition, M.-C.W.; Methodology, B.-H.W.; Project administration, Y.-C.H. and W.-C.C.; Software, Y.-L.C.; Supervision, W.-C.C. and M.-C.W.; Validation, M.-C.W.; Writing—original draft, Y.-C.H. and W.-C.C.; Writing—review & editing, W.-C.C. and M.-C.W.

Funding: This work was supported by National Science Council of the Republic of China (ROC), Taiwan (Grant no. 106-2221-E-020-025-MY2).

Conflicts of Interest: The authors declare no conflict of interest.

References

1. Guariguata, L.; Whiting, D.R.; Hambleton, I.; Beagley, J.; Linnenkamp, U.; Shaw, J.E. Global estimates of diabetes prevalence for 2013 and projections for 2035. *Diabetes Res. Clin. Pract.* **2014**, *103*, 137–149. [CrossRef] [PubMed]

2. Huang, Y.; Wang, X.; Wang, J.; Wu, F.; Sui, Y.; Yang, L.; Wang, Z. *Lactobacillus plantarum* strains as potential probiotic cultures with cholesterol-lowering activity. *J. Dairy Sci.* **2013**, *96*, 2746–2753. [CrossRef] [PubMed]

3. Panwar, H.; Calderwood, D.; Gillespie, A.L.; Wylie, A.R.; Graham, S.F.; Grant, I.R.; Green, B.D. Identification of lactic acid bacteria strains modulating incretin hormone secretion and gene expression in enteroendocrine cells. *J. Funct. Foods* **2016**, *23*, 348–358. [CrossRef]

4. Barus, T.; Wati, L.; Suwanto, A. Diversity of protease-producing *Bacillus* spp. from fresh Indonesian tempeh based on 16S rRNA gene sequence. *HAYATI J. Biosci.* **2017**, *24*, 35–40. [CrossRef]

5. Behloul, N.; Wu, G. Genistein: A promising therapeutic agent for obesity and diabetes treatment. *Eur. J. Pharmacol.* **2013**, *698*, 31–38. [CrossRef] [PubMed]

6. Jeleń, H.; Majcher, M.; Ginja, A.; Kuligowski, M. Determination of compounds responsible for tempeh aroma. *Food Chem.* **2013**, *141*, 459–465. [CrossRef] [PubMed]

7. Haron, H.; Ismail, A.; Shahar, S.; Azlan, A.; Peng, L.S. Apparent bioavailability of isoflavones in urinary excretions of postmenopausal Malay women consuming tempeh compared with milk. *Int. J. Food Sci. Nutr.* **2011**, *62*, 642–650. [CrossRef] [PubMed]

8. Ahmad, A.; Ramasamy, K.; Majeed, A.B.A.; Mani, V. Enhancement of β-secretase inhibition and antioxidant activities of tempeh, a fermented soybean cake through enrichment of bioactive aglycones. *Pharm. Biol.* **2015**, *53*, 758–766. [CrossRef] [PubMed]

9. Zhang, X.M.; Zhang, Y.B.; Chi, M.H. Soy protein supplementation reduces clinical indices in type 2 diabetes and metabolic syndrome. *Yonsei Med. J.* **2016**, *57*, 681–689. [CrossRef] [PubMed]

10. Feizollahzadeh, S.; Ghiasvand, R.; Rezaei, A.; Khanahmad, H.; Hariri, M. Effect of probiotic soy milk on serum levels of adiponectin, inflammatory mediators, lipid profile, and fasting blood glucose among patients with type II diabetes mellitus. *Probiotics Antimicrob. Proteins* **2017**, *9*, 41–47. [CrossRef] [PubMed]

11. Gandhi, G.R.; Stalin, A.; Balakrishna, K.; Ignacimuthu, S.; Paulraj, M.G.; Vishal, R. Insulin sensitization via partial agonism of PPARγ and glucose uptake through translocation and activation of GLUT4 in PI3K/p-Akt signaling pathway by embelin in type 2 diabetic rats. *Biochim. Biophys. Acta* **2013**, *1830*, 2243–2255. [CrossRef] [PubMed]

12. Matthews, D.R.; Hosker, J.P.; Rudenski, A.S.; Naylor, B.A.; Treacher, D.F.; Turner, R.C. Homeostasis model assessment: Insulin resistance and β-cell function from fasting plasma glucose and insulin concentrations in man. *Diabetologia* **1985**, *28*, 412–419. [CrossRef] [PubMed]

13. Holben, W.E.; Williams, P.; Saarinen, M.; Särkilahti, L.K.; Apajalahti, J.H.A. Phylogenetic analysis of intestinal microflora indicates a novel Mycoplasma phylotype in farmed and wild salmon. *Microb. Ecol.* **2002**, *44*, 175–185. [CrossRef] [PubMed]

14. Ramu, R.; Shirahatti, P.S.; Zameer, F.; Dhananjaya, B.L.; Prasad, N. Assessment of in vivo antidiabetic properties of umbelliferone and lupeol constituents of banana (*Musa* sp. var. Nanjangud Rasa Bale) flower in hyperglycaemic rodent model. *PLoS ONE* **2016**, *11*, e0151135.

15. Lebovitz, H.E. Postprandial hyperglycaemic state: Importance and consequences. *Diabetes Res. Clin. Pract.* **1998**, *40*, S27–S28. [PubMed]

16. Ali, A.A.; Velasquez, M.T.; Hansen, C.T.; Mohamed, A.I.; Bhathena, S.J. Modulation of carbohydrate metabolism and peptide hormones by soybean isoflavones and probiotics in obesity and diabetes. *J. Nutr. Biochem.* **2005**, *16*, 6993–6999. [CrossRef] [PubMed]

17. Park, S.; Kim, D.S.; Kim, J.H.; Kim, J.S.; Kim, H.J. Glyceollin-containing fermented soybeans improve glucose homeostasis in diabetic mice. *Nutrition* **2012**, *28*, 204–211. [CrossRef] [PubMed]

18. Himsworth, H.P. Diabetes mellitus: Its differentiation into insulin-sensitive and insulin-insensitive types. *Lancet* **1936**, *227*, 127–130. [CrossRef]

19. Yalow, R.S.; Berson, S.A. Plasma insulin concentrations in nondiabetic and early diabetic subjects: Determinations by a new sensitive immuno-assay technic. *Diabetes* **1960**, *9*, 254–260. [CrossRef] [PubMed]

20. Kahn, C.R.; Flier, J.S.; Bar, R.S.; Archer, J.A.; Gorden, P.; Martin, M.M. The syndromes of insulin resistance and acanthosis nigricans: Insulin-receptor disorders in man. *N. Engl. J. Med.* **1976**, *294*, 739–745. [CrossRef] [PubMed]

21. Olefsky, J.; Farquhar, J.W.; Reaven, G. Relationship between fasting plasma insulin level and resistance to insulin-mediated glucose uptake in normal and diabetic subjects. *Diabetes* **1973**, *22*, 507–513. [CrossRef] [PubMed]

22. Kolterman, O.G.; Insel, J.; Saekow, M.; Olefsky, J.M. Mechanisms of insulin resistance in human obesity: Evidence for receptor and postreceptor defects. *J. Clin. Investig.* **1980**, *65*, 1272–1284. [CrossRef] [PubMed]

23. Howard, G.O.; Leary, D.H.; Zaccaro, D.; Haffner, S.; Rewers, M.; Hamman, R. Insulin sensitivity and atherosclerosis. *Circulation* **1996**, *93*, 1809–1817. [CrossRef] [PubMed]

24. Yip, J.; Facchini, F.S.; Reaven, G.M. Resistance to insulin-mediated glucose disposal as a predictor of cardiovascular disease. *J. Clin. Endocrinol. MeTab.* **1998**, *83*, 2773–2776. [CrossRef] [PubMed]

25. Park, S.C.; Hwang, M.H.; Kim, Y.H.; Kim, J.C.; Song, J.C.; Lee, K.W. Comparison of pH and bile resistance of Lactobacillus acidophilus strains isolated from rat, pig, chicken, and human sources. *World J. Microbiol. Biotechnol.* **2006**, *22*, 35–37. [CrossRef]
26. Danielson, A.D.; Peo, E.R., Jr.; Shahani, K.M.; Lewis, A.J.; Whalen, P.J.; Amer, M.A. Anticholesteremic property of Lactobacillus acidophilus yogurt fed to mature boars. *J. Anim. Sci. Technol.* **1989**, *67*, 966–974. [CrossRef]
27. Liong, M.T.; Shah, N.P. Effects of a Lactobacillus casei synbiotic on serum lipoprotein, intestinal microflora, and organic acids in rats. *J. Dairy Sci.* **2006**, *89*, 1390–1399. [CrossRef]
28. Choi, M.S.; Jung, U.J.; Yeo, J.K.; Kim, M.J.; Lee, M.K. Genistein and daidzein prevent diabetes onset by elevating insulin level and altering hepatic gluconeogenic and lipogenic enzyme activities in non-obese diabetic (NOD) mice. *Diabetes Metab. Res. Rev.* **2008**, *24*, 74–81. [CrossRef] [PubMed]
29. Ding, M.; Pan, A.; Manson, J.E.; Willett, W.C.; Malik, V.; Rosner, B. Consumption of soy foods and isoflavones and risk of type 2 diabetes: A pooled analysis of three US cohorts. *Eur. J. Clin. Nutr.* **2016**, *70*, 1381. [CrossRef] [PubMed]
30. Mezei, O.; Banz, W.J.; Steger, R.W.; Peluso, M.R.; Winters, T.A.; Shay, N. Soy isoflavones exert antidiabetic and hypolipidemic effects through the PPAR pathways in obese Zucker rats and murine RAW 264.7 cells. *J. Nutr.* **2003**, *133*, 1238–1243. [CrossRef] [PubMed]
31. Park, S.A.; Choi, M.S.; Cho, S.Y.; Seo, J.S.; Jung, U.J.; Kim, M.J. Genistein and daidzein modulate hepatic glucose and lipid regulating enzyme activities in C57BL/KsJ-db/db mice. *Life Sci.* **2006**, *79*, 1207–1213. [CrossRef] [PubMed]
32. Lee, J.S. Effects of soy protein and genistein on blood glucose, antioxidant enzyme activities, and lipid profile in streptozotocin-induced diabetic rats. *Life Sci.* **2006**, *79*, 1578–1584. [CrossRef] [PubMed]
33. Kwon, D.Y.; Daily, J.W.; Kim, H.J.; Park, S. Antidiabetic effects of fermented soybean products on type 2 diabetes. *Nutr. Res.* **2010**, *30*, 1–13. [CrossRef] [PubMed]
34. Anandharaj, M.; Sivasankari, B.; Santhanakaruppu, R.; Manimaran, M.; Rani, R.P.; Sivakumar, S. Determining the probiotic potential of cholesterol-reducing Lactobacillus and Weissella strains isolated from gherkins (fermented cucumber) and south Indian fermented koozh. *Res. Microbiol.* **2015**, *166*, 428–439. [CrossRef] [PubMed]
35. Erkkilä, S.; Petäjä, E. Screening of commercial meat starter cultures at low pH and in the presence of bile salts for potential probiotic use. *Meat Sci.* **2000**, *55*, 297–300. [CrossRef]
36. Tsai, Y.T.; Cheng, P.C.; Fan, C.K.; Pan, T.M. Time-dependent persistence of enhanced immune response by a potential probiotic strain Lactobacillus paracasei subsp. paracasei NTU 101. *Int. J. Food Microbiol.* **2008**, *128*, 219–225. [CrossRef] [PubMed]
37. Panasevich, M.R.; Schuster, C.M.; Phillips, K.E.; Meers, G.M.; Chintapalli, S.V.; Wankhade, U. Soy compared with milk protein in a Western diet changes fecal microbiota and decreases hepatic steatosis in obese OLETF rats. *J. Nutr. Biochem.* **2017**, *46*, 125–136. [CrossRef] [PubMed]
38. Shankardass, K.; Chuchmach, S.; Chelswick, K.; Stefanovich, C.; Spurr, S.; Brooks, J. Bowel function of long-term tube-fed patients consuming formulae with and without dietary fiber. *J. Parenter. Enteral. Nutr.* **1990**, *14*, 508–512. [CrossRef] [PubMed]
39. Schneider, S.M.; Pouget, I.; Staccini, P.; Rampal, P.; Hebuterne, X. Quality of life in long-term home enteral nutrition patients. *Clin. Nutr.* **2000**, *19*, 23–28. [CrossRef] [PubMed]
40. Cabré, E. Fibre supplementation of enteral formula-diets: A look to the evidence. *Clin. Nutr.* **2004**, *1*, 63–71. [CrossRef]
41. Meier, R.; Gassull, M.A. Consensus recommendations on the effects and benefits of fibre in clinical practice. *Clin. Nutr.* **2004**, *1*, 73–80. [CrossRef]
42. Hofman, Z.; Van Drunen, J.D.E.; De Later, C.; Kuipers, H. The effect of different nutritional feeds on the postprandial glucose response in healthy volunteers and patients with type II diabetes. *Eur. J. Clin. Nutr.* **2004**, *58*, 1553. [CrossRef] [PubMed]
43. Read, N.W. Diarrhee motrice. *Clin. Gastroenterol.* **1986**, *15*, 657–686. [PubMed]
44. Russell, W.R.; Hoyles, L.; Flint, H.J.; Dumas, M.E. Colonic bacterial metabolites and human health. *Curr. Opin. Microbiol.* **2013**, *16*, 246–254. [CrossRef] [PubMed]
45. Topping, D.L.; Clifton, P.M. Short-chain fatty acids and human colonic function: Roles of resistant starch and nonstarch polysaccharides. *Physiol. Rev.* **2001**, *81*, 1031–1064. [CrossRef] [PubMed]

46. Fukuda, S.; Toh, H.; Hase, K.; Oshima, K.; Nakanishi, Y.; Yoshimura, K.; Taylor, T.D. Bifidobacteria can protect from enteropathogenic infection through production of acetate. *Nature* **2011**, *469*, 543–547. [CrossRef] [PubMed]

47. Maslowski, K.M.; Vieira, A.T.; Ng, A.; Kranich, J.; Sierro, F.; Yu, D. Regulation of inflammatory responses by gut microbiota and chemoattractant receptor GPR43. *Nature* **2009**, *461*, 1282. [CrossRef] [PubMed]

48. Hara, H.; Haga, S.; Aoyama, Y.; Kiriyama, S. Short-chain fatty acids suppress cholesterol synthesis in rat liver and intestine. *J. Nutr.* **1999**, *129*, 942–948. [CrossRef] [PubMed]

49. Hughes, S.A.; Shewry, P.R.; Gibson, G.R.; McCleary, B.V.; Rastall, R.A. In vitro fermentation of oat and barley derived β-glucans by human faecal microbiota. *FEMS Microbiol. Ecol.* **2008**, *64*, 482–493. [CrossRef] [PubMed]

50. Arora, T.; Sharma, R.; Frost, G. Propionate. Anti-obesity and satiety enhancing factor? *Appetite* **2011**, *56*, 511–515. [CrossRef] [PubMed]

51. Lin, H.V.; Frassetto, A.; Kowalik, E.J.; Nawrocki, A.R.; Lu, M.M.; Kosinski, J.R. Butyrate and propionate protect against diet-induced obesity and regulate gut hormones via free fatty acid receptor 3-independent mechanisms. *PLoS ONE* **2012**, *7*, e35240. [CrossRef] [PubMed]

52. Schneider, S.M.; Girard-Pipau, F.; Anty, R.; van der Linde, E.G.; Philipsen-Geerling, B.J.; Knol, J. Effects of total enteral nutrition supplemented with a multi-fibre mix on faecal short-chain fatty acids and microbiota. *Clin. Nutr.* **2006**, *25*, 82–90. [CrossRef] [PubMed]

53. Clarkson, T.B. Soy, soy phytoestrogens and cardiovascular disease. *J. Nutr.* **2002**, *132*, 566S–569S. [CrossRef] [PubMed]

54. Lichtenstein, A.H.; Jalbert, S.M.; Adlercreutz, H.; Goldin, B.R.; Rasmussen, H.; Schaefer, E.J. Lipoprotein response to diets high in soy or animal protein with and without isoflavones in moderately hypercholesterolemic subjects. *Arterioscler. Thromb. Vasc. Biol.* **2002**, *22*, 1852–1858. [CrossRef] [PubMed]

55. Matsumoto, K.; Watanabe, Y.; Yokoyama, S.I. Okara, soybean residue, prevents obesity in a diet-induced murine obesity model. *Biosci. Biotechnol. Biochem.* **2007**, *71*, 720–727. [CrossRef] [PubMed]

56. Otieno, D.O.; Shah, N.P. Endogenous β-glucosidase and β-galactosidase activities from selected probiotic micro-organisms and their role in isoflavone biotransformation in soymilk. *J. Appl. Microbiol.* **2007**, *103*, 910–917. [CrossRef] [PubMed]

57. Suzuki, T.; Hara, H. Role of flavonoids in intestinal tight junction regulation. *J. Nutr. Biochem.* **2011**, *22*, 401–408. [CrossRef] [PubMed]

58. Kim, M.H.; Park, J.S.; Jung, J.W.; Byun, K.W.; Kang, K.S.; Lee, Y.S. Daidzein supplementation prevents non-alcoholic fatty liver disease through alternation of hepatic gene expression profiles and adipocyte metabolism. *Int. J. Obes.* **2011**, *35*, 1019. [CrossRef] [PubMed]

59. Begley, M.; Gahan, C.G.; Hill, C. The interaction between bacteria and bile. *FEMS Microbiol. Rev.* **2005**, *29*, 625–651. [CrossRef] [PubMed]

60. Kakiyama, G.; Pandak, W.M.; Gillevet, P.M.; Hylemon, P.B.; Heuman, D.M.; Daita, K. Modulation of the fecal bile acid profile by gut microbiota in cirrhosis. *J. Hepatol.* **2013**, *58*, 949–955. [CrossRef] [PubMed]

61. Ridlon, J.M.; Kang, D.J.; Hylemon, P.B.; Bajaj, J.S. Bile acids and the gut microbiome. *Curr. Opin. Gastroenterol.* **2014**, *30*, 332. [CrossRef] [PubMed]

62. Islam, K.S.; Fukiya, S.; Hagio, M.; Fujii, N.; Ishizuka, S.; Ooka, T. Bile acid is a host factor that regulates the composition of the cecal microbiota in rats. *Gastroenterology* **2011**, *141*, 1773–1781. [CrossRef] [PubMed]

63. Zhang, M.; Hang, X.; Fan, X.; Li, D.; Yang, H. Characterization and selection of Lactobacillus strains for their effect on bile tolerance, taurocholate deconjugation and cholesterol removal. *World J. Microbiol. Biotechnol.* **2008**, *24*, 7–14. [CrossRef]

64. Begley, M.; Hill, C.; Gahan, C.G. Bile salt hydrolase activity in probiotics. *Appl. Environ. Microbiol.* **2006**, *72*, 1729–1738. [CrossRef] [PubMed]

65. Nagata, Y.; Ishiwaki, N.; Sugano, M. Studies on the mechanism of antihypercholesterolemic action of soy protein and soy protein-type amino acid mixtures in relation to the casein counterparts in rats. *J. Nutr.* **1982**, *112*, 1614–1625. [CrossRef] [PubMed]

66. El-Gawad, I.A.A.; El-Sayed, E.M.; Hafez, S.A.; El-Zeini, H.M.; Saleh, F.A. The hypocholesterolaemic effect of milk yoghurt and soy-yoghurt containing bifidobacteria in rats fed on a cholesterol-enriched diet. *Int. Dairy J.* **2005**, *15*, 37–44. [CrossRef]

67. Imaizumi, K.; Hirata, K.; Zommara, M.; Sugano, M.; Suzuki, Y. Effects of cultured milk products by Lactobacillus and Bifidobacterium species on the secretion of bile acids in hepatocytes and in rats. *J. Nutr. Sci. Vitaminol.* **1992**, *38*, 343–351. [CrossRef] [PubMed]

68. Gudbrandsen, O.A.; Wergedahl, H.; Liaset, B.; Espe, M.; Berge, R.K. Dietary proteins with high isoflavone content or low methionine-glycine and lysine-arginine ratios are hypocholesterolaemic and lower the plasma homocysteine level in male Zucker fa/fa rats. *Br. J. Nutr.* **2005**, *94*, 321–330. [CrossRef] [PubMed]

69. Ni, W.; Yoshida, S.; Tsuda, Y.; Nagao, K.; Sato, M.; Imaizumi, K. Ethanol-extracted soy protein isolate results in elevation of serum cholesterol in exogenously hypercholesterolemic rats. *Lipids* **1999**, *34*, 713–716. [CrossRef] [PubMed]

70. Cao, Y.; Ma, Z.; Zhang, H.; Jin, Y.; Zhang, Y.; Hayford, F. Phytochemical properties and nutrigenomic implications of yacon as a potential source of prebiotic: Current evidence and future directions. *Foods* **2018**, *7*, 59. [CrossRef] [PubMed]

71. Okarter, N.; Liu, R.H. Health benefits of whole grain phytochemicals. *Crit. Rev. Food Sci. Nutr.* **2010**, *50*, 193–208. [CrossRef] [PubMed]

72. Wang, C.Y.; Wu, S.J.; Fang, J.Y.; Wang, Y.P.; Shyu, Y.T. Cardiovascular and intestinal protection of cereal pastes fermented with lactic acid bacteria in hyperlipidemic hamsters. *Food Res. Int.* **2012**, *48*, 428–434. [CrossRef]

73. Lazaridou, A.; Biliaderis, C.G. Molecular aspects of cereal β-glucan functionality: Physical properties, technological applications and physiological effects. *J. Cereal Sci.* **2007**, *46*, 101–118. [CrossRef]

74. Ooi, L.G.; Liong, M.T. Cholesterol-lowering effects of probiotics and prebiotics: A review of in vivo and in vitro findings. *Int. J. Mol. Sci.* **2010**, *11*, 2499–2522. [CrossRef] [PubMed]

75. Bäckhed, F.; Ley, R.E.; Sonnenburg, J.L.; Peterson, D.A.; Gordon, J.I. Host-bacterial mutualism in the human intestine. *Science* **2005**, *307*, 1915–1920. [CrossRef] [PubMed]

76. Yusof, N.; Hamid, N.; Ma, Z.F.; Lawenko, R.M.; Mohammad, W.M.Z.W.; Collins, D.A.; Lee, Y.Y. Exposure to environmental microbiota explains persistent abdominal pain and irritable bowel syndrome after a major flood. *Gut Pathog.* **2017**, *9*, 75. [CrossRef] [PubMed]

77. Sáez, C. Gut Microbiota May Improve Sugar Metabolism in Humans. 2016. Available online: http://www. gutmicrobiotaforhealth.com/en/gut-microbiota-may-improve-sugar-metabolism-in-humans/ (accessed on 11 February 2016).

78. De Filippo, C.; Cavalieri, D.; Di Paola, M.; Ramazzotti, M.; Poullet, J.B.; Massart, S. Impact of diet in shaping gut microbiota revealed by a comparative study in children from Europe and rural Africa. *Proc. Natl. Acad. Sci. USA* **2010**, *107*, 14691–14696. [CrossRef] [PubMed]

79. Pan, X.D.; Chen, F.Q.; Wu, T.X.; Tang, H.G.; Zhao, Z.Y. Prebiotic oligosaccharides change the concentrations of short-chain fatty acids and the microbial population of mouse bowel. *J. Zhejiang Univ. Sci. B* **2009**, *10*, 258–263. [CrossRef] [PubMed]

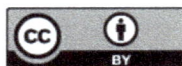

nutrients

MDPI

Article

Combination of Aronia, Red Ginseng, Shiitake Mushroom and Nattokinase Potentiated Insulin Secretion and Reduced Insulin Resistance with Improving Gut Microbiome Dysbiosis in Insulin Deficient Type 2 Diabetic Rats

Hye Jeong Yang [1], Min Jung Kim [1], Dae Young Kwon [1], Da Sol Kim [2], Ting Zhang [2], Chulgyu Ha [3] and Sunmin Park [2,*]

[1]   Research Division of Food Functionality, Korean Food Research Institutes, Wanjoo 55365, Korea; yhj@kfri.re.kr (H.J.Y.); kmj@kfri.re.kr (M.J.K.); dykwon@kfri.re.kr (D.Y.K.)
[2]   Department of Food and Nutrition, Obesity/Diabetes Center, Hoseo University, Asan 31499, Korea; tpfptm14@daum.net (D.S.K.); zhangting92925@gmail.com (T.Z.)
[3]   Department of Bioprocess Technology, Bio Campus Korea Polytechnic, Nonsan 32943, Korea; hckue@kopo.ac.kr
*   Correspondence: smpark@hoseo.edu; Tel.: +82-41-540-5345

Received: 12 June 2018; Accepted: 17 July 2018; Published: 23 July 2018

Abstract: The combination of freeze-dried aronia, red ginseng, ultraviolet-irradiated shiitake mushroom and nattokinase (AGM; 3.4:4.1:2.4:0.1) was examined to evaluate its effects on insulin resistance, insulin secretion and the gut microbiome in a non-obese type 2 diabetic animal model. Pancreatectomized (Px) rats were provided high fat diets supplemented with either (1) 0.5 g AGM (AGM-L), (2) 1 g AGM (AGM-H), (3) 1 g dextrin (control), or (4) 1 g dextrin with 120 mg metformin (positive-control) per kg body weight for 12 weeks. AGM (1 g) contained 6.22 mg cyanidin-3-galactose, 2.5 mg ginsenoside Rg3 and 244 mg β-glucan. Px rats had decreased bone mineral density in the lumbar spine and femur and lean body mass in the hip and leg compared to the normal-control and AGM-L and AGM-H prevented the decrease. Visceral fat mass was lower in the control group than the normal-control group and its decrease was smaller with AGM-L and AGM-H. HOMA-IR was lower in descending order of the control, positive-control, AGM-L, AGM-H and normal-control groups. Glucose tolerance deteriorated in the control group and was improved by AGM-L and AGM-H more than in the positive-control group. Glucose tolerance is associated with insulin resistance and insulin secretion. Insulin tolerance indicated insulin resistance was highly impaired in diabetic rats, but it was improved in the ascending order of the positive-control, AGM-L and AGM-H. Insulin secretion capacity, measured by hyperglycemic clamp, was much lower in the control group than the normal-control group and it was improved in the ascending order of the positive-control, AGM-L and AGM-H. Diabetes modulated the composition of the gut microbiome and AGM prevented the modulation of gut microbiome. In conclusion, AGM improved glucose metabolism by potentiating insulin secretion and reducing insulin resistance in insulin deficient type 2 diabetic rats. The improvement of diabetic status alleviated body composition changes and prevented changes of gut microbiome composition.

Keywords: aronia; ginseng; mushroom; pancreatectomy; type 2 diabetes; gut microbiome; insulin secretion

1. Introduction

The prevalence of type 2 diabetes is markedly increasing in Asian countries, including Korea and reached 8.7% of the Asian population by 2014; it is expected to reach 12–5% by 2025 [1]. This is associated with ethnic differences in the etiology of type 2 diabetes [1]. Type 2 diabetes generally develops as a consequence of the imbalance between insulin resistance and insulin secretion [2]. When insulin resistance increases due to obesity, inflammation, oxidative stress, aging, less physical activity, etc., insulin secretion is elevated to overcome insulin resistance and to maintain normoglycemia. Increased inflammation and oxidative stress may accelerate the development of type 2 diabetes especially in Asians. However, Asians are more susceptible to type 2 diabetes under the insulin resistant condition since their insulin secretory capacity and β-cell mass are low [3]. The Westernization of diets mostly elevate insulin resistance in Asians which that is not compensated due to low insulin secretion capacity. Thus, Westernization of diets can increase the prevalence of type 2 diabetes in many cases although obesity is much less in Asian than Caucasians.

Type 2 diabetes is prevented and treated by reducing insulin resistance and increasing insulin capacity in both Asians and non-Asians, although the disease has a somewhat different etiology in Asians than non-Asians. Asians with type 2 diabetes are usually not obese, although they are insulin resistant [3]. Thus, the proper animal model for Asian type 2 diabetes needs to be non-obese, have lower insulin secretion capacity, and higher insulin resistance than the non-diabetic rats. Partially pancreatectomized rats are an optimal model for studying Asian type 2 diabetes [4]. They have about 60% insulin secretion capacity and about 50% of the pancreatic mass of the rats with intact pancreas [4]. The Px rats gradually develop insulin resistance. A high fat diet accelerates the increase of insulin resistance in Px rats [5]. Anti-diabetic interventions for Asians can be examined for improvements in both insulin resistance and insulinotropic activity in Px rats fed with a high fat diet [6].

Previous studies have supported that the gut microbiome produces microbial metabolites including short-chain fatty acids (SCFAs), bile acids (BAs) and lipopolysaccharides (LPS) that modulate host glucose metabolism, mainly in the liver [7]. This is called the gut liver axis. These metabolites directly influence metabolic diseases including type 2 diabetes [7]. Low-grade peripheral inflammation also promotes the development of type 2 diabetes. Patients with a low bacterial α- diversity in the gut microbiome are at greater risk of metabolic diseases than are patients with high α-diversity [8]. Herbs rich in fiber, polyphenols and polysaccharides increase the abundance of the phylum *Bacteroidetes,* and genera *Akkermansia, Bifidobacteria, Lactobacillus, Bacteroides* and *Prevotella* [7]. However, it reduces the number of phylum *Firmicutes* and *Firmicutes/Bacteroidetes* ratio in the intestines. It is well known that some herbal compounds improve glucose metabolism by modulating insulin resistance and insulin secretion. The changes in some of the microbial metabolites from consuming plant compounds are correlated with changes to the gut microbiome that modulate glucose metabolism [9].

Aronia melanocarpa, red ginseng and shiitake mushroom have been reported to improve glucose metabolism. Aronia and its anthocyanins have anti-inflammatory and antioxidant properties that improve insulin sensitivity and prevent type 2 diabetes [10]. Red ginseng and ginsenoside Re, Rb1, and Rb2, its active ingredients, have demonstrated an antidiabetic action in in vitro, animal, and clinical studies [11–14]. Ultraviolet-irradiated shiitake mushroom (Lentinus edodes), polysaccharides, has antioxidant activity and it is a good source for vitamin D (V-D) in humans [5]. The dosage of 100–400 mg shiitake mushroom/kg bw is effective for anti-oxidant properties because it increases the content of the reduced form of glutathione, but at higher dosages it has an adverse effect on immunity [15]. Anti-diabetic effects of V-D are still controversial. V-D may exert anti-diabetic activity by improving insulin secretion and insulin sensitivity [5]. However, some placebo-controlled clinical studies of vitamin D administration have not shown that it improves insulin release and sensitivity [16]. Type 2 diabetes increases the thrombotic risk to develop cardiovascular diseases [17]. Although nattokinase has not been shown shown to possess anti-diabetic activity, it is reported to improve blood flow by inhibiting platelet aggregation and thrombosis to reduce cardiovascular events [18]. The water or ethanol extracts of aronia, red ginseng and shiitake mushroom have been well studied, but the whole foods, including dietary fiber, may be better for inducing changes to the gut microbiome that influence glucose metabolism.

Insulin resistance and β-cell function and mass are associated with increased oxidative stress and inflammation [1,10,19]. Aronia and shiitake mushrooms improve insulin resistance [5,10], red ginseng potentiates β-cell function and mass [11], and nattokinase prevents thrombosis [18]. The combination of aronia, red ginseng, shiitake mushroom and nattokinase, which have anti-oxidative and anti-inflammatory properties, may alleviate type 2 diabetic symptoms and its complications. However, its direct effects on anti-diabetic activity such as insulin resistance and insulin secretion have not been examined. The relationship between anti-diabetic activity and the gut microbiome is also not well characterized. We hypothesized that the combination of freeze-dried aronia, red ginseng, ultraviolet-irradiated shiitake mushroom and nattokinase would prevent or reverse insulin resistance, improve insulin secretion, and help normalize serum glucose levels, due to changes in the gut microbiome. We tested this hypothesis in Px rats, a non-obese type 2 diabetic animal model.

2. Materials and Methods

2.1. Preparation of the Product and Analysis of Ingredients

Each of aronia, red ginseng, and shiitake mushroom was washed, dried at room temperature, freeze-dried, and powdered. Freeze-dried Aronia, red ginseng, shitake mushroom and nattokinase were mixed with the ratio of (3.4:4.1:2.4:0.1) (Chakreis, AGM) and Chakreis was generously provided by YD Nutraceuticals Ltd. (Yongin-si, Korea). The dosages were determined by considering preliminary studies and previous studies [10,12,13,15,16,18]. The freeze-dried powder mixture was used for the animal study. The mixture was extracted with in distilled water at 95 °C for 12 h and the extracts were centrifuged at 10,000× g at 4 °C for 20 min. The supernatants were lyophilized in a freeze-dryer.

For measuring indicative components in the mixture, it was extracted with methanol and lysophilized. The extracts were dissolved in methanol, and a syringe filter was used to remove undissolved contents. The contents of ginsenoside Rg, cyanidin-galactoside, cyanidin-glucoside and cyanidin-arabinoside in the extract were measured were analyzed by high performance liquid chromatography using a Luna C18 column (4.6 mm × 250 mm; ID, 5 μm). The mobile phase solvents were acetonitrile and 0.1% formic acid in water (6:4, vol:vol) with isocratic elution at a flow rate of 1 mL/min, 40 °C in-column temperature, and UV detection at 270 nm. We used ginsenoside Rg, cyanidin-galactose, cyanidin-glucose and cyanidin-arabinoside as standards to quantify the sample.

The β-glucan contents of shitake mushroom were sequentially digested with digestion enzymes by incubating in lower temperature for 2 h. The enzymes used to digest the shitake mushroom were amylase (20 units, pH 6.9) at 20 °C, cellulase (50 units, pH 5.0) at 37 °C, protease (10 units, pH 7.5) at 37 °C, and amyloglucosidase (70 units, pH 4.8) at 60 °C. The digested shiitake mushroom was mixed with 95% ethanol and the mixture was left at 4 °C for 12 h. The mixture was centrifuged at 10,000 rpm for 10 min and water was added into the precipitates. Sulfuric acid was added (1:5) into the diluted precipitate. The mixture was left at room temperature for 20 min and the optical density was measured at 470 nm. Glucose solution was used as a standard.

2.2. Animals and Ethics

Eight-week-old male Sprague–Dawley rats (weight, 218 ± 23 g) were housed individually in stainless steel cages in a controlled environment (23 °C; 12-h light/dark cycle). All surgical and experimental procedures were performed according to the guidelines of the Animal Care and Use Review Committee of Hoseo University, Korea (HUACUC-17-57). The rats underwent a 90% pancreatectomy using the Hosokawa technique [20] or received a sham pancreatectomy (sham) under anesthesia induced by intramuscular injection of a mixture of ketamine and xylazine (100 and 10 mg/kg body weight, respectively). The pancreatectomized (Px) rats exhibited characteristics of type 2 diabetes (random glucose levels >180 mg/dL), whereas the sham rats did not [20,21].

2.3. Experimental Design

A total of 40 Px rats were assigned randomly to the following four groups, which differed according to diet: (1) 1 g dextrin/kg bw (negative-control) (2) 0.5 g AGM/kg bw, (3) 1 g AGM/kg bw, and (4) 120 mg/kg bw metformin (positive-control). Each group included 10 Px rats. The sham-operated rats were given 1 g dextrin/kg bw for normal-control (*n* = 10). All experimental animals were given free access to water and a high-fat diet containing either the assigned extracts or dextrin for 12 weeks. The high-fat diet was a modified semi-purified AIN-93 formulation for experimental animals [22] that consisted of 42% carbohydrate, 15% protein, and 43% fat. The major carbohydrate, protein, and fat sources were starch and sugar, casein (milk protein), and lard (CJ Co., Seoul, Korea), respectively.

2.4. Body Composition Measurement

After calibrating a dual-energy X-ray Absorptiometer (DEXA; Norland pDEXA Sabre; Norland Medical Systems Inc., Fort Atkinson, WI, USA) with a phantom supplied by the manufacturer, the body compositions of the rats were measured at the 7th week of the experimental period. The animals were anesthetized with ketamine and xylazine (100 and 10 mg/kg bw, respectively), and laid in a prone position, with the posterior legs maintained in external rotation with tape. The hip, knee, and ankle articulations were in 90° flexion. Upon the completion of scanning, lean mass was determined in the leg and hip using the DEXA instrument equipped with the appropriate software for the assessment of bone density in small animals [22]. Similarly, the fat mass was measured in the leg and abdominal areas using the DEXA instrument.

2.5. Glucose Homeostasis

Overnight fasted serum glucose levels, food intake, and body weights were measured every week. An oral glucose tolerance test (OGTT) was performed at the 7th week in overnight-fasted animals by orally administering 2 g glucose/kg body weight [23]. Blood samples were taken by tail bleeding at 0, 10, 20, 30, 40, 50, 60, 70, 80, 90, and 120 min after glucose loading. The serum insulin levels were determined at 0, 20, 40, 90, and 120 min. The averages of the total areas under the curves for the serum glucose and insulin concentrations were calculated using the trapezoidal rule. At 3 days after OGTT, an intraperitoneal insulin tolerance test (IPITT) was conducted after the food was removed for 6 h. The serum glucose levels were measured every 15 min for 90 min after an intraperitoneal injection of insulin (0.75 U/kg body weight). Serum glucose and insulin levels were analyzed with a Glucose Analyzer II (Beckman Coulter, Palo Alto, CA, USA) and rat Ultrasensitive insulin kit (Crystal Chem, Elk Grove Village, IL, USA), respectively.

2.6. Hyperglycemic Clamp and Cerebral Blood Flow

Catheters were surgically implanted into the right carotid artery and left jugular vein in all rats after 7 weeks of treatment and anesthetization with ketamine and xylazine. A hyperglycemic clamp was performed in 10 free-moving and overnight-fasted rats/group after 5–6 days of implantation to determine insulin secretion capacity, as described previously [20,24,25]. During the clamp, glucose was infused to maintain a serum glucose level of 5.5 mM above baseline, and serum insulin level was measured at designated times. After the clamp, the rats were freely provided food and water for 2 days and then deprived of food for 16 h the next day. After anesthesia with a mixture of ketamine and xylazine, the rats were placed in a stereotaxic device with a midline incision of the scalp exposing the periosteum. A small pore was made with a drill in the right lateral ventricle with stereotaxic coordinates: 1.0 mm posterior, 6 mm lateral, 3.7 mm ventral to bregma. A Doppler flow probe was placed on the cerebral vein and blood flow was measured continuously with Laser Doppler Flowmetry (LDF100C-1, BIOPAC Systems, Inc., Goleta, CA, USA) for 10 min.

After measuring cerebral blood flow regular human insulin (5 U/kg body weight; Humulin; Eli Lilly, Indianapolis, IN, USA) was injected through the inferior vena cava. The rats were euthanized by decapitation 10 min later, and tissues were collected rapidly, frozen in liquid nitrogen, and stored at −70 °C for further experiments. Insulin resistance was determined using the homeostasis model assessment estimate of insulin resistance (HOMA-IR) and calculated using the following equation: HOMA-IR = fasting insulin (μIU/mL) × fasting glucose (mM)/22.5. Lipid profiles in the circulation were measured using colorimetry kits from Asan Pharmaceutical (Seoul, Korea).

2.7. Immunohistochemistry

Five rats from each group were injected with BrdU (100 μg/kg body weight) after 6 weeks of treatment. The rats were anesthetized intraperitoneally 6 h post-injection with a mixture of ketamine and xylazine, and the brain and pancreas were dissected immediately, perfused with saline and a 4% paraformaldehyde solution (pH 7.2) sequentially, and post-fixed with the same fixative overnight at room temperature [24].

Two serial 5-μm paraffin-embedded tissue sections were selected from the seventh or eighth sections to avoid counting the same islets twice when measuring β-cell area, BrdU incorporation, and apoptosis, were determined as described previously using an immunohistochemistry method [24]. Endocrine β-cells were identified by applying guinea pig anti-insulin and rabbit anti-glucagon antibodies to the sections. Pancreatic β-cell area was measured by examining all non-overlapping images in two insulin-stained sections from each rat at 10× magnification with a Zeiss Axiovert microscope (Carl Zeiss Microimaging, Thornwood, NY, USA). Pancreatic β-cell mass, individual β-cell size, β-cell proliferation by BrdU incorporation, and apoptotic β-cell were measured as described previously [24].

2.8. Next Generation Sequencing of the Gut Microbiome

The gut microbiome composition was measured from feces of each rat by analyzing metagenome sequencing using next-generation sequencing [26]. Bacterial DNA was extracted from the samples of each rat using a Power Water DNA Isolation Kit (MoBio, Carlsbad, CA, USA) according to the manufacturer's instructions. Each library was prepared using polymerase chain reaction (PCR) products according to the GS FLX plus library prep guide. The emPCR, corresponding to clonal amplification of the purified library, was carried out using the GS-FLX plus emPCR Kit (454 Life Sciences, Branford, CT, USA). Libraries were immobilized onto DNA capture beads. The library-beads were added to the amplification mix and oil, and the mixture was vigorously shaken on a Tissue Lyser II (Qiagen, Valencia, CA, USA) to create "micro-reactors" containing both amplification mix and a single bead. The emulsion was dispensed into a 96-well plate and the PCR amplification program was run with 16S universal primers in the FastStart High Fidelity PCR System (Roche, Basel, Switzerland) according to the manufacturer's recommendations. Sequencing of bacterial DNA in the feces was performed by the Macrogen Ltd. (Seoul, Korea) by a Genome Sequencer FLX plus (454 Life Sciences) as previously reported.

2.9. Statistical Analyses

All data are expressed as means ± standard deviations, and all statistical analyses were performed using SAS ver. 9.1 (SAS Institute, Cary, NC, USA). Significant differences among the control, AGM-L, AGM-H, positive-control and normal-control animal groups were identified with one-way analyses of variance. Significant differences in the main effects among the groups were detected using post-hoc Tukey's tests. A *p*-value <0.05 was considered significant.

3. Results

3.1. Contents of Anthocyanins and Ginsenoide Rg3

Aronia mainly contained cyanidin-galactoside, but also and cyanidin-glucoside, and cyanidin-arabinoside, whereas red ginseng had mostly ginsenoside Rg3 (2.5 mg/g sample). Shiitake mushroom contained 244 mg β-glucans/g sample (Table 1).

3.2. Body Composition

Body weight gains for 11 weeks were higher in the normal-control group than the control group whereas the positive-control and AGM-H increased body weight more than the control group but less than the normal-control ($p < 0.05$). Unlike body weight gain, food intake was not significantly different among the groups. Food efficiency decreased in the control group compared to the normal-control group and its reduction was prevented by AGM-H the most ($p < 0.05$). Epididymal and retroperitoneal fat contents and visceral fat mass, were much lower in the control group than the normal-control group (Table 2). The visceral fat mass was higher in the AGM-L and AGM-H groups than the positive-control group ($p < 0.05$), but it was not significantly different between the control and positive-control groups (Table 2). Thus, less increase of body weight and fat mass might be associated with urinary glucose loss.

Table 1. The contents of ingredients in the mixture.

	Contents (mg/g Powder)
C3-Galactoside	6.22
C3-Glucoside	0.33
C3-Arabinoside	1.53
Total Anthocyanin	8.08
Ginsenoside Rg3	2.5
β-glucan	244

Table 2. Energy metabolism and visceral fat mass.

	Normal-Control (*n* = 10)	Control (*n* = 10)	Positive-Control (*n* = 10)	AGM-L (*n* = 10)	AGM-H (*n* = 10)
Body weight gain for 10 week (g)	283 ± 10.5 [a]	144 ± 10.7 [b]	169 ± 11.8 [b]	156 ± 19.1 [b]	155 ± 13.0 [b]
Food intake (g/day)	14.4 ± 1.0 [a]	15.1 ± 0.8 [a]	15.0 ± 1.0 [a]	13.4 ± 1.5 [b]	12.3 ± 1.5 [b]
Food efficiency	0.30 ± 0.01 [a]	0.15 ± 0.01 [d]	0.18 ± 0.12 [c]	0.19 ± 0.03 [c]	0.22 ± 0.02 [b]
Epididymal fat pads (g)	6.7 ± 0.7 [a]	3.0 ± 0.4 [c]	2.9 ± 0.3 [c]	3.8 ± 0.5 [b]	3.3 ± 0.4 [c]
Retroperitoneal fat mass (g)	8.1 ± 0.8 [a]	3.6 ± 0.5 [c]	3.8 ± 0.5 [c]	4.3 ± 0.6 [b,c]	5.0 ± 0.7 [b]
Visceral fat (g)	14.8 ± 1.6 [a]	6.7 ± 0.9 [c]	6.7 ± 0.8 [c]	8.1 ± 1.0 [b]	8.3 ± 1.0 [b]

Food efficiency: daily energy intake/daily weight gain × 100. Values are means ± standard deviation. The test product was the mixture of free-dried aronia, red ginseng, mushroom and nattokinase. Px rats fed a high fat diet supplemented with (1) 0.5 g mixture/kg bw/day (AGM-L), (2) 1 g mixture/kg bw/day (AGM-H), (3) 1 g dextrin/kg bw/day (control), or (4) metformin (120 mg/kg body weight; positive-control) for 12 weeks. Sham-operated rats (normal-control) fed the same diet of control. [a,b,c,d] Values on the same row with different superscripts were significantly different at $p < 0.05$.

BMD in the lumbar spine and femur was much lower in the control group than the normal-control group whereas AGM-L and AGM-H prevented the decrease of BMD as much as the positive-control group ($p < 0.05$; Figure 1A). LBM showed a similar pattern of BMD. LBM exhibited a lower value in the control group than the normal-control and AGM-L and AGM-H protected against the decrease of LBM as much as the positive-control group ($p < 0.05$; Figure 1B). Fat mass also showed the similar tendency to LBM (Figure 1C).

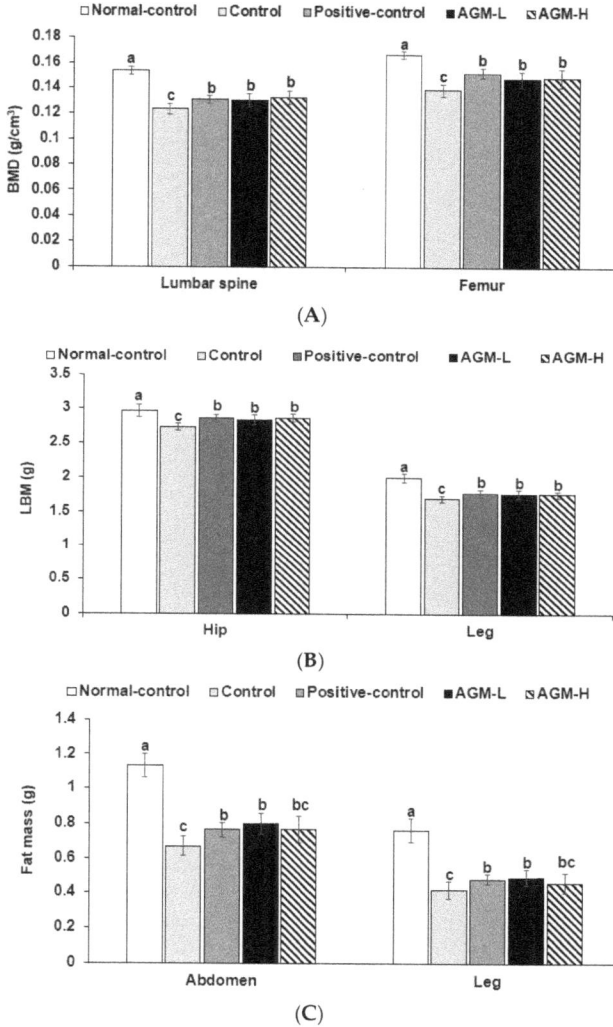

Figure 1. Bone mineral density (BMD), lean body mass (LMB) and fat mass (FM) at the end of experiment. Px rats were fed a high fat diet supplemented with aronia, red ginseng, shiitake mushroom, and nattokinase powders (1) 0.5 g mixture/kg bw/day (AGM-L), (2) 1 g mixture/kg bw/day (AGM-H), (3) 1 g dextrin/kg bw/day (control), or (4) metformin (120 mg/kg body weight; positive-control) for 12 weeks. Sham rats fed the same diet of control. BMD (**A**) in the lumbar spine and femurs, LBM (**B**) of the hip and legs and FM of the abdomen and legs (**C**) were measured by DEXA. Each bar and error bar represents the mean $\pm$ SD (n = 10 of each group). [a,b,c] Different superscripts on the bars represent significant differences at $p < 0.05$.

3.3. Glucose Metabolism

Overnight-fasting serum glucose levels in the control group were higher than those in the normal-control group indicating the diabetic conditions of the control group, and AGM-L and AGM-H decreased the serum glucose levels at fating states ($p < 0.05$; Table 3). Overnight serum insulin levels were lower in the control group than in the normal-control group. As calculated from serum glucose and insulin levels at fasting state, HOMA-IR, an index of insulin resistance, was higher in the control group than in the normal-control (Table 3). AGM-L and positive-control group showed a similar HOMA-IR, and AGM-H was lowered the most ($p < 0.05$). Mean cerebral blood flow was lower in the control than normal-control and it was not significantly different between the control and positive-control. However, AGM-L and AGM-H protected against the decrease in cerebral blood flow in Px rats and the levels in AGM-L were similar to normal-control.

Table 3. Serum glucose and insulin levels at fasting states and insulin resistance.

	Normal-Control ($n = 10$)	Control ($n = 10$)	Positive-Control ($n = 10$)	AGM-L ($n = 10$)	AGM-H ($n = 10$)
Serum glucose at fasting state (mM)	5.4 ± 0.5 [d]	9.8 ± 0.6 [a]	8.4 ± 0.6 [b]	8.1 ± 0.7 [b]	7.2 ± 0.5 [c]
Serum insulin at fasting state (ng/mL)	3.78 ± 0.36 [a]	2.83 ± 0.32 [c]	3.55 ± 0.35 [a,b]	3.27 ± 0.34 [b]	3.23 ± 0.36 [b]
HOMA-IR	5.4 ± 0.6 [d]	9.8 ± 1.0 [a]	8.4 ± 0.9 [b]	8.1 ± 0.8 [b]	7.2 ± 0.8 [c]
Urinary glucose	-	++++	+++	++	+
Mean cerebral blood flow (mm/s)	657 ± 45 [a]	405 ± 42 [c]	424 ± 45 [c]	643 ± 65 [a]	571 ± 67 [b]

+, ++, +++, ++++ higher amount of urinary glucose detection with more +. ⁻ No detection of urinary glucose. Values are means ± standard deviation. The test product was the mixture of free-dried aronia, red ginseng, mushroom and nattokinase. Px rats fed a high fat diet supplemented with (1) 0.5 g mixture/kg bw/day (AGM-L), (2) 1 g mixture/kg bw/day (AGM-H), (3) 1 g dextrin/kg bw/day (control), or (4) metformin (120 mg/kg body weight; positive-control) for 12 weeks. Sham-operated rats (normal-control) fed the same diet of control. [a,b,c,d] Values on the same row with different superscripts were significantly different at $p < 0.05$.

Cerebral blood flow was much lower in the control group than the normal-control group and positive-control did not improve blood flow compared to the control. However, AGM-L and AGM-H prevented the decrease and the level in the AGM-L group was similar to the normal-control group.

The OGTT revealed that glucose tolerance was highly impaired in the control group compared to the normal-control group and it was improved by metformin in the positive-control group (Figure 2A). AGM-L and AGM-H improved the glucose tolerance better than the positive-control but the improvement did not return it to normal-control group values ($p < 0.05$; Figure 2A). AUC of serum glucose levels during OGTT in the first phase was much higher in the control group than the normal-control group whereas AGM-L and AGM-H decreased the AUC of serum glucose levels ($p < 0.05$; Figure 2B). In the second phase of OGTT, AUC of serum glucose concentrations were much higher in the control group than in the normal-control group and AGM-L prevented the increase (Figure 2B). AGM-H increased the 2nd part of the serum insulin levels in comparison to the control but it was not significantly different (Figure 2C).

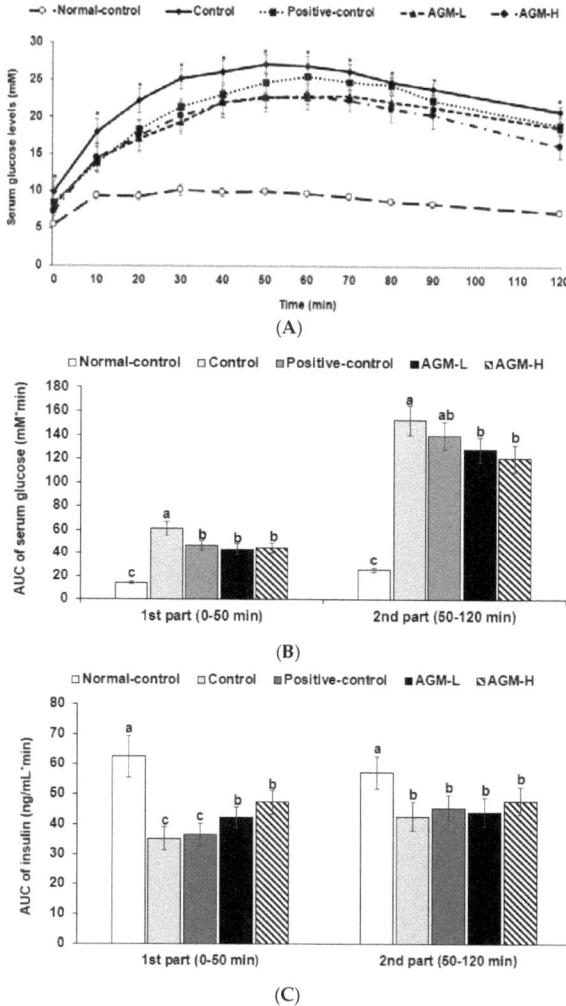

Figure 2. Serum glucose and insulin levels and area under the curve (AUC) of serum glucose and insulin during oral glucose tolerance test (OGTT). Px rats were fed a high fat diet supplemented with aronia, red ginseng, shiitake mushroom, and nattokinase powders (1) 0.5 g mixture/kg bw/day (AGM-L), (2) 1 g mixture/kg bw/day (AGM-H), (3) 1 g dextrin /kg bw/day (control), or (4) metformin (120 mg/kg body weight; positive-control) for 12 weeks. Sham rats fed the same diet of control. Changes of serum glucose levels (**A**) were measured after orally giving 2 g of glucose/kg body weight. The average of the area under the curve (AUC) of glucose (**B**) and insulin (**C**) during the first part (0–40 min) and second part (40–120 min) of OGTT. Each dot and bar and error bar represent the mean ± SD (n = 10 of each group). * Significantly different among the groups at each time point at $p < 0.05$. [a,b,c] Different superscripts on the bars represent significant differences at $S < 0.05$.

3.4. Insulin Tolerance

At 6 h after food deprivation, serum glucose levels were much higher in the control group than the normal-control group and the levels were lowered in the descending order of the control, positive-control, AGM-L and AGM-H ($p < 0.05$; Figure 3A). After insulin injection, serum glucose levels decreased until 60 min in all groups and the levels were almost maintained in all groups except the control group. The AUC of serum glucose concentrations were much higher in the control than in the normal-control in the 1st and 2nd phase (Figure 3B). AGM-L and AGM-H markedly decreased serum glucose levels during the 1st phase and the levels at the 2nd phase was similar to the normal-control group ($p < 0.05$; Figure 3B). Thus, AGM-L and AGM-H improved insulin tolerance in comparison to the control.

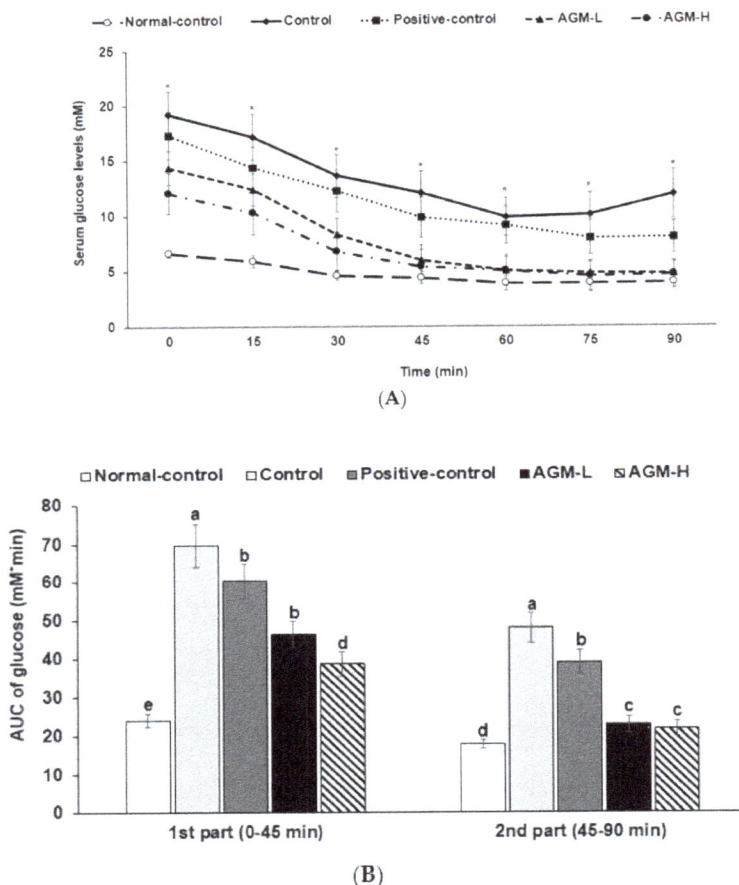

(A)

(B)

Figure 3. Changes of serum glucose concentrations during the intraperitoneal insulin tolerance test (IPITT). Px rats were fed a high fat diet supplemented with aronia, red ginseng, shiitake mushroom, and nattokinase powders (1) 0.5 g mixture/kg bw/day (AGM-L), (2) 1 g mixture/kg bw/day (AGM-H), (3) 1 g dextrin /kg bw/day (control), or (4) metformin (120 mg/kg body weight; positive-control) for 12 weeks. Sham rats fed the same diet of the control. IPITT was conducted with intraperitoneal injection of 0.75 IU insulin/kg body weight and measured serum glucose concentrations in blood collected from the tail every 15 min for 90 min. Changes of serum glucose levels were measured during IPITT (**A**). The average of the area under the curve (AUC) of glucose (**B**) during the first part (0–45 min) and second part (45–120 min) of IPITT. Each dot and bar and error bar represents the mean $\pm$ SD ($n = 10$ of each group). * Significantly different among the groups at each time point at $p < 0.05$. [a,b,c,d] Different superscripts on the bars represent significant differences at $p < 0.05$.

3.5. Hyperglycemic Clamp

Serum insulin levels were much lower in the control group than normal-control group for 90 min after glucose challenge ($p < 0.05$; Figure 4A). Serum insulin levels exhibited the 1st (0–10 min) and 2nd (60–90 min) phases in all groups. The AUC of 1st and 2nd phases of serum insulin levels increased in AGM-L the most whereas AGM-H elevated the AUC 1st and 2nd phases more than the control but less than the AGM-L ($p < 0.05$; Figure 4B). Glucose infusion rates during hyperglycemic clamp were much lower in the control group than the normal-control group whereas AGM-H prevented the decrease in Px rats, but the levels were less than the normal-control ($p < 0.05$; Table 4). AGM-H showed a higher glucose infusion rates and the levels were higher than the positive-control group ($p < 0.05$). Insulin sensitivity in the hyperglycemic state markedly decreased in the control group compared to the normal-control group and it was higher in the ascending order of control, AGM-H, positive-control and AGM-L ($p < 0.05$; Table 4).

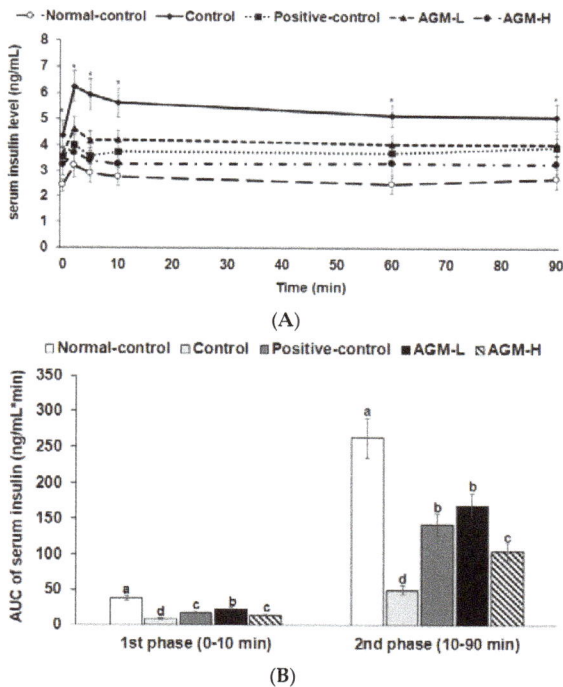

(A)

(B)

Figure 4. Insulin secretion during hyperglycemic clamp. Px rats were fed a high fat diet supplemented with aronia, red ginseng, shiitake mushroom, and nattokinase powders (1) 0.5 g mixture/kg bw/day (AGM-L), (2) 1 g mixture/kg bw/day (AGM-H), (3) 1 g dextrin /kg bw/day (control), or (4) metformin (120 mg/kg body weight; positive-control) for 12 weeks. Sham rats fed the same diet of the control. Hyperglycemic clamp was conducted in conscious, free moving, and overnight fasted rats to measure glucose-stimulated insulin secretion. As exogenous glucose was infused into jugular vein to make approximately 5.5 mM above overnight fasted serum glucose levels, serum insulin levels were measured at 0, 2, 5, 10, 30, 60, 90 and 120 min (**A**). The average of the area under the curve (AUC) of serum insulin levels (**B**) during the first part (0–10 min) and second part (10–90 min) during hyperglycemic clamp (**B**). Each dot and bar and error bar represents the mean $\pm$ SD ($n = 10$ of each group). * Significantly different among the groups at each time point at $p < 0.05$. [a,b,c,d] Different superscripts on the bars represent significant differences at $p < 0.05$.

Table 4. Glucose metabolism during hyperglycemic clamp.

	Normal-Control (*n* = 10)	Control (*n* = 10)	Positive-Control (*n* = 10)	AGM-L (*n* = 10)	AGM-H (*n* = 10)
Serum glucose levels at 60 min (mM)	9.8 ± 0.9 [c]	17.7 ± 1.4 [a]	14.6 ± 1.7 [b]	15.1 ± 1.6 [b]	15.1 ± 1.1 [b]
Serum glucose levels at 90 min (mM)	9.9 ± 0.9 [c]	18.3 ± 1.7 [a]	15.6 ± 1.7 [b]	15.2 ± 1.3 [b]	14.6 ± 1.2 [b]
Serum insulin levels at 2 min (ng/mL)	6.2 ± 0.6 [a]	3.2 ± 0.5 [d]	4.0 ± 0.4 [c]	4.6 ± 0.5 [b]	3.7 ± 0.4 [c]
Serum insulin levels at 60 min (ng/mL)	5.1 ± 0.4 [a]	2.5 ± 0.4 [d]	3.7 ± 0.3 [b,c]	4.1 ± 0.5 [b]	3.3 ± 0.6 [c]
Glucose infusion rates (umol/kg bw/min)	59.4 ± 3.9 [a]	26.1 ± 2.8 [d]	35.6 ± 3.9 [c]	32.8 ± 4.4 [c]	43.9 ± 3.9 [b]
Insulin sensitivity at hyperglycemic state (μmol glucose min−1 100 g−1 per μmol insulin/L)	33.3 ± 3.9 [a]	19.8 ± 2.4 [d]	25.8 ± 2.9 [c]	23.4 ± 2.6 [c]	28.9 ± 3.3 [b]

Values are means ± standard deviation (*n* = 10 of each group). The test product was the mixture of free-dried aronia, red ginseng, mushroom and nattokinase. Px rats fed a high fat diet supplemented with (1) 0.5 g mixture/kg bw/day (AGM-L), (2) 1 g mixture/kg bw/day (AGM-H), (3) 1 g dextrin /kg bw/day (control), or (4) metformin (120 mg/kg body weight; positive-control) for 12 weeks. Sham-operated rats (normal-control) fed the same diet of the control. [a,b,c,d] Values on the same row with different superscripts were significantly different at *p* < 0.05.

3.6. Pancreatic β-cell Mass, Proliferation, and Apoptosis

Pancreatic β-cell area is calculated by the number and individual size of β-cells. The increased number of β-cells improves diabetic status. However, individual β-cell size increases with β-cell hypertrophy that is associated with increased insulin resistance. Pancreatic β-cell area was higher in the control group than the normal-control group, but individual β-cell size was higher in the control group than in the normal-control group (*p* < 0.05; Table 5). AGM-H increased pancreatic β-cell area with smaller individual sized beta-cells, demonstrating that AGM-H increased β-cell number (Table 5). Pancreatic β-cell mass, calculated by multiplying β-cell area by pancreatic weight, was much lower in the control group than the normal-control group. Pancreatic β-cell mass increased in the ascending order of the control, positive-control, AGM-L, and AGM-H (*p* < 0.05; Table 5).

Table 5. The modulation of islet morphometry in the pancreas section.

	Normal-Control (*n* = 5)	Control (*n* = 5)	Positive-Control (*n* = 5)	AGM-L (*n* = 5)	AGM-H (*n* = 5)
β-cell area (%)	5.5 ± 0.7 [c]	6.3 ± 0.8 [b]	6.8 ± 0.8 [a,b]	6.9 ± 0.8 [a,b]	7.6 ± 0.9 [a]
Individual β-cell size (μm²)	185 ± 23 [c]	239 ± 26 [a]	209 ± 23 [b]	206 ± 25 [b]	189 ± 22 [b,c]
Absolute β-cell mass (mg)	33.4 ± 2.9 [a]	17.9 ± 1.9 [d]	22.4 ± 2.6 [c]	23.7 ± 2.9 [c]	28.8 ± 3.5 [b]
BrdU+ cells (% BrdU+ cells of islets)	0.72 ± 0.09 [c]	0.84 ± 0.09 [b]	0.89 ± 0.11 [b]	0.90 ± 0.12 [b]	1.04 ± 0.12 [a]
Apoptosis (% apoptotic bodies of islets)	0.64 ± 0.07 [a,b]	0.70 ± 0.09 [a]	0.66 ± 0.07 [a,b]	0.65 ± 0.07 [a,b]	0.59 ± 0.07 [b]

Values are means ± standard deviation. The test product was the mixture of free-dried aronia, mushroom and nattokinase. Px rats fed a high fat diet supplemented with (1) 0.5 g mixture/kg bw/day (AGM-L), (2) 1 g mixture/kg bw/day (AGM-H), (3) 1 g dextrin /kg bw/day (control), or (4) metformin (120 mg/kg body weight; positive-control) for 12 weeks. Sham-operated rats (normal-control) fed the same diet of the control. [a,b,c,d] Values on the same row with different superscripts were significantly different at *p* < 0.05.

The β-cell number is balanced by β-cell proliferation and β-cell apoptosis. The control rats exhibited a higher β-cell apoptosis than the positive-control rats and AGM-H decreased β-cell apoptosis (*p* < 0.05; Table 5). The β-cell proliferation was lower in the control group than the normal-control group. AGM-H increased the β-cell proliferation (*p* < 0.05; Table 5). Therefore, AGM-H increased β-cell mass by elevating β-cell proliferation and decreasing β-cell apoptosis.

3.7. Gut Microbiome

Community composition of the gut microbiota was compared with both total and shared operational taxonomic units among the groups by analysis of molecular variance (AMOVA). The AMOVA test revealed significant differences between the fecal bacterial communities among the groups (*p* < 0.01). Principal coordinate analysis (PCoA) illustrates the clustering of gut bacterial community (Figure 5A). Normal-control and control showed a significant separation of gut microbiota. AGM-L and AGM-H also had separate gut microbiota clustering from control but they overlapped with the normal-control. However, positive-control exhibited a similar pattern to that of the control group (Figure 5A). These results indicated that diabetes modulated the composition of gut microbiome and AGM prevented the modulation of gut microbiome.

The bacterial distribution was different among the groups at the phylum and order levels (Figure 5B,C). The major bacteria were *Firmicutes*, *Bacteriodetes*, *Proteobacteria*, *Actinobacteria*, and *Deferribacteres* at the phylum level. The percentage of *Firmicutes* was higher in the control group than the normal-control group and AGM-L and AGM-H reduced its percentage (Figure 5B). In contrast to *Firmicutes*, the percentage of *Bacteroidetes* was lower in the control than the normal-control and it increased with AGM-L and AGM-H ($p < 0.05$; Figure 5B). The percentages of *Proteobacteria*, *Actinobacteria*, and *Deferribacteres* were not altered by diabetic status and AGM supplementation (Figure 5B). The bacteria community was different among the groups in order level more than the phylum level. The percentage of *Bacteroidales* was much lower in the control than the normal-control and it was increased by AGM-L and AGM-H (Figure 5C). The percentages of *Erysipelotrichales* and *Clostridiales* were higher in the control than the normal-control and they were decreased by AGM-L and AGM-H. AGM-L increased the percentage of *Desulfovibrionales* ($p < 0.05$; Figure 5C). Thus, AGM-L modulated gut microbiome to make it similar to the normal-control.

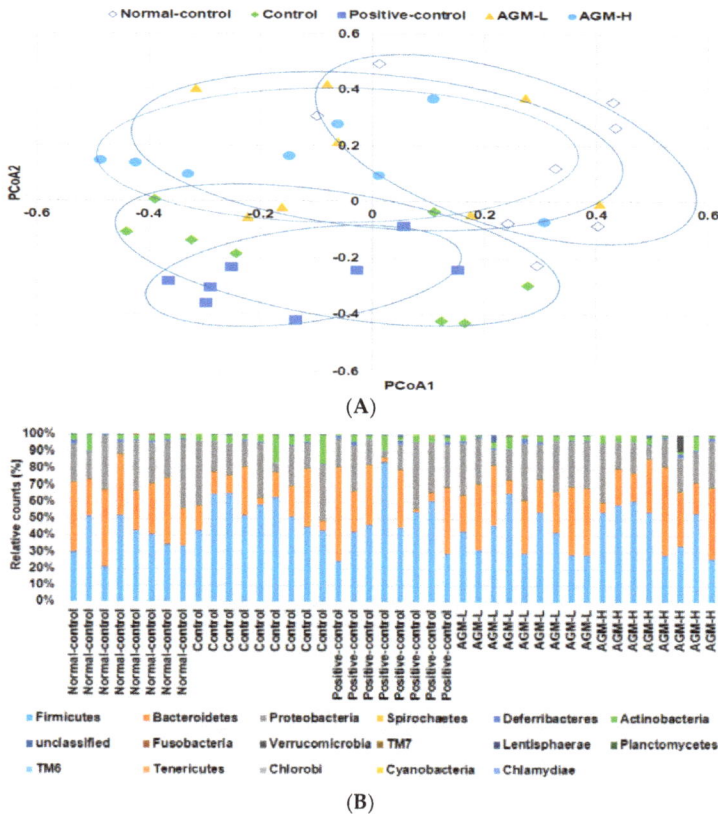

Figure 5. *Cont.*

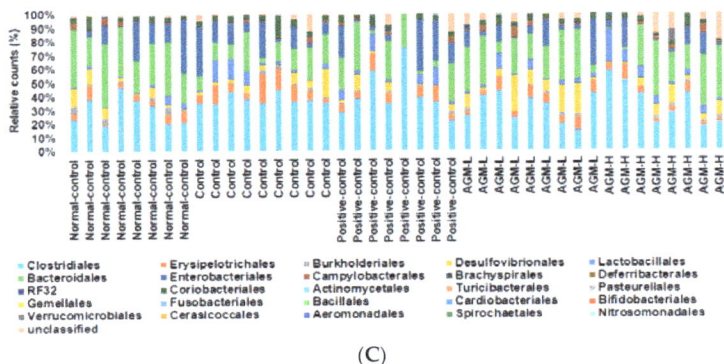

(C)

Figure 5. The profiles of gut microbiomes Px rats were fed a high fat diet supplemented with aronia, red ginseng, shiitake mushroom, and nattokinase powders (1) 0.5 g mixture/kg bw/day (AGM-L; *n* = 8), (2) 1 g mixture/kg bw/day (AGM-H; *n* = 8), (3) 1 g dextrin/kg bw/day (control; *n* = 8), or (4) metformin (120 mg/kg body weight; positive-control; *n* = 8) for 12 weeks. Sham rats were fed the same diet as the control (*n* = 8). At the end of experimental periods feces were collected and the bacterial DNA was analyzed. The fecal bacterial community was shown in principal coordinate analysis (PCoA) (**A**). Proportion of taxonomic assignments [Phylum (**B**) and Order (**C**)] for gut microbiomes was analyzed.

4. Discussion

Aronia, red ginseng and ultraviolet-irradiated shiitake mushroom have been reported to influence glucose metabolism. Based on a previous study, freeze-dried aronia, red ginseng, ultraviolet-irradiated shiitake mushroom and nattokinase were mixed at the ratio of 3.4:4.1:2.5:0.1 and the anti-diabetic activity was examined by assessing its efficacy for improving insulin sensitivity and potentiating insulin secretion in non-obese type 2 diabetic rats (Px rats). Px rats fed high fat diets, a well-established model of Asians type 2 diabetes, were used as the animal model for investigating the efficacy of the mixture in the present study. The Px rats had hyperglycemia due to increased insulin resistance and decreased insulin secretion. We used whole food not extracts since the gut microbiome is influenced by dietary fiber in the ingredients and anthocyanins can be easily degraded due to high temperature during extraction. Aronia, red ginseng, ultraviolet-irradiated shiitake mushroom and nattokinase contain different effective components such as anthocyanins, ginsenoside and β-glucan with vitamin D [27–29]. The major ingredients are known to be beneficial for alleviating type 2 diabetic symptoms and they are not overlapped between the plants. Thus, the efficacy of the mixture was examined for anti-diabetic activity in the present study.

Hyperglycemia develops when there is insufficient insulin secretion to compensate for insulin resistance. Insulin resistance is due to the impairment of insulin signaling by inflammation, oxidative stress and other factors. Elevated reactive oxygen species (ROS) and proinflammatory cytokines are also associated with impaired insulin signaling and β-cell function, with increasing β-cell apoptosis [30]. The decrease in ROS and proinflammatory cytokines alleviates the diabetic symptoms [29,31]. Hyperglycemia also reduces blood flow, which increases cardiovascular events [32]. The mixture of *Aronia melanocarpa*, red ginseng and mushroom is a good combination for anti-diabetic activity. *Aronia melanocarpa* extracts are rich in anthocyanins that suppress the production of ROS and proinflammatory cytokines [33,34]. Furthermore, aronia extracts prevent hyperglycemia by inhibiting α-glucosidase activity in the small intestines, by their ROS scavenging in humans and animal models [35,36]. Red ginseng can complement the anti-diabetic activity of aronia. Ginsenosides in red ginseng are known to prevent insulin resistance by activating insulin signaling in cells, animals and humans [11–13,28]. Red ginseng enhances insulin secretion and increases the pancreatic β-cell mass, which has hypoglycemic effects [14]. A systematic review and meta-analysis of randomized controlled clinical trials demonstrates that ginseng modestly, but significantly, improved fasting blood glucose in non-diabetic and diabetic patients but it does not change hemoglobin A1c and plasma insulin levels [37]. However, Reeds et al. [28] reported that ginseng and ginsenoside Re do not improve insulin sensitivity and β-cell function in obese type 2 diabetic patients. The ginsenosides are not detected in the blood after ginseng and ginsenoside Re treatment due to poor systemic bioavailability of ginsenosides [28]. Shiitake mushroom, which is rich in β-glucans and vitamin D, also has anti-diabetic activities [5,38,39]. β-glucan changes the gut microbiome and may be associated with improving insulin sensitivity. β-glucan mainly reduces insulin resistance to improve glucose metabolism [39]. Koreans have low levels of 25-OH-cholecalciferol in the blood, indicating vitamin D insufficiency that may affect glucose homeostasis with decreasing lean body mass [40,41]. Hyperglycemia increases platelet aggregation and thrombose formation that elevate the susceptibility to cardiovascular events [32]. Nattokinase is reported to suppress thrombosis [17,18]. The present study showed that AGM improved cerebral blood flow to as much as the normal-control. Since serum glucose levels in AGM were higher than the normal-control, the improvement of cerebral blood flow was associated with the factors beyond serum glucose levels. Nattokinase might be involved in the increase of cerebral blood flow in AGM. Therefore, the combination of aronia, red ginseng, shiitake mushroom and nattokinase may have a potent ant-diabetic activity and reduce the diabetic complications such as cardiovascular events. We decided to investigate the anti-diabetic activity of the combination treatment in Px rats. The present study showed that AGM-L and AGM-H improved glucose tolerance by improving insulin sensitivity in a dose-dependent manner, but AGM-L potentiated glucose-stimulated insulin secretion more than AGM-H. Thus, the combination supplementation alleviated the diabetic symptoms in Px rats.

The present study also showed that Px changed the body composition in comparison to the normal-control rats: Body weight and body fat were lower in Px rats compared to the normal-control rats due to increased urinary glucose loss. Fat mass was lower in the Px rats than the normal-control rats and both AGM-L and AGM-H suppressed the decrease in fat mass, but the fat mass of the AGM-L and AGM-H groups was still much lower than that of the normal-control. The suppression of fat mass loss was associated with the reduction of urinary glucose loss. The decrease of fat mass was not prevented as much as the urinary glucose loss. That may be associated with the properties of aronia and ginseng to suppress body fat synthesis and to increase skeletal muscle mass [42–44]. Furthermore, Px rats had lower BMD in the lumbar spine and femur and lower LBM in the hip and leg in comparison to the normal-control. These results suggested that the decrease of BMD is associated with lower insulin sensitivity and insulin secretion in diabetic rats. Sufficient insulin release promotes osteoblast activity by binding to insulin receptors in insulin insufficient states [45]. When osteoblasts are activated, osteocalcin is released from the bone and it binds to osteocalcin receptors that are highly expressed in pancreatic β-cells [45]. V-D is weakly correlated with osteocalcin [46] and it may not be involved in osteocalcin activity in insulin signaling. The activation of osterocalcin receptor by binding with osteocalcin promotes β-cell proliferation to improve β-cell function when glucose levels are elevated [47,48]. However, the osteocalcin effect on insulin resistance is still controversial [49,50]. In addition, BMD is associated with peroxisome proliferator-activated receptor (PPAR)-γ activation [41]. Skeletal muscle mass is reduced by decreasing anabolic signaling in the myocytes [51]. Ginsenosides in ginseng are reported to activate the PPAR-γ pathway to improve insulin sensitivity in various tissues [52,53]. The AGM-L inhibited the decrease of BMD and LBM, indicating that the inhibition by AGM was associated with the improvement of insulin sensitivity and potentiating insulin secretion. A potential limitation of the study is stress induced by multiple invasive procedures. However, the stress effects were mitigated by separating invasive procedures by at least one week to allow recovery from the stress. A unique aspect of this study was the use whole herbs instead of their extracts since the gut microbiome plays an important role in host metabolism of energy, glucose and lipids [54]. Dietary fiber works as food for gut microbes which produce short-chain fatty acids [54]. Dietary fibers in lyophilized aronia, red ginseng and shiitake mushroom may improve the composition and richness of the gut microbiome to establish eubiosis. However, another limitation of this study was not to include an AGM extract group in this study. The involvement of the gut microbiome in the development and progression of metabolic diseases is well recognized. Qin et al. has reported that several *Clostridium* species are increased in type 2 diabetes, and butyrate-producing bacteria are decreased [55]. Our preliminary study demonstrated that metabolism of β-glucan produced propionate and butyrate more than dextrin by 3.5 and 2 folds in vitro. However, the effects of dietary fiber in aronia and red ginseng on the microbiome were not examined. The present study also showed that *Clostridales* and *Erysipelorichales*, which are included in the *Fircumicultes.* was higher in the control than the normal-control but AGM decreased them. These changes in the gut microbiome might be associated with modulating the production of propionate and butyrate to influence gut-brain axis [56]. However, metformin treatment, the positive-control, did not alter the *Fircumicutes* although it improved glucose tolerance in the present study. Previous studies have shown that metformin modulates the gut microbiota composition by increasing the growth of some bacteria, such as *Akkermansia muciniphila*, *Escherichia* spp. or *Lactobacillus* and by decreasing the levels of some other bacteria such as *Intestinibacter* [57]. However, metformin treatment has adverse effects such as diarrhea, nausea, heartburn and gas and it may negatively influence the gut microbiome. Further study is needed to elucidate the metformin effect on gut dysbiosis. The present study showed that AGM had a beneficial effect on gut dysbiosis caused by type 2 diabetes: AGM inhibited the increase of *Clostridales* and increased *Bacterioidales* in the type 2 diabetic rats. Therefore, AGM improved glucose metabolism and prevented gut dysbiosis.

5. Conclusions

Hyperglycemia caused gut dysbiosis by increasing *Fircumicultes*, and AGM protected against gut dysbiosis. AGM improved glucose metabolism and lipid profiles in insulin insufficient type 2 diabetic rats, with Asian type 2 diabetes. The improved glucose metabolism protected against the decrease in BMD. Thus, AGM may be useful for preventing type 2 diabetes in Asians.

Author Contributions: S.P.; M.J.K.; D.Y.K. participated in designing the study and writing the manuscript. M.J.K.; H.J.Y., T.Z. and C.H. conducted biochemical experiments. M.J.K. and H.J.Y. quantified individual components of herbs. D.S.K. participated by conducting the animal study.

Funding: Ministry of Food, Agriculture, Forestry and Fisheries and the Korea Science and Engineering Foundation at 2017, Main Research Program (E0150302-04) of the Korea Food Research Institute (KFRI) and the National Research Council of Science & Technology (NST) grant by the Korea government (MSIT) (No. CAP-16-07-KIOM).

Conflicts of Interest: The authors declare that they have no competing interests.

References

1. Yuan, H.; Li, X.; Wan, G.; Sun, L.; Zhu, X.; Che, F.; Yang, Z. Type 2 diabetes epidemic in East Asia: A 35-year systematic trend analysis. *Oncotarget* **2018**, *9*, 6718–6727. [CrossRef] [PubMed]
2. DeFronzo, R.A.; Ferrannini, E.; Groop, L.; Henry, R.R.; Herman, W.H.; Holst, J.J.; Hu, F.B.; Kahn, C.R.; Raz, I.; Shulman, G.I.; et al. Type 2 diabetes mellitus. *Nat. Rev. Dis. Primers* **2015**, *1*, 15019. [CrossRef] [PubMed]
3. Kim, D.S.; Kim, B.C.; Daily, J.W.; Park, S. High genetic risk scores for impaired insulin secretory capacity doubles the risk for type 2 diabetes in asians and is exacerbated by western-type diets. *Diabetes Metab. Res. Rev.* **2018**, *34*. [CrossRef] [PubMed]
4. Yang, H.J.; Kim, M.J.; Kwon, D.Y.; Kim, D.S.; Lee, Y.H.; Kim, J.E.; Park, S. Anti-diabetic activities of *Gastrodia elata* blume water extracts are mediated mainly by potentiating glucose-stimulated insulin secretion and increasing beta-cell mass in non-obese type 2 diabetic animals. *Nutrients* **2016**, *8*, 161. [CrossRef] [PubMed]
5. Park, S.; Kim, D.S.; Kang, S. Vitamin D deficiency impairs glucose-stimulated insulin secretion and increases insulin resistance by reducing PPAR-gamma expression in nonobese type 2 diabetic rats. *J. Nutr. Biochem.* **2016**, *27*, 257–265. [CrossRef] [PubMed]

6. Park, S.; Kim, D.S.; Kang, S.; Moon, B.R. Fermented soybeans, Chungkookjang, prevent hippocampal cell death and beta-cell apoptosis by decreasing pro-inflammatory cytokines in gerbils with transient artery occlusion. *Exp. Biol. Med.* **2016**, *241*, 296–307. [CrossRef] [PubMed]

7. Lyu, M.; Wang, Y.F.; Fan, G.W.; Wang, X.Y.; Xu, S.Y.; Zhu, Y. Balancing herbal medicine and functional food for prevention and treatment of cardiometabolic diseases through modulating gut microbiota. *Front. Microbiol.* **2017**, *8*, 2146. [CrossRef] [PubMed]

8. Wen, L.; Duffy, A. Factors influencing the gut microbiota, inflammation, and type 2 diabetes. *J. Nutr.* **2017**, *147*, 1468s–1475s. [CrossRef] [PubMed]

9. Brunkwall, L.; Orho-Melander, M. The gut microbiome as a target for prevention and treatment of hyperglycaemia in type 2 diabetes: From current human evidence to future possibilities. *Diabetologia* **2017**, *60*, 943–951. [CrossRef] [PubMed]

10. Wedick, N.M.; Pan, A.; Cassidy, A.; Rimm, E.B.; Sampson, L.; Rosner, B.; Willett, W.; Hu, F.B.; Sun, Q.; van Dam, R.M. Dietary flavonoid intakes and risk of type 2 diabetes in US men and women. *Am. J. Clin. Nutr.* **2012**, *95*, 925–933. [CrossRef] [PubMed]

11. Park, S.; Ahn, I.S.; Kwon, D.Y.; Ko, B.S.; Jun, W.K. Ginsenosides Rb1 and Rg1 suppress triglyceride accumulation in 3T3-L1 adipocytes and enhance beta-cell insulin secretion and viability in min6 cells via pka-dependent pathways. *Biosci. Biotechnol. Biochem.* **2008**, *72*, 2815–2823. [CrossRef] [PubMed]

12. Lee, H.J.; Lee, Y.H.; Park, S.K.; Kang, E.S.; Kim, H.J.; Lee, Y.C.; Choi, C.S.; Park, S.E.; Ahn, C.W.; Cha, B.S.; et al. Korean red ginseng (*Panax ginseng*) improves insulin sensitivity and attenuates the development of diabetes in Otsuka Long-Evans Tokushima fatty rats. *Metabolism* **2009**, *58*, 1170–1177. [CrossRef] [PubMed]

13. Park, S.H.; Oh, M.R.; Choi, E.K.; Kim, M.G.; Ha, K.C.; Lee, S.K.; Kim, Y.G.; Park, B.H.; Kim, D.S.; Chae, S.W. An 8-wk, randomized, double-blind, placebo-controlled clinical trial for the antidiabetic effects of hydrolyzed ginseng extract. *J. Ginseng Res.* **2014**, *38*, 239–243. [CrossRef] [PubMed]

14. Kim, H.Y.; Kim, K. Regulation of signaling molecules associated with insulin action, insulin secretion and pancreatic beta-cell mass in the hypoglycemic effects of Korean red ginseng in Goto-Kakizaki rats. *J. Ethnopharmacol.* **2012**, *142*, 53–58. [CrossRef] [PubMed]

15. Grotto, D.; Bueno, D.C.; Ramos, G.K.; da Costa, S.R.; Spim, S.R.; Gerenutti, M. Assessment of the safety of the shiitake culinary-medicinal mushroom, lentinus edodes (agaricomycetes), in rats: Biochemical, hematological, and antioxidative parameters. *Int. J. Med. Mushrooms* **2016**, *18*, 861–870. [CrossRef] [PubMed]

16. Wagner, H.; Alvarsson, M.; Mannheimer, B.; Degerblad, M.; Östenson, C.G. No Effect of high-dose vitamin D treatment on β-cell function, insulin sensitivity, or glucose homeostasis in subjects with abnormal glucose tolerance: A randomized clinical trial. *Diabetes Care* **2016**, *39*, 345–352. [CrossRef] [PubMed]

17. Westein, E.; Hoefer, T.; Calkin, A.C. Thrombosis in diabetes: A shear flow effect? *Clin. Sci.* **2017**, *131*, 1245–1260. [CrossRef] [PubMed]

18. Fujita, M.; Hong, K.; Ito, Y.; Fujii, R.; Kariya, K.; Nishimuro, S. Thrombolytic effect of nattokinase on a chemically induced thrombosis model in rat. *Biol. Pharm. Bull.* **1995**, *18*, 1387–1391. [CrossRef] [PubMed]

19. O'Keefe, J.H.; Gheewala, N.M.; O'Keefe, J.O. Dietary strategies for improving post-prandial glucose, lipids, inflammation, and cardiovascular health. *J. Am. Coll. Cardiol.* **2008**, *51*, 249–255. [CrossRef] [PubMed]

20. Hosokawa, Y.A.; Hosokawa, H.; Chen, C.; Leahy, J.L. Mechanism of impaired glucose-potentiated insulin secretion in diabetic 90% pancreatectomy rats. Study using glucagonlike peptide-1 (7-37). *J. Clin. Investig.* **1996**, *97*, 180–186. [CrossRef] [PubMed]

21. Islam, M.S.; Wilson, R.D. Experimentally induced rodent models of type 2 diabetes. *Methods Mol. Biol.* **2012**, *933*, 161–174. [PubMed]

22. Reeves, P.G.; Nielsen, F.H.; Fahey, G.C., Jr. Ain-93 purified diets for laboratory rodents: Final report of the american institute of nutrition ad hoc writing committee on the reformulation of the ain-76a rodent diet. *J. Nutr.* **1993**, *123*, 1939–1951. [CrossRef] [PubMed]

23. Park, S.; da Kim, S.; Kang, S. *Gastrodia elata* blume water extracts improve insulin resistance by decreasing body fat in diet-induced obese rats: Vanillin and 4-hydroxybenzaldehyde are the bioactive candidates. *Eur. J. Nutr.* **2011**, *50*, 107–118. [CrossRef] [PubMed]

24. Choi, S.B.; Jang, J.S.; Park, S. Estrogen and exercise may enhance beta-cell function and mass via insulin receptor substrate 2 induction in ovariectomized diabetic rats. *Endocrinology* **2005**, *146*, 4786–4794. [CrossRef] [PubMed]

25. Dobbins, R.L.; Szczepaniak, L.S.; Myhill, J.; Tamura, Y.; Uchino, H.; Giacca, A.; McGarry, J.D. The composition of dietary fat directly influences glucose-stimulated insulin secretion in rats. *Diabetes* **2002**, *51*, 1825–1833. [CrossRef] [PubMed]

26. Park, S.; Kim, D.S.; Kang, E.S.; Kim, D.B.; Kang, S. Low dose brain estrogen prevents menopausal syndrome while maintaining the diversity of the gut microbiomes in estrogen-deficient rats. *Am. J. Physiol. Endocrinol. Metab.* **2018**, *315*, E99–E109. [CrossRef] [PubMed]

27. Kamweru, P.K.; Tindibale, E.L. Vitamin d and vitamin d from ultraviolet-irradiated mushrooms (review). *Int. J. Med. Mushrooms* **2016**, *18*, 205–214. [CrossRef] [PubMed]

28. Reeds, D.N.; Patterson, B.W.; Okunade, A.; Holloszy, J.O.; Polonsky, K.S.; Klein, S. Ginseng and ginsenoside re do not improve beta-cell function or insulin sensitivity in overweight and obese subjects with impaired glucose tolerance or diabetes. *Diabetes Care* **2011**, *34*, 1071–1076. [CrossRef] [PubMed]

29. Banjari, I.; Misir, A.; Savikin, K.; Jokic, S.; Molnar, M.; De Zoysa, H.K.S.; Waisundara, V.Y. Antidiabetic effects of *Aronia melanocarpa* and its other therapeutic properties. *Front. Nutr.* **2017**, *4*, 53. [CrossRef] [PubMed]

30. Newsholme, P.; Cruzat, V.F.; Keane, K.N.; Carlessi, R.; de Bittencourt, P.I., Jr. Molecular mechanisms of ROS production and oxidative stress in diabetes. *Biochem. J.* **2016**, *473*, 4527–4550. [CrossRef] [PubMed]

31. Pahwa, R.; Jialal, I. Hyperglycemia induces toll-like receptor activity through increased oxidative stress. *Metab. Syndr. Relat. Disord.* **2016**, *14*, 239–241. [CrossRef] [PubMed]

32. Tang, W.H.; Stitham, J.; Gleim, S.; Di Febbo, C.; Porreca, E.; Fava, C.; Tacconelli, S.; Capone, M.; Evangelista, V.; Levantesi, G.; et al. Glucose and collagen regulate human platelet activity through aldose reductase induction of thromboxane. *J. Clin. Investig.* **2011**, *121*, 4462–4476. [CrossRef] [PubMed]

33. Rugina, D.; Diaconeasa, Z.; Coman, C.; Bunea, A.; Socaciu, C.; Pintea, A. Chokeberry anthocyanin extract as pancreatic beta-cell protectors in two models of induced oxidative stress. *Oxid. Med. Cell. Longev.* **2015**, *2015*, 429075. [CrossRef] [PubMed]

34. Zhu, W.; Jia, Q.; Wang, Y.; Zhang, Y.; Xia, M. The anthocyanin cyanidin-3-O-beta-glucoside, a flavonoid, increases hepatic glutathione synthesis and protects hepatocytes against reactive oxygen species during hyperglycemia: Involvement of a cAMP-PKA-dependent signaling pathway. *Free Radic. Biol. Med.* **2012**, *52*, 314–327. [CrossRef] [PubMed]

35. Yamane, T.; Kozuka, M.; Konda, D.; Nakano, Y.; Nakagaki, T.; Ohkubo, I.; Ariga, H. Improvement of blood glucose levels and obesity in mice given aronia juice by inhibition of dipeptidyl peptidase iv and alpha-glucosidase. *J. Nutr. Biochem.* **2016**, *31*, 106–112. [CrossRef] [PubMed]

36. Simeonov, S.B.; Botushanov, N.P.; Karahanian, E.B.; Pavlova, M.B.; Husianitis, H.K.; Troev, D.M. Effects of aronia melanocarpa juice as part of the dietary regimen in patients with diabetes mellitus. *Folia Med.* **2002**, *44*, 20–23.

37. Shishtar, E.; Sievenpiper, J.L.; Djedovic, V.; Cozma, A.I.; Ha, V.; Jayalath, V.H.; Jenkins, D.J.; Meija, S.B.; de Souza, R.J.; Jovanovski, E.; et al. The effect of ginseng (the *Genus panax*) on glycemic control: A systematic review and meta-analysis of randomized controlled clinical trials. *PLoS ONE* **2014**, *9*, e107391. [CrossRef] [PubMed]

38. Maschio, B.H.; Gentil, B.C.; Caetano, E.L.A.; Rodrigues, L.S.; Laurino, L.F.; Spim, S.R.V.; Jozala, A.F.; Dos Santos, C.A.; Grotto, D.; Gerenutti, M. Characterization of the effects of the shiitake culinary-medicinal mushroom, lentinus edodes (agaricomycetes), on severe gestational diabetes mellitus in rats. *Int. J. Med. Mushrooms* **2017**, *19*, 991–1000. [CrossRef] [PubMed]

39. Jeong, S.Y.; Kang, S.; Hua, C.S.; Ting, Z.; Park, S. Synbiotic effects of beta-glucans from cauliflower mushroom and *Lactobacillus fermentum* on metabolic changes and gut microbiome in estrogen-deficient rats. *Genes Nutr.* **2017**, *12*, 31. [CrossRef] [PubMed]

40. Lee, B.K.; Park, S.; Kim, Y. Age- and gender-specific associations between low serum 25-hydroxyvitamin d level and type 2 diabetes in the Korean general population: Analysis of 2008–2009 Korean national health and nutrition examination survey data. *Asia Pac. J. Clin. Nutr.* **2012**, *21*, 536–546. [PubMed]

41. Park, S.; Ham, J.O.; Lee, B.K. A positive association of vitamin d deficiency and sarcopenia in 50 year old women, but not men. *Clin. Nutr.* **2014**, *33*, 900–905. [CrossRef] [PubMed]

42. Lee, H.M.; Lee, O.H.; Kim, K.J.; Lee, B.Y. Ginsenoside Rg1 promotes glucose uptake through activated AMPK pathway in insulin-resistant muscle cells. *Phytother. Res.* **2012**, *26*, 1017–1022. [CrossRef] [PubMed]

43. Shin, S.S.; Yoon, M. Korean red ginseng (*Panax ginseng*) inhibits obesity and improves lipid metabolism in high fat diet-fed castrated mice. *J. Ethnopharmacol.* **2018**, *210*, 80–87. [CrossRef] [PubMed]

44. Sikora, J.; Broncel, M.; Markowicz, M.; Chalubinski, M.; Wojdan, K.; Mikiciuk-Olasik, E. Short-term supplementation with *Aronia melanocarpa* extract improves platelet aggregation, clotting, and fibrinolysis in patients with metabolic syndrome. *Eur. J. Nutr.* **2012**, *51*, 549–556. [CrossRef] [PubMed]
45. Liang, J.; Lian, S.; Qian, X.; Wang, N.; Huang, H.; Yao, J.; Tang, K.; Chen, L.; Li, L.; Lin, W.; et al. Association between bone mineral density and pancreatic beta-cell function in elderly men and postmenopausal women. *J. Endocr. Soc.* **2017**, *1*, 1085–1094. [CrossRef] [PubMed]
46. Buranasinsup, S.; Bunyaratavej, N. The Intriguing Correlation between Undercarboxylated Osteocalcin and Vitamin D. *J. Med. Assoc. Thail.* **2015**, *98*, S16–S20.
47. Sabek, O.M.; Nishimoto, S.K.; Fraga, D.; Tejpal, N.; Ricordi, C.; Gaber, A.O. Osteocalcin Effect on Human β-Cells Mass and Function. *Endocrinology* **2015**, *156*, 3137–3146. [CrossRef] [PubMed]
48. Kover, K.; Yan, Y.; Tong, P.Y.; Watkins, D.; Li, X.; Tasch, J.; Hager, M.; Clements, M.; Moore, W.V. Osteocalcin protects pancreatic beta cell function and survival under high glucose conditions. *Biochem. Biophys. Res. Commun.* **2015**, *462*, 21–26. [CrossRef] [PubMed]
49. Gower, B.A.; Pollock, N.K.; Casazza, K.; Clemens, T.L.; Goree, L.L.; Granger, W.M. Associations of total and undercarboxylated osteocalcin with peripheral and hepatic insulin sensitivity and β-cell function in overweight adults. *J. Clin. Endocrinol. Metab.* **2013**, *98*, E1173–E1180. [CrossRef] [PubMed]
50. Choi, H.J.; Yu, J.; Choi, H.; An, J.H.; Kim, S.W.; Park, K.S.; Jang, H.C.; Kim, S.Y.; Shin, C.S. Vitamin K2 supplementation improves insulin sensitivity via osteocalcin metabolism: A placebo-controlled trial. *Diabetes Care* **2011**, *34*, e147. [CrossRef] [PubMed]
51. Lecka-Czernik, B. Diabetes, bone and glucose-lowering agents: Basic biology. *Diabetologia* **2017**, *60*, 1163–1169. [CrossRef] [PubMed]
52. Gao, Y.; Yang, M.F.; Su, Y.P.; Jiang, H.M.; You, X.J.; Yang, Y.J.; Zhang, H.L. Ginsenoside Re reduces insulin resistance through activation of PPAR-gamma pathway and inhibition of TNF-alpha production. *J. Ethnopharmacol.* **2013**, *147*, 509–516. [CrossRef] [PubMed]
53. Mollah, M.L.; Kim, G.S.; Moon, H.K.; Chung, S.K.; Cheon, Y.P.; Kim, J.K.; Kim, K.S. Antiobesity effects of wild ginseng (*Panax ginseng* C.A. Meyer) mediated by PPAR-gamma, GLUT4 and LPL in ob/ob mice. *Phytother. Res.* **2009**, *23*, 220–225. [CrossRef] [PubMed]
54. Zhao, L.; Zhang, F.; Ding, X.; Wu, G.; Lam, Y.Y.; Wang, X.; Fu, H.; Xue, X.; Lu, C.; Ma, J.; et al. Gut bacteria selectively promoted by dietary fibers alleviate type 2 diabetes. *Science* **2018**, *359*, 1151–1156. [CrossRef] [PubMed]
55. Forslund, K.; Hildebrand, F.; Nielsen, T.; Falony, G.; Le Chatelier, E.; Sunagawa, S.; Prifti, E.; Vieira-Silva, S.; Gudmundsdottir, V.; Pedersen, H.K.; et al. Disentangling type 2 diabetes and metformin treatment signatures in the human gut microbiota. *Nature* **2015**, *528*, 262–266. [CrossRef] [PubMed]
56. Perry, R.J.; Peng, L.; Barry, N.A.; Cline, G.W.; Zhang, D.; Cardone, R.L.; Petersen, K.F.; Kibbey, R.G.; Goodman, A.L.; Shulman, G.I. Acetate mediates a microbiome-brain-β-cell axis to promote metabolic syndrome. *Nature* **2016**, *534*, 213–217. [CrossRef] [PubMed]
57. Rodriguez, J.; Hiel, S.; Delzenne, N.M. Metformin: Old friend, new ways of action-implication of the gut microbiome? *Curr. Opin. Clin. Nutr. Metab. Care* **2018**, *21*, 294–301. [CrossRef] [PubMed]

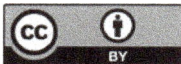

MDPI
St. Alban-Anlage 66
4052 Basel
Switzerland
Tel. +41 61 683 77 34
Fax +41 61 302 89 18
www.mdpi.com

Nutrients Editorial Office
E-mail: nutrients@mdpi.com
www.mdpi.com/journal/nutrients

www.ingramcontent.com/pod-product-compliance
Lightning Source LLC
Chambersburg PA
CBHW051714210326
41597CB00032B/5479